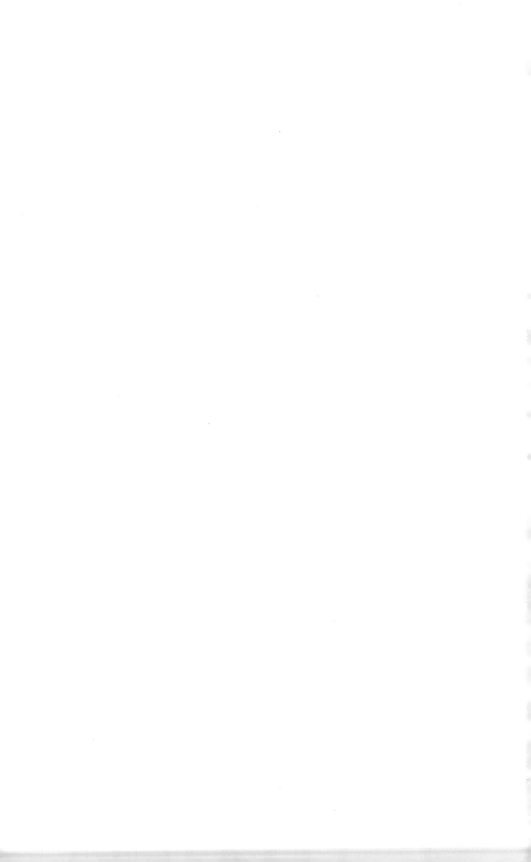

# Maternal and Child Health

## Programs, Problems, and Policy in Public Health

### Second Edition

Editor

**Jonathan B. Kotch, MD, MPH, FAAP**

The University of North Carolina at Chapel Hill
Chapel Hill, North Carolina

**JONES AND BARTLETT PUBLISHERS**

*Sudbury, Massachusetts*

BOSTON    TORONTO    LONDON    SINGAPORE

*World Headquarters*

| Jones and Bartlett Publishers | Jones and Bartlett Publishers | Jones and Bartlett Publishers |
|---|---|---|
| 40 Tall Pine Drive | Canada | International |
| Sudbury, MA 01776 | 2406 Nikanna Road | Barb House, Barb Mews |
| 978-443-5000 | Mississauga, ON L5C 2W6 | London W6 7PA |
| info@jbpub.com | CANADA | UK |
| www.jbpub.com | | |

Cover Images: Main: © Photos.com, Bar: © LiquidLibrary, © Alamy Images, © Photos.com

Jones and Bartlett's books and products are available through most bookstores and online booksellers. To contact Jones and Bartlett Publishers directly, call 800-832-0034, fax 978-443-8000, or visit our website www.jbpub.com.

Substantial discounts on bulk quantities of Jones and Bartlett's publications are available to corporations, professional associations, and other qualified organizations. For details and specific discount information, contact the special sales department at Jones and Bartlett via the above contact information or send an email to specialsales@jbpub.com.

**Production Credits**
Executive Editor: Michael Brown
Production Director: Amy Rose
Production Editor: Susan Schultz
Editorial Assistant: Kylah McNeill
Marketing Manager: Matthew Payne
V.P., Manufacturing and Inventory Control: Therese Bräuer
Composition: Auburn Associates, Inc.
Text Design: Anne Spencer
Cover Design: Kristin E. Ohlin
Printing and Binding: Malloy, Inc.
Cover Printing: Malloy, Inc.

**Library of Congress Cataloging-in-Publication Data**

Maternal and child health: programs, problems, and policy in public health/editor, Jonathan B. Kotch. —2nd ed.
    p.; cm.
Includes bibliographical references and index.
ISBN 0-7637-3171-4 (casebound)
1. Child health services—United States. 2. Maternal health services—United States.
[DNLM: 1. Child Health Services—United States. 2. Maternal Health Services—United States. 3. Child Welfare—United States. 4. Maternal Welfare—United States. WA 310 M4245 2005] I. Kotch, Jonathan.
RJ102.M26 2005
362.1'9892'000973—dc22

                                                                                    2004026193

Printed in the United States of America
09 08 07 06 05    10 9 8 7 6 5 4 3 2 1

# Table of Contents

# Contributors

**Greg R. Alexander, MPH, ScD**
Professor and Chair
Department of Maternal and
   Child Health
School of Public Health
The University of Alabama at
   Birmingham
Birmingham, Alabama

**Trude Bennett, MSW, DrPH**
Associate Professor
Department of Maternal and
   Child Health
School of Public Health
The University of North Carolina
   at Chapel Hill
Chapel Hill, North Carolina

**Shelah Bloom, MA, SM, ScD**
Research Assistant Professor
Department of Maternal and
   Child Health
School of Public Health
The University of North Carolina
   at Chapel Hill
Chapel Hill, North Carolina

**Dorothy C. Browne, MSW,
   MPH, DrPH**
Professor and Director
Center for Health Disparities
   Solutions
Public Health Program
Morgan State University
Baltimore, Maryland

**Theresa Chapple**
Master's Student
Department of Maternal and
   Child Health
School of Public Health
The University of North Carolina
   at Chapel Hill
Chapel Hill, North Carolina

**George Cole, MSW, DrPH**
Clinical Assistant Professor
School of Social Work
Senior Research Associate
Jordan Institute for Families
The University of North Carolina
   at Chapel Hill
Chapel Hill, North Carolina

**Larry Crum, PhD**
Health, Social, & Economics
  Research
Research Triangle Institute
Research Triangle Park,
  North Carolina

**Sian Curtis, MSc, PhD**
Research Associate Professor
Department of Maternal and
  Child Health
School of Public Health
Director, Measure Evaluation
  Project
Carolina Population Center
The University of North Carolina
  at Chapel Hill
Chapel Hill, North Carolina

**Janice M. Dodds, EdD, RD**
Professor
Department of Maternal and
  Child Health and Nutrition
School of Public Health
The University of North Carolina
  at Chapel Hill
Chapel Hill, North Carolina

**Anita M. Farel, MSW, DrPH**
Clinical Professor
Department of Maternal and
  Child Health
School of Public Health
The University of North Carolina
  at Chapel Hill
Chapel Hill, North Carolina

**Jody M. Greene, M.S.**
Research Sociologist
Health, Social, and Economics
  Research
Research Triangle Institute
Research Triangle Park, North
  Carolina

**Catherine A. Hess, MSW**
Adjunct Associate Professor of
  Health Policy,
George Washington University
  School of Public Health and
  Health Services
Senior Associate, Johns Hopkins
  University Bloomberg School of
  Public Health
Health Policy Consultant
1722 Seaton Place
Washington, District of Columbia

**Vijaya Hogan, MPH, DrPH**
Clinical Associate Professor
Department of Maternal and
  Child Health
School of Public Health
The University of North Carolina
  at Chapel Hill
Chapel Hill, North Carolina

**Russell S. Kirby, PhD, MS,
  FACE**
Professor and Vice Chair
Department of Maternal and
  Child Health
School of Public Health
The University of Alabama at
  Birmingham
Birmingham, Alabama

**David Knopf, LCSW, MPH**
Clinical Social Worker
Department of Pediatric Social
　Work
Children's Hospital at the
　University of California, San
　Francisco, and
Assistant Clinical Professor of
　Pediatrics
Division of Adolescent Medicine
　and the National Adolescent
　Health Information Center
Department of Pediatrics
School of Medicine
University of California, San
　Francisco
San Francisco, California

**Jonathan B. Kotch, MD, MPH**
Professor and Associate Chair for
　Graduate Studies
Department of Maternal and
　Child Health
School of Public Health
The University of North Carolina
　at Chapel Hill
Chapel Hill, North Carolina

**Milton Kotelchuck, MPH, PhD**
Professor and Chair
Department of Maternal and
　Child Health
School of Public Health
Boston University
Boston, Massachusetts

**Barbara Laraia, RD, MPH, PhD**
Research Assistant Professor
Department of Nutrition
School of Public Health
The University of North Carolina
　at Chapel Hill
Chapel Hill, North Carolina

**Lewis Margolis, MD, MPH**
Associate Professor
Department of Maternal and
　Child Health
School of Public Health
The University of North Carolina
　at Chapel Hill
Chapel Hill, North Carolina

**C. Arden Miller, MD**
Professor and Chair Emeritus
　Department of Maternal and
Child Health
　School of Public Health
　The University of North
Carolina at Chapel Hill
　Chapel Hill, North Carolina

**Mary D. Peoples-Sheps, MS,
DrPH**
Director, Public Health Programs
Associate Professor, Department of
　Health Services Research,
　Management, and Policy
College of Public Health and
　Health Professions
University of Florida
Gainesville, Florida

**Donna J. Petersen, MHS, ScD**
Dean
College of Public Health
University of South Florida
Tampa, Florida

**Herbert B. Peterson, MD, FACOG**
Professor and Chair
Department of Maternal and
Child Health
School of Public Health
The University of North Carolina
at Chapel Hill
Chapel Hill, North Carolina

**Linda Piccinino, MPS (ID)**
Associate
Abt Associates Inc.
Bethesda, Maryland

**Elizabeth Sutherland**
Doctoral Student
Department of Maternal and
Child Health
School of Public Health
The University of North Carolina
at Chapel Hill
Chapel Hill, North Carolina

**Joseph Telfair, DrPH, MSW/MPH**
Associate Professor
Department of Maternal and
Child Health
School of Public Health
The University of Alabama at
Birmingham
Birmingham, Alabama

**Amy Tsui, MA, PhD**
Professor
Population and Family Health
Sciences Department
Director
The Bill and Melinda Gates
Institute for Population and
Reproductive Health
Bloomberg School of Public
Health
Johns Hopkins University
Baltimore, Maryland

**Anjel Vahratian, MPH, PhD**
Research Investigator
Department of Obstetrics and
Gynecology
School of Medicine
The University of Michigan at
Ann Arbor
Ann Arbor, Michigan

**Martha S. Wingate, DrPH**
Assistant Professor
Department of Health Care
Organization and Policy
School of Public Health
University of Alabama at
Birmingham
Birmingham, Alabama

**B. Cecelia Zapata, MPH, DrPH**
Director
Affirmative Action and
Institutional Diversity
Bates College
Lewiston, Maine

# Foreword

As we reach the tenth anniversary of the International Conference on Population and Development held in Cairo during 1994, we reflect on the global commitment to improving reproductive health that emerged from that forum. That commitment included the concept that reproductive health is not only the absence of disease or infirmity but also the presence of well-being, and that it embraced the recognition that reproductive health is a basic human right. Realizing this commitment will be central to achieving our global goals in improving maternal and child health (MCH). Although there is much to celebrate today, much is yet to be done to achieve these goals. We live in a world where maternal deaths are rare in most of the developed world but one in which every minute of every hour of every day a woman dies in a developing country from pregnancy or childbirth. We live in a world where infant deaths are rare in most of the developed world but one in which approximately 30,000 children less than 5 years old die each day in developing countries—with two thirds of these deaths being preventable if proven, effective interventions were available to the children and mothers who need them.

Thus, the challenges that we noted 7 years ago in the first edition of this book remain, and it is imperative that we train the MCH leaders of tomorrow to meet these challenges. The Institute of Medicine[1] issued a report in 2002 in which it recommended that "schools of public health should embrace as a primary educational mission the preparation of individuals for positions of senior responsibility in public health practice, research, and training." We hope that this text will make a meaningful contribution toward that objective.

---

[1]Gebbie, K., Rosenstock, L., & Lyla, M. (2002). *Who will keep the public healthy? Educating public health professionals for the 21st century.* Washington DC: National Academies Press.

This second edition also addresses a second recommendation of the Institute of Medicine: "to emphasize the importance and centrality of the ecological approach." This is reflected in the updates and enhancements to chapters from the first edition and in the addition of three new chapters on program monitoring and performance appraisal, evaluation research, and advocacy and policy development. This introductory text shares our approach at University of North Carolina at Chapel Hill to teaching MCH with a larger audience and brings together the cycle of MCH, including reproductive health, maternal and infant health, and child and adolescent health, with a more global and ecological perspective. I am proud to invite you to join the effort to achieve "optimal health and well-being for all children and women of reproductive age."

*H.B. Peterson*

# Introduction

Women, children, and families have had their ups and downs in the 7 years since the first edition of this textbook was published. Infant mortality went up, but so did low birth weight rates. Teen pregnancy went down, but so did child physical activity. Insurance coverage among children went up despite the fact that private insurance coverage declined. This is, of course, because Medicaid and the State Child Health Insurance Program are picking up the slack (and then some).[1]

During the course of writing and editing, I had the pleasure of discussing and corresponding with Dr. Greg Alexander, Chair of the Department of Maternal and Child Health of the School of Public Health, University of Alabama at Birmingham. We had each discovered on our own that there was no definition of maternal and child health (MCH) in the first edition of *Maternal and Child Health: Programs, Problems, and Policy in Public Health*. Greg was gracious enough to share his definition:

> *MCH is the professional and academic field that focuses on the determinants, mechanisms and systems that promote and maintain the health, safety, well-being, and appropriate development of children and their families in communities and societies, in order to enhance the future health and welfare of society and subsequent generations.*[2,3]

---

[1]Child Trends DataBank. (2004). *Health care coverage.* Available September 28, 2004, from: http://childtrendsdatabank.org/indicators/26HealthCareCoverage.cfm

[2]Alexander, G.R., Petersen, D., Pass, M.A., Chadwick, C, & Slay M. (n.d.). *MCH public health milestones No. XII: Philosophy of maternal and child health.* Available September 29, 2004, from: http://www.soph.uab.edu/mchcontent.asp?ID=587

[3]Alexander, G.R. (2004). Maternal and child health (MCH). *Encyclopedia of health care management.* CA: Sage Publications.

I would characterize this definition as linear; that is, it starts with "determinants, mechanisms and systems" and ends with the "future health and welfare of society," a goal that no one can argue with. I prefer a more circular approach, captured in Figure 1, a contribution of the late Earl Siegel and affectionately known to his students as "Siegel's Circles." One can hop on board this life-cycle-go-round at any point and find common ground with colleagues in women's health, perinatal health, reproductive health, and children's health. The means that achieving optimal health and well-being for all children and women of reproductive age is just as important as the end.

MCH is a profession rather than a discipline. It is a big tent that is characterized by a multidisciplinary cast of characters who share a commitment to a vulnerable population. Although a source of strength, the focus on a specific population rather than on a theory or method can pose a threat. The lack of a unifying theoretical paradigm can be a weakness in an academic setting, placing MCH training programs on the defensive. Are MCH departments and professional training programs turning out generations of practitioners, or are they graduate departments that are cloning future faculty and MCH researchers?

The answer, of course, is that they are both, for academic researchers and MCH practitioners each contribute, in their own ways, to the shared

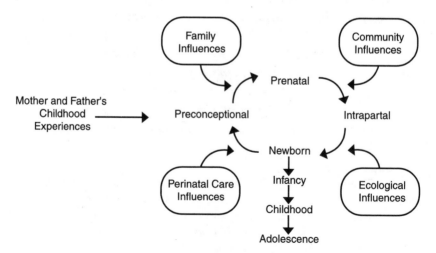

**FIGURE 1** A Longitudinal/Life Cycle Perspective of Child Health and Development

goal of improving the health status of women, children, and families. In doing so, MCH borrows from many health and social science disciplines, but increasingly, MCH is developing a set of knowledge and skills of its own. It was as recently as 1993, for example, that the Association of Schools of Public Health and the Association of Teachers of Maternal and Child Health (1993) developed the first set of competencies that MCH training programs across the country are striving to implement.[4] These have been revised in February 2001.[5]

This book is an attempt to present, in a consolidated form, the way that one such MCH training program, the Department of Maternal and Child Health of the School of Public Health of the University of North Carolina at Chapel Hill (UNC-CH), approaches the task of educating Master's students in the core material that is necessary for entering the field of MCH. With few exceptions, all of the contributors to this edited volume are faculty (current or former), students, or alumni of UNC-CH. By and large, the chapters correspond with courses that students at UNC-CH must take to satisfy the requirements of the Master of Public Health degree or the Master of Science in Public Health degree in MCH. As such, the scope of this book is not intended to be comprehensive, nor is any individual topic pursued in depth. Rather, this book is an introduction to MCH for students, hopefully with some prior health training or experience, approaching formal training in MCH for the first time.

The structure of the book is straightforward. The first two chapters, which cover children's rights, justice, advocacy, and MCH history, provide the ethical and philosophical underpinnings without which MCH would be a mechanical exercise at best. The chapter on families provides background to the changing social context affecting the health and development of all children. The next five chapters follow the developmental cycle, beginning with family planning and proceeding through maternal and infant health, preschool, school age, and adolescent health. In these

[4]Association of Teachers of Maternal and Child Health/Association of Schools of Public Health-MCH Council. (1993, November). *Competencies for education in maternal and child health*. Arlington, VA: National Center for Education in Maternal and Child Health.
[5]Association of Teachers of Maternal and Child Health. (2001, February). *Maternal and child health competencies*. Available September 29, 2004, from: http://www.atmch.org/mchcomps.pdf.

chapters, to the extent possible, the authors have followed a similar, but not identical, outline, from demography to history to epidemiology, programs, policy, and current or future issues.

The next chapters deal with issues that crosscut the developmental stages of the previous five chapters and are more idiosyncratic in structure as befits the various topics—health disparities, women's health, children with special needs, nutrition, and international MCH. Finally, the last five chapters present the public health skills that no MCH professional should leave home without, namely, research, planning, evaluation (new), advocacy (new), and program monitoring and performance appraisal (new). Although necessarily succinct, these chapters should inspire readers to seek hands-on experience to complement the didactic presentations herein.

As with any edited text, there are bound to be a variety of styles, but the faculty of the UNC-CH Department of MCH and the other contributors have provided material of uniformly high quality, making my job as editor that much easier. It is a credit to the department, both to those currently in residence and to those who have since moved on, that such a book can be produced almost entirely from within.

Because the focus of the book is on how MCH is taught at UNC-CH (with additional contributions from colleagues at other institutions), there are many important areas that, in another format, would deserve chapters, indeed entire books, of their own. Injuries, children's environmental health, HIV/AIDS, immunizations, dental public health, mental health, and other key public health issues overlap with core MCH areas and are discussed, to a greater or lesser extent, within one or more chapters. Nevertheless, none of these topics is unique to MCH. To do them justice, one would have to call on the skills of disciplines such as health behavior, epidemiology, health policy and management, environmental science, etc. In fact, this is exactly how courses in these areas are offered at UNC, sometimes with and sometimes without MCH faculty participation. There are only so many of us to go around.

At the end of the day, we hope that we have produced a readable introduction to MCH problems, programs, and policies for the beginning graduate student. If some of our readers go on to careers that promote and protect the health of women and children, then this effort will have been a success.

*Jonathan B. Kotch*

# Foundations of Maternal and Child Health

# CHAPTER 1

# Children's Rights, Distributive Justice, and Advocacy in Maternal and Child Health

*Lewis Margolis, George Cole, and Jonathan Kotch*

*Remember, that the human being is the most important of all products to turn out. I am eagerly anxious to do everything I can to wake up our people to the need of protecting the soil, protecting the forests, protecting the water; but first and foremost, protect the people. If you do not have the right kind of citizens in the future, you cannot make any use of the natural resources. Protect the children—protect the boys; still more, protect the girls; because the greatest duty of this generation is to see to it that the next generation is of the proper kind to continue the work of this nation.*
(President Theodore Roosevelt, 1911)

## INTRODUCTION

In 1988, the Institute of Medicine (IOM) published *The Future of Public Health*, a study and critique of the state of the public health field, accompanied by recommendations to enhance its effectiveness as the nation

moves into the 21st century. The authors of the report articulated a definition of public health with three components: the mission, the substance,
and the organizational framework. The mission was defined as "the fulfillment of society's interest in assuring the conditions in which people can be
healthy" (IOM, 1988, p. 40). The substance was defined as "organized
community efforts aimed at the prevention of disease and promotion of
health" (IOM, 1988, p. 41). The organizational framework of public
health encompasses "both activities undertaken within the formal structure of government and the associated efforts of private and voluntary
organizations and individuals" (IOM, 1988, p. 42). Each component of
this definition reflects the central dynamic or tension in the field of public
health, that is, balancing the rights of individuals to pursue their private
interests with the needs of communities to control the hazards that
inevitably arise when groups of people pursue those interests (Beauchamp
& Steinbock, 1999; Gostin, 2000; Jennings, Kahn, Mastroianni, &
Parker, 2003).

It is only since the evolution of the recognition of children as individuals with interests and rights, potentially separate from those of their parents, that communities and nations have justified and conferred special
protections and benefits on children through assorted public health, welfare, and education programs. In the United States, for example, the early-
20th-century movement to ban child labor recognized that a child's right
to an education was in conflict with the rights of employers to use child
labor and the rights of parents ·to insist that their children go to work,
especially if the family needs the income. Today's child advocates continue
the tradition that argues that children should never be treated as means to
an end. Rather, optimal health, growth, and development in childhood
are ends in themselves. This chapter explores ethical principles underlying
maternal and child health and relates those principles to advocacy for
services on behalf of mothers and children.

# RIGHTS

Rights are defined as valid claims (Feinberg, 1978) that imply a reciprocal
duty. Such claims must be validated by rules obligating someone to
respond. In the case of moral rights, such claims must be validated by
moral rules. Similarly, legal rights are validated by legal rules. Although

moral rights may make claims on religion and social conscience, only legal rights are enforceable by the legal apparatus of the state.

Rights are classified as positive or negative according to whether reciprocating a claimed right may require the transfer of resources. Therefore, positive rights are also referred to as subsistence rights or welfare rights, requiring some people to give up something of economic value in order to satisfy the legitimate claims of others. Negative rights, on the other hand, are option rights or rights of forbearance. A positive right is a right to something tangible, whereas a negative right is a right to be left alone.

Philosophers have argued about which came first, positive or negative rights. Historically, negative rights appeared in the US Constitution and the French Declaration of the Rights of Man before positive rights were codified in the United Nations' charter and the constitution of the Soviet Union, but Bandman (1977) claimed that logically some assurance of human subsistence must have preceded liberty, citing the biblical tale of the gleaners, who benefited from the moral obligation to leave behind some produce in the fields after the harvest.

The distinction between positive and negative rights may not always be clear-cut, especially in the case of children. For example, the Bill of Rights of the US Constitution articulates negative rights in that Congress is prohibited from passing laws that restrict the freedom of speech and freedom of assembly and the free exercise of religion. These are rights to be left alone, not rights to economic resources. The ability of children, however, to exercise negative rights is, more so than for adults, a direct function of education, housing, nourishment, and health care. Satisfying children's valid claims to these goods and services would involve their recognition by society as positive rights. Positive and negative rights are enumerated in the United Nations Convention on the Rights of the Child (Melton, 1991), ratified by the United Nations in 1989. Examples of positive rights are rights to

- The highest attainable standard of health and access to medical services
- Access to information and material from a diversity of sources
- An adequate standard of living
- Education
- Leisure, play, and participation in cultural and artistic activities

Examples of negative rights are rights to:

- Respect for parents or guardians to provide direction to the child in the exercise of his or her rights
- Legal protection against arbitrary or unlawful interference with privacy, family, home, or correspondence or attacks on honor and reputation
- Freedom of association
- Express an opinion in matters affecting the child and to have that opinion heard
- Practice any belief

Obligations to satisfy rights may clash with one another. For example, participation in cultural activities may conflict with the right to practice any belief. Respect for parents to provide direction may conflict with access to information.

The issue of children's rights is further complicated by the fact that they cannot make claims on their own behalf. In other words, if children are to have rights at all, someone else must claim those rights for them. In fact, a child's first claims are against its own parents, and the rights of parents in their own child derive from a prior duty to satisfy the legitimate needs of that child (Blackstone, 1968). Unlike the case with adults' rights, which requires a reciprocal obligation on the part of another, a parent's right in a child requires an obligation on the part of that same parental rights holder. "Parents' rights" therefore imply "parents' duties." Parents who do not satisfy their child's need for subsistence and, indeed, for love and affection as well, risk losing their rights in that child, as in the case of the state's removal of a neglected child from his or her home. A parent, however, has not been required to act in the best interests of the child until recent history. Many ancient cultures codified aspects of the parent–child relationship by institutionalizing the absolute authority of the parent. Greek city-states condoned infanticide and even required it in the case of unwanted, illegitimate, and deformed children. In classical Sparta, a defective child could be thrown from a cliff without penalty. In the Roman Empire, a father had absolute legal authority over the life and death of his children (and, for that matter, his wife). In Egypt, the Middle East, China, and the Scandinavian countries, children were routinely sold into slavery or if without value on the open market, strangled, drowned, "thrown from a high place," or abandoned. European laws supported the right of parents to use lethal force in controlling adolescents, who were sometimes flogged or even executed for disobedience. Unwanted European newborns were discarded without penalty. There are accounts of infants left to die on trash heaps and dung heaps or buried alive in the foundations of bridges and buildings for "good luck" (DeMause, 1974; Leiby, 1976; Williams, 1983).

Children were not even depicted in archival art until after the 11th century. The historian Barbara Tuchman has written that medieval illustrations show people in every contemporary human activity—making love and dying, sleeping and eating, being in bed and in the bath, praying, hunting, dancing, plowing, participating in games and in combat, trading, traveling, reading and writing—yet rarely with children. When children did appear, they were portrayed as miniature adults in adult clothing. The concept of childhood as a developmental continuum simply did not exist, and children were pushed into adulthood as quickly as possible. Tuchman surmises that it just was not worth investing in individuals who were apt to die before they could actively participate in the adult struggle to survive. "Owing to the high infant mortality rate of the times, estimated at one or two in three, the investment of love in a young child may have been so unrewarding that by some ruse of nature . . . it was suppressed. Perhaps also the frequent childbearing put less value on the product. A child was born and died and another took its place" (Tuchman, 1978, p. 50).

Intermittently, children come under official protection. The Code of Hammurabi made it a crime for a mother to murder her newborn, and Tiberius ordered the death penalty for those caught sacrificing children to non-Roman gods. In 13th-century England, sleeping parents smothered so many infants that it was made illegal to "bed with a swaddling child" (Pfohl, 1976; Williams, 1983). Furthermore, by the 16th century, there was a dawning recognition of the unique identity and developmental status of children. Christian reformers such as Martin Luther had for some time advocated for social concern and intervention, and there was a trend among contemporary secular philosophers and commentators to romanticize childhood. However, in the main, children were regarded as innately evil little adults or the playthings of adults. There are accounts from the medical literature of injuries resulting from the popular pastime of "child tossing," and the violent control of children by parents continued largely unabated (DeMause, 1974; Williams, 1983). Since the promulgation of Elizabethan Poor Laws, English tradition has vested ultimate guardianship over those incapable of acting on their own behalf in the sovereign (i.e., the king or queen). In the United States, the states, rather than the federal government, have this power. Hence, the states are ultimately responsible for public education, child welfare, and child protection. The early 20th century saw the passage of a number of child welfare and child labor laws during what has since become known as the Progressive Era in US history. When enacted at the federal level, some of these, such as the National Child Labor Law, ultimately were declared unconstitutional. Although subsequently enacted during the depression of the 1930s, in 1918, the Supreme Court ruled that the federal government had no jurisdiction to intervene in a decision (to make a child go to school instead of work) best left to parents (*Hammer v. Dagenhart*, 1918).

Nevertheless, the children's rights movement continued to gain momentum. The 1930 White House Conference on Children promulgated the Children's Charter, which declared, among other things, that every child should have "health protection from birth through adolescence, including: periodic health examinations and, where needed, care of specialists and hospital treatment; regular dental examinations and care of the teeth; protective and preventive measures among communicable diseases; the insuring of pure food, pure milk, and pure water" (US Department of Health, Education, and Welfare, 1976). Recent US Supreme Court decisions established certain constitutional rights of children, such as the right to due process in adult court (*Kent v. US*, 1966) and the same rights as adults in criminal court (*In Re Gault*, 1967), rights that even parents may not overrule (*Planned Parenthood of Central Missouri v. Danforth*, 1976).

Legislation at the federal level has recognized some rights of children. Child abuse and neglect legislation, for example, establishes that children must be protected from abuse and that parents may be prosecuted for failing to provide necessary food, clothing, shelter, education, medical care, and even love and affection, as determined by state governments (Child Abuse Treatment and Prevention Act, 1973). Protection from abuse corresponds with a negative right, whereas protection from neglect corresponds with the child's positive right to subsistence. Other rights established at the federal level include the right to a free, public education for all handicapped children (Education for All Handicapped Children Act, 1975) and the right to a barrier-free environment for children and adolescents with disabilities, as found in the Americans with Disabilities Act (1990).

Satisfying positive rights to, for example, health care or education requires the expenditure of resources. In the face of limited resources, societies need rules for the fair allocation of resources. Such rules are called the principles of distributive justice.

## THEORIES OF JUSTICE

From the perspective of social policy, it is necessary to justify taking or redistributing resources legitimately earned by one person in order to purchase health care or any other good for another, or in this case, for the child of another. For the purposes of analyzing and assessing distributive justice for children, it is useful to consider two basic theories of justice (for an excellent discussion of ethical frameworks for professionals, see Applebaum & Lawton, 1990). One theory is based on the principle of utility that Jeremy Benthem and John Stuart Mill developed. This theory assumes that individuals act to maximize their own happiness or utility. A just allocation of resources within a community, therefore, derives from the calculation and balancing of positive and negative utilities for each of the individuals in the group. If the total of the positive utilities or benefits exceeds the total of the negative utilities or costs, then that allocation is deemed to be just or fair. Utilitarian theory is the basis for cost–benefit analysis as a common and powerful tool in policy analysis.

In the United States, the market is the mechanism for maximizing utility. To the extent that it rewards effort, merit, and social contribution, the market is the primary determinant of how health care resources are allocated (Arrow, 1963; Epstein, 1997). Economists note, however, that under certain circumstances, markets may not be the most efficient way to distribute resources. For example, markets may result in a distribution of income and other resources that leave some individuals incapable of meeting their needs (Stiglitz, 2000). Under such circumstances, the distributive principle of need argues that people who are ill or even at-risk of becoming ill should have access to more medical care resources (Beauchamp & Childress, 2001; Buchanan, 1984). Public support for health insurance for the poor through the Medicaid program, supplemental security income for the disabled, or targeted services for children with special health care needs may be considered examples of redistribution of health care according to the principle of need. Another condition that leads to market failure is that of public goods, items for which it does not cost anything for an additional individual to participate in the benefits, and it is impossible to exclude individuals from the benefits. Although children represent the products of private reproductive decisions and parents reap the benefits of children—pleasure, support in old age—to some extent, all members of a community benefit from children. Children grow up to be economically productive, cultivating the resources needed to produce the goods and services that sustain societies in general. Therefore, another justification for redistributing resources to children or to families with children is that as public goods the market may not allocate to them very efficiently.

A second basic theory, articulated by Immanuel Kant, is based on rules or duties. Unlike utilitarian theory that focuses on the consequences of resource allocation, Kant's focus is on fundamental duties. Kant asserted, "Act in such a way that you treat humanity, whether in your own person or in the person of any other, never simply as a means, but always at the same time as an end" (Applebaum & Lawton, 1990, p. 16). Kantian theory would emphasize individual need or perhaps merit as allocation principles.

Building on the work of Kant, Rawls (1969), in *A Theory of Justice*, described a thought experiment to explain one way that fair rules of distributive justice might be derived. In the "original position," rational adults come together behind a "veil of ignorance" for the sole purpose of making the rules that govern the distribution of goods and benefits. In such a position, with the decision makers ignorant of their statuses and roles in society, Rawls posited that all would agree with the following: that basic political liberties would be guaranteed, that desirable statuses and roles would be equally accessible to all, and that unequal distribution of resources would be tolerated to the extent that such inequalities benefit the least well off. One implication of this theory, however, is that it is necessary to take resources from those that are "well off"; that is, the effort of some individuals would be used as a means to make others better off, an apparent contradiction with the Kantian view.

Rawls' formulation provides one test of social policy: Does such policy benefit the least well off? Take the case of infant mortality. For as long as race/ethnicity has been recorded for infant mortality, a marked disparity has existed between white and black rates of infant death. Nevertheless, the rates for both groups have consistently declined, suggesting that the medical, social, and public health resources affecting infant mortality have been distributed in a just manner.

Building on the work of Rawls, Green (1976) argued that society cannot withhold from children their fair share of health care resources. Because children are not considered "rational" from a developmental and legal perspective, they cannot participate in the original position. What would then be a child's "fair share?" Certainly a child's fair share of health care can be no less than that necessary for him or her to grow and develop to be able to exercise fully those political liberties and human rights guaranteed to all.

The assertion of rights is not sufficient to assure that children's rights are satisfied. Inequities in the distribution of decision-making authority, economic resources, and information among different segments of a population behoove individuals and organizations to act as advocates for children in order to articulate their needs and interests, especially in the presence of opposition. Advocates attempt to influence the legislative, administrative processes of society to make children's rights a reality. We now turn to consideration of advocacy for mothers and children.

# CHILD ADVOCACY

## *Defining Advocacy*

Definitions of child advocacy, developed largely in the 1970s and 1980s, characterize the contemporary child advocate as operating at three levels:

1. On the individual or case level, an advocate is a person acting on behalf of a child . . . a defender, protector, mediator, supporter, investigator, negotiator, monitor, promoter, enabler, and/or counselor (Fernandez, 1980). Individual or case advocacy is the process of challenging an organization on behalf of an individual, a process in which an individual or group attempts to obtain more responsive, adequate, and effective services for a child or a family.

2. On the organizational level, an advocate is a person or group attempting to alter and monitor legislative, budgetary, and administrative processes and, at times, monitor professionals and professionalism (Kahn & McGowan, 1972).

3. Systems or class advocacy is the process of reforming an organization or a system to benefit a group of people, cases, or users of the organization or system. Class advocacy may begin with action on behalf of one individual and then move its focus to all members of a class of cases. Often, individuals with similar motivations for case advocacy organize in order to take advantage of the power of numbers and combined resources. Advocacy on behalf of a class is often precipitated by an event with broad public exposure and emotional impact. For example, a fundamental change in Medicaid policy occurred in the early 1980s when the mother of Katie Beckett was able to impress on President Reagan the outrageous expenses resulting from the regulation that children with special health care needs be hospitalized for certain services when those same services could be provided less expensively and often more humanely at home (Roberts & Considine, 1997).

As discussed previously here, because children have special developmental and physical needs (that to a greater or lesser degree have been translated into positive rights by different communities and cultures), the fundamental value for child advocates would seem to be that goods and services ought to be distributed on the basis of need (Margolis & Salkind, 1996). Some organizations translate that value into *child saving*, emphasizing children's incompetence and vulnerability, and the role of assistance from the community or state. A second, albeit related, advocacy promotes *parents as savers*, arguing for policies that enable parents to address the vulnerabilities and thereby meet the needs of children. Others are *child liberators*, who argue for policies that ensure the independence and autonomy of children, assuming that children have the right as well as the capability to determine and act on their own needs. Others, however, advocate for *parental rights*, believing that the private domain of the family is the only appropriate arena in which to meet the needs of children.

The list of organizations engaged in child advocacy is not only long but also extremely diverse in the goals that they promote and the principles on which they are based. Private, nonprofit organizations devoted almost exclusively to advocacy include groups such as the Children's Defense Fund and the National Association for Child Advocates. Organizations such as the March of Dimes, with broad missions involving community service, research, and education, also frequently play substantial advocacy roles. Professional organizations such as the American Academy of Pediatrics or the American Public Health Association, particularly through its Maternal and Child Health Section, allocate time and resources to advocacy for mothers and children. Religious or church-based organizations also support advocacy efforts. A cursory search on the Internet generates dozens of organizations of multiple political and philosophical views engaged in advocacy on behalf of mothers and children.

The role of governments—whether federal, state, or local—in advocacy is problematic. Clearly, agency social workers or attorneys engaged in child protection are charged with the responsibility for individual children as case advocates. At the systems level, however, governmental advocacy is more controversial. The Centers for Disease Control and Prevention, for example, has supported advocacy institutes to teach individuals to influence policies regarding the use of tobacco by youth. These same institutes are roundly criticized by other government officials whose constituencies depend on the production and sale of tobacco products! The 1970 White House Conference on Children called for a formal system of child advocacy (White House Conference, 1971). Quoting from the final report, "This Forum believes independent representation for children, a *system of child advocacy* (emphasis added), is urgently needed and should be immediately created" (White House Conference, 1971, p. 390). Citing such basic child needs as parental care, a secure home, moral guidance, proper nutrition, health, discipline, and education, the forum observed that "government should be responsive to these needs" (White House Conference, 1971, p. 389). Among its recommendations were a cabinet-level Department of Children and Youth, a National Advisory Council on Child Advocacy, an Office of Child Advocacy (specifically recommended for immediate establishment) within the new department, federally funded state advisory councils on child advocacy, and local advocacy boards, funded by the state councils, which would hire full-time, salaried child advocates to be responsible for children in a specific geographic region. Although these recommendations were never implemented, states and communities around the country have set up child advocacy agencies at the state and local levels.

## Steps in the Child Advocacy Process

Child advocates may pursue a number of strategies that are neither mutually exclusive nor restricted to a particular order. Strategies include educating policy makers and citizens, lobbying for legislation and/or regulation, and adjudicating when rights or interests cannot be satisfied. Some advocates would add demonstrating on behalf of children as well.

Informed and strategic use of the media is today a necessary component of successful public education on behalf of children's causes. A successful public information campaign may be targeted to increased use of bicycle helmets, higher immunization rates, or reduction in adolescent cigarette smoking. An educational activity that may be the most important component of the advocate's armamentarium is the education of policy makers. Such an educational strategy, when exercised by the leadership of formal public health organizations, is part of public health's policy development function. Indeed, as the IOM (1988, p. 119) envisioned, public health leadership includes "communication skills; knowledge of and skills in the public decision process, including its political dimensions; and the ability to marshal constituencies for effective action."

As history and experience demonstrate, linking education with policy change at the legislative or regulatory levels can be more effective than public information campaigns alone. For example, seat belts and child auto safety restraints had been technologically feasible for decades before states began requiring their use. Before legislation, the percentage of child passengers using child auto safety restraints was in the teens. Today, in states such as North Carolina with vigorous enforcement of legislative mandates and loaner programs for poor families coupled with media campaigns, child auto safety restraint use may be as high as 80%.

Many large Maternal and Child Health (MCH)-related organizations have published handbooks and guides to effective advocacy (Children's Defense Fund, 1991; Michigan Council for Maternal and Child Health, n.d.). In 1981, the American Academy of Pediatrics produced an advocacy handbook for its state chapters (Government Affairs Committee, 1981). This manual outlines a strategic process for advocates to follow. Effective advocacy begins with identifying simple, specific, achievable objectives that "should benefit children directly and pediatricians indirectly, if at all" (Government Affairs Committee, 1981, p. 4). Next, advocates should develop data. Although data alone will not convince legislators, good data are necessary both to convince legislators and to gain the support of ancillary groups. Access to data enhances the credibility of advocates. Earning a reputation as a source of reliable information may lead to legislators and policy makers approaching the advocate for answers on the next child health issue.

Moving from a good idea and good data to a bill requires choosing an author to sponsor the legislation. One should select a legislator with authority and a place on the appropriate legislative committee. Working with or through a constituent from that legislator's home district, arrange a meeting, preceded by a letter outlining the proposal. Work with that legislator's staff to determine the feasibility of the proposal and the best ways to link the proposal with the legislator's personal interests. Once the meeting has taken place, assuming that the legislator agrees, the staff then provides the technical support necessary for crafting the most appropriate language for the legislation.

With a proposal for legislation and a secured sponsor, recruiting allies to the cause is a necessary next step. Natural allies for child advocacy are parent/teacher associations, junior leagues, March of Dimes chapters, state and local child advocacy councils, city/county boards of health, and educators. These allies can be key to marshaling additional constituent support at the local level for generating letters and phone calls and testifying at hearings. Coalitions of child advocacy groups can remain organized after the passage of the bill both for monitoring implementation and for developing a legislative agenda for the future.

Success in the legislative arena does not guarantee the changes necessary for children to realize the benefits. Advocacy involves continuing involvement during the rule-making process. Advocates must now turn their attention to the administrative department charged with the responsibility of implementing the law. In order to influence and monitor the implementation of regulations that put the legislation into effect, meetings with administrative staff may be necessary. Proposed regulations must be publicized with an adequate period for public comment. Advocates need to keep the sponsoring legislator(s) informed of the implementation process, especially if it is not going well. Lapses in effective advocacy at this stage may be part of the reason for the failure of early and periodic screening, diagnosis, and treatment to reach more than 39% of eligible children (Hill, 1992), given the administrative decision to place primary responsibility for the program in the reimbursement-minded federal Medicaid agency rather than the public health–oriented Title V agency.

In contrast, active advocacy through the Consumer Product Safety Commission has resulted in numerous regulatory bans of dangerous products such as unsafe toys, infant cribs with entrapment and strangulation hazards, and three-wheel all-terrain vehicles. In contrast to the popular impression of regulations as illegitimate violations of personal liberties, much public health regulation has enjoyed widespread public support. The most conspicuous examples come from auto safety regulation, but even in an era of suspicion of government, clean air and water regulations and even regulation of handguns and of access to tobacco products by minors can be successful, if opposition by well-funded special interests can be matched by the organized activities of child and public health advocates.

Regulatory authority for public health, as is the case for many other governmental functions in the United States, is divided among the three levels: federal, state, and local. Although most public health regulation resides at the state level, each level of government has a role to play. Advocates, therefore, need to be active at each level. Although the federal government is legitimately involved in actions and services that are in the public interest of the entire nation, especially in the case of conditions that do not respect state boundaries, it is at the state level that responsibility for assessment, assurance, and policy development is vested unless specifically assumed by the federal government. Child advocates with a national agenda may find the strategy of working up from the state level desirable. There are many examples of advocacy at the local level that not only succeeded in improving the health of children but also became precedents for action at the state level. The American Academy of Pediatrics has been a consistent supporter of legislative initiatives on behalf of children and families for over 65 years. Many of its successes can be traced to the advocacy activities of state pediatric societies. Among the triumphs at the state level that went on to become nation-wide policy are health insurance coverage for newborns, child auto safety seat legislation, and vaccine liability legislation. In the case of preventing tap water burns, Dr. Murray Katcher, former Director of Maternal and Child Health for Wisconsin, and his colleagues (1989) started advocating for regulating the maximum setting of hot water heaters at 120°F in Wisconsin. After a few other states joined ranks with Wisconsin, hot water heater manufacturers voluntarily agreed to a national standard that set the maximum temperature of new hot water heaters at the factory. Manufacturers realized that it would be in their best interest to have a single standard rather than 50 different standards, and advocates achieved a success without resorting to federal regulation. Importantly, many policy and program decisions having to do with public schools are made at the local level.

In addition to educational and legislative/regulatory strategies, advocates can attempt to secure the rights or interests of mothers and children through the judicial process. Numerous advocacy victories have been won in court when legislatures were immovable. Some of these, in the areas of juvenile justice and reproductive health, have already been alluded to. A good example from the area of children with special health care needs is the case of the Pennsylvania suit by parents, which resulted in a ruling guaranteeing free public education for all handicapped children (*Pennsylvania Association for Retarded Children v. Pennsylvania*, 1971). It was only *after* this landmark ruling that Congress passed the Education for All Handicapped Children Act (see Chapter 11).

# THE FUTURE

As argued by Preston (1984), the older population, in contrast to children, has three willing cohorts of advocates for their interests—older persons themselves, the adult children of the older population who want assistance in the care of their parents, and the adult children of the older persons who see themselves as eventually becoming old and needing assistance. In order to realize the promise of children's rights, a change needs to be made in the political perspectives of how to maximize the value of children (Kopelman & Palumbo, 1997).

Richard Titmuss (1975), the architect of the British National Health Service, has described three models of social policy that reflect the spectrum of political views at play in discussions of the well-being of children and families. One, the Residual Welfare Model, postulates that there are two legitimate ways to meet people's needs—through the family and through the free market. When one or the other breaks down, social institutions temporarily provide the necessary resources to individuals. Under this model, "the object of the welfare state is to teach people to do without it," and beneficiaries are expected to accept society's judgment that in some way or ways they have failed. This view prevailed in the passage of welfare reform in 1996. As described in Chapter 2, the transformation of welfare in the United States from an entitlement to a more incentive-based system has been associated with a marked decline in the proportion of children in poverty, especially those children at greatest risk of poverty (Blank & Haskins, 2001; Finegold & Wherry, 2004).

The second model, Industrial Achievement-Performance, exemplified by the former communist societies and currently represented by North Korea and Cuba, currently garners little political support in the United States. This model offers the social welfare system as an adjunct to the economy. Benefits are putatively distributed on the basis of need, but political decisions end up allocating welfare benefits based on one's status in the civil service or military bureaucracy.

Third, Titmuss describes the Industrial-Redistributive model, which offers universalistic services outside of the market economy. Resources are distributed according to the principle of equity based on need, that is, disproportionately more social benefits are allocated to the least well off. Under this model, social welfare is not viewed as short-term charity for individuals, but as an instrument of a social policy that provides for the needs of society as a whole. For Titmuss, this orientation is exemplified by the National Health Service itself, although this respected institution in Great Britain has been the object of continuous political debate, especially as Britain grapples with the same challenges to health care—aging population, increasing use of technology, and medical cost inflation—that are at play in the United States (Klein, 2001). Most west European countries, in one way or another, have created social policies that recognize access to basic health care and other welfare benefits as a right of all citizens, especially pregnant women and children (Miller, 1987). At the same time, Europe has begun to struggle with the demands and distortions that are created by universal entitlements in an aging population (Specter, 1998). Generous support for the older population in Europe and the United States is based on the view that their social contributions entitle them to societal benefits, without consideration for the population base and economic policies needed to sustain such benefits, a cause of growing political debate.

The future of the children is dependent on active and vibrant advocacy that articulates the unique value that the children's cause brings to political and economic analysis and policy development. In addition to their unique economic dimensions, children lack the developmental maturity to advocate for themselves. For these reasons, children are often excluded from the design and implementation of the very policies that affect them, making advocates essential. Promoting justice for children by distributing resources based on children's needs and by defining and securing rights for children is the central role that advocates play in policy debates. Not only should advocacy skills be taught to and practiced by public health officials but also, in turn, they should encourage the development of advocacy skills in the communities and among the parents with whom they work.

# REFERENCES

Americans with Disabilities Act, US Code Vol. 104, sec. 12101. Pub. L. 101-336 (1990).

Applebaum, D., & Lawton, S.V. (1990). *Ethics and the professions.* Englewood Cliffs, NJ: Prentice Hall.

Arrow, K. (1963). Uncertainty and the welfare economics of medical care. *The American Economic Review, 53,* 941–973.

Bandman, B. (1977). Some legal, moral, and intellectual rights of children. *Educational Theory, 17,* 169–178.

Beauchamp, T., & Childress, J.F. (2001). *Principles of biomedical ethics.* New York: Oxford University Press.

Beauchamp, D., & Steinbock, B. (Eds.). (1999). *New ethics for the public's health.* New York: Oxford University Press.

Blackstone, W. (1968). Blackstone on children and the rights and duties of parents. In G. Abbott (Ed.), *The child and the state: Legal status in the family, apprenticeship and child labor* (Vol. 1, pp. 9–13). New York: Greenwood Press.

Blank, R., & Haskins, R. (Eds.). (2001). *The new world of welfare.* Washington, DC: Brookings Institution Press.

Buchanan, A. (1984). The right to a decent minimum of health care. *Philos Public Aff 13,* 54–78.

Child Abuse Treatment and Prevention Act, Pub. L. 93-247 (1973).

Children's Defense Fund. (1991). *An advocate's guide to lobbying and political activity for nonprofits: What you can and can't do.* Washington, DC: Author.

DeMause, L. (1974). The evolution of childhood. In L. deMause (Ed.), *The history of childhood.* New York: Psychohistory Press.

Education for All Handicapped Children Act. Pub. L. 94-142 (1975).

Epstein, R. (1997). *Mortal peril: Our inalienable right to health care?* Reading, MA: Addison Wesley Publishing Company.

Feinberg, J. (1978). Rights. In T. Beauchamp & L. Walters (Eds.), *Contemporary Issues in Bioethics* (pp. 38–43). Encino, CA: Dickerson Publishing Co.

Fernandez, H.C. (1980). *The child advocacy handbook.* New York: The Pilgrim Press.

Finegold, K., & Wherry, L. (2004). *Race, ethnicity, and economic well-being: Snapshots of America's Families* (No. 19). Washington, DC: Urban Institute.

Gostin, L. (2000). *Public health law: Power, duty, restraint.* Berkeley, CA: University of California Press.

Government Affairs Committee, American Academy of Pediatrics. (1981). *Pediatricians and the legislative process: A potent prescription for children.* Washington, DC: American Academy of Pediatrics, Office of Government Liaison.

Green, R. (1976). Health care and justice in contract theory perspective. In R.M. Veatch & R. Branson (Eds.), *Ethics and health policy.* Cambridge, MA: Ballinger.

*Hammer v. Dagenhart,* 247 US Reports 251, 268 (1918).

Hill, I.T. (1992). The role of Medicaid and other government programs in providing medical care for children and pregnant women. *Future of Children, 2,* 134–153.

*In Re Gault,* 387 US 1 (1967).

Institute of Medicine. (1988). *The future of public health.* Washington, DC: National Academy Press.

Jennings, B., Kahn, J., Mastroianni, A., & Parker, L. (Eds.). (2003). *Ethics and public health: Model curriculum.* Rockville, MD: Health Services and Resources Administration.

Kahn, A., & McGowan, S. (1972). *Child advocacy: Report of a national baseline study.* Washington, DC: Columbia University School of Social Work and US Department of Health, Education and Welfare, Office of Child Development, Children's Bureau (HEW Publication #OCD 7318).

Katcher, M.L., Landry, G.L., & Shapiro, M.M. (1989). Liquid crystal thermometer use in Pediatric office counseling about tap water burn prevention. *Pediatrics, 83,* 766–771.

*Kent v. US,* US 383 541, 16 LE 2d 84, 86 S. Ct. 1045 (1966).

Klein, R. (2001). What's happening to Britain's national health service? *New England Journal of Medicine, 345,* 305–308.

Kopelman, L., & Palumbo, M. (1997). The US health care delivery system: Inefficient and unfair to children. *American Journal of Law and Medicine, 28,* 319–337.

Leiby, J. (1976). History of social welfare. In Minahan A. (Ed.), *Encyclopedia of Social Work* (18th ed., Vol. 1). Silver Spring, MD: National Association of Social Workers.

Margolis, L.H., & Salkind, N.J. (1996). Parents as advocates for their children. *Journal for a Just and Caring Education, 2,* 103–120.

Melton, G.B. (1991). Preserving the dignity of children around the world: The UN Convention on the rights of the child. *Child Abuse and Neglect, 15,* 343–350.

Michigan Council for Maternal and Child Health. (n.d.). *From vision to action: A citizens' guidebook to grass roots advocacy.* Lansing, MI: Michigan Council for Maternal and Child Health.

Miller, C.A. (1987). *Maternal health and child survival.* Washington, DC: National Center for Clinical Infant Programs.

*Pennsylvania Association for Retarded Children v. Pennsylvania,* 334 F. Supp. 1257 E. D. Pa (1971).

Pfohl, S.J. (1976). The "discovery" of child abuse. *Social Problems, 24,* 310–323.

*Planned Parenthood of Central Missouri v. Danforth,* 428 US 52, 96 S. Ct. 2831 (1976).

Preston, S.H. (1984). Children and the elderly: Divergent paths for America's dependents. *Demography, 21,* 435–457.

Rawls, J. (1969). *A theory of justice.* Cambridge, MA: Harvard University Press.

Roberts, B.S., & Considine, B.G. (1997). Public policy advocacy. In H.M. Wallace, J.C. MacQueen, R.F. Biehl, & J.A. Blackman (Eds.), *Mosby's resource guide to children with disabilities and chronic illness* (pp. 162–171). St. Louis, MO: Mosby.

Roosevelt, T. (1971). The conservation of childhood. In R. Bremner (Ed.), *Children and Youth in America* (Vol. 2, pp. 653–654). Washington, DC: American Public Health Association.

Specter, M. (1998, July 10). Population implosion worries a graying Europe. *New York Times.*

Stiglitz, J. (2000). *Economics of the public sector.* New York: W. W. Norton.

Titmuss, R. (1975). Social policy: An introduction. New York: Pantheon Books.

Tuchman, B.W. (1978). *A distant mirror.* New York: Alfred A. Knopf.

US Department of Health, Education and Welfare, Office of Child Development, Children's Bureau, National Center on Child Abuse and Neglect. (1976). Child abuse and neglect: An overview of the problem. In *The Problem and Its Management* (Vol. 1). Washington, DC: Author.

White House Conference on Children. (1971). *Report to the President.* Washington, DC: US Government Printing Office.

Williams, G.J.R. (1983). Child protection: A journey into history. *Journal of Clinical Child Psychology, 12,* 236–243.

# CHAPTER 2

# Historical Foundations of Maternal and Child Health

*Lewis Margolis, George Cole, and Jonathan Kotch*

> *These questions of child health and protection are a complicated problem requiring much learning and action. And we need have great concern over this matter. Let no one believe that these are questions which should not stir a nation; that they are below the dignity of statesman or governments. If we could have but one generation of properly born, trained, educated, and healthy children, a thousand other problems of government would vanish.*
> (Herbert Hoover, 1931)

## INTRODUCTION

Policy development to address the needs of mothers and children has played out in the unique political and social context of the United States. Three attributes in particular have influenced and continue to influence the development of maternal and child health (MCH) policies. One attribute is federalism, that is, the fact that there are two major governmental entities—federal and state—that vie for influence within the structure outlined in the US Constitution. This federal state relationship is further complicated by the fact that there are thousands of county and city jurisdictions, each of which relates to both the federal government and its own state. The relative influence of these partners has waxed and waned since the onset of local and state government interest in the population of mothers and children at the close of the 19th century.

A second attribute is the independent judiciary that has served as the interpreter and upholder of the basic values infused in the Constitution. Although the interpretation of certain constitutional limits has varied over the years, any given legislative action must pass judicial muster. The third attribute of the US political and social scene is the high value placed on individualism, the free enterprise economic system, and the concomitant and dominant role of the private sector. Governmental influence in many spheres of life in the United States is generally justified in response to market failures rather than as a fundamental aspect of the social framework (Epstein, 2003; Gostin & Blocke, 2003).

This chapter characterizes three phases in the development of US health policy for mothers and children. First, the chapter reviews the origins of local, state, and federal participation in health care for mothers and children. Next, the discussion focuses on the emergence of the federal government as a major force in public MCH program development, with particular attention to the federal role in addressing equity. The chapter then concludes with consideration of the current political efforts to return power and responsibility for MCH policies, once again, to the states. Table 2–1 presents a chronology of the development of MCH services in the United States.

# ORIGINS OF GOVERNMENTAL PARTICIPATION IN THE CARE OF MOTHERS AND CHILDREN

These attributes of social policy began to interact in prominent ways with regard to mothers and children after the Civil War. A series of developments prompted increased attention to the particular needs of children as distinct from adults. In the field of medicine, Dr. Abraham Jacobi and others began to articulate that the therapeutic needs of children differed from those of adults. Developments in the field of sanitation provided new understanding of determinants of infant mortality (Meckel, 1990). Fundamental discoveries in bacteriology and the prevention and control

**Table 2-1  Chronology of MCH Services in the United States**

| | |
|---|---|
| 1855 | Founding of the Children's Hospital of Philadelphia |
| 1869 | State board of health established in Massachusetts |
| 1879 | Formation of a Section on Diseases of Children of the American Medical Association |
| 1888 | The American Pediatric Society founded to promote scientific inquiry into children's diseases |
| 1893 | First milk station established in New York City |
| 1904 | National Child Labor Committee organized to monitor effects of child labor on health and development |
| 1907 | First Bureau of Child Hygiene established in New York City |
| 1909 | First White House Conference on Children called by President Theodore Roosevelt |
| 1912 | Congress established the Children's Bureau |
| 1921 | First Maternity and Infancy Act (Sheppard-Towner) |
| 1930 | American Academy of Pediatrics founded |
| 1935 | Social Security Act, including grants to states for aid for dependent children and maternal and child welfare (Titles IV and V, respectively), enacted |
| 1943 | Emergency Maternity and Infant Care Act |
| 1944 | Association of Maternal and Child Health Programs founded as the Association of Directors of State and Territorial Maternal and Child Health and Crippled Children Services |
| 1951 | American College of Obstetricians and Gynecologists founded |
| 1954 | Special appropriation to MCH programs for community services for children with mental retardation |
| 1963 | Special project grants for Maternity and Infant Care |
| 1965 | Title XVIII (Medicare) and Title XIX (Medicaid) added to the Social Security Act; amendments to Title V establish maternity care and children's projects; first Neighborhood Health Center grant awarded |
| 1967 | Office of Child Development created as a home for Head Start; functions of the Children's Bureau distributed among four federal agencies |
| 1968 | Amendments to Title V and Title XIX authorizing the creation of Early and Periodic Screening, Diagnosis, and Treatment |
| 1972 | Special Supplemental Food Program for Women, Infants, and Children established |
| 1974 | Child Abuse Prevention and Treatment Act enacted |
| 1981 | Maternal and Child Health Services Block Grant amendments to Title V enacted |
| 1984 | Beginning of a series of amendments to expand access to Medicaid |
| 1989 | Title V amended to increase accountability |
| 1991 | Healthy Start funded in 15 communities |
| 1996 | The Personal Responsibility and Work Opportunity Reconciliation Act |
| 1997 | Title XXI (State Child Health Insurance Program) added to the Social Security Act |

of infectious diseases provided a dramatic opportunity to demonstrate the possibilities of preventing infant deaths (Lesser, 1985). Although the discovery of the "germ theory" of disease gave public health a technological base, it became clear that prevention was not simply a medical research issue. Effective health promotion also demanded social mechanisms, the most important of which was public health education (Tratner, 1974).

In 1874, Henry Bergh, founder of the New York Society for the Prevention of Cruelty to Animals, personally intervened on behalf of a child who had been physically abused, bringing her situation to the attention of local authorities in New York City. Outrage over the absence of laws to protect children from such treatment prompted New York and other cities to enact laws prohibiting child cruelty and giving private agencies police authority to intervene in abusive situations (Williams, 1983). In New York, the new Society for the Prevention of Cruelty to Children assumed this responsibility.

Throughout history, children have been expected to provide menial or hazardous labor for their parents. The intense industrialization of the late 19th century drew many children into factories and mines, raising the concerns of child advocates and social reformers about the effects of working conditions on the health and education of children. Industrialization led to the creation of labor-intensive, low-paid jobs in mills, mines, and factories. Coupled with the high Civil War mortality experienced by working-aged males, especially in the South, this situation resulted in the widespread employment of children in a number of out-of-home occupations (Schmidt & Wallace, 1988). By 1900, one in six 10- to 15-year-olds was employed, 40% in industry, 60% in agriculture, and children as young as 7 years were employed in poor or hazardous work environments (Schmidt & Wallace, 1988).

In 1916 the Keating–Owen Act prohibited interstate commerce of goods produced by children. This legislation was controversial because of the necessity for children from poor families to work, and it was overturned by the US Supreme Court in a 1918 case, *Hammer v. Dagenhart*, from textile-producing North Carolina (Berger & Johansson, 1980). It was not until the Depression forced unemployed adults to take jobs previously reserved for children that child labor was permanently constrained (Miller, 1988).

As immigrants poured into cities seeking new opportunities, the unmet health and educational needs of their children, as well as the potential threat to public health through the transmission of infectious diseases, became the subject of concern for reformers and politicians. The institutionalization of vital records keeping provided the first real evidence of the social impact of infant mortality. Infant death records revealed that in the United States in 1900, infant mortality averaged 150 per 1,000 births and was as high as 180/1,000 in some industrial cities and claimed as many as 50% of the infants that had been abandoned or orphaned to the foundling hospitals that proliferated as a result of urbanization and immigration (Schmidt & Wallace, 1988). In this context, late 19th and early 20th-century social workers and public health officials joined forces. As social workers recognized that poverty and social dislocation engendered ill health and that ill health caused poverty by creating economic burdens, they used their particular skills to combat poverty by promoting good health. They mobilized the lay leaders and residents of the community for the control of disease (Tratner, 1974). For example, recognizing the risk to infants of consuming spoiled milk, and the heightened risk for poor infants because of the lack of adequate storage facilities, public health advocates urged municipalities and private individuals to fund milk stations where poor families could collect fresh milk (Grotberg, 1977).

The evolving concept of childhood as a "special" period of growth, socialization, and development provided a rational context for advocacy, whereas child labor, infant mortality, and child maltreatment provided highly visible targets for reform. A coalition of female reformers, the driving force behind the women's suffrage movement, lent energy, motivation, and "critical mass" to the ranks of settlement house workers, social workers, and public health nurses engaged in child advocacy. The first Bureau of Child Hygiene was established in 1907 in New York City under the leadership of Dr. S. Josephine Baker. She had entered the New York City Health Department after prejudice against female physicians had limited her ability to advance in academic medicine and private practice (Baker, 1994). One of the main strategies undertaken by Baker was to send public health nurses to visit the tenement homes of newborn babies in order to educate mothers about how to care for their new infants. The bureau became involved in the care of school children, the supervision of midwives, and the regulation of children's institutions.

The convergence of social, economic, and political forces at the turn of the century resulted in the call for a federal role in promoting, if not assuring, the well-being of children. In 1909, President Theodore Roosevelt convened the first White House Conference on Children. Emerging from the conference were calls for service programs and financial aid to protect the home environment and recommendations that the federal government take responsibility for gathering information on problems of infant and child health and welfare (Lesser, 1985; Schmidt & Wallace, 1988; Skocpol, 1992; Tratner, 1974). These recommendations gave rise to the Mother's Aid Movement and the American Association for the Study and Prevention of Infant Mortality. The former group drew attention to the benefits of keeping children in the family while pointing out the detrimental effects of dehumanizing institutions. The latter group drew attention to the unacceptably high rate of infant deaths (Lesser, 1985; Schmidt & Wallace, 1988; Tratner, 1974).

With advocacy from education, psychology, medicine, public health, labor, and social work, and over the opposition of groups opposing federal meddling in the private domain of parents, Congress followed another of the conference's recommendations and enacted legislation establishing the Children's Bureau. Legislation for such an agency had been first introduced in 1906, but intense debate centering on the question of whether child welfare was a federal or state responsibility stalled its passage until 1912. Assigned to the Department of Commerce and Labor, reflecting the roots of the bureau in concern over labor conditions for children, the act charged the Children's Bureau to "investigate and report . . . upon all matters pertaining to the welfare of children and child life among all classes of our people, and . . . especially investigate the questions of infant mortality, the birth rate, orphanages, juvenile courts, desertion, dangerous occupations, accidents and diseases of children, employment, and legislation affecting children in the several States and Territories" (US Congress, 1912). The tension between public and private responsibility for children was reflected in the legislation that stated, "No official, or agent, or representative of said bureau shall, over the objection of the head of the family, enter any house used exclusively as a family residence."

Under the leadership of its first chief, Julia Lathrop, the Children's Bureau embarked on an active repertoire of investigations into the conditions of children. For example, the bureau conducted a longitudinal study of the relationship between income and infant mortality (Lathrop, 1919). Other studies addressed child labor, working mothers, children's nutrition, services for crippled children, and juvenile delinquency. In 1915, as the result of bureau studies that concluded that birth registration is "the starting point for the reduction of infant mortality by identifying infants at risk for health problems, or dying," the National Birth Registry was established.

Although the mandate of the bureau was to investigate and report, its leaders began to develop a legislative agenda to address identified problems. In 1918, Representative Jeanette Rankin of Montana introduced legislation to provide federal funds to the states to establish preventive health programs for mothers and infants (Wilson, 1989). This legislation was strongly supported by the suffragettes but was opposed by the medical community because it would place responsibility for a health care program under the "nonmedical" Children's Bureau (Lesser, 1985). In the midst of the debate over the legislation, the Second White House Conference on Children in 1919 issued recommendations for minimum standards of MCH care.

By 1920, sponsorship of the bill was assumed by Senator Morris Sheppard of Texas and Representative Horace Towner of Iowa. Subsequently, partially in recognition that the United States was not doing particularly well in responding to problems of maternal and infant health and partially out of fear of a feminine voting bloc backlash, Congress passed the Maternity and Infancy Act (also known as the Sheppard-Towner Act) in November 1921 (Schmidt & Wallace, 1988).The Sheppard-Towner Act authorized grants paid "to the several States for the purpose of cooperating with them in promotion the welfare and hygiene of maternity and infancy as hereinafter provided" (Bremner, 1970). Under the act, each state that elected to receive these funds was required to establish a child welfare or child hygiene agency, representing the first federal effort to develop a MCH infrastructure within the states. The monies were allocated as a grant in two parts. Under the first part, each state received an equal share of a $480,000 appropriation. Under the second part, totaling $1,000,000, each state received $5,000, plus an amount proportionate to that state's population in the census of 1920. States were required to match the funds provided under the second part of the act. Funds were distributed in response "to detailed plans for carrying out the provisions of this Act within such State." Although the Sheppard-Towner Act did not regulate the content of these plans beyond "promoting the welfare and hygiene of maternity and infancy," the legislation was quite explicit in what states were not permitted to do.

Continuing the attention to individual liberty instilled in the Children's Bureau authorization, the act asserted the following:

> No official, agent, or representative of the Children's Bureau shall by virtue of this Act have any right to enter any home over the objection of the owner thereof, or to take charge of any children over the objection of the parents, or either of them, or of the person standing *in loco parentis* or having custody of such child. Nothing in this Act shall be construed as limiting the power of a parent or guardian or person standing *in loco parentis* to determine what treatment or correction shall be provided for a child or the agency or agencies to be employed for such purpose. Second, states were not permitted to spend monies on buildings or payment of any maternity or infancy pension, stipend, or gratuity.

The Congressional debate over the Sheppard-Towner Act replicated the heated encounters that occurred over the establishment of the Children's Bureau. On one side were those who argued for a federal role in promoting the welfare of mothers and children. This argument was presented in economic terms, that is, that the federal government plays a role in agricultural and commercial activities in order to promote economic development and that children represent no less valuable a resource. The opposition to Sheppard-Towner was argued on several grounds. Some were opposed to any governmental role, that is, interference, in the relationship between children and their parents. In this view, the family was a private domain, and the responsibility for children resided with their parents or local family members or charities. Another source of opposition was organized medicine through the American Medical Association (AMA). Exploiting the uncertainty and fear stemming from the Communist revolution in Russia in 1917, the AMA decried the law as an "imported socialistic scheme unsuited to our form of government." Furthermore, the AMA sought to protect practitioners from what was perceived as the potential for governmental interference or control over the practice of medicine, despite the fact that Sheppard-Towner support for primary care (as opposed to preventive care) was expressly forbidden. Furthermore, the bill was also assailed by conservatives as "a move toward eliminating racial discrimination" because it required services to be available to all citizens. When it was reconsidered in 1929, the Maternity and Infancy Act was defeated (Schmidt & Wallace, 1988).

The debate within the AMA over Sheppard-Towner spawned the birth of the American Academy of Pediatrics (Hughes, 1980). During the 1922 meeting of the AMA, the Pediatric Section debated and endorsed Sheppard-Towner, concluding that it was in the best interests of mothers and children. The AMA House of Delegates, however, not only condemned the act, but also repudiated the Pediatric Section for its endorsement without the approval of the governing House. Recognizing that the AMA was not prepared to speak for the welfare of children, pediatricians met over the next 8 years and finally convened the first meeting of the American Academy of Pediatrics in Detroit in 1930, becoming a powerful and consistent supporter of MCH policies and programs (Lesser, 1985; Schmidt & Wallace, 1988).

The Sheppard-Towner Act passed handily in 1921, in part because of uncertainty over how newly enfranchised women would vote. Passage of this legislation was the first national political issue to follow the passage the previous year of the 19th amendment, granting women the right to vote. Another factor that facilitated its passage was the effort to assuage organized medicine by emphasizing the preventive nature of this legislation in an attempt to avoid a conflict with the private practice of medicine. Whereas physicians were viewed as the appropriate source of care for sick infants and parturient women, the educational and screening activities envisioned in the bill were presented as complements and enhancements of traditional medical care. Nevertheless, opposition intensified throughout the 1920s. Physicians began to recognize the competitive potential that the provision of preventive services had for the development of their practices. Opposition also grew within the Catholic Church, fearful of a governmental role in the provision of historically church-based charitable services. A third source of protest came from within the Public Health Service, annoyed at the dissemination of health services through this program of the Department of Commerce and Labor. As a result, the act was not renewed after 1929. In succumbing, the Maternity and Infancy Act established the hegemony of both the medical community and the medical model in MCH policy development and established the publicly funded use of private providers as the preferred method of health care delivery.

The accomplishments of the Sheppard-Towner Act were reviewed in the Eighteenth Annual Report of the Children's Bureau. Birth registration increased from 30 states, covering 72% of the births in 1922, to 46 states, representing 95% of the population. By 1920, child hygiene bureaus had been established in 28 states, 16 of them in 1919 alone, as a result of Children's Bureau leadership. After the implementation of the act, another 19 states established such bureaus. Hundreds of maternal and/or child health consultation centers were established, often in conjunction with local health agencies. Even after expiration of the appropriation, 19 states continued to fund the efforts implemented under the act.

## THE EMERGENCE OF THE FEDERAL GOVERNMENT IN COMMUNITY ASSESSMENT, POLICY DEVELOPMENT, AND ASSURANCE FOR MOTHERS AND CHILDREN

With the descent into the Great Depression in 1929, many states and local communities were confronted by the challenge of rising health needs in the face of catastrophic levels of unemployment and devastated budgets as state and local governments witnessed the decimation of their tax bases. State programs for indigent parents and children existed, but without Maternity and Infancy Act funds, health services for mothers and infants were drastically reduced. By 1934, "23 states appropriated virtually no MCH funds" for such services (Lesser, 1985, p. 592). The Depression impoverished 40% of the population, including a good number of citizens of good moral credentials. Therefore, the link between indigency and immorality was weakened.

After his election in 1932, President Franklin D. Roosevelt recommended legislation designed to provide temporary assistance to the "deserving" poor and ongoing economic insurance to those who were making it but might need help in the future (Guyer, 1987). He charged the Economic Security Committee to address "security for men, women and children . . . against several of the great disturbing factors of life—especially those which relate to unemployment and old age" (Grotberg, 1977, p. 87). Consultation with Grace Abbott and other representatives of the Children's Bureau resulted in the incorporation of bureau plans into the Social Security Act of 1935. The Bureau proposed three major sets of activities: (1) aid to dependent children, (2) welfare services for children needing special care, and (3) MCH services including services for crippled children. These were incorporated into the Social Security Act, enacted on August 14, 1935 (Hutchins, 1994). Title IV provided cash payments to mothers who had lost fathers' support for their children. Responsibility for this title was given to the newly created Social Security Board, rather than the Children's Bureau. Title V consisted of four parts. Part 1, Maternal and Child Health Services, represented an expansion of the programs established under the Sheppard-Towner Act. Part 2, Services for Crippled Children, enabled states to improve services for locating crippled children and "for providing medical, surgical, corrective, and other services and care, and facilities for diagnosis, hospitalization, and aftercare, for children who are crippled or who are suffering from conditions which lead to crippling" (US Congress, 1935, p. 631). Part 3, Child-Welfare Services, enabled states to provide services for "the protection and care of homeless, dependent, and neglected children, and children in danger of becoming delinquent" (US Congress, 1935, p. 633). Part 4, Vocational Rehabilitation, enabled states to strengthen programs of vocational rehabilitation of the physically disabled, although the administration of this part was not under the Children's Bureau.

A broad base of public support existed for the child health, welfare, and economic security components of the Social Security Act. Support for Titles IV and V was especially strong, with leading women's organizations of the country present at the Congressional hearings to express their support. Opposition to Titles IV and V, which might have been expected given the history of the Maternity and Infancy Act, did not materialize. The AMA was preoccupied with the broader issue of blocking any possibility of national health insurance (Witte, 1963).

Unlike Title IV, which was an entitlement, funding for Title V was discretionary and had several components. One set of funds sent an equal share to each state. A second set was distributed on the basis of live births and required a dollar for dollar match. A third set of funds was allocated based on financial need and the number of live births, without a required match. Finally, Crippled Children's funds provided an equal share as well as an allotment based on the number of children served, building an incentive to locate and treat children. The secretary retained up to 15% of the appropriation for training, research, and demonstrations, including Special Projects of Regional and National Significance (SPRANS).

The onset of World War II created a new challenge in addressing the health needs of mothers and children. With the mobilization of millions of soldiers, many military wives who dislocated from their homes were in need of maternity care. Although the bureau attempted to provide support for medical care and hospitalization of these women through Title V funds, the amounts were inadequate. In 1943, Congress appropriated additional funds for the Emergency Maternity and Infant Care Program. These funds, allocated from general revenues and distributed through the states with no required match, paid for medical care for the wives of servicemen in the lowest four pay grades. By the time the program was phased out in 1949, it had provided care in 1.5 million maternity cases, approximately one of every seven births in the United States at its peak (Grotberg, 1977).

Federal initiatives after World War II were rather limited. Although Title V secured and encouraged the development of MCH agencies within state health departments, the federal government directed its efforts mainly at the support of research and services for particular diseases. For example, the Crippled Children's Program adopted many conditions beyond the orthopedic problems that were the first targets of its programs. Epilepsy, congenital and rheumatic heart disease, hearing impairments, premature newborn care, and other conditions were incorporated into state programs (Lesser, 1985).

Also after the Second World War, the Children's Bureau began a slow but steady decline from its position of prominence in the national health and welfare arena. At its founding in 1912, the director of the bureau reported directly to the Secretary of Commerce and Labor and then, after the department split in 1913, to the Secretary of Labor. Although arguments were raised about the appropriateness of the bureau within Labor as opposed to the Public Health Service, the early leaders of the bureau maintained its leadership role in a wide range of maternal and child interests. During the 1930s, consideration was given to dividing the health, education, and welfare activities of the bureau among various agencies, but the political pressure both within and outside the federal bureaucracy was not sufficient to effect this change until the late 1940s. The bureau was moved to the newly created Federal Security Administration in 1945. Although it did retain control, temporarily, of the various grant-in-aid programs that it had developed and administered, this move marked the beginning of the decline of the influence of the Children's Bureau.

# SOCIAL ACTIVISM, EQUITY, AND THE DEVELOPMENT OF MATERNAL AND CHILD HEALTH POLICY IN THE 1960S

## Special Projects Under Title V of the Social Security Act

President Kennedy's interest in mental retardation, stirred in part by the efforts of his parents to provide for their mentally retarded daughter, provided the bureau with the opportunity to launch new initiatives. Arguing that mental retardation could be prevented, in part, by adequate prenatal care, the administration developed a program of special grants through Title V. Different from the traditional Bureau focus on preventive services, these maternity and infant care (M & I) projects, authorized by PL 88-156 in 1963, were designed to provide comprehensive services including prenatal, intrapartum, and postpartum medical care and hospitalization. By 1969, 53 projects had served 100,000 impoverished women and their infants nationwide (Lesser, 1985). Not only did the scope of supported activities change with the introduction of these projects, but also the administration of bureau activities changed. Rather than allocating funds through state health agencies, the bureau distributed M & I funds directly to the service agencies. Furthermore, funds for these demonstration projects could be allocated to private, nonprofit institutions. Comparable projects for children and youth (C & Y) were inaugurated in 1965. By 1969, 58 C & Y Projects had provided preventive and primary medical care to 335,000 children (Lesser, 1985). Funded as "demonstration" projects, the M & I projects in particular reported notable improvements in infant health (Sokol, Woolf, Rosen, & Weingarden, 1980). Special projects for neonatal intensive care, family planning, and dental care followed. The M & I and C & Y projects expanded in number during the 1960s and early 1970s but were never extended beyond their demonstration status to become the general policy.

## Public Health and Child Protection

The period from 1960 to 1974 was much like the earlier era of social reform in its public expression of social malcontent and institutional mistrust. Civil rights advocates established that otherwise disenfranchised adults and children had rights that could be enforced by legal and administrative means. Furthermore, by gaining legal access to bureaucratic decision making, those same advocates challenged the complacency of professionals who purportedly "served" disenfranchised adults and children.

At the same time, medical and public health professionals were challenged to reconsider the relationship of child health and social phenomena. In 1946, John Caffey, a pediatric radiologist, published an article describing traumatic long bone fractures in infants. In 1953, an article by Silverman, also a radiologist, discussed the possibility that such fractures might be parent induced. In 1955, Wooley and Evans concluded that infants suffering from repeated fractures often come from homes with aggressive, immature, or emotionally ill adults. In 1957, Caffey recapitulated his earlier findings, adding a commission to physicians to consider parental abuse when diagnosing injured infants (Pfohl, 1976).

However, it was not until 1962, with the publication of Henry Kempe's article, "The Battered Child Syndrome," that the phenomenon of physically abused children seen in the nation's hospitals caught the attention of child health professionals and the public everywhere. "The Battered Child Syndrome" challenged the belief that parental abuse "was a deplorable fact of antiquity." It also documented the medical community's unwillingness to implicate parents in diagnosing abuse (Pfohl, 1976; Williams, 1983).

The public health community's response to Kempe's "discovery" of child abuse was immediate and dramatic, and within a decade, child protection had become a national priority. In 1962, the Children's Bureau prepared and disseminated a model child abuse reporting law, and the Social Security Amendments of 1962 required each state to make child welfare services available to all children, including the abused child. In 1963, 18 bills to protect abused children were introduced in Congress, 11 of which passed, and "throughout the 1960s and into the early 1970s, states developed or expanded their capacities to investigate and treat reports of child abuse." By 1967, all states had child abuse reporting laws (Pfohl, 1976; Williams, 1983).

In 1973, widely publicized hearings were chaired by Senator Walter Mondale (Democrat from Minnesota) on proposed legislation to establish federal leadership in child protection. In 1974, with the support of virtually every children's advocacy group and the AMA, the Child Abuse Prevention and Treatment Act was passed, creating a structure for responding to the problem of child maltreatment much like the original

Children's Bureau had been a structure for responding to MCH needs (Williams, 1983).

### Title XVIII (Medicare) and Title XIX (Medicaid)

Culminating three decades of debate over the nature of the federal role in providing health insurance, Congress enacted Medicare, Title XVIII of the Social Security Act, in 1965. Unique among industrialized nations with compulsory health insurance, the United States limits its coverage to the older population. Medicare provides coverage for short-term hospitalization and medical services. Hospitalization is financed through employment taxes, and physician services are financed jointly through premiums (approximately 25% of the actuarial cost) and general federal revenues (the remaining cost). Unlike Title V, states play no role in the financing, administering, or standard setting for this program.

Because the political struggle over the federal role in health care was waged in the arena of Medicare, the accompanying legislation to establish Medicaid, a program of health insurance assistance for the poor, was shielded from controversy. Enacted as Title XIX of the Social Security Act, the structure of the Medicaid program built on earlier federal support to the states for low-income older persons. Although an entitlement like Medicare, the Medicaid program involves joint federal–state financing and state development of standards within guidelines established by the federal government. A third characteristic of Medicaid (a characteristic that has gradually changed through a series of alterations during the 1980s) was the linkage of eligibility for Medicaid to eligibility for Aid for Families with Dependent Children (AFDC). Consistent with the state–federal partnership, criteria for welfare eligibility are established by the states so that state welfare regulations have a direct effect on eligibility for the federal Medicaid program. The welfare eligibility requirement severely limited eligibility for Medicaid. As Davis and Schoen (1978) noted in *Health and the War on Poverty*, a majority of states limited AFDC to families without a father in the home. The income and assets requirements further limited access to the program. For example, in 1985, the cutoff for eligibility for Medicaid ranged among states from a low of only 16% of the federal poverty income guidelines to 97% (Rosenbaum & Johnson, 1986).

Soon after the implementation of Medicaid, it became apparent that its focus on acute medical care rather than preventive services impeded its effectiveness for children. Social Security amendments submitted by

President Lyndon Johnson in 1967 modified Medicaid and Title V Crippled Children's programs to include a new benefit, the Early and Periodic Screening, Diagnosis, and Treatment (EPSDT) program. Building on language in the original Crippled Children's legislation of 1935, the EPSDT program has been described as "potentially the most comprehensive child health care program the government had ever undertaken" (Foltz, 1975, p. 35). The program called for specific services such as physical and developmental exams, vision and hearing screening, appropriate laboratory tests, dental referral, immunizations, and payment for other services covered by each state's Medicaid program. Furthermore, the services had to be provided according to a periodicity schedule consistent with reasonable standards of care. Finally, states were expected actively to enroll Medicaid-eligible children into their programs.

Unfortunately, the implementation of EPSDT was slowed by several issues. First, the program was cobbled together through changes in programs (Medicaid and Title V) with different missions and different bureaucracies. In particular, the Medicaid program was anchored in the welfare system with its restrictive eligibility criteria, impairing the ability of this bold screening, referral, and treatment program to reach broad groups of children in need. Second, the costs of such an ambitious screening and treatment program were daunting to the states that were required to pay for these new services under the shared financing structure of Medicaid. As Rosenbaum and Johnson (1986) have emphasized, however, the main obstacle to the successful implementation of EPSDT as a program to address the preventive health needs of poor children was the fact that the proportion of poor children who were Medicaid eligible remained low.

In spite of the limitations of the Medicaid program, it did increase access to medical care for poor children. According to a review conducted by the Office of Technology Assessment (US Congress, 1988) and published in *Healthy Children: Investing in the Future*, children with Medicaid were similar to middle-income insured children with regard to general check-ups and immunizations. Furthermore, Medicaid recipients with health problems were more likely to have seen a physician than were uninsured children. Although use of services increased for Medicaid recipients, the sites of care tended to be public health clinics, emergency rooms, and hospital outpatient departments rather than private physician offices (Orr & Miller, 1981), resulting in the further evolution of a dual system of health care. Studies of the effectiveness of EPSDT in particular suggest that participation in the program decreased the likelihood of referral for specialized care over time (Irwin & Conroy-Hughes, 1982; Keller, 1983). Other studies confirm that this screening and prevention program has not achieved the goals originally envisioned. For example, a review of California's screening program indicated that 30% of the children under one enrolled in Medicaid reported a preventive service, and only 65% of children aged 1 to 4 years were up to date on their immunizations (Yudkowsky & Fleming, 1990).

## Neighborhood/Community Health Centers

Although Medicaid quickly became the financial underpinning of medical services for poor mothers and children, several additional health programs arose out of the political and social activism of the early 1960s. The Economic Opportunity Act of 1964 established the Office of Economic Opportunity. Recognizing medical care as only one of many determinants of health, the Office of Economic Opportunity funded a series of Neighborhood Health Centers. Although these centers provided comprehensive medical services, including prevention and treatment of physical and mental conditions, their mission was much broader. The Neighborhood Health Centers provided employment opportunities in their low-income catchment areas and served as the focus for other community and economic development activities. In addition to the broad service mandate, several other characteristics made these centers a unique approach to health services for the poor. For example, independent of state and local governments, the centers were supposed to be governed by boards of community members. Furthermore, services were supposed to be without cost to the users.

A key administrative and political aspect of these centers was that their federal support came directly to the local community organizations that had solicited the funds. Unlike the Title V program and Medicaid that allocated funds to states and required a state match, the establishment of Neighborhood Health Centers enabled federal policy makers to leap over potential state level bureaucratic impediments to addressing local conditions as well as social and political attitudes and prejudices that had disenfranchised the poor people who needed the services provided by these health centers (Sardell, 1988).

As political support for the War on Poverty declined with the election of Richard Nixon in 1968, the legislative base for Neighborhood Health Centers changed. As Sardell (1988) noted, the centers achieved their own authorization under PL 94-63 and were renamed Community Health Centers. Unfortunately, attempts to rationalize the administration and oversight of the centers through the delineation of two types of financial support for (1) required and (2) supplemental services resulted in disproportionate emphasis on required, traditional medical services in contrast to the supplemental services such as health education, social services, and outreach. The appeal of the infrastructure established by the centers was strong, however, and Congress has occasionally appropriated funds for special infant mortality initiatives by them.

### Special Supplemental Food Program for Women, Infants, and Children

Created in 1972, the Special Supplemental Food Program for Women, Infants, and Children (WIC) has become a fundamental component of government support for mothers and children. This discretionary program provides supplemental food, nutrition education, and access to medical care. Under eligibility guidelines established by the federal government and through federally appropriated funds, states distribute food (or coupons for selected, nutritious foods) to low-income pregnant women, nursing mothers, and infants and children considered at nutritional risk. The key economic risk factor is family income under 185% of the federal poverty level. WIC has been associated with health improvements reflected in decreased rates of low birth weight (Rush, Sloan, Leighton, Alvir, Horvitz, Seaver, Garbowski, et al., 1988) and anemia (Yip, Bintin, Fleshood, & Trowbridge, 1987). From a services perspective, there has been difficulty in incorporating WIC into other MCH programs. As indicated later here in the discussion of major policy changes in the 1980s, administrative efforts are underway to make the supplemental food program a more cohesive part of services for mothers and children. For example, studies of the linkage of the provision of WIC services with immunization have, not surprisingly, shown marked improvement in immunization rates (Kotch & Whiteman, 1982) and use of dental services (Lee, Rozier, Kotch, Norton, & Vann, 2004).

### Head Start

Just as Community Health Centers provided sites around which to organize efforts to address the more far-reaching determinants, the period of early childhood offered a time during which key social and economic influences might be altered to promote the later well-being of children. Project Head Start was launched as a summer program in 1965 to provide an intellectually stimulating and healthful environment for preschool children in centers established for that purpose. Proposed for 100,000 children, the popularity was such that over 560,000 children enrolled during that first summer. In spite of controversy over the intellectual benefits of Head Start, this federal effort has grown steadily since its inception. An often overlooked impact of Head Start has been its effect on health. In a review of Head Start studies, Ron Haskins (1989), then a staff analyst with the Committee on Ways and Means of the House of Representatives, noted that children attending Head Start were "more likely to get medical and dental exams, speech and developmental assessments, nutrition evaluations, and vision and hearing screenings." Furthermore, Head Start programs are well-targeted toward poor children and provide many jobs as teachers and staff for low-income community members.

With the implementation of Head Start, the Children's Bureau met its functional, if not legislative, demise. The focus of bureau responsibilities had become increasingly in the area of welfare, even though the actual administration of AFDC fell within the purview of another agency. As reviewed by Steiner (1976), there was reluctance to assign a prominent and potentially substantial initiative such as Head Start to the Children's Bureau. Secretary of Health, Education, and Welfare Robert Finch, lacking strong political support for the Children's Bureau, delegated Head Start to a newly created Office of Child Development, also assigning the Children's Bureau, a shell of its former self, to this newly created office. The Title V Maternal and Child Health and Crippled Children's programs were assigned to the Health Services and Mental Health Administration of the Public Health Service. Child Welfare Services and the Juvenile Delinquency Service were assigned to the Social and Rehabilitation Service (Hutchins, 1994). What remained of the Children's Bureau was left with its responsibilities limited to that of a clearinghouse for agency information about children's health and welfare.

## REDEFINING THE ROLES OF STATES

The election of Ronald Reagan as President in 1980 was followed by changes in Title V and Medicaid. As part of the Reagan effort to decrease the size of the federal government, reduce federal spending for social programs, and return power to the states, many categorical grants were combined into a series of block grants. The initial proposal by the president was to create two health block grants, converting 11 health services grants and 15 preventive health programs, respectively. Negotiations with Congress resulted in the consolidation of 21 programs into four health block grants: (1) alcohol, drug abuse, and mental health; (2) primary care; (3) preventive health; and (4) MCH.

The Maternal and Child Health Services Block Grant consolidated seven programs: Maternal and Child Health Services and Crippled Children's Services under Title V, Supplemental Security Income Disabled Children's Services, Hemophilia, Sudden Infant Death Syndrome, Prevention of Lead-Based Paint Poisoning, Genetic Disease, and Adolescent Health Services. Federal regulations covering the content of the programs in this block grant were minimal, permitting states to establish their own priorities. Funding for the block grant was reduced from $454.9 million in fiscal year 1981 to $373.7 million in fiscal year 1982, under the rationale that reduced federal regulation would enable states to undertake these activities more efficiently (Peterson, Bovbjerg, Davis, Davis, & Durman, 1986). States were permitted, however, to transfer other block grant funds into the MCH block grant, although transfers of funds from MCH were prohibited. As the decade progressed, Congress increased MCH Block Grant funding to a high of $527 million by 1986 (Guyer, 1987). Political forces in the 104th Congress threatened to cut the 1997 appropriation for Title V by 50%, but MCH advocates succeeded in reducing the proposed reduction to 1%.

The allocation formula for Title V funds with the Maternal and Child Health Services Block Grant as their current incarnation has undergone several revisions. The initial formula described previously here was altered in 1963 when Congress authorized that project grants could be distributed directly to local health agencies and various public and nonprofit organizations, providing the funding base for the Maternity and Infant Care Projects and the Children and Youth Projects mentioned previously. As described by Klerman (1981) in her lucid review of the development of Title V, Congress decided in 1967 to reallocate these special project funds back into the basic formula grant. States were required to have a "Program of Projects" in M & I care, neonatal intensive care, family planning, health of C & Y, and dental health of children, although by no means was the intent or expectation that these were to extend statewide, beyond the "demonstration" mode. Funds were provided to assure that each state undertook these required programs, but states with large urban populations were at risk of receiving smaller allocations than they had received under the previous scheme. The section 516 allotment was added to assure that no state received less through the formula grants than it had received through its previous formula and project grants.

With the creation of the Maternal and Child Health Services Block Grant in 1981, the allocation formula was again based on previous allocations under the categorical programs. States were held "harmless" in that they would receive the same proportion of funds as under the prior legislation. As excess funds became available, they were to be distributed on the basis of the low income population, but as the General Accounting Office (GAO) noted, in 1990, 90% of the MCH block grants were allocated on the basis of their previous allocations, rather than adjustments for the low-income population. In a provocative study of allocation, the US GAO (1992) examined what allocations would look like if done on the basis of three simple "at-risk" indicators—proportion of low birth-weight children, proportion of children living in poverty, and proportion of the state's population under the age of 21 years (compared with the US population). The GAO determined that 14% of the block grant funds would shift from lower risk to higher risk states, with decreases in 37 states and increases in 14.

The Medicaid program also was the object of major change in 1981. Mothers and children were directly affected by adverse changes in the eligibility requirements for AFDC. Because eligibility for AFDC was the major criterion for participation in Medicaid, a loss of AFDC meant a loss of Medicaid coverage, resulting in a decline in the proportion of poor people covered by Medicaid early in the 1980s.

Changes in Title V and Medicaid during the 1980s reflected the ongoing tension between the White House, controlled by Republicans, and the Congress, controlled by Democrats. The back-to-back economic recessions of 1979 through 1982 were accompanied by deterioration in several fundamental MCH indicators. For example, although the national infant mortality rate continued to decline, several states experienced increases or plateauing rates. The proportion of children covered by health insurance declined. Pressured by governors and advocates for mothers and children, Congress turned to the Medicaid program as the structure on which to address some of the glaring gaps in health services for mothers and children. The budget reconciliation process produced the changes shown in Table 2–2. In 1986, Congress severed the link between AFDC and Medicaid by permitting states to enroll pregnant women in Medicaid whose incomes were up to 100% of the federal poverty level even if their incomes were greater than the state income limit. The 1989 Omnibus Budget Reconciliation Act (OBRA) was noteworthy in that it set a national floor for Medicaid eligibility. By April 1990, states were required to extend Medicaid coverage to all pregnant women and children up to the age of 6 years with family incomes below 133% of the federal poverty level.

The Medicaid expansions of the 1980s were effective in increasing access to care for poor pregnant women and children. As Cartland, McManus, and Flint (1993) have reported, Medicaid added 5 million recipients, half of whom were children. In 1990, 7% of the children enrolled in Medicaid were recipients as a result of the expansions of the

---

**Table 2–2  Changes in Medicaid Eligibility During the 1980s**

| | |
|---|---|
| 1984 | Required states to provide Medicaid coverage to single pregnant women, women in two-parent unemployed families, and all children born after September 30, 1983, if their incomes would have made them eligible for AFDC, according to each state's income guidelines. |
| 1985 | Required states to provide Medicaid coverage to all remaining pregnant women with family incomes below each state's AFDC eligibility levels and immediate coverage of all children under the age of 5 years with AFDC-level income or below. |
| 1986 | Allowed states to cover pregnant women, infants up to 1 year old, and on an incremental basis, children up to 5 years old living in families with incomes above the state's AFDC income levels, but below 100% of the federal poverty level effectively severing the link between AFDC eligibility and Medicaid eligibility. Also permitted states to make pregnant women presumptively eligible for prenatal care after application and permitted states to eliminate the assets tests for poverty-related eligible pregnant women and children, allowing shortened application forms. |
| 1987 | Permitted states to increase the upper limit on income for pregnant women and infants up to 1 year old from 100 to 185% of the FPL. |
| 1989 | Required states to provide Medicaid coverage to all pregnant women and children up to the age of 6 years with family incomes below 133% of the FPL by April 1990. |
| 1990 | Increase eligibility level for pregnant women and infants to 185% of the FPL for children ages 1 to 6 years to 133% of the FPL. |

1980s. The proportion of recipients as a result of AFDC eligibility decreased from 90% in 1979 to 72% in 1990, although this population accounted for 29.8% of the increased costs in contrast to 26.8% by the expansion children. The remaining increased costs were accounted for by children not receiving cash assistance (19.4%) and medically needy (24.0%).

The OBRA of 1989 also mandated changes in the design and implementation of the Maternal and Child Health Services Block Grant. States were required to allocate 30% of the their funds to children's preventive/primary care services and 30% to children with special health care needs.[1] For appropriations greater than $600 million, 12.75% was set aside for four targeted initiatives. One set of initiatives expanded maternal and infant home visiting programs as well as enhanced the abilities of states to provide a range of health and social services using the "one-stop shopping" model. A second set of initiatives was aimed at increasing the participation of obstetricians and pediatricians in Medicaid. Third, monies were directed at the enhancement of rural projects for the care of pregnant women and infants and the development of MCH centers at nonprofit hospitals. The fourth targeted area was to expand outpatient and community-based services (including child care) for children with special health needs. Furthermore, the act required states to undertake a statewide needs assessment and formulate a plan for the use of Title V funds that was based on the identified needs. In addition to these specific MCH mandates to improve access to care, OBRA 1989 directed the secretary of Health and Human Services to develop a uniform, simple application for use by Medicaid, Maternal and Child Health, WIC, Head Start, Migrant and Community Health Centers, and Health Care Programs for the Homeless. A final initiative to promote accessibility required state Title V agencies to coordinate their activities with Medicaid. For example, state Title V agencies were expected to work with Medicaid agencies to achieve specified enrollment goals for the EPSDT program.

OBRA 1989 mandated changes to hold states and the Maternal and Child Health Bureau more accountable for the Block Grant expenditures.

---

[1]During the 1980s, the name of the Crippled Children's Program was changed to Children With Special Health Care Needs to reflect the multifaceted aspects of care for these children.

Annual reports were required to address progress toward their state goals, particularly as linked to the goals articulated in *Healthy People 2000* (US Department of Health and Human Services, 1991). Required reporting elements included a variety of MCH health status indicators by class of individuals (pregnant women, infants up to 1 year old, children with special health care needs, and other children less than 22 years of age), provider information, and the numbers served as well as health insurance status, including enrollment to Medicaid. The secretary is also required to provide the House Energy and Commerce and Senate Finance Committees with detailed summaries of states' annual reports, a compilation of national MCH data by health status indicators (including an assessment of progress toward *Healthy People 2000* goals), and detailed results of each Special Projects of Regional and National Significance project.

Concern over infant mortality, particularly the persistence of areas of strikingly high rates, prompted President George Bush to launch a targeted infant mortality initiative of substantial size. The Healthy Start program, administered by the Maternal and Child Health Bureau, selected 15 communities (13 urban and 2 rural) and provided over $200 million dollars annually to facilitate community-driven approaches to infant mortality reduction. Building on the lessons of Sheppard-Towner and M & I projects, Healthy Start has provided social and educational interventions as well as medical services. Employment of community members as outreach workers reflects economic development as yet another component of this substantial initiative. Beginning in 1998, the initiative was expanded so that by 2002, 96 federally funded Healthy Start projects were addressing infant mortality through perinatal health, border health, interconceptional care, perinatal depression, and family violence services with a budget reduced in scale to approximately $97 million. In 2000, Mathematica Policy Research, Inc., completed its evaluation of the first 15 Healthy Start projects, noting associations with improved adequacy of prenatal care, lower preterm birth rates, decreased low and very low birthweight rates only in selected sites, and infant morality rates that declined significantly, but of the same magnitude as comparable communities (Devaney, Howell, McCormick, & Moreno, 2000).

Since the inception of Title V in 1935, there have been three major motivations behind federal involvement in health services for children. Arising out of the Great Depression, Title V was the first in a series of federal initiatives that attempted to address inequities in health outcomes and services. With the globalization of the economy in the 1970s and 1980s, the motivation shifted to a recognition that a healthy workforce was needed in order to remain competitive. Although Medicaid expansions certainly addressed inequities, the broadening of eligibility represented a strategy to invest in the health of the potential workforce. As health care costs continued to grow at an alarming rate, with Medicaid and Medicare in particular escalating at annual rates of 21% and 10%, respectively, the motivating force behind health care reform became cost control. Bill Clinton's election to the Presidency in 1992 was motivated, in part, by a growing concern over access to health care, particularly as escalating costs impeded the abilities of employers to offer health care as a benefit, state governments to finance Medicaid and other state health care programs, and individuals to purchase needed care.

Soon after his election, President Clinton proposed the Health Security Act, a sweeping reorganization of the health care system. The primary goal was to ensure that every citizen would have access to health insurance. Stemming from the work of Enthoven and Kronick (1989), the proposal promoted the concept of managed competition, with a substantial federal role. Large "accountable health partnerships," consisting of providers of health services (physicians, hospitals, etc.) and managers of payment systems (insurance companies, large health maintenance organizations), would compete with one another to offer packages of services to those who pay for services (employers, governments, and individuals). The "managed" part reflects the imposition of standardized packages of services and in some models the requirement that all populations be served. The "competition" takes place among the partnerships, as they would adjust their prices (and to some degree their packages of services within the established guidelines) in order to attract those who pay for services. As Iglehart (1993, p. 1220) explained, "Managed competition is price competition, but the price it focuses on is the annual premium for comprehensive health care services, not the price for each service." Each partnership was required to provide several "packages" from which consumers might choose on the basis of price. The packages were required to include one choice that was without cost to the consumer, for example, a health maintenance organization HMO in which costs could be strictly controlled. Other packages could include the equivalent of fee-for-service options in which consumers could choose among physicians, but they would bear the additional cost through premiums.

The complexity of the Health Security Act and the timing of its consideration leading up to the 1994 midterm Congressional elections resulted in the defeat of this initiative. The 1994 elections were a watershed in national and local politics in that the Republicans gained the majority in the House of Representatives for the first time in 50 years and regained the majority in the Senate, which they had maintained from 1981–1986. No Republican incumbent governors lost re-election bids, and Republicans ended up controlling 31 states. Acting on the belief that the role of the federal government must be reduced and that responsibility for health and welfare should return to states and even local communities, the Republicans proposed an end to the entitlement status for AFDC and Medicaid, creating instead block grants to the states to address these issues as they deemed appropriate.

In August of 1996, after 2 years of raucous debate, President Clinton signed into law "The Personal Responsibility and Work Opportunity Reconciliation Act of 1996 (PRWORA)" (P.L. 104-193). This comprehensive reform made welfare a transition to work, enhanced child support enforcement programs, required unmarried teen mothers to live with parent(s) and remain in school, and limited eligibility for noncitizens (Blank & Haskins, 2001). AFDC, the individual cash entitlement, was repealed and replaced with a block grant, Temporary Assistance to Needy Families (TANF), allowing states the flexibility to convert welfare from a cash assistance program to a jobs program. The block grant also provided an incentive to states to assist individuals in the transition from dependence on a government subsidy to reliance on work, because unlike previous policy efforts to encourage work, work requirements were imposed on the state programs. For example, most participants were limited to 2 consecutive years of assistance and 5 years of lifetime assistance, although 20% of the caseload (e.g., people with disabilities) was exempt from this requirement. The legislation also incorporated sanctions, particularly financial penalties, for states that failed to meet the work requirements. Although the number of families in receipt of AFDC and then TANF benefits has declined from 4,415,000 at the signing of the law in August of 1996 to 2,032,157 in June of 2003 (Administration for Children and Families, 2004), the scholarly and policy debates about how to measure the effects of this fundamental change in welfare policy continue (Blank & Haskins, 2001). As of the spring of 2004 Congress had failed to reauthorize PRWORA, and thus, this legislation, scheduled for reauthorization in 2002, continues under the regulations and financial commitments of the original 1996 bill.

In contrast to the successful effort to convert welfare to a block grant, removing the entitlement to cash welfare, parallel proposals to change the entitlement to Medicaid continue to be debated. By 2002, Medicaid expenditures totaled $259 billion. Overall, the states are responsible for 43% of Medicaid costs, with state contributions ranging from 50% for the wealthier states to 23% for the poorer states (GAO, 2003). Annual growth of total Medicaid spending reached 27.1% in 1990–1992, subsided to a more modest 3.2% rate of growth in 1995–1997, but has gradually accelerated to 12.8% in 2002 (Smith, Ellis, Gifford, & Ramesh, 2002). As an entitlement, Medicaid requires states to generate the funds to cover eligible individuals, thus potentially impinging on discretionary expenditures in state budgets. From the perspective of mothers and children, however, it is important to examine Medicaid expenditures through the lens of Figure 2–1 and Figure 2–2: children comprise approximately 50% of the population of Medicaid recipients but consume only 18% of the expenditures. Coverage of children and pregnant women accounts for a small component of Medicaid's financial demands on state budgets.

Given the large and growing impact of Medicaid on state budgets, governors and state legislatures vigorously opposed the reform of Medicaid

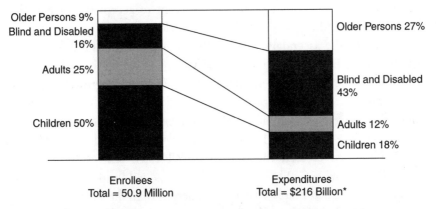

Enrollees
Total = 50.9 Million

Expenditures
Total = $216 Billion*

*Expenditure distribution based on CBO data that includes only spending on services and excludes DSH, supplemental provider payments, vaccines for children, and administration.
Source: Kaiser Commission estimates based on CBO and OMB data, 2003.

**FIGURE 2–1** Medicaid Enrollees and Expenditures by Enrollment Group, 2002.

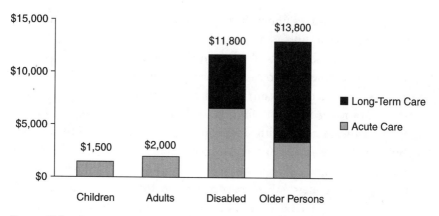

Source: Kaiser Commission based on CBO and Urban Institute estimates, 2003.

FIGURE 2–2 Medicaid Expenditures Per Enrollee by Acute and Long-Term Care, 2002

from an entitlement to a discretionary block grant, with the likely limitation on federal funds inherent in a discretionary grant (Iglehart, 2003). Medicaid has become the infrastructure for many components of the health system—health care for the poor, medically needy, and other vulnerable individuals; long-term care for the older population; and maintenance of hospitals and other organizations that serve the population of those eligible for Medicaid—so that even in the face of the fiscal pressures created by the entitlement, states are reluctant to accept the managerial freedom that would be associated with a block grant.

In spite of the ascendancy of the Republicans in the House and the Senate and their assertion of a political view that would limit the implementation of new major federal expenditures, there was a growing consensus on the appropriateness of providing health insurance to low-income children who were not eligible for Medicaid, even after the expansions that had taken place during the 1990s. As part of the Balanced Budget Act of 1997, Congress created the State Child Health Insurance Program (SCHIP) to provide $40 billion in additional federal funds over a 10-year period, with a match that is 30% more generous than the Medicaid match. Established as Title XXI of the Social Security Act, SCHIP reflected the prevailing view that responsibility for design and implementation of programs should rest with the states by allowing states to pursue one of three basic options: (1) create a separate child health program, (2) expand Medicaid eligibility, or (3) develop a combination of new insurance and

Medicaid expansion. Of the estimated 11 million children without health insurance in 1998, approximately 39.5% were eligible for Medicaid but had not been enrolled; 25.3% had incomes above that required for Medicaid or the new SCHIP insurance, and the remaining 35.2% became the focus of a new health insurance effort. As of July 2002, 16 states had developed separate SCHIP programs, 15 expanded Medicaid, and 19 adopted a combination (Mann, Rowland, & Garfield, 2003). By 2002, the number of uninsured children had declined to approximately 9.2 million (approximately 12% of children under the age of 19 years), with approximately 23.5% covered by Medicaid or SCHIP (Kaiser Commission on Medicaid and the Uninsured, 2003a). For low-income children, however, 25% of children in families with incomes less than 100% of the poverty level and 17% with incomes less than 199% of the poverty level remained without insurance (Kaiser Commission on Medicaid and the Uninsured, 2003b).

The election of George W. Bush in 2000 aligned both the Presidency and Congress under the Republicans for the first time in nearly 50 years. Ironically, this alignment resulted in the largest expansion of federal entitlements since the passage of Medicare and Medicaid in 1965, with the creation of the Medicare drug benefit under the Medicare Prescription Drug Improvement and Modernization Act (P.L. 108-173). Originally budgeted at $409.8 billion for the 10-year period from 2004 to 2013, estimates from the Medicare actuaries and the Office of Management of Budget subsequent to the bill's passage and signature in December of 2003 were as high as $534 billion (Pear & Andrews, 2004). As an entitlement, the fiscal effects created by the demand for drugs will likely create extraordinary pressure on the entire federal budget in general, especially the discretionary health and social service programs that affect so many families (Iglehart, 2004).

## CONCLUSION

As we enter the 21st century, the population of US mothers and children remains at the center of the same debate that raged over the establishment of the Children's Bureau at the beginning of the 20th century. On one side are those that argue that children represent a community resource, a type of public good, the support of which is a responsibility of all citizens. On the other side are those who assert that the care and nurturance of children, although a community resource, are most effectively undertaken by families and their immediate communities. Interestingly, the same debate with regard to the other large dependent population—older persons—seems to have been answered in 1935, again in 1965, and once again in 2003. Namely, it is the federal government, rather than the states, to which we assign responsibility for the older population. Furthermore, benefits for older persons—Social Security Old Age and Survivors Benefits, Medicare (and the new drug benefit)—are entitlements and are not subject to the same uncertainty of discretionary programs such as Title V, TANF, and the new SCHIP.

With the implementation of TANF as block grants, particularly the elimination of the categorical entitlements to income support for poor, dependent children, states have assumed more responsibility for assuring minimum health and welfare services for children. Although state and local governments are indeed "closer" to the people that they serve, it is the federal government through the Congress and the Supreme Court that has traditionally articulated and enforced children's rights to the special services and protections that are the prerequisites of their healthy growth and development. With the devolution of responsibility to the states, it remains to be seen who will assure, and to what degree, that all children, the most vulnerable and innocent among us, receive the social and health benefits that they need to become productive members of society (Nathan, 1996).

# REFERENCES

Administration for Children and Families. (2004). *Change in TANF caseloads.* Retrieved from http://www.acf.dhhs.gov/news/stats/case-fam.htm.

Baker, J.P. (1994). Women and the invention of well child care. *Pediatrics, 94,* 527–531.

Berger, L., & Johansson, S.R. (1980). Child health in the workplace: The Supreme Court in *Hammer v. Dagenhart* (1918). *J Health Politics, Policy and Law, 5,* 81–97.

Blank, R., & Haskins, R. (2001). *The new world of welfare.* Washington, DC: Brookings Institution Press.

Bremner, R.H. (1970). *Children and youth in America.* Cambridge, MA: Harvard University Press.

Cartland, J.D.C., McManus, M.A., & Flint, S.S. (1993). A decade of Medicaid in perspective: What have been the effects on children? *Pediatrics, 91,* 287–295.

Davis, K., & Schoen, C. (1978). *Health and the war on poverty.* Washington, DC: Brookings Institution.

Devaney, B., Howell, E., McCormick, M., & Moreno, L. (2000). *Reducing infant mortality: Lessons learned from healthy start.* Princeton, NJ: Mathematica Policy Research.

Enthoven, A., & Kronick, R. (1989). A consumer-choice health plan for the 1990s. *New England Journal of Medicine, 320,* 29–37.

Epstein, R. (2003). Let the shoemaker stick to his last. *Perspectives in Biology and Medicine, 46,* S138–S159.

Foltz, A. (1975). The development of ambiguous federal policy: Early and Periodic Screening, Diagnosis and Treatment (EPSDT). *Milbank Memorial Fund Quarterly, 53,* 35–64.

General Accounting Office. (2003, July). *Medicaid formula: Differences in funding ability among states often are widened* (GAO-03-620). Washington, DC: Author.

Gostin, L.O., & Blocke, M.G. (2003). *Perspectives in Biology and Medicine, 46,* S160–S175.

Grotberg, E. (1977). *200 Years of children.* Washington, DC: US Department of Health, Education, and Welfare.

Guyer, B. (1987). [Title V: An overview of its evolution and roles]. Unpublished paper.

Haskins, R. (1989). Beyond metaphor. *American Psychologist, 44,* 274–282.

Hoover, H. (1931). *White house conference on child health and protection.* New York: Century Company.

Hughes, J.G. (1980). *American Academy of Pediatrics: The first 50 years.* Elk Grove Village, IL: American Academy of Pediatrics.

Hutchins, V. (1994). Maternal and Child Health Bureau: Roots. *Pediatrics, 94,* 695–699.

Iglehart, J.K. (1993). Managed competition. *New England Journal of Medicine, 328,* 1208–1212.

Iglehart, J.K. (2003). The dilemma of Medicaid. *New England Journal of Medicine, 348,* 2140–2148.

Iglehart, J.K. (2004). The new Medicare prescription-drug benefit: A pure power play. *New England Journal of Medicine, 350,* 826–833.

Irwin, P., & Conroy-Hughes, R. (1982). EPSDT impact on health status: Estimates based on secondary analysis of administratively generated data. *Medical Care, 20,* 216–234.

Kaiser Commission on Medicaid and the Uninsured. (2003a). *Coverage in America: 2002 Data update.* Washington, DC: Henry J. Kaiser Foundation.

Kaiser Commission on Medicaid and the Uninsured. (2003b). *Uninsured: A Primer.* Washington, DC: Henry J. Kaiser Foundation.

Keller, W. (1983). Study of selected outcomes of the EPSDT program in Michigan. *Public Health Reports, 28,* 110–118.

Klerman, L. (1981). Title V The Maternal and Child Health and Crippled Children's Services Section of the Social Security Act: Problems and opportunities. In Select Panel for the Promotion of Child Health (Ed.), *Better health for our children: A national strategy* (DHHS [PHS] Publication No. 79-55071). Washington, DC: US Department of Health and Human Services.

Kotch, J.B., & Whiteman, D. (1982). Effect of the WIC program on children's clinic activity in a local health department. *Medical Care, 20,* 691–698.

Lathrop, J. (1919). Income and infant mortality. *American Journal of Public Health, 19,* 270–274.

Lee, J.Y., Rozier, R.G., Kotch, J.B., Norton, E.C., & Vann, W.F. Jr. (2004). The effects child WIC participation on use of oral health services. *American Journal of Public Health, 94,* 772–777.

Lesser, A.J. (1985). The origin and development of maternal and child health programs in the United States. *American Journal of Public Health, 75,* 590–598.

Mann, C., Rowland, D., & Garfield, R. (2003). Historical overview of children's health care coverage. *Future of Children, 13,* 31–53.

Meckel, R. (1990). *"Saving babies": American public health and the prevention of infant mortality.* Baltimore, MD: The Johns Hopkins University Press.

Miller, C.A. (1988). Development of MCH services and policy in the United States. In: H.M. Wallace, G.M. Ryan, Jr., & A. Oglesby (Eds.), *Maternal and child health practices* (3rd ed.). Oakland, CA: Third Party Publishing Co.

Nathan, R. (1996). The "devolution revolution." *Rockefeller Institute Bulletin.* Albany, NY: The Nelson A. Rockefeller Institute of Government.

Orr, S.T., & Miller, C.A. (1981). Utilization of health services by poor children since advent of Medicaid. *Medical Care, 19,* 583–590.

Pear, R., & Andrews, E. (2004, February 2). *White house says Congressional estimate of new Medicare cost was too low.* New York: New York Times.

Peterson, G.E., Bovbjerg, R.R., Davis, B.A., Davis & Durman. (1986). *The Reagan Block Grants: What Have We Learned?* Washington, DC: Urban Institute Press.

Pfohl, S.J. (1976). The "discovery" of child abuse. *Social Problems, 24,* 310–323.

Rosenbaum, S., & Johnson, K. (1986). Providing health care for low-income children: Reconciling child health goals with child health financing realities. *Milbank Quarterly, 64,* 442–478.

Rowland, D. (2003). Medicaid: Issues and challenges: Testimony for the Committee on Energy and Commerce. Available from: http://energycommerce. house.gov/108/hearings/10082003hearing1103/rowland1735.htm.

Rush, D., Sloan, N.L., Leighton, J., Alvir, J.M., Horvitz, D.G., Seaver, W.B., Garbowski, G.C., Johnson, S.S., Kulka, R.A., Holt, M., et al. (1988). The national WIC evaluation: Evaluation of the special supplemental food program for women, infants, and children. *American Journal of Clinical Nutrition, 48,* 389–519.

Sardell, A. (1988). *The US experiment in social medicine.* Pittsburgh, PA: University of Pittsburgh Press.

Schmidt, W.M., & Wallace, H.M. (1988). The development of health services for mothers and children in the US. In H.M. Wallace, G.M. Ryan, Jr., & A. Oglesby (Eds.), *Maternal and child health practices* (3rd ed.). Oakland, CA: Third Party Publishing Co.

Skocpol, T. (1992). *Protecting soldiers and mothers: The political origins of social policy in the US.* Cambridge, MA: Harvard University Press.

Smith, V., Ellis, E., Gifford, K., & Ramesh, R. (2002). *Medicaid spending growth: Results from a 2002 survey.* Washington, DC: Kaiser Family Foundation.

Sokol, R.J., Woolf, R.B., Rosen, M.G., & Weingarden, K. (1980). Risk, antepartum care, and outcome: impact of a maternity and infant care project. *Obstetrics & Gynecology, 56,* 150–156.

Steiner, G. (1976). *The children's cause.* Washington, DC: Brookings Institution.

Tratner, W.I. (1974). The public health movement: from poor laws to welfare state. In: *A history of social welfare in America.* New York: The Free Press.

US Congress. (1912). *An act to establish in the Department of Commerce and Labor a bureau to be known as the Children's Bureau.* 37 US Statutes 79.

US Congress. (1935). Grants to states for maternal and child welfare. *Social Security Act.* 49 US Statutes 633, Title V.

US Congress, Office of Technology Assessment. (1988). *Healthy children: Investing in the future* (OTA-H-345). Washington, DC: US Government Printing Office.

US Department of Health and Human Services. (1991). *Healthy people 2000: National health promotion and disease prevention objectives* (DHHS Publication No. [PHS] 91-50212). Washington, DC: Author.

US General Accounting Office. (1992, April). *Maternal and child health: Block grant funds should be distributed more equitably* (GAO/HRD-92-5). Washington, DC: Author.

Williams, G.J.R. (1983). Child protection: A journey into history. *Journal of Clinical Child Psychology, 12,* 236–243.

Wilson, A.L. (1989). Development of the US federal role in children's health care: A critical appraisal. In L. Kopelman & J. Moskop (Eds.), *Children and health care.* Dordrecht: Kluwer Academic Publishers.

Witte, E.E. (1963). *The development of the Social Security Act.* Madison, WI: University of Wisconsin Press.

Yip, R., Bintin, F., Fleshood, L., & Trowbridge, F.L. (1987). Declining prevalence of anemia among low income children in the US. *Journal of the American Medical Association, 258,* 1619–1623.

Yudkowsky, B., & Fleming, G. (1990). Preventive health care for Medicaid children. *Health Care Financing Review, Suppl,* 89–96.

# CHAPTER 3

# Families and Health

*Joseph Telfair*

> *The life of a man is a circle from childhood to childhood, and so it is in everything where power moves. Our tepees were round like the nests of birds, and these were always set in a circle, the nation's hoop, a nest of many nests, where the Great Spirit meant for us to hatch our children.*
> (Neihardt, 1975)

## INTRODUCTION

Historical and ethical concerns with the needs of children are inextricably linked with the family, the social institution most basic to the study and practice of maternal and child health (MCH). A family has been defined as a small, usually kinship-structured group, whose key function is nurturant socialization (Reiss & Lee, 1988). In contrast to the theory that the extended family was the prevalent structure in preindustrial society, in the United States, the predominant family system has always been the nuclear family (i.e., social positions of husband–father, wife–mother, and offspring). Relationships with extended kin had importance, but as mobility of families has increased, accessibility to these relationships has decreased.

The nuclear family, or more appropriately the "nuclear household" (Hareven, 1984), has been the definitive unit of analysis in the social scientific study of kinship relationships of the past several centuries. Much of what we know about the social health and overall well-being of children has come from these household studies, which have portrayed the family as the foundation for understanding human social development in modern US society.

The family is an institution beneficial to both individuals and society; however, it is an institution that is under great stress from the significant changes that have taken place in recent times. The increase in single-parent units, the intensification of economic hardships, the exacerbation of racial divisions, and the rise in rates of divorce and separation are all changes that are shaking the foundation of families as we have come to know them.

With the current political emphasis on "family values" connoting the more idealized "traditional" family unit, it has become necessary for practitioners in the field of MCH to develop an empirical understanding of the reality of the composition of the family in the United States today. It is of value in MCH practice to recognize that as a system-level foundation for social development, a healthy, nurturing family is essential to a child's as well as a parent's normal physical, emotional, and social development. Consistent, supportive relationships as well as adequate nutrition, safe environments, and healthy lifestyles are as important to the well-being of children and parents as timely access to appropriate medical care (Center for the Future of Children, 1992; Van Dyck & Hogan, 2003).

This chapter describes the characteristics of current American families. As part of these descriptions, there is a discussion of health and health service issues (including emerging trends) as they affect families and whether these services meet their needs. Emerging trends in family services are also examined. For a very thorough review of the topics examined in this chapter, the reader is referred to the edited text by Wallace, Green, and Jaros (2003), *Health and Welfare for Families in the 21st Century* (2nd ed.).

# FAMILY TRENDS IN THE HISTORICAL CONTEXT

## *World War I and World War II*

Until World War I, the United States was primarily a society of farms and small towns with a few big urban centers. In these early communities, the typical form of household structure was the nuclear family. These were family units consisting of parents and their children, of a childless couple, or of one parent and children. Interestingly, the most important distinguishing feature of the nuclear family was the absence of extended kin. The nuclear *family* (discussed previously here) should not, however, be seen as identical to the nuclear *household*, as the latter may have included nonrelatives (Hareven, 1984; Laslett & Wall, 1972).

By the time of the 1920 US census, the majority of the US population had shifted from rural to urban areas (*World Almanac*, 1990). Before World War II, the nuclear household served the economic purpose of members working together on the farm (in rural areas) or in family businesses or for others (in urban areas). Adult children tended to live near their parents, creating communities with multigenerational kinship ties. There was a continuity of shared values and prescribed family roles. For example, men were seen as the major wage earners, and women remained at home, if possible, with the responsibility of rearing the children. Furthermore, because of the values of close family bonds, mutual support, and the overall well-being of the community, the care of poor children and families was not always seen as a responsibility to be shared by the community and the government. However, the impact of World War II on the economic and social structure of America brought significant change to kinship and community relationships on the one hand and government responsibilities on the other.

The continuing urbanization of America during and after World War II led to many changes that significantly affected the family unit and its functional roles and responsibilities. The increased mobility of families over the last 3 decades, spurred by the need to seek employment wherever it could be found, led to less spatial and temporal continuity and communal security (McNally, 1980). Furthermore, the lure of opportunity and the need to survive within a rapidly changing society have led to a redefinition of the role of family members and to a new understanding of family structure and family life.

## American Family Composition

The makeup of American families has changed significantly since the end of World War II. There has been an increase in the total number of households from 91.9 million in 1990 to 105 million households in 2000. The trend over the last 30 years has been a slowed growth rate in the number of households per year. The majority of the households were married couples at 54.5 million, followed by the second most common household with people living alone (27.2 million). Family households increased by 11% from 64.5 million in 1990 to 71.8 million in 2000.

The proportion of children living with two parents has decreased in each decade since 1960. Single-mother families increased from 3 million in 1970 to 10 million in 2000, whereas the number of single-father families grew from 393,000 to 2 million. In 1970, 12% of family households were headed by single mothers compared with 1% headed by single fathers. In 2000, the proportions of single mother households grew to 26% and single fathers to 5%. This trend illustrates a shift in our society from two-parent to one-parent family households, with a larger proportion of births occurring for unmarried women when comparing the 1990s to the 1960s and 1970s. These one-parent households are an outgrowth of several factors, including the delaying of marriage, which increases the likelihood of a nonmarital birth, and the increasing divorce rate of married couples with children. These trends affect a number of programs and policies, which in turn have an overall effect on the well-being of children in these one-parent households through changes in work and family life.

In the early 1990s, an increase of children living in grandparent households occurred. In 2000, the Current Population Survey (CPS) determined that 4 million children (5% of all children) lived with a grandparent. Only 14% of children living with a grandparent had both mother and father living with them also. Forty-five percent of children who lived with grandparents lived with a mother and no father, whereas 6% living with grandparents lived also with a father and no mother. The other 35% lived with their grandparents only (US Bureau of the Census, 2000). Grandparents play a huge role in many children's lives. Even with one parent present, 10% of children who lived with a single mother and 8% of children living with a single father were living in a household headed by a grandparent. Children who live with grandparents without a parent present (30%) are two times as likely to live in family that is below the poverty level when compared with children who live with both grandparents and a parent (15%) (US Bureau of the Census, 2000). This trend also affects both health insurance coverage and public assistance, with a twofold difference found when comparing children living with grandparents with and without parents present. These trends illustrate how the pools of resources from parents are a primary source for economic well-being for children (Current Population Reports, 2004; Fields, 2003).

Another noteworthy trend in the US families is the growing number of blended, extended, and cohabiting parents. Blended families are created when remarriages result in stepparents living in the household with their children from previous marriages (in 1996, 17% of all children lived in blended families). Extended families are created when a child lives with at least one parent and someone other than his or her own parents or siblings, often an additional relative (in 1996, 14% of all children lived in extended families). Cohabitating parent–child families are defined as such when the children's parent is living with at least one nonrelated adult of the opposite sex. This person may or may not be the biological parent of the child (in 1996, 5% of all children were living with one parent and their partner (US Bureau of the Census, 2000).

## Family and Household Size

The trend toward smaller families and households began with the end of the postwar baby boom in the mid-1960s and has continued to the present, reaching in 1990 a level of 2.63 persons per household, on average, and 3.17 persons per family. By the year 2000, the average number in a household declined to 2.62 and the average number in a family to 3.14. The most significant changes in household size occurred in the smallest and largest households. Smallest (households with one to two persons) increased from 46% to 59% of all households and largest (households with five or more persons) decreased from 21% to 10% of all households. The average sizes of households and families have declined in the last decade because there are fewer children per family, more one-parent families, a growing number of persons living alone, and a growing number couples choosing to delay having children or not have them at all (US Bureau of the Census, 2000; Ventura, 2003).

During the last 30 years, the percentage of families with children less than 18 years old present declined. In 2000, there were 72 million family households and 76 million family groups. Of the 76 million family groups in 2000, 21% had children less than 6 years old, and 12 million of the 76 million were maintained by one parent (Fields & Casper, 2001). The additional family groups were largely related subfamilies (3 million) with 571,000 additional unrelated subfamilies. In 1970, there were 3.8 million one-parent family groups, only 13% of the 29.6 million families with children at that time. In 2000, 37 million family groups with children were counted; 12 million of these were one-parent families, and 10 million were headed by women (Fields & Casper, 2001).

Between 1970 and 2000, the proportion of two-parent family groups has declined for whites, blacks, and persons of Hispanic origin (who may be of any race), whereas father–child and mother–child family groups have increased. The proportion of mother–child family groups has increased most dramatically because of the rise in divorce and births outside of marriage. There is a higher proportion of births to women who never married. In 2000, 59.5 million or 27.1% of the 221 million people 15 years old and older in the United States were never married. The number of female-headed family households with no husband present but with own children rose from 6 million in 1990 to 7.6 million in 2000 (Fields & Casper, 2001).

In 2000, 16.5 million children were living with a single mother, but 1.8 million of these lived in a household with their mother and her unmarried partner. Children who lived with a single father (3.3 million) were much more likely to be living in the house with his unmarried partner. In 1990, 32% of children were living in homes in which the mother never married. This varied by the race of the child, with 53% of black children, 37% of Hispanic children, and 22% of white children living in family households with never-married mothers between the ages of 14 and 44 years (Lugaila, 1992; US Bureau of the Census, 2000). Several factors have affected the trend in our society for the shift from two-parent to one-parent households; one factor is illustrated with the increasing rate of births to unmarried women from 1970 from 26.4 per 1,000 to 45.2 per 1,000 live births to unmarried women aged 15–44 years in 2000 (Ventura, 2003). Possible reasons for the increase for all races have been noted as follows (Donovan, 1995):

1. Increasing sexual activity at earlier ages
2. Decreasing social stigma toward out-of-wedlock birth
3. The only positive relationships in the woman's life being those with the male partner and the baby

## Marriage, Divorce, and Remarriage

In the decades since World War II, changes in the social and technologic fabric of American society have led to dramatic challenges and changes for families. Opportunities for women to delay (choosing to marry at a later age) or not pursue marriage as the path to having a family have increased dramatically. These opportunities were the result of the changing social perceptions of the role of women. The chance for many more women to pursue higher education and careers rose significantly between 1960 and 1990. Married-couple families dropped from 87% in 1970 to 82% in 1980, 79% in the first quarter of 1990 to 52.8% in 2000 (US Bureau of the Census, 1990, 2000). Between 1970 and 1990, the overall marriage rate has had a decrease from a rate of 76% of all women 15 years of age and older in 1970 to 52.3% of women 15 years of age and older in 1992 (Rawlings, 1993). For both men and women, the median ages at first marriage were lowest in the mid-1950s and have been rising since (Lugaila, 1992). In 1970, the median age for marriage for men was 23.2 years and for women was 20.8 years. In 2000, the average age for first marriage increased to 26.8 years for men and 25.1 years for women. In 2000, never-married people accounted for 31% of men and 25% of women over 15 years of age. This is an increase since 1970 from 28% and 22%, respectively (Fields & Casper, 2001).

Over the past 3 decades, the increasing median age for first marriage and increasing divorce rates (which became level in the 1990s) caused a great demographic shift in the status of marriage in the US population. Larger numbers of Americans in 2000 were never married or divorced than in 1970, resulting in a decline in the numbers currently married. Just as age at first marriage has been rising, so are the proportions of men and women who have never married. Increases have occurred for each 5-year age group between ages of 20 and 34 years in the proportions who have never married. For women, only 23% had never married in 1960 compared with 63% in 1990. For men, 53% had never married in 1960 compared with 79% in 1990 (Fields & Casper, 2001).

Change in social mores and the attenuation of some of the earlier taboos against single parenthood and divorce has allowed both to become more socially acceptable. The discarding of traditional social constraints and the availability of medical methods of contraception led to more acceptance of cohabitation without marriage. There was less bias against pregnancy out of wedlock and a trend for single mothers to keep their babies rather than placing them for adoption or in long-term child care homes (Schorr & Schorr, 1988). Divorce rates have increased since 1921, with the sharpest increases occurring from the mid 1960s to the late 1970s (Lugaila, 1992; Schorr & Schorr, 1988). The rate of divorce dramatically rose over the last 3 decades from approximately 15% of all marriages in 1960 to a rate of approximately 50% of all marriages in 1990 (i.e., 4.6 of every 10 marriages ends in divorce), and the children of these divorces typically live in one-parent families (Lugaila, 1992). The divorce rate for men over 15 years of age in 1990 was 8.8% and for women 11.7%. By 2000, the divorce rate for both sexes had risen slightly to 10.1% for men and 12.6% for women. According to the marital status report by US Bureau of the Census, the highest rate of divorce is among the age group of 45 to 54 years for both men (15%) and women (18%). The rate for women is higher because of the fact that women tend to remarry at a lower rate than men. Asians have the lowest divorce rate when compared with whites, African Americans, American Indians and Alaska Natives, Native Hawaiians, or other Pacific Islanders. An overall increase occurred for divorce in the United States from 1950 to 2000 among persons aged 25 to 34 years from 2% to 6% for men and from 3% to 9% for women.

Similarly, a high percentage of remarriages fail. In 1991, 37% of remarriages versus 30% first marriages failed. Studies suggest that children growing up in divorced families and in stepfamilies have greater difficulties in social relationships, achievement, and behavioral adjustment (Hetherington & Jodl, 1994). Researchers caution, however, that the results of these studies have small effect sizes and diversity in outcome. There is considerable variation in the balance of risk and protective factors within family structures, and individual and policy decisions should not be based on these findings alone (Amato, 1994).

Of children living with two parents in 1996, 88% lived with both biological mother and father, and 9% lived with a stepparent (US Bureau of the Census, 2000). The vast majority of these stepfamily situations consist of a biological mother and a stepfather combination because children usually remain with their mother after divorce. In the case of unmarried parents, the children also usually remain with the mother. In 1990, the majority of children living with one parent were living with a parent who was divorced or whose spouse was absent (either separated or living elsewhere). The proportion living with a widowed parent declined during the past 30 years from 20% to 4.3%. The proportion of children in one-parent families who lived with a never-married mother increased from 7% in 1970 to 32% in 1990 and 43% in 2000 (Fields & Casper, 2001).

Finally, the increased availability of artificial insemination technology and the number of states allowing adoption by same-sex couples provided many single women the chance to have a family without a commitment to marriage. At the same time, the development of an effective oral contraceptive and the initiation of public policy allowing the use of tax funds to support family planning clinics gave couples the opportunity to avoid pregnancy. Both of these trends have contributed to the increasing proportion of children living with single, never-married mothers.

## Family Income and Employment

The median family income increased by 104% during the 26 years between 1947 and 1973. The median income of married-couple families increased by 115%. Despite these fluctuations and the increase in wives' labor force participation, by 1990, the median income for all families was only 6% more than in 1973, and the median income for married-couple families was only 11% greater than in 1973. Among families with female householders and no spouse present, the median family income grew by 37% between 1947 and 1973 but increased only by 5% between 1973 and 1990. In 1989, the median family income was $33,585. In 1992, the median family income was $31,553. In 1993, the median family income was $31,241, and in 2000, the median family income was $48,196. This illustrates an increase in median family income of approximately $17,000 over the past 7 years (Current Population Survey, 2001). The current (1999) median family income differs by race: Asians at $33,144, whites at $53,356, Hispanics at $34,397, and blacks at $33,255 (Kids Count, Annie E. Casey Foundation, 2000 Census).

The official poverty rate for children has fluctuated since the early 1980s. It reached a high of 22% in 1993, decreased to 16% in 2000, and has remained stable since that time (Federal Interagency Forum on Child Health and Family Statistics, 2003). In 2001, more children lived in families with relatively medium incomes (33%) than in other income groups; 22% lived in relatively low income families, and 29% lived in relatively high-income families (US Bureau of the Census, 2002). However, the percentage of children living in families with relatively medium incomes fell from 41% in 1980 to 33% in 2001, whereas the percentage of children living in families with relatively high incomes rose from 17 to 29% during that same period (Federal Interagency Forum on Child Health and Family Statistics, 2003). In contrast the percentage of children living in families experiencing extreme poverty rose from 7% in 1980 to 10% in 1992 and has steadily decreased to 7% in 2001 (US Bureau of the Census, 2002). The rates of low relative income varied significantly by race. For whites, the proportion of relatively low-income families increased from 13% in

1969 to 15% in 1989; for Hispanics, the increase was from 33% in 1979 to 38% in 1989 (1969 numbers were not available), and for blacks, the increase was from 42% in 1974 to 44% in 1989 (1969 numbers were not available) (US Bureau of the Census, 1991b). More recent statistics suggest the same pattern. The low-income rate is much higher for black or Hispanic children than for white, non-Hispanic children. In 2001, 9% of white, non-Hispanic children lived in poverty compared with 30% of black children and 27% of Hispanic children (Federal Interagency Forum on Child Health and Family Statistics, 2003).

### Women in the Workforce

An increasing number of women have entered the work force since 1950. The percentage of married mothers with children less than 18 years old in the work force in 1960 was less than 30%, in 1970 the number was 40%, in 1990 was 59%, and in 2000 was 74%. The percentage of married mothers with children aged 6 to 17 years who were employed rose from less than 30% in 1960 to 49% in 1970 and to 74% in 1990 (Lugaila, 1992). These data indicate that labor force participation by married women is increasing, especially for those women with children less than 6 years old. Between 1970 and 1990, among married women with pre-school children in the home, the proportion of those in the labor force doubled from 30% in 1970 to 59% in 1990. Furthermore, by 1990, 74% of all married women with school-age children were in the labor force (Lugaila, 1992). According to the 2000 US Census, 63.9% of all people aged 16 years and older were in the labor force. This was an increase from 1990 of 13.5 million people. Labor force participation among women had also increased between 1990 and 2000 (57 in every 100 to 58 in every 100 women), respectively. Women in 2000 were more likely than men to be outside the workforce (30% women outside to 18.1% of men) (Clark & Weismantle, 2003).

### Parents in the Workforce

Among married-couple families with children in 1990, the proportion in which both the husband and wife worked was 70%. A slight decrease occurred between 1990 and 2002, with 68.7% of all children having both parents in the workforce (Fields, 2003). In 71% of single-mother families and 85% of single-father families with children ages 6 to 17 years, the custodial parent is working (Departments of Education and Justice, 2000).

In 2002, only 7% of all US households consisted of married couples with children in which only the husband worked. Dual-income families with children made up more than two times as many households. Even families with two incomes and no children outnumbered the traditional family by almost two to one (US Bureau of the Census, 2002). Married couple families with children are more likely to have mothers out of the work force than fathers (Fields, 2003).

## Means-Tested Cash Assistance

In the year 2002, almost a third of all children lived in families with incomes below $30,000, and 17% were in families below 100% of poverty. Public assistance was received by 5% of children, and 11% received food stamps. In comparison, 49% of all children lived in families with incomes of $50,000 per year or more, and 29% were in families with $75,000 per year.

In 1990, among poor married-couple families with children, 27% received means-tested cash assistance,[1] but 78% had one or more members who worked to earn wages or salaries (Baugher, 1993). Poor female-headed households with children, on the other hand, were more likely to have received means-tested cash assistance than to have one or more members with income earned through work (67% vs. 49%). Of the total income of poor families, approximately 80% was received from these two sources. The remaining 20% of total income for poor families with children came from other sources, such as Social Security.

## Poverty

Families with children under 18 years of age experienced a decline in poverty from 20.3% in 1959 to 10.8% in 1966. Between 1966 and 1979, the poverty rate remained within 2.5 percentage points of this previous low, varying from 10.8% to 13.3%. Poverty estimates based on the current definition date back to the early 1960s. The poverty rate fell dramatically during the 1960s from 22.2% in 1960 to 12.1% in 1969. From 1970 to 1978, changes in poverty were relatively small, with the poverty rates ranging between 12.6% in 1970 and 11.7% in 1979. The poverty rate in 1983 (15.2%) was the highest since 1965. Although the poverty rate in 1991

---

[1]Means-tested cash assistance includes public assistance or welfare payments and SSI.

(14.2%) was lower than that more recent peak, it remained well above the 1978 level of 11.4%, a recent low point (US Bureau of the Census, 1994). The official poverty rate rose from 11.7% in 2001 to 12.1% in 2002. The number in poverty increased also by 1.7 million people to 34.6 million in 2002. Child poverty rates have dropped over a quarter in the last 10 years, but this decline stopped in 2001. The US economy has been in a downward trend as of this writing, which often results in policy changes that affect programs for families in low-income levels. Presently, the federal poverty level (2003) for a two-parent family of four is $18,400, and the US child poverty rate is higher than those of most other large industrialized nations, frequently two to three times higher.

### Poverty and Race

During the period from 1965 to 1990, white families had the lowest poverty rates (14% in 1965 to 12% in 1990), and black families had the highest poverty rates (40% in 1965 to 38% in 1990[2]). In 1980, the poverty rate for all families with children rose to 14.7%, and between 1981 and 1990, the poverty rate for families with children varied from 15.5% to 17.9%, respectively (Baugher, 1993; Lugaila, 1992). In 1990, 16.4% of families (all races with children under 18 years old) were below the poverty level, and in 2002, 13.9% were below the poverty level among all races (US Bureau of the Census, 2002). Almost half of all families in poverty are white. A little more than a quarter of the families are black. Slightly less than a quarter are Hispanic, and the remainder are Asian or from other groups. However, when poverty rates are examined by race/ethnicity, whites are less likely than other groups to be poor. In fact, black and Hispanic families are about three times more likely to live in poverty than white families (Federal Interagency Forum on Child Health and Family Statistics, 2003).

### Poverty, Race, and Marital Status

Despite a decrease in overall poverty rates since 1966, poverty rates for white, black, and Hispanic married-couple families with children have been much lower than corresponding poverty rates for female-headed families with children, from 17% in 1959 to 8% in 1990 for all married-couple families with children versus from 60% in 1959 to 45% in 1990

---

[2]Estimates are for all white and all black families during this time period.

for female-headed families with children (Lugaila, 1992; US Bureau of the Census, 1990, 1991b). Within these two family types, however, the poverty rates for blacks and Hispanics have been substantially higher than for whites. For example, from 1975 to 1990, the poverty rate for married-couple families has remained stable at 8%, whereas the poverty rate for black married couples has remained stable at 15% (US Bureau of the Census, 1991a[3]). In addition, in 1991, 40.9% of all poor families were maintained by a married couple, whereas 54% were headed by a female householder, with no spouse present. In contrast women maintained only 12.7% of nonpoor families. After leveling off in the early 1980s, the proportion of female-householder families among all poor families has grown from 48.1% in 1985 to 54.1% in 1991. Furthermore, in 1991, female-headed households constituted 78.3% of all poor black families compared with 45.7% of poor Hispanic-origin families and 28.4% of poor white families (Baugher, 1993).

## Poverty and Educational Attainment

CPS reports track educational level's improvement since 1947. The CPS reports that over four fifths of all adults by the year 2000 had at least completed high school. One in four of these adults had attained a bachelor's degree or higher. Eighty-eight percent of white non-Hispanics were high school graduates. Blacks increased to 79%, narrowing the difference among high school graduates between whites and blacks. Asian and Pacific Islanders had the greatest proportion of college graduates. When comparing races among ages 25 and older, Hispanics were the least likely to complete high school or college, although this improved from 51% to 57% since 1989. In contrast, Asian/Pacific Islanders had 44% with college degrees or higher compared with 28% of white non-Hispanics, 17% of blacks, and 11% of Hispanics in the 25 years and older age group (US Bureau of the Census, 2000).

In 1990, white, black, and Hispanic-origin family householders aged 25 years and over with higher educational attainments were each less likely to live in poverty, but within educational levels, the poverty rates for blacks and Hispanics were much greater than for whites. For example, for

---

[3]The exception in both cases is the increase in the rate of poverty for all families by 5 percentage points from 1975 to 1985.

high school graduates, the rate of poverty for Hispanic families was 15%. That for white families was 7% and for black families was 26%. However, the overall poverty rate for white, black, and Hispanic families with at least a high school education fell in 1990 to 9%.

**Poverty and Work Status**

During the most recent era of welfare reform, the percentage of poor children in working families increased steadily between 1995 and 2000 from 32% to 43% before decreasing to 40% in 2001. This illustrates a trend reversal that occurred during a period when recession resulted in a loss of jobs in the US economy as a whole. This recent decline happened during a period when child poverty remained constant at 16% overall. These trends are also evident for children living in single-mother families. Among all children, the percentage living in working poor families has stayed constant at 6% to 7%.

Only one third of poor children have at least one parent in the household employed full-time, full-year compared with seven of eight nonpoor children. Among poor children, those living with families with two parents were much more likely to have a parent employed full-time, full-year than children living with only their mother or father (54% compared with 19% and 29% in 2001). White non-Hispanic children are more likely to have at least one parent employed full-time, full-year than either Hispanic or black non-Hispanic children (84% vs. 73% and 65%, respectively). Among children living in two-parent and father-only families, there is no difference between children less than 6 years old and older children in the percentage who have at least one parent employed full-time, full year. For those in single-mother families, however, the difference is substantial, at 38% for those under the age of 6 years versus 53% for those ages 6 to 17 years.

## Assistance Programs

Preliminary survey results of the Survey of Program Dynamics suggest that levels of participation in Food Stamps, housing assistance, energy assistance, and free or reduced-price school lunches declined significantly between 1993 and 1996 for all household types, including married-couple households with children and for other family households with children. Individuals in other family households with children were more likely to participate in these noncash benefit programs than their married-couple counterparts in 1996. Changes in the welfare system precipitated by the Personal Responsibility and Work Opportunity Reconciliation Act of 1996, which replaced the Aid for Families of Dependent Children (AFDC) program with the Temporary Assistance for Needy Families Program (TANF) (Barr, Lee, & Benjamin, 2003). Although individuals in married-couple households with children were less likely to participate in these programs than those in other family households with children, their relative decline in receipt of Food Stamps and housing assistance between 1993 and 1996 was greater. The two groups experienced similar declines in receipt of energy assistance and free or reduced-price lunches between 1993 and 1996. This has been accelerated with the passage of the welfare law enacted in 1996. That is, the number of individual welfare recipients declined by 56%, and the number of families has decreased by 52%, respectively, since 1996 (Parrott, 2002). In 2002, 2.1 million families received cash assistance through TANF (Administration for Children and Families, 2002). In 2002, approximately 5 million individuals and 2 million families received TANF benefits, a decline of 5% and 4%, respectively, from 2001 (US Department of Health and Human Services, 2002). Interestingly, relatives caring for children comprised 9% of the TANF caseload in 2001.

## Child Care

Every day, three of five children under school age are in child care (Children's Defense Fund, 2004). The increased number of parents in the workforce led to schools and other institutions (e.g., child care) taking on more of the responsibility for caring for children. The increase in labor force participation among mothers with preschool children was not limited to mothers with older preschoolers. In 1976, the proportion of women with children less than 1 year old who were in the labor force was only 31%. However, the rapid increase in the proportion of women with infants and children under 1 year of age, jumping to 59% in 1999, has produced a corresponding increase in the demand for child care for children under the age of 1 year. Among the 49 million children living at home with both parents, 29 million had both parents in the work force. Fourteen million children living with father only and 2 million with mother only had their custodial parents in the work force. Fourteen million children lived with a single mother, and greater than 75% of these single mothers were working.

In 1997, 63% of the 19.6 million children under the age of 5 years were in some form of child care on a regular basis. Forty one percent of the children under 5 years old were cared for by a relative with 35% cared for by a nonrelative. Approximately one fifth of these children were cared for in child-care facilities (Smith, 2002). Families with preschoolers who are in poverty with employed mothers use relative care more often than child-care centers. Among preschoolers in general, there is a higher proportion of 3–4 year olds in child-care centers than 1–2 year olds. This is may suggest a relationship with age and preparation for school (Smith, 2002).

School-aged children of employed mothers numbered 23.4 million in 1997, and 62% of all children in grade school have employed mothers with whom they are living. Just 6% of these children (5–14 years old) are cared for in organized facilities; the difference lies in the rate of children enrolled in school (84%). Nineteen percent of the school-aged children took care of themselves without adult supervision, and 17% attended enrichment activities outside of school hours (Smith, 2002).

The cost of child care is significant. In 1997, 51% of the 12.1 million preschoolers living with mothers paid $67 a week on average in child care payments. The average cost per week for families paying for child care services was $49 with the last Survey of Income and Program Participation, an increase of $8 per week since 1991. School-aged children were not as likely to have paid child care as the under 5-year-old preschoolers, and the cost of child care per week is also lower for grade-school children (Smith, 2002).

There are 34.2 million children less than 15 years old who have regular child-care arrangements; of these, 5% receive assistance in paying for this care. The assistance sources are often the government, their parent's employer, their other parent, or another source. Preschoolers are more likely to receive assistance (7%) when compared with grade school-aged children (4%). Although 812,000 children under the age of 15 received assistance from the government in 1997, this is directly related to one's economic level. Nine percent of preschoolers in poverty receive this kind of assistance compared with only 5% living just above poverty and only 1% of those preschoolers at 200% of poverty. Children receiving TANF (15%) are recipients of government assistance for child care. A relationship may exist, with the TANF families having the needed connections to access this kind of assistance for child care (Smith, 2002). Disparities exist in the cost of child care by income level and poverty status among children, where a poor family with a working mother pays an average of $52 a week compared with nonpoor families who pay an average of $77 per week. Poor families (20%) spend roughly three times the amount of nonpoor families (7%) of their budgets on child care. There has been a persistent difference in poor and nonpoor families from 1987–1997 (Smith, 2002).

### Health Insurance Coverage

Health insurance coverage for children rose slightly during the late 1990s, reaching 88% by 2000 and staying at that level in 2001 and 2002. In the late 1990s, health care insurance coverage for children increased somewhat from 85% in 1996 through 1998 to 88% in 2000 and has remained stable through 2002. Children's health insurance coverage comes from two major sources: private insurance companies and the government. Medicaid coverage for children increased from 20% in 2000 to 24% in 2002 (Mills & Shailesh, 2003). The percentage of children with private insurance decreased from 71% in 2000 to 68% in 2001, remaining at 68% in 2002.

Hispanic children are much less likely than other children to have health insurance coverage. In 2002, only 77% of Hispanic children had health insurance coverage compared with 88% of Asian-only children, 86% of black-only children, and 92% of white, non–Hispanic-only children. According to a recent article in *The Future of Children* (Holahan, Dubay, & Kenney, 2003), a lack of awareness of eligibility, language barriers, enrollment problems, and fear of repercussions for using publicly funded insurance may partially explain why more Hispanic children are uninsured.

In 2002, 79% of children in single-father families and 86% of children in single-mother families had health insurance coverage compared with 90% of children with married-couple families. The likelihood of being covered by health insurance increases with income. In 2002, 95% of children living in families with incomes of $75,000 or more were covered by health insurance. In contrast, only 81% of children in families with incomes of under $25,000 were covered. US citizens, whether native born or naturalized, are more likely than are noncitizens to have health insurance coverage. The health insurance coverage rates in 2002 for US citizens were 90% for native-born citizens and 81% for naturalized citizens compared with only 59% for noncitizens under the age of 18 years. In general, children belonging to economically advantaged groups are the most likely to have private health insurance, which is largely employment based, whereas children in economically disadvantaged groups are the most likely to have government health insurance, which is most often Medicaid, a needs-tested program.

Private health insurance covered 68% of all children in 2002. Private health insurance coverage is most common among white non-Hispanic only children (79%), children in married-couple families (77%), and children in families with incomes of $75,000 and over (92%). Private health insurance is least common among Hispanic children (43%), black-only children (50%), children in single-mother families (45%), and noncitizens (37%). Although Medicaid covers only about 24% of the entire population of children, it covers 62% of poor children. Among poor children, Medicaid coverage is highest for black children (70%) and is substantially lower for white non-Hispanics only, Hispanics and Asian or Pacific Islanders only, with 57%, 61%, and 51%, respectively, receiving coverage (Child Trends, 2003).

In 1990, poor families with children were twice as likely as nonpoor families with children not to be covered by private or public health insurance at any given time during the year (22% vs. 11%) (Lugaila, 1992; Short, 1993; US Bureau of the Census, 1991b). Among nonpoor families with children, those in female-headed household families were about twice as likely as those in married-couple families not to be covered by health insurance at any given time during the year (17% vs. 9%). The reverse held true for poor families with children. It should be noted that some families with children covered by health insurance during 1990 had coverage for only part of the year. Hence, the proportions of families with children not covered at any given time (or at all) during the year, and discussed here, are certainly smaller than the proportions that did not have coverage for the full year. In addition, families with children who did not have health insurance coverage may also differ in the extent to which specific health care costs were fully, partially, or not paid by their health insurance (Short, 1993). Between 1987 and 1991, approximately 22.2 million children had no health insurance during some part of each year (Flint, 1992; Short, 1993). In contrast to what many believe, access to health care is not primarily a problem of the poor. The majority of uninsured children live in two-parent families, in which at least one parent is employed full time and earns an income above the poverty line (Foley, 1991). Seventy percent of the uninsured have family incomes above the poverty level (Darman, 1992).

At the end of 1990, 87% of Americans were covered at a given point in time by health insurance of all types. Government health insurance, which consists primarily of Medicaid but includes several other sources of coverage such as the State Child Health Insurance Program, covered 27% of all children in 2002 (Holahan, Dubay, & Kenney, 2003). Approximately six in eight of all insured persons were covered by private insurance. Stable full-time employment improved the chances of having continuous coverage (Short, 1993). From mid-1987 to the end of 1990, only 14% of those who worked full time—35 hours or more per week—for all 28 months experienced lapses in coverage. In contrast, 43% of those who spent a month or more without a job experienced a lapse in health insurance coverage (Short, 1993). Furthermore, taking into account the changing system of employer-provided dependent coverage, Newson and Harvey (1994) point out the following:

> Currently, 60% of all Americans obtain insurance through their own or a family member's employment. This arrangement, however, is seriously threatened. Employers concerned with rising health care costs are either dropping dependent health insurance, reducing the benefit packages, or increasing the employee's share of the premium for dependent coverage. In 1980, 72% of medium- and large-sized firms paid the full cost of health insurance for their workers, and 51% paid the full cost of dependent coverage. By 1991, fully paid individual insurance dropped to 45% of firms, and family coverage to 23%. While employer-provided health insurance is declining, even plans that do cover dependents often fail to meet the health care needs of children, which are not the same as those of adults. Most child health services are provided in an ambulatory setting, and services rendered in such a setting are often not covered by health insurance. Because health insurance plans tend to be designed for adults, children's needs are often addressed inadequately. (pp. 11–12)

Therefore, there is continuing concern that as a result of the current health care reform climate, poor and nonpoor families with children are at risk of having no source of health insurance for their dependents (US Department of Health and Human Services, 2001).

# COMMUNITY SERVICES

## Historical Background

The most basic social agency available in almost every US community today is the tax-supported public welfare agency. However, voluntary nonprofit agencies have played an important role in the history and current provision of social services in the United States. Because of the greater need, they have flourished mainly in urban areas. Nonetheless, the public welfare agency remains the one resource available nationwide.

The public welfare system of the United States is based on the English poor laws of the 17th century, which placed the responsibility for care of the needy on the local community and stated that the income of persons receiving assistance should not be greater than the lowest income of a self-sufficient person (Reisch, 1995). In the United States, public welfare was administered entirely by local and state agencies until the Social Security Act was passed in 1935. The reason for this change was that there was great inequity in criteria for eligibility and benefits across states. Nevertheless, the belief that the state or local community is better situated to assess the need and benefits for dependent persons, and the use of a means test to determine that need, form the basis for much of current welfare reform policies. Thus, the United States' welfare system is founded on the Residual Welfare Model (described in Chapter 1), and there is still adherence to some of these principles, whereas England and other western European countries have adopted the principles of the Industrial Redistributive Model of social welfare (Kahn, 1973).

In the 18th and early 19th century, the American welfare system also used institutional care for the older population, chronically ill, and dependent children, for example, almshouses and orphanages. With the industrial revolution and the wave of immigration, private agencies were developed to help people in their own homes. The Community Organization Societies, which developed into today's Family Service Agencies, and Children's Aid Societies (antecedents of United Way), were major resources offering financial assistance as well as other services in kind. With the onset of the Great Depression in the 1930s, private organizations found that they were unable to meet the financial needs of the masses of unemployed persons. After the passage of the Social Security Act, private agencies made the policy decision not to provide income maintenance but to provide only counseling and supplementary services. In turn, the original Social Security Act provided only financial assistance, not services (Meyer, 1995).

The Social Security Act established the responsibility of the federal government to provide funds to all states for the support of certain groups and the policy of entitlement, that is, that all persons who met eligibility criteria were entitled to benefits (Reisch, 1995). Originally, the Social Security Act provided funds for three groups in the population: the aged (Old Age Assistance), the blind (Aid to the Blind), and dependent children (Aid to Dependent Children [ADC]). In 1950, a third group, disabled persons (Aid to the Permanently and Totally Disabled), was added. These programs were administered by the states. That is, under general federal guidelines, states established eligibility criteria and benefits. In answer to complaints about the wide variation in benefits according to the economic status of a state, Old Age Assistance, Aid to the Blind, and Aid to the Permanently and Totally Disabled were "federalized" in 1974 under a program named Supplemental Security Income (SSI) (Meyer, 1995). It is administered directly by the Social Security Administration whose primary responsibility is to (1) set eligibility criteria, (2) establish a basic measure of income maintenance, and (3) mail checks directly to recipients. States can supplement the amount of SSI benefit. States that gave higher benefits before 1974 were required to supplement the new federal level in order to remain at that level (Meyer, 1995).

The ADC program originally provided benefits only for the children; however, in 1950, funds for the caretaker in the family were added, and the name was changed to AFDC. It has not been "federalized" as were the other programs because of the moral and political feelings expressed by communities toward the population group served by this program. "To qualify for assistance, a child in a single parent household must be deprived of support because the parent is deceased, continually absent from the home, or suffering a mental or physical incapacity that is expected to last more than 30 days. Under limited conditions, a two-parent family can receive aid if principal wage earner is unemployed even with support from other service programs" (Abramovitz, 1995). In 1935, one of the goals of the Social Security Act was to remove from the labor pool economically dependent persons, thus freeing employment opportunities for the able bodied. In the beginning, mothers of dependent children continued to work because they were not included as recipients of the ADC benefits. They were included in 1950 because of the culture of that era. That is, it was believed to be better for the development of children if the mother remained at home to care for them. Also, the role of women as homemakers was encouraged as a means of removing women from the labor pool after World War II in order to increase opportunities for returning veterans.

The demographics of AFDC also changed between 1935 and 1990. The AFDC program subsumed the population previously served by Mothers Pensions programs, which states had initiated as a result of the 1909 White House Conference on Children. These programs were focused primarily on widows who otherwise would have had to place their children in orphanages. The proportion of widows with children was high under the original ADC program but diminished as this group became eligible for survivors' benefits under the Social Security insurance program. Currently, the children in the AFDC caseload are primarily those of divorced, separated, or never-married women. The average monthly AFDC family caseload for calendar year 1992 was 4,829,000, up 8.1% from the preceding year (US Department of Health and Human Services, Social Security Administration, 1994). The AFDC recipient count averaged 13,773,000 in 1992. In 1992 payments to AFDC recipients totaled $21.66 billion, an increase of $725.3 million or 3.5% above 1991 (US Department of Health and Human Services, Social Security Administration, 1994). However, the average monthly payment per family was down $16.73 (–4.3%) to $373.71 for 1992 from the 1991 level of $390.44 (Abramovitz, 1995; US Department of Health and Human Services, Social Security Administration, 1994).

The role of public welfare agencies in providing social services not only to its own beneficiaries but also to the general population has varied in recent years. Beginning in 1956, the federal government offered to match a certain percentage of state funds spent on counseling, rehabilitation, and other direct services to persons receiving public welfare benefits. These services were always perceived as services to individual cases for purposes of rehabilitation and control. In the 1960s, in the era of the War on Poverty and the Great Society, there was more of an interest among academicians and policy makers in dealing with the problem of social dependency on a systems basis (Reisch, 1995). A leader in the systems approach was Dr. Alfred J. Kahn, Professor at the Columbia University School of Social Work, who was influenced by the work of Titmuss cited in Chapter 1. He believed that a function of public welfare was the socialization and development of society, regardless of the economic status of individuals. His ultimate goal was the Industrial Redistributive Model, but as an intermediate phase, he recommended that governmental units be responsible for providing "social utilities," that is, services that are needed to meet emerging needs and are generally accepted as representing social infrastructure (Kahn, 1973). Public social utilities may be divided into those available at user options (e.g., museums, community centers) and others by user status (child care, centers for the aged). He stresses that the user is a citizen, not a client or patient (Kahn, 1973).

This concept of public welfare offering services to all citizens was incorporated in to Title XX of the Social Security Act passed in 1975. The services of information and referral, family planning, and protective services for children and the aged were provided to all families regardless of income. Other developmental services were available to people with incomes up to 115% of a state's median income; persons with 80% to 115% of the state's median income paid a sliding fee for services. Title XX legislation led to many innovative programs with a preventive approach. However, it was an open-ended appropriation. In the 1980s, it was placed in a block grant with all other provisions for social services under the Social Security Act, and a cap was placed on appropriations (Reisch, 1995). Current programs are more limited.

The history of child welfare services for the protection and enhancement of the lives of children has a history similar to income maintenance. Services, such as they were, were provided by the local judicial and welfare system with use of institutional care. Private nonprofit, including religious, agencies developed protective and custodial care. Until the 1930s, these varied according to the state and locality. The child welfare provisions under Title V of the Social Security Act required each state to have a statewide agency that is responsible for public child welfare services. Originally administered by the Children's Bureau, this program offered mainly guidance and staff training in foster care, adoption, maternity homes, child-care centers, homemaker services, etc. Its relatively small budget was used to try to upgrade the quality of staffs of public child welfare agencies, providing funds for the employment of social workers with master's degrees. It did not provide funds for the payment of foster care or to assist adoptive parents. Studies in the 1970s, which tracked children through their experiences in foster care, documented the inadequacy of foster homes, the agencies' tendencies to "lose children" and not to provide continuous service to the child. It also found that if children were not returned to their parents within their first 2 years in foster care they were likely never to be returned. These findings resulted in the Child Welfare and Adoption Assistance Act in the 1980s. Federal funds were appropriated for payment of foster care. Agencies were required to establish registers and tracking systems. Plans had to be made to review cases by the time the child was in foster care for 18 months to see whether there was potential for the child to be returned to his or her parents or plans made for his placement in an adoptive home. Funds were provided to assist adoptive parents with the cost of care of children with special needs.

The original placement of Child Welfare Services and MCH services in the Children's Bureau was a felicitous one in that the two programs had so many areas of mutual concern, such as services to unwed mothers, standards for foster homes, adoption, child care centers, and homemaker services. During the 1960s, they both received funds to expand services for mentally retarded children. The Social Work Section of MCH was able to work closely with the social workers in the Child Welfare Division on these issues (Kadushin, 1980). Since 1973, when Child Welfare Services was transferred to the Administration for Children and Families and MCH was transferred to the Public Health Service, these two programs have had to collaborate through interagency committees.

When initiated in 1935 the Social Work Section of the Children's Bureau was concerned mainly with the program for children with special health care needs (then called the Crippled Children's Program) because many of the states had incorporated social work positions into their clinical services. The impetus for the development of social work positions in state MCH agencies came with the initiation of the Program of Projects in the 1960s. Because of the nature of the programs, the federal administrators of MCH services always insisted on the multidisciplinary approach. Social work positions were created in state health departments to give guidance and supervision to the social workers employed in the special projects. After the end of the Program of Projects with the initiation of block grants to the states in the 1980s, state-level positions for public health social workers remained important in assessing the impact of health and social policy on the health status and social needs of low income families. For example, data gathered by public health social workers in the southeastern states regarding rates of premature birth and infant death occurring to women not eligible for Medicaid were used in the development of legislation for the expansion of Medicaid to include married women and women with incomes up to 185% of poverty. The provision of payment for case-management services to Medicaid patients led to an increase in the number of social work positions in local public health departments providing MCH services (Schmidt & Wallace, 1994; Watkins, 1993). These public health social workers provide information about and referral to other community resources as well as counseling and follow-up. They work closely with other community agencies in developing new resources for families as well as working to change policies that may serve as barriers. The current trend for states to assign the Medicaid population to managed-care programs is leading to a reduction of the availability of public health social work and other "wrap-around" services, which facilitate the accessibility and effectiveness of medical care for low-income populations.

## Current Issues

Decreasing support for public social welfare services and the proposal to fund Medicaid through block grants to the states threaten the health and social resources available to young low-income families. Politicians expressing the need to "reform the welfare system" are referring to the AFDC program, as other dependent populations are now covered by the SSI Program. The negative atmosphere that surrounded the AFDC program was for two major reasons. One was that the more socially acceptable group of women, that is, widows, is now cared for by Survivors Insurance, which leaves the politically unacceptable group of divorced, separated, and unmarried women as the primary recipients of AFDC. This group of women is targeted for "reform" despite the fact that their numbers reflect social phenomena, which is occurring in all economic groups. Second, the recipients are perceived negatively because of their high rate of unemployment. Today, greater numbers of women work outside the home, and thus, AFDC recipients are seen as not meeting society's expectations, even though the early intention of the AFDC program was precisely to enable mothers to stay home and raise their children. Since the passage of Family Support legislation in 1988, recipients whose children are over 3 years of age have been required to participate in the Job Opportunity and Basic Skills program. However, these efforts have not led to any greater numbers obtaining employment. Current proposals have a more punitive approach, that is, cutting benefits if the woman does not return to work within a certain time limit (e.g., 2 years) or if she has additional children while receiving benefits.

Legislation passed in 1996 (Personal Responsibility and Work Opportunity Reconciliation Act; US Congress, 1996) replaced AFDC with

TANF and gave administration of TANF to the states with minimal federal guidelines, reduced funds, employment requirements, and time limits on assistance, ending entitlements for those most in need. Now there is the question whether state legislatures will be willing to raise taxes to replace lost federal revenue and to meet the new demands of the law (training, employment, child care, etc.). The resources of private organizations are inadequate and too unevenly distributed to meet nationwide needs. Efforts to help recipients enter employment or return to school require training programs and provision of child-care services that are not guaranteed by the new legislation.

The proposal to fund Medicaid through block grants to the states would lead to similar problems of inequity in criteria for eligibility and benefits. Mothers and children excluded from TANF assistance may find they are also excluded from a state's Medicaid program. Although converting Medicaid to a block grant was originally considered as part of the welfare reform legislation of 1996, it was omitted from the final version of PL 104-193.

The increase in acquired immunodeficiency syndrome, drug abuse, and family violence has placed a great strain on child welfare agencies (Reiss & Lee, 1988). Children in these families often have to be removed from these threatening environments temporarily or permanently. There are insufficient qualified foster homes to meet this demand. A high proportion of caseworkers in child welfare agencies has not had formal social work training and is given responsibility for solving problems in family relationships far beyond their abilities. Turnover in staff is frequent, and children in care often become lost in the system. Also, the policy that a decision must be made to either return the child to his or her biological parents or place him or her in a permanent adoptive home after 18 months in foster care often leads to the child's being returned to the original hazardous environment. Current approaches to remedying this situation include closer case management and monitoring, crisis and long-term family counseling, parental life-skill training, and permanency planning that involves the family's biological and "other kinship/support network."

## CONCLUSION

American family life has changed dramatically during the past 3 decades. Age at first marriage for women has increased, as has age at first pregnancy for married women. Since 1970, small families with one or two children increased sharply as a proportion of all families with children. In contrast, there are high rates of divorce and births to unmarried mothers, which are largely responsible for the growing proportion of families headed by single, mostly female, parents. These families are a heterogeneous group in terms of income, education, employment, and race. However, black and Hispanic-origin families are disproportionately represented (Cunningham & Hahn, 1994). Thus, given the continuing high levels of divorce and premarital childbearing, the proportion of children living with a lone parent doubled between 1970 and 1990, reaching approximately 25% (Lugaila, 1992).

There was an increase in the proportion of women in general, particularly mothers, participating in the labor force since 1970. This increase in mothers in the labor force corresponded with the increased need for child care, especially for children under 5 years old. Furthermore, in 1990, nearly 30% of married-couple families had both spouses working year round. Also, the number of parents with at least some college education increased during the 1970s and 1980s. Despite the increases in mothers and married couples in the labor force and higher educational attainment of parents, the overall median family income was only 6% above what it was in 1970. This increase was so small predominantly because of the rise in single-parent households.

The disparity in poverty rates between married and unmarried has increased, with unmarried women being far more likely to have incomes below the poverty level or to be receiving public assistance than married women. Similarly, the disparity in poverty rates between employed and unemployed women with children has also increased. As with many other demographic trends over the last 30 years, blacks and Hispanic-origin women and children were disproportionately represented among the ranks of the poor. The latter is particularly poignant as blacks have much lower median family incomes and higher rates of poverty than whites with similar educational attainment and patterns of work (Lugaila, 1992). The lack of health insurance coverage is often noted as a problem for poor children living in mother-only families, but even among children living in married-couple families, the proportion not covered by health insurance anytime during 1990 was 9% for the nonpoor and 3% for the poor.

Stable family relationships and adequate financial support are essential for the healthy development of children. In the United States, changes in family structure and in the economic system are weakening supports for families. Current social systems, such as public assistance, tax-supported medical care, and child welfare services are being questioned and restructured, possibly placing some families at risk. Public health professionals in the field of MCH are challenged with the tasks of assessing the impact of these proposed changes on the health status of families with children and initiating policies and programs that will promote and protect their well-being.

Acknowledgment: The author thanks Beth Johns for her help in the preparation of this chapter.

## REFERENCES

Abramovitz, M. (1995). Aid to families with dependent children. In Edwards, R.L. (Editor-in-Chief), *Encyclopedia of Social Work* (Vol. 1, 19th ed., pp. 183–194). Washington, DC: National Association of Social Workers.

Administration for Children and Families. (2002). *Temporary assistance for needy families: Total number of families and recipients April–June 2002.* Washington, DC: US Department of Health and Human Services.

Amato, P.R. (1994). The implications of research findings on children in stepfamilies. In A. Booth & J. Dunn (Eds.), *Stepfamilies: Who benefits? Who does not?* (pp. 81–88). Hillsdale, NJ: Lawrence Erlbaum Associates.

Barr, D.A., Lee, P.R., & Benjamin, A.E. (2003). Health care and health care policy in changing world. In H.M. Wallace, G. Green, & K.J. Jaros (Eds.), *Health and welfare for families in the 21st century* (pp. 26–42). Mississauga, Ontario, Canada: Jones and Bartlett Publishers.

Baugher, E. (1993). Population profile of the US 1993: Poverty. In U.S. Bureau of the Census, *Current population reports: Population characteristics* (Special Studies Series P-23, No. 185). Washington, DC: US Department of Commerce, Economics and Statistics Administration, Bureau of the Census.

Center for the Future of Children. (1992, winter). *US health care for children* (Vol. 2, No. 2). Los Altos, CA: The David and Lucille Packard Foundation.

Children's Defense Fund. (2004). The State of America's Children, Washington, DC: Author.

Child Trends. (2003). *Health care coverage.* Available from: www.childtrendsdata bank.org/indicators/26healthcarecoverage.cfm

Clark, S.L., & Weismantle, M. (2003, August). *Employment status 2000, census 2000 brief.* US Department of Commerce, Economics and Statistical Administration, US Bureau of the Census, Washington, DC.

Cunningham, P.J., & Hahn, B.A. (1994). The changing American family: Implication for children's health insurance coverage and the use of ambulatory care services. *The Future of Children, 4,* 24–42.

Current Population Reports, Income, Poverty, and Health Insurance Coverage in the United States: 2003. (August 2004). Available at http://www.census.gov/prod/2004pubs/p60-226.pdf

Current Population Survey Annual Demographic Survey. (2001, March Supplement). Available from: http://ferret.bls.census.gov/macro/032002/health/h08_000.htm

Darman, R. (1992, January 17). *Comprehensive health reform: Observations about the problem and alternative approaches to solution* (p. 6). Washington, DC: Testimony before the US House of Representatives, Committee on Ways and Means.

Departments of Education and Justice. (2000). *Working for children and families: Safe and smart after-school programs.* Available from: www.sedl.org/pubs/fam95/resourceguide

Donovan, P. (1995). *The politics of blame: Family planning, abortion, and the poor.* New York: Alan Guttmacher Institute.

Federal Interagency Forum on Child Health and Family Statistics. (2003). *America's children: Key national indicators of well-being, 2003.* Washington, DC: US Government Printing Office.

Fields, J. (2003, June). *Children's living arrangements and characteristics: March 2002, population characteristics.* US Department of Commerce, Economics and Statistics Administration, US Census Bureau, Demographic Programs, Washington, DC.

Fields, J., & Casper, L.M. (2001, June). *America's families and living arrangements: 2000, Current Population Reports.* US Department of Commerce, Economics and Statistics Administration, US Census Bureau, Demographic Programs, Washington, DC.

Flint, S. (1992). *Decline in uninsured children registered in 1990: Child health financing report* (Vol. IX, No. 1, p. 5). Elk Grove Village, IL: American Academy of Pediatrics.

Foley, J.D. (1991). *Uninsured in the United States: The nonelderly population without health insurance: Analysis of the March 1990 current population survey* (Special Report SR-10). Washington, DC: Employee Benefit Research Institute.

Hareven, T.K. (1984). Themes in the historical development of the family. In R.D. Parke (Ed.), *The review of child development* (Vol. 7, pp. 137–178). Chicago, IL: The University of Chicago Press.

Hetherington, E.M., & Jodl, K.M. (1994). Stepfamilies as settings for child development. In A. Booth & J. Dunn (Eds.), *Stepfamilies: Who benefits? Who does not?* (pp. 55–80). Hillsdale, NJ: Lawrence Erlbaum Associates.

Holahan J., Dubay L., & Kenney G. (2003). Which children are still uninsured and why. *The Future of Children, 13,* 68–70.

Kadushin, A. (1980). *Child welfare services* (3rd ed.). New York: Macmillan Publishing.

Kahn, A.J. (1973). *Social policy and social services.* New York: Random House.

Kids Count. Annie E. Casey Foundation. 2000 Census. http://www.aecf.org/kids count/census/

Laslett, P., & Wall, R. (1972). *Households and families in past times*. Cambridge, UK: Cambridge University Press.

Lugaila, T. (1992). Households, families, and children: A 30-year perspective. *Current population reports: Population characteristics* (Special Studies Series P-23, No. 181). Washington, DC: US Department of Commerce, Bureau of the Census.

McNally, S.J. (1980). Historical perspectives on the family. In J.R. Miller & E.H. Janosik (Eds.), *Family focused care* (pp. 16–30). New York: McGraw-Hill Book.

Meyer, D. (1995). Supplemental Security Income. In Edwards, R.L. (Editor-in-Chief), *Encyclopedia of social work* (Vol. 3, 19th ed.). Washington, DC: National Association of Social Workers.

Mills, R.J., & Shailesh, B. (2003). *Health insurance coverage in the United States: 2002*. Current Population Reports, P60-223. Washington DC: US Census Bureau.

Neihardt, J. (1975). *Black Elk speaks* (p. 165). New York: Pocket Books.

Newson, G., & Harvey, B. (1994). Assuring access to health care. In H.M. Wallace, R.P. Nelson, & P.J. Sweeney (Eds.), *Maternal and child health practices* (4th ed., pp. 11–17). Oakland, CA: Third Party Publishers.

Parrott, S. (2002). *The TANF-related provisions in the president's budget*. Washington, DC: Center on Budget and Policy Priorities.

Rawlings, S. (1993). Population profile of the US 1993: households and families. In U.S. Bureau of the Census, *Current population reports: Population characteristics* (Special Studies Series P-23, No. 185). Washington, DC: US Department of Commerce, Bureau of the Census.

Reisch, M. (1995). Public social services. In Edwards, R.L. (Editor-in-Chief), *Encyclopedia of social work* (Vol. 3, 19th ed., pp. 1982–1991). Washington, DC: National Association of Social Workers.

Reiss, I., & Lee, G. (1988). *Family systems in America*. New York: Holt, Rinehart and Winston.

Schmidt, W.M., & Wallace, H.M. (1994). The development of health services for mothers and children in the US. In H.M. Wallace, R.P. Nelson, & P.J. Sweeney (Eds.), *Maternal and child health practices* (4th ed., pp. 103–119). Oakland, CA: Third Party Publishers.

Schorr, L., & Schorr, D. (1988). *Within our reach: Breaking the cycle of disadvantage*. New York: Anchor Doubleday.

Short, E. (1993). Population profile of the US 1993: Health insurance. In U.S. Bureau of the Census, *Current population reports: Population characteristics* (Special Studies Series P23, No. 185). Washington, DC: US Department of Commerce, Bureau of the Census.

Smith, K. (2002, July). Who's minding the kids? Child care arrangements: Spring 1997, Current Population Reports, Household Economic Studies, US Department of Commerce.

US Bureau of the Census. (1990). How we are changing: Demographic state of the nation: 1990. In U.S. Bureau of the Census, *Current Population Reports* (Special Studies Series P-23, No. 170). Washington, DC: US Department of Commerce.

US Bureau of the Census. (1991a). Poverty in the US: 1990. In U.S. Bureau of the Census, *Current Population Reports* (Consumer Income Series P-60, No. 175). Washington, DC: US Department of Commerce.

US Bureau of the Census. (1991b). Trends in relative income: 1964–1989. *Current population reports* (Consumer Income Series P-60, No. 177). Washington, DC: US Government Printing Office.

US Bureau of the Census. (1994). Demographic state of the nation: 1995. In U.S. Bureau of the Census, *Current Population Reports* (Special Studies Series P-23, No. 188). Washington, DC: US Department of Commerce, Bureau of the Census.

US Bureau of the Census. (2000). *Population profile of the United States: 2000, from birth to seventeen: The living arrangements of children, 2000.* US Department of Commerce, Bureau of the Census. Available from: http://www.census.gov/population/pop-profile/2000/chap06.pdf

US Bureau of the Census. (2002). *Age, sex, household relationship, race and Hispanic origin: Poverty status of people by selected characteristics in 2001* (Table 1). Washington, DC: Census Bureau.

US Congress. (1996). *Personal Responsibility and Work Opportunity Reconciliation Act,* Public Law 104-193.

US Department of Health and Human Services. (2001). *Trends in the well-being of America's children and youth 2001.* Office of the Assistant Secretary for Planning and Evaluation. Tables HC 1.1.A and HC 1.1.C. Available from: http://aspe.hhs.gov/hsp/01trends/contents.htm#HC (see Tables HC 1.1.A and HC 1.1.C).

US Department of Health and Human Services. (2002, November 1). *Welfare caseloads continue downward trends* (press release). Washington, DC: Author.

US Department of Health and Human Services, Social Security Administration. (1994, August). Annual statistical supplement. *Social Security Bulletin,* SSA Pub. No. 13-71700.

Van Dyck, P., & Hogan, M.D. (2003). Health and social care of women, children, youth and families. In H.M. Wallace, G. Green, & K.J. Jaros (Eds.), *Health and welfare for families in the 21st century* (pp. 5–25). Boston, MA: Jones and Bartlett Publishers.

Ventura, S.J. (2003). Demographic factors affecting fertility patterns in the United States. In H.M. Wallace, G. Green, & K.J. Jaros (Eds.), *Health and welfare for families in the 21st century,* (pp. 52–70). Boston, MA: Jones and Bartlett Publishers.

Wallace, H.M., Green, G., & Jaros, K.J. (Eds.). (2003). *Health and welfare for families in the 21st century* (2nd ed., pp. 5–25). Boston, MA: Jones and Bartlett Publishers.

Watkins, E. (1993). The history of maternal and child health: The role of public health social workers. In J.J. Fickling (Ed.), *Social problems with health consequences: Program design, implementation, and evaluation.* Proceedings of the 1990 Bi-Regional Conference for Public Health Social Workers in Regions IV and VI. Columbia, SC: College of Social Work, University of South Carolina.

*World Almanac and Book of Facts 1990* (p. 551). (1990). New York: Pharos Books.

# Determinants of Health and Health Services: The Developmental Cycle

# CHAPTER 4

# Family Planning

*C. Arden Miller, Linda Piccinino, and Amy Tsui*

> "*A sustainable United States is one where all Americans have access to family planning and reproductive health services . . .*"
> President's Council for Sustainable Development, *Sustainable America: A New Consensus for the Prosperity, Opportunity and a Healthy Environment for the Future, 1996*

## INTRODUCTION

The next section of this textbook groups chapters according to the maternal and child health (MCH) developmental cycle and appropriately begins with a discussion of family planning, organized programs to enable individual management of fertility. Family planning represents a key component of reproductive health services in the United States and elsewhere. Emphasis here features needs and programs in the United States.

Although contraceptive use has increased in the United States, so too has the percentage of births that are unwanted. At the same time, in real dollars, public spending on contraceptive services through Title X of the Public Health Service Act declined by 72% between 1980 and 1992, although Medicaid has risen in prominence as the primary federal financing mechanism (Poole & Hawkins, 1999). This chapter presents some of the history of the family planning movement not covered in Chapter 2 and reviews the status of family planning services in the United States in terms of their availability and barriers to their access. It also describes current and past levels and trends of contraceptive practice, the characteristics of users, the methods adopted, and sources of services. The likely future of family planning in the United States is discussed in terms of critical policy issues that prevent the population of the United States from achieving the status of an appropriately contracepting society. The chapter concludes with a call to reinforce commitment to the public financing of family planning services in the United States, even as the trend toward privatization of services continues.

Clarification of terms is appropriate in this chapter. *Unintended* or *unplanned pregnancies* include those that are unwanted and those that are mistimed. *Unwanted pregnancies* and *unwanted childbearing* occur among women who report that they never intended to give birth or to continue childbearing. *Mistimed pregnancies* occur among women who report that they at some time in the future intended to bear one or more children but not at the time this pregnancy occurred. Data on these issues are based on surveys that in part require recall of intent, a procedure with a degree of uncertainty among some women and their partners.

As of 1995, the latest year for which national data are available, almost one half of women 15–44 years of age in the United States have experienced at least one unplanned pregnancy (Henshaw, 1998). Approximately one half of all pregnancies (approximately 3 million) in the United States are unintended. Another half of these unintended pregnancies end in abortion. Approximately 40% of all live births are the result of unintended pregnancies, a proportion that may have since increased (Institute of Medicine, 1995). The proportion is higher among women in poverty, those never married, and those 18 to 24 years old. Approximately 28% of births are the result of mistimed pregnancies, and another 12% are births from unwanted pregnancies. The consequences of these circumstances are dire for many women and children and underscore a pressing need for more effective programs of family planning (Kost & Forrest, 1995).

# BACKGROUND

Efforts to control fertility date from earliest recorded history. Egyptian papyri recommend the insertion of a vaginal suppository containing crocodile's dung and honey mixed with sodium carbonate, or the insertion of acacia tips. Soranos, a Greek physician writing in the second century, advised that for the prevention of conception, coitus should be avoided during critical times in the menstrual cycle. Other suggested methods included anointing the cervix with astringent materials or closing the *os uteri* with cotton (Major, 1954). The contraceptive effect of *coitus interruptus* has been known since antiquity. By an account in Genesis, Onan, required by tribal custom to sleep with his deceased brother's widow but not wishing to establish a collateral family line, chose to spill his seed on the ground. Through history, various penile sheaths, often from strips of linen or animal membranes, have been tried as contraceptives.

The prevailing motivations for promoting access to contraception have changed from time to time. Concern for the well-being of unwanted children is one of them. Boswell (1988) estimated that from antiquity through the Renaissance, approximately one quarter of liveborn children were abandoned. Some of these children survived but many did not. Medieval chronicles report a harvest of infant corpses yielded by rivers such as the Nile and the Arno. Child abandonment was not a socially reprehensible method for coping with unwanted fertility. Rousseau, the noted 18th-century French philosopher, wrote without apparent shame or regret that he abandoned all five of his children. It was a practice that not many theologians condemned, except for risk of committing the grave sin of incest by inadvertently having sexual relations with a previously abandoned daughter or son (Boswell, 1988).

Circumstances in the United States through the early decades of this century can be interpreted as evidence of socially sanctioned infanticide. Nearly every large city accommodated a foundling hospital, often with convenient provision for depositing unwanted infants. The mortality rates in those hospitals approached 90% (English, 1984). During the same period, upper class French women boarded their unplanned infants with peasant families, a practice with a comparably high mortality rate (Klaus, 1993).

## SUPPORTIVE RATIONALE

Some less stark considerations relate to unplanned childbearing. Infants and children have better survival rates, and survivors are healthier if they are born to mothers who are not at the extremes of the childbearing age span, if there is spacing of 2 years between births, and if family size is limited. Unwanted childbearing poses health burdens beyond those that can be attributed to social and economic characteristics of the mother. For an unwanted pregnancy, the mother is less likely to seek prenatal care and is more likely to expose the fetus to harmful substances such as tobacco and alcohol. The child of an unwanted conception is more likely to be of low birth weight, to die in the first year of life, and to be abused. Kost, Landry, and Darroch (1998) studied more than 11,000 births from two 1988 national surveys in which the planned status of pregnancies was known and found a higher probability of negative outcomes, such as low birth weight or prematurity, early well-baby care and breastfeeding, for unintended than planned pregnancies. The risks and outcomes for a mistimed conception are of a similar nature but of lesser magnitude (Institute of Medicine, 1995).

Concern about the effects of unwanted, mistimed, or excessive childbearing on the health of women has been conspicuous in the policy dynamics of family planning programs in this century. Childbearing and parenthood are low risk and rewarding experiences for people who want them. The risks and rewards become adverse for women at the extreme of childbearing years, women experiencing short interpregnancy intervals, women with health problems such as diabetes or hypertension, women with multiple pregnancies, and those women whose pregnancies are unwanted or mistimed. The adversities are biological, psychological (depression), economic, and social. Educational and career prospects for women are curtailed by unplanned childbearing. Women whose pregnancies are unwanted or mistimed are four times as likely as women with a planned pregnancy to be physically abused by their husband or partner (Gazmararian et al., 1995).

Maternal deaths from major complications of pregnancy (uncontrolled bleeding, blood clots to the lungs, and toxemia with high blood pressure and convulsions) are concentrated among fourth and higher order births and among very young women and those in the upper ranges of the childbearing years. These hazards are minimized among women given access to family planning.

When women have access to contraceptive services, they have reduced likelihood of resorting to dangerous illegal abortions for control of fertility. Under safe conditions, induced abortion is a low-risk procedure—with even fewer complications than childbearing. When access to abortion is limited, many women resort to unsafe procedures in order to avert pregnancy. Accurate data on illegal procedures are not readily available, but some estimates place the total number of illegal abortions the world over to be in the range of 20 million each year. Associated deaths are estimated to number over 70,000, nearly one fifth of the half million maternal deaths that occur annually worldwide (Mundigo & Indriso, 1998).

During the early years of this century, Margaret Sanger worked as a public health nurse in the poorest sectors of New York City where she confronted appalling evidence of the plight of women caught in lives of excessive and unwanted fertility. She began promoting family planning, a cause that attracted many followers. Her work led to the formation of The Family Planning Federation, an organization that sponsored family planning clinics in nearly every community in the United States and in many other countries. It continues under the name of Planned Parenthood Federation of America, as one of this country's largest organized providers of family planning services.

The eugenics theme has played a part in the promotion of family planning. In the early decades of this century, the view developed that society would be improved if only the "right" people were encouraged to propagate. This view today is greatly diminished but is not entirely absent. Voices from developing countries and from minority populations in the United States sometimes charge that the promotion of family planning is a covert expression of genocidal intent.

Concern about overpopulation has been a strong motivating force for family planning, especially in densely populated countries such as China, India, Indonesia, and Bangladesh. Malthus was one of the earliest (1798) analysts to point out that the growth of a population could outstrip resources to support it. This consideration figured prominently in the United States during the 1970s when public programs to enable access to family planning, both domestically and internationally, were greatly expanded. As rational as the population theme may be in support of family planning, it is not now a strong influence in this country, Europe, or other countries that have passed through the fertility transition. The size of the population of the United States would be stable if it were not for immigration. Historically, some countries have been more concerned about too little population than too much. Nationalistic rivalries in Europe during the late 19th and early 20th centuries caused many countries to adopt pronatalist policies, which offered strong inducements for childbearing, even among unmarried women (Klaus, 1993). These inducements and supportive services formed the basis for protections that contribute to favorable pregnancy outcomes and that persist to this day.

Feminists currently provide the strongest advocacy for abortion rights. Their concern is fortified by data on the health and well-being of women, but the cause is largely argued on the basis of human rights, an argument that the political process has thus far upheld even in a climate of increasing contention. Proponents maintain that women are entitled to sexual fulfillment that is free from the risk of unintended pregnancy. Denial of pregnancy prevention services is interpreted by some voices as a form of social control over women by a male-dominated society. Advocacy for abortion services, for family planning, and for family planning services for poor women remains an urgent policy priority for workers in MCH.

## SOCIAL AND POLITICAL CONTEXT

Public health workers are apt to find the supportive rationale for family planning so compelling that countervailing forces are underestimated. These forces are considerable. In 1873, Anthony Comstock, secretary of the New York Society for the Suppression of Vice, induced Congress to pass an act prohibiting the use of the mails for obscene matter. Any content dealing with sex education or family planning was declared pornographic and was prohibited under provisions of the act. Comstockery (George Bernard Shaw's term) found even more stringent expression in various state laws. Margaret Sanger was arrested a number of times for lecturing and distributing pamphlets on family planning. As recently as the 1940s, an obstetrician in Connecticut was jailed for prescribing contraceptives for a married woman.

The tenets of nearly every organized religion are construed by some as supportive of family planning. Conversely, nearly every organized religion produces other voices that raise opposition. For many decades, the Catholic Church has been the strongest force in opposition. The official position of the church is supportive of family planning except by "unnatural" means. These include all currently available methods of contraception that are most effective. The "natural" methods approved by the church include periodic abstinence and breastfeeding, which tends to delay ovulation in some women. These methods have some effectiveness on a population-wide basis, but they are all high risk for individual couples who seek protection from unwanted childbearing. It is not surprising, as a consequence, that Catholic women in the United States have a rate of abortion 22% higher than Protestant women (Jones et al., 2002b).

Women of all ages, socioeconomic circumstances, religions, and races may find it necessary to have an abortion when faced with an unwanted pregnancy.

Withdrawal from intercourse before ejaculation is another "natural" method of attempted contraception. The annual failure rate for withdrawal is 26%, which means that 26 of 100 women will experience a pregnancy while using this method. Practicing this method over 3 years produces a cumulative failure rate of 54%. More than one half of such contraceptors will have an unwanted pregnancy.

The social reforms of the 1960s (e.g., Medicare, Medicaid, Head Start, the War on Poverty) included a prevailing attitude that family planning and population policy were appropriate matters for government action (Rosoff, 1988). Presidents Kennedy (the nation's only Catholic president) and Johnson spoke frequently in support of government-sponsored family planning programs. Support was bipartisan. President Nixon declared, "No American woman should be denied access to family planning assistance because of her economic conditions. I believe, therefore, that we should establish as a national goal the provision of family planning services . . . to all who want but cannot afford them" (Rosoff, 1988, p. 313). Former presidents Truman and Eisenhower served as honorary co-chairmen of Planned Parenthood Federation of America. As part of the War on Poverty, the MCH provisions of the Social Security Act were required to allocate to family planning a minimum of 6% of available funds and to offer services to "all appropriate cases." Congressman George Bush lent his support to a national program of government support for family planning clinics. Before the 1980s, he also supported the Supreme Court's decision of 1973, which protected a woman's constitutional right to abortion. Abortion remains a procedure not generally regarded as an appropriate method of family planning in the United States (unlike some countries in Eastern Europe) except as an alternative to be considered when contraception fails.

In 1970, Congress enacted Title X of the Public Health Service Act, which provided funds and implementation authority for a nationwide program of family planning clinics for poor women. Under this act, teenage women were generally eligible for services regardless of their parents' resources. The program expanded rapidly throughout the 1970s.

The political climate began to change toward the end of the decade. In 1976, Congress prohibited the use of Medicaid funds to pay for abortions. Aspirants to elective office began to reassess their positions supportive of family planning. Controversy over abortion grew as a conspicuous political issue. These changes were driven by the growing influence of a conservative political coalition given finance and voice by a Christian fundamentalist movement. The movement garnered support from a growing radio and television audience for charismatic media evangelists.

The election of Ronald Reagan to the presidency in 1980 marked a watershed in government policy. He omitted family planning funds from all of his budgets and spoke energetically in opposition to abortion. The "right to life," formulated around the abortion issue, became confusedly linked with negative attitudes toward family planning. As vice-president, George H.W. Bush changed his position on both abortion and family planning.

During each year in the next decade and a half, a Democratic-majority Congress succeeded in restoring funds to Title X, holding them only to the 1981 funding level. After considering inflation, however, real financial support for the program dwindled by 72%. This decrease was only partially offset by increases in Medicaid funding for family planning services (Daley & Gold, 1993). The election of a Republican Congress in 1994, strongly beholden to ultraconservative influences, brought new threats to the existence of public supported programs for family planning. The current Republican administration under President George W. Bush has shown little enthusiasm for family planning and actively promotes the practice of abstinence before marriage.

The issue is not easily resolved. A strongly articulated view holds that easy access to contraception, especially for teenagers, has promoted irresponsible behavior, increasing early and extramarital sexual activity and, paradoxically, an increase in extramarital teenage childbearing. It is true that during the 1970s and 1980s more teenagers were engaging in sexual intercourse at earlier ages than in previous years (Alan Guttmacher Institute, 1995). It is also true that many difficult-to-measure influences other than access to contraception were brought to bear during those years. Ubiquitous media programming and advertising, often with provocative sexual content, and sexual maturation at younger ages are among the possible factors contributing to intercourse at earlier ages.

An opposing view holds that access to contraception is not the problem but is in fact the solution. It is certainly true that during the 1980s programs to promote "just say no," generously financed during the Reagan administration, did not reverse trends in sexual behavior. It is also true that teenage fertility in this country has been at a stable level for many decades, increasing only slightly during the late 1980s and decreasing again in the mid-1990s. The problem appears larger than it really may be because older women have reduced their fertility so much more than young women, resulting in an increased proportion of newborns with teenage mothers.

Few good studies are available to resolve this controversy to everyone's satisfaction. Many public health workers are attracted by the findings of a controlled study by Zabin et al. (1986) on the influence of a school-linked program of counseling and clinical services that included contraception. The onset of the age of first intercourse by participants in the study population was delayed by 13 months. More such studies are needed. This one suggests that when young people have information and related clinical services, their behavior becomes more responsible than without them. Experience from other industrialized nations is relevant. Many of them provide school-based sex education beginning at young ages and access to contraception when teenagers choose to become sexually active. Under these circumstances, the average age of first intercourse is no younger than in the United States, but teenage pregnancy and abortion rates are much lower (Jones et al., 1988). The US experience with teenage pregnancy prevention programs includes very few judged to be effective (for a review, see Frost & Forrest, 1995).

## METHODS OF FAMILY PLANNING

Readers who are not thoroughly familiar with the physiology of sexual maturation, menstruation, and childbearing are urged to take time to study these processes with a standard text of physiology. Understanding the successes, failures, indications, and possible complications of various contraceptives is not possible without knowledge, for example, of the hormonal orchestration of reproduction. Some of the most widely used contraceptives manipulate female hormonal balances.

Successful family planning programs make available a variety of methods. No one of them is entirely satisfactory for all women or for all circumstances. Most women make use of different methods at different stages of their reproductive history. Condoms or diaphragms may be useful for relationships that are intermittent. A daily contraceptive pill may

be convenient for stable, continuing partnerships, and surgical sterilization may be chosen when plans for family formation are completed.
Surgical sterilization, more often female than male, is the most commonly
used method of contraception in the United States. Latex (and, more
recently, polyurethane) condoms and diaphragms are also useful for protection against sexually transmitted diseases (STDs).

Some methods rely on preventing the union of the ovum and sperm
in normally ovulating women. Such methods include periodic abstinence (often identified as the rhythm method because it attempts to confine coitus to phases of the menstrual cycle when the woman is presumed
not to be ovulating) and withdrawal, or onanism, when the male discon-
tinues vaginal penetration before ejaculation. More effective methods of
preventing union between ovum and sperm provide barriers such as the
male and female condom, diaphragm, or cervical cap (the last infre-
quently used).

One of the most widely used contraceptive methods prevents ovulation
by replacing the woman's normal hormonal cycle with an imposed one by
means of a daily sequence of oral hormonal pills. The method is highly
effective, but it requires diligence to remember to take the pills according
to the prescribed schedule. Lapses reduce effectiveness; guidance on how
to correct for lapses has no firm scientific basis. This problem is averted by
adaptations of the hormonal method, such as the provision of the replacement hormones in a long-acting injection, effective for several months, or
in subcutaneous implants, which can be effective for up to 5 years. If during this period a couple desires to conceive, the implants can be removed
and fertility restored. In the last few years, contraceptive hormonal
patches have become available that also are nonpermanent methods, but
somewhat like the pill, these patches require that the user change the
patch on a weekly basis.

Various chemical agents can deactivate the sperm and hence prevent
conception. These agents are prepared as vaginal foams, creams, gel strips,
or jellies to be inserted into the vagina before intercourse or more commonly to be used in conjunction with other methods, such as the
diaphragm or the condom.

The mode of action of some methods is not precisely known. For
example, some models of the intrauterine device (IUD) may not actually
prevent fertilization but act by disrupting implantation of the conceptum
in the uterine wall. This matter has relevance to some people who take a

microscopic view of a "right to life," charging that the device is not a contraceptive but an abortifacient. This view is contradicted when chemical agents, such as copper, are incorporated into the IUD. This is a highly effective method that acts by chemical, as well as by mechanical, means. IUDs currently available in the United States are contraceptives, not abortifacients (Sivin, 1989).

A postcoital "morning after" regimen for taking certain oral contraceptive pills can also avert pregnancy. This method is widely used in Europe and already widespread in many other countries, available both by prescription and over the counter or "behind the counter" (i.e., requiring counseling at the point of purchase by a trained health professional). The morning-after pill is also available in the United States; however, its use is not much promoted, and its availability is not known to many sexually active couples. In recent years, the contraceptive pill has been publicized as a means of "emergency contraception" for women having unprotected intercourse in the past 72 hours (Ellertson, 1996). Although four fifths of family planning clinics offer emergency contraceptive pills (ECPs) on site, only 18% of them provided the method to more than 20 women in 1998 (Finer et al., 2001). Jones et al. (2002a) estimated that ECP use prevented as many as 51,000 abortions in 2000. In view of the nearly 8 million women reporting condoms as their contraceptive method, emergency contraception presents an important and reassuring option (Trussell et al., 2004).

Surgical sterilization by ligating the fallopian tubes or by severing the vas deferens is a choice elected by many individuals who have no further desire for family formation. The method is rarely ineffective, but it has the disadvantage of being almost irreversible if circumstances change and a couple desires a pregnancy.

The current and future focus of contraceptive research and development has expanded to include male methods (e.g., male pill and vas deferens clips, in addition to condoms and vasectomy). Although the nature of the male reproductive biology is often thought to limit contraceptive development for men, recent research on cellular and molecular events show some promising directions (Harrison & Rosenfield, 1996). At the behavioral level, much can be learned about the prevalence and use of selected male methods from the findings of Cycle 6 (2002) of the National Survey of Family Growth (Mosher et al., 2004).

Approximately 90% of women at risk of unintended pregnancy use a contraceptive at least some of the time. The methods they choose are

shown in Table 4–1. The most frequently used methods (surgical sterilization and the pill) require a medical visit. (In many countries, the pill is
available without a medical prescription.) Also, the use patterns change
rapidly, particularly in response to concerns about STDs. For people who
are not in a stable monogamous relationship, the use of latex or polyurethane condoms is strongly recommended as the best protection next to
abstinence to prevent venereal infection, including human immunodeficiency virus. Hormonal and other nonbarrier methods are not protective
against venereal disease (STDs).

Use patterns also change rapidly in response to fear of complications.
All of the methods described have greater health benefits than health risks
that are rare, but in past years, with a regime of higher dose hormonal pills
than those now in use, some women experienced uncomfortable side
effects. An IUD, the Dalkon Shield, no longer manufactured, caused serious pelvic complications in some women. That experience has con-

**Table 4–1** Contraceptive Prevalence in the United States: 1982–2002
and 2002 Total Users

| Method | Contraceptive Prevalence Among Women 15–44 Years | | | 2002 | |
| | 1982 | 1995 | 2002 | Number of Users (in Thousands) | Percentage of Users |
| --- | --- | --- | --- | --- | --- |
| Sterilization | 19.0 | 24.8 | 22.4 | 13,800 | 36.2 |
| Tubal | 12.9 | 17.8 | 16.7 | 10,289 | 27.0 |
| Vasectomy | 6.1 | 7.0 | 5.7 | 3,511 | 9.2 |
| Pill | 15.6 | 17.3 | 18.9 | 11,679 | 30.6 |
| Implant | NA | 0.8 | 0.8 | 458 | 1.2 |
| Injectable | NA | 1.9 | 3.3 | 2,023 | 5.3 |
| IUD | 4.0 | 0.5 | 1.3 | 763 | 2.0 |
| Diaphragm | 4.5 | 1.2 | 0.2 | 115 | 0.3 |
| Condom | 6.7 | 13.1 | 11.1 | 6,870 | 18.0 |
| Periodic abstinence | 2.1 | 1.5 | 0.9 | 611 | 1.6 |
| Withdrawal | 1.1 | 1.9 | 2.5 | 1,527 | 4.0 |
| Other methods | 2.7 | 1.1 | 0.6 | 344 | 0.9 |
| Total | 55.7 | 64.2 | 61.9 | 38,109 | 100.0 |

*Definition of abbreviation:* NA = not applicable.
Source: Mosher et al. (2004).

tributed to the unpopularity in the United States of all IUDs, among both users and providers.

Use patterns also respond to changes in contraceptive technology. Some of the most effective means of contraception have been available for only a few decades. Among female users between 1982 and 2002, reliance on sterilization increased from 34.1% to 36.1%. Hormonal pill use declined from 28.0% to 26.9% in 1995 but rose to 30.6% in 2002. IUD use decreased from 7.1% to a negligible 0.8% in 1995 and 2.0% in 2002, and diaphragm use decreased from 8.1% to 0.3%. Reliance on periodic abstinence dropped from 3.9% in 1982 to 1.6% in 2002. Among users, between 1982 and 2002 condom use increased from 12.0% to 20.4% (Piccinino & Mosher, 1998). Changes in use patterns occurred in response to recent approved access to long-acting injectable and implanted hormonal contraceptives. Net change in condom use since 1988 has not been dramatic despite educational campaigns urging protection against acquired immunodeficiency syndrome.

Malcolm Potts (1988) emphasized that women in the United States, compared with those in other developed countries, are inefficient contraceptors. Contributing factors include limitations in the United States on contraceptive information and services as well as restrictions on the methods available. The choices available to European women are greater and include easy access to postcoital contraceptives, a wider range of IUDs, and injectable or implanted contraceptives, only recently approved for use in the United States. Darroch et al. (2001) confirmed these disparities also exist for American teens compared to European teenagers.

The effectiveness of different family planning methods varies greatly. Failure rates for 1988 and 1995 of the most widely used methods are indicated in Table 4–2. Even for the most protective methods, the failure rates are substantial unless usage conforms perfectly to guidance. Failure rates are calculated only for the first year of use. As noted earlier, when failures are accumulated over multiple years of the reproductive life span, they are greatly increased. This circumstance is alarmingly confirmed by the finding that almost half of unintended pregnancies occur among women who are attempting some form of reversible contraception (Institute of Medicine, 1995). This dismal record helps explain this country's high abortion rate. One in four pregnancies is terminated by induced abortion, one in two among pregnant teenagers. Improving this record suggests the need for more effective contraception.

**Table 4–2** First-Year (12-month) Contraceptive Failure Rates,*
1988 and 1995

| Method | 1988 | | 1995 | |
|---|---|---|---|---|
| | Perfect Use | Typical Use | Total | Corrected[†] |
| No method (chance) | 85.0 | 85.0 | | |
| Spermicides | 3.0 | 30.0 | 16.6 | 28.2 |
| Sponge | 8.0 | 24.0 | NA | NA |
| Withdrawal | 4.0 | 24.0 | 20.1 | 26.0 |
| Periodic abstinence | 9.0 | 19.0 | 20.2 | 21.8 |
| Cervical cap | 6.0 | 18.0 | } 9.2 | } 13.2 |
| Diaphragm | 6.0 | 18.0 | | |
| Condom (male) | 2.0 | 16.0 | 9.7 | 14.9 |
| Pill | 1.0 | 6.0 | 7.3 | 8.5 |
| IUD | 0.8 | 4.0 | NA | NA |
| Injectables | 0.3 | 0.4 | 2.8 | 3.5 |
| Tubal sterilization | 0.2 | 0.5 | NA | NA |
| Vasectomy | 0.1 | 0.2 | NA | NA |
| Implants | 0.04 | 0.05 | 1.8 | 2.0 |

*Estimated percentage of women experiencing an unintended pregnancy in the first year of use.
[†]Corrected for underreporting.
*Definition of abbreviation:* NA = not applicable.
Source: 1988 Data are reprinted from Facts in Brief (1993). 1995 Data are from Fu et al. (1999) (Table 1).

# FAMILY PLANNING PROVIDERS

Most users of reversible contraceptives obtain them from private physicians or managed-care organizations. Little is known about the scope or quality of those services. Approximately one user in three obtains services from a family planning clinic; the proportion is much higher for poor people, teenagers, and minority populations. A great deal is known about those clinics and their users. Accurate data are available on family planning agencies in the United States and their funding sources in 1997 (Frost et al., 2001; Frost, 2001). Those studies show that

- 3,117 agencies provided family planning services in 7,206 clinics, a level that has held steady since 1994.

- Annually, some 6.6 million women obtain contraceptive services from these providers, approximately 40% of those estimated to need publicly funded services.
- Health departments operate 40% of the clinic sites; community health centers, 21%; Planned Parenthood affiliates, 13%; and 26% by hospitals or other agencies.
- Three fifths of the agencies received Title X funding for family planning services.
- Most sites offer family planning services in clinic sessions devoted specifically to that purpose.
- Planned Parenthood clinics serve on average twice the number of clients as the next largest provider (2,074 clients per Planned Parenthood clinic compared with 1,319 clients at hospital clinics).
- Eighty-five percent of counties in the United States had one or more publicly funded family planning clinics.

Most family planning clinics offer a great deal more than a range of contraceptives. A recent study (Finer et al., 2001) found that 9 in 10 agencies offer the pill, condom, and injectable, and 4 in 5 offer ECPs, up from 38% in 1995. A usual cluster of services would include pregnancy testing; screening for breast and cervical cancer; screening and treatment for STDs; screening for hypertension, anemia, and kidney disease; infertility and genetic counseling; abortion; and sometimes prenatal and postpartum care. This extensive array of services has led some analysts to suggest that family planning clinics should become comprehensive primary health care centers for women. In truth, family planning clinics are now the only or major source of health care for many women of reproductive age. The prospect of expanding the role of family planning clinics has some appeal, but it presents many problems. Among them is funding. Family planning is a low-cost service. As other more expensive services draw on the same resources, the family planning mission is diluted. A case can be made that the cause of family planning can best be served, as in many countries, by narrowly focused programs that strive for the widest possible participation of the population in need, leaving provision of other appropriate services to other providers.

The funding issue is central to consideration of the family planning mission. The most important single funding source for clinics is the federal Title X program, which contributes support to three fifths of the agencies. The Fiscal Year 2004 appropriations bill, signed into law early in 2004, provides $280 million in Title X funding, $15 million more than the Presidential budget request. More than half of all family planning provider agencies receive some support from Title X; more than four fifths receive Medicaid funding, and 85% take in client fees. An important funding source for 43% of the agencies is MCH block grants from state and local governments. When considering all providers, not just the public clinics, the funding role of Medicaid and client fees increases appreciably. Other fee income and private contributions are minor sources of support, as is Social Services block grants (Finer et al., 2001).

The number of women who received their most recent family planning services at a publicly subsidized clinic, according to clinic reported data, was 6.6 million in 1997 (Frost et al., 2001). Based on 1995 survey data, nearly 60 million women aged 15 to 44 years in the United States obtained contraceptive or other reproductive services in the past year, 17% of whom accessed them at a publicly funded family planning clinic (Frost, 2001). Title X clinics are especially important sources of care for low-income women, single and young women ages 15 to 24 years, where more than half of those obtaining services fall into these categories. Moreover, 70% of those at risk for an unintended pregnancy reported Title X family planning clinics as their primary source for reproductive health care.

Since the 1980s, family planning clinics have been caught in a squeeze between increased demand for more costly services and reduced funding (Donovan, 1991). As a result, some clinics have had to resort to increased fee income with resultant threats to nonpaying clients for services. Gold and Daley (1991) estimated that after adjusting for inflation public support for contraceptive services and supplies diminished by one third during the 1980s. Frost et al. (2001) reported a high clinic turnover between 1994 and 1997.

## NEEDS AND PROSPECTS

The fact that a high proportion of sexually active people practice contraception at least part of the time suggests that the need for it is widely known. The fact that such a high proportion of pregnancies is unintended and that the abortion rate is so high also suggests that the effective practice of contraception is poorly understood and that use of family planning services is insufficient. Use is especially low among women in households with incomes below 200% of poverty. For some women, access to family planning can be an expensive procedure, not always covered by health insurance, especially for young women and those of low income. Waiting times for an appointment at family planning clinics have lengthened as clinic resources have shrunk. The need for a renewed national effort to enable planned childbearing is well established (Grason et al., 1999; Institute of Medicine, 1995).

Ever since the second Nixon administration in the early 1970s, a policy theme has gained strength to diminish the role of government, especially at the federal level, and to privatize as many public programs as possible. This theme has found expression, along with the political power to implement it, in the mid-1990s, with Congressional intent to make draconian cuts in the federal budget. Title X has been slated for elimination, or failing that, being folded into the MCH Block Grant. At the very best, this alternative would place public family planning at the uncertain discretion of different state governments. In many states, Planned Parenthood Federation affiliates, major providers of clinic services, would be shunted out of the funding stream. In other states, services in the public clinics would face serious political constraints. A consistent national policy and funding source for family planning would be lost. No strong private initiative shows promise of replacing it. What traditionally has been regarded as a public good now becomes an individual responsibility.

Threats and uncertainties come from another direction. The Clinton administration's health care reform proposal provided for everyone to be enrolled in a managed care plan that would offer all indicated personal health services. The reform was initially proposed for legislative action, which failed, but the managed care movement gained strength without it. Favorable experience with managed care rests largely on the record of early models of Health Maintenance Organizations, which ordinarily enrolled working families and which provided services financed at a fixed per capita rate.

Enrollees who had the resources and inclination could opt out of the program to purchase selected services from other providers. The new managed care plans are of a different sort. For the most part, they are not providers of services, but financial intermediaries for services that are rendered under contract with a variety of providers. Enrollees increasingly are low-income people, often Medicaid recipients, who are locked into the system without resources to purchase services independent of the plan.

The inclination and expertise of these plans to render family planning services is largely unknown. There was even controversy over whether some providers (such as Catholic hospitals) may refuse to include family planning services under circumstances (such as "conscience clauses") when beneficiaries' choices of alternative providers were limited. Prospects for availability of family planning services through managed care plans should not be underestimated, however. Service priorities under managed care will be driven by considerations of cost, if not profit. Nearly all methods of averting unwanted childbearing, including abortion, are less costly than maternity care (Trussell et al., 1995). For this reason, insurance companies that do not explicitly cover the costs of abortion will sometimes do so if asked. Still, financing abortions is a less appealing prospect than preventing unplanned pregnancies.

The need for family planning clinics to continue functioning outside managed care plans, or under contract with them, is an ongoing concern. Only one in five family planning agencies in 1995 had a Medicaid managed care contract. One study found women reporting themselves as uninsured in order to continue to obtain family planning care from their preferred provider (Rosenbaum et al., 1994). No matter how the issue is resolved, there is room here for expert influence from public health. Gold and Sonenfield (1999) also encouraged focusing efforts at the state level, wherein key programs such as the Temporary Aid to Needy Families and State Children's Health Insurance Program have included some coverage for family planning services. Insofar as managed care plans are currently influenced by standards that define benefits, they are framed around consideration of cost to enable employers to purchase economical plans on behalf of employees and their families. Standards for Medicaid-managed care are evolving and present barriers to access of contraceptive services from family planning clinics. A strong influence protective of user interests has not yet coalesced.

Standards for family planning, well established in Planned Parenthood clinics, need to be developed for managed care plans. A pressing commitment for public health workers would be to define those standards, see to their incorporation into managed care benefits and contracts, arrange to participate in quality review, develop data systems that enable accountability and outcome evaluations, train personnel capable of performing these tasks, and monitor the quality and outcome of services. The institutionalization of quality care standards for family planning under managed care, drawing from the long experience of publicly funded clinics, is of utmost importance. Nothing in the history of this country suggests that the family planning needs of the population are likely to be met without the strongest possible advocacy.

## REFERENCES

Alan Guttmacher Institute. (1995). The U.S. family planning program faces challenges and change. *Issues in brief.* Washington, DC: Alan Guttmacher Institute.

Boswell, J. (1988). *The kindness of strangers.* New York: Pantheon.

Daley, D., & Gold, R.B. (1993). Public funding for contraceptive, sterilization and abortion services, fiscal year 1992. *Family Planning Perspectives, 25,* 244–251.

Darroch, J., Singh, S., Frost, J.J., & The Study Team. (2001). Differences in teenage pregnancy rates among five developed countries: The roles of sexual activity and contraceptive use. *Family Planning Perspectives, 33,* 244–250, 281.

Donovan, P. (1991). Family planning clinics: Facing higher costs and sicker patients. *Family Planning Perspectives, 23,* 198–203.

Ellertson, C. (1996). History and efficacy of emergency contraception: Beyond Coca-Cola. *Family Planning Perspectives, 28,* 44–48.

English, P.C. (1984). Pediatrics and the unwanted child in history: Foundling homes, disease and the origins of foster care in New York City, 1860 to 1920. *Pediatrics, 73,* 699–711.

Finer, L., Darroch, J.E., & Frost, J.J. (2001). U.S. agencies providing publicly funded contraceptive services in 1999. *Perspectives on Sexual and Reproductive Health, 34,* 15–24.

Frost, J.J. (2001). Public or private providers? U.S. women's use of reproductive health services. *Family Planning Perspectives, 33,* 4–12.

Frost, J.J., & Forrest, J.P. (1995). Understanding the impact of effective teenage pregnancy prevention programs. *Family Planning Perspectives, 27,* 188–195.

Frost, J.J., Ranjit, N., Manzella, K., Darroch, J.E., & Audam, S. (2001). Family planning clinic services in the United States: Patterns and trends in the late 1990s. *Family Planning Perspectives, 33,* 113–122.

Fu, H., Darroch, J.E., Haas, T., & Ranjit, N. (1999). Contraceptive failure rates: New estimates from the 1995 National Survey of Family Growth. *Family Planning Perspectives, 31,* 56–63.

Gazmararian, J.A., Adams, M.A., Saltzman, L.E., Jonson, C.H., Bruce, F.C., Marks, M.S., & Zahniser, S.C. (1995). The relationship between pregnancy intendedness and physical violence in mothers of newborns. *Obstetrics and Gynecology, 85,* 1031–1038.

Gold, R.B., & Daley, D. (1991). Public funding of contraceptive, sterilization and abortion services, fiscal year 1990–1991. *Family Planning Perspectives, 23,* 204–211.

Gold, R.B., & Sonenfield, A. (1999). Family planning funding through four federal-state programs, FY1997. *Family Planning Perspectives, 31,* 176–181.

Grason, H., Hutchins, J., & Silver, G. (1999). *Charting a course for the future of women's and perinatal health: Vol. II, Reviews of Key Issues.* Baltimore, MD: Women's and Children's Health Policy Center, Johns Hopkins School of Public Health and Maternal and Child Health Bureau, Department of Health and Human Services.

Harrison, P., & Rosenfield, A. (Eds.). (1996). *Contraceptive research and development.* Washington, DC: National Academy Press.

Henshaw, S. (1998). Unintended pregnancy in the United States. *Family Planning Perspectives, 30,* 24–29, 46.

Institute of Medicine. (1995). *The best intentions: Unintended pregnancy and the well-being of children and families.* Washington, DC: National Academy Press.

Jones, E.F., et al. (1988). Unintended pregnancy, contraceptive practice and family planning services in developed countries. *Family Planning Perspectives, 20,* 53–67.

Jones, R., Darroch, J.E., & Henshaw, S.K. (2002a). Contraceptive use among U.S. women having abortions in 2000–2001. *Perspectives in Sexual and Reproductive Health, 34,* 294–303.

Jones R., Darroch, J.E., & Henshaw, S.K. (2002b). Patterns in the socioeconomic characteristics of women obtaining abortions in 2000–2001. *Perspectives in Sexual and Reproductive Health, 34,* 226–235.

Klaus, A. (1993). *Every child a lion: The origins of maternal and infant health policy in the United States and France, 1890–1920.* Ithaca, NY: Cornell University Press.

Kost, K., & Forrest, J.D. (1995). Intention status of U.S. births in 1988: Differences by mothers' socioeconomic and demographic characteristics. *Family Planning Perspectives, 27,* 11–17.

Kost, K., Landry, D., & Darroch, J. (1998). The effects of pregnancy planning status on birth outcomes and infant care. *Family Planning Perspectives, 30,* 223–230.

Major, R.H. (1954). *A history of medicine* (Vol. 1). Springfield, IL: Charles C. Thomas.

Mosher, W., Martinez, G.M., Chandra, A., Abma, J.C., & Willson, S. (2004). Use of contraception and use of family planning services in the United States: 1982–2002. *Advance data from vital and health statistics, no. 350.* Hyattsville, MD: National Center for Health Statistics.

Mundigo, A., & Indriso, C. (1998). *Abortion in the developing world.* London: Zed Books.

Piccinino, L., & Mosher, W. (1998). Trends in contraceptive use in the United States: 1982–1995. *Family Planning Perspectives, 30,* 4–10, 46.

Poole, V., & Hawkins, M. (1999). Pregnancy planning and unintended pregnancy. In *Charting a course for the future of women's and perinatal health: Vol.*

*II, Reviews of Key Issues* (pp. 81–102). Baltimore, MD: Women's and Children's Health Policy Center, Johns Hopkins School of Public Health and Maternal and Child Health Bureau, Department of Health and Human Services.

Potts, M. (1988). Birth control methods in the U.S. *Family Planning Perspectives, 20*, 288–296.

Rosenbaum, S., Shin, P., Mauskopf, A., Funk, K., Stern, G., & Zuvekus, A. (1994). *Beyond the freedom to choose: Medicaid, managed care and family planning.* Washington, DC: George Washington University Center for Health Policy Research.

Rosoff, J. (1988). The politics of birth control. *Family Planning Perspectives, 20*, 312–320.

Sivin, I. (1989). IUDs are contraceptives, not abortifacients: A comment on research and belief. *Studies in Family Planning, 20*, 355–359.

Trussell, J., Leveque, J.A., Koenig, J.D., London, R., Borden S., Henneberry, J., LaGuardia, K.D., Stewart F., Wilson, T.G., Wysocki, S., & Strauss, M. (1995). The economic value of contraception: A comparison of 15 methods. *American Journal of Public Health, 85*, 494–503.

Trussell, J., Ellertson, C., Stewart, F., Raymond, E.G., & Shochet, T. (2004). [Emergency contraception: A cost-effective approach to preventing unintended pregnancy.] Unpublished manuscript.

Zabin, L.S., Hirsch, M.B., Smith, E.A., Streett, R. & Hardy, J.B. (1986). Evaluation of a pregnancy prevention program for urban teenagers. *Family Planning Perspectives, 18,* 119–126.

# CHAPTER 5

# Mothers and Infants

*Trude Bennett and Milton Kotelchuck*

> *At the present time medical schools do not prepare students for the work of preventing infant mortality. . . . In short, preventive pediatrics must be taught. This becomes possible only when it is a required course based upon the present-day needs of the community. To be successful the preventive work in pediatrics must have a foundation in the knowledge that the faulty social structure is at the basis of many of the ills that are thrust upon infant flesh. (Wile, 1910)*
>
> *I am 37 years old and I am so worried and filled with perfect horror at the prospects ahead. So many of my neighbors die at giving birth to their children. I have a baby 11 months old in my keeping now, whose mother died. When I reached their cabin last Nov. it was 22 below zero, and I had to ride 7 miles horse back. She was nearly dead when I got there, and died after giving birth to a 14 lb. boy. (Mrs. A-C-P, 1916)*

## INTRODUCTION

At the beginning of the 20th century, childbirth was still a life-threatening event for women in the United States. The risk of death to mothers and infants was substantial, and the available information and treatments were not adequate to assuage women's fears. Although the uneven distribution of risks has always placed disadvantaged groups in greatest jeopardy, the tragedy of a maternal or infant death elicits universal sympathy. Dr. Sara

**113**

Josephine Baker, who became director of the New York City Bureau of Child Hygiene in 1908, coined the slogan "No Mother's Baby is Safe Until Every Mother's Baby Is Safe" (Wertz & Wertz, 1982, p. 228). A pamphlet published by the United States Children's Bureau in 1913 proclaimed, "The infant death rate is the truest index of the welfare of any community" (Bremner, 1971, p. 966).

Infant deaths remain a widely used indicator of the general health and well-being of society. Infant mortality continues to plague developing countries at alarming rates, exacting significant social and economic costs and curtailing overall life expectancy. Although both maternal and infant mortality have been markedly reduced in this country, major racial and socioeconomic disparity persists as a gauge of social inequality. The relatively poor international ranking of the United States in infant mortality has been a source of national embarrassment. The last 2 decades have seen a great deal of effort targeted toward lowering the US infant mortality rate, especially toward reducing the extremely high death rates of African American infants. The maternal and child health (MCH) community has focused on equalizing the life circumstances of mothers and the life chances of infants as a starting point toward greater social equity in the United States.

This chapter provides an overview of reproductive outcomes that are used as health indicators for mothers and infants. Definitions are provided, and epidemiologic trends and salient policy issues are briefly discussed. The notion of reproductive risk is explored and its usefulness examined in relationship to the defined outcomes. The chapter concludes with a review of current interventions in the field and some of the controversies that we face in setting program and policy priorities in the search for equity.

# OUTCOMES

## Definitions

Formal efforts to study the health of populations began in Europe and the United States in the 1840s with the development of vital statistics systems in which the state, as opposed to the church, began to record births and deaths. The well-being of children has always been recognized as critical to a society's vitality and continuity, and the measurement of early death has been an important topic from the beginning of birth registration systems. In an era with no vaccinations or cures for infectious childhood diseases, the first efforts to examine the health of a state's youngest citizens focused on deaths of children under 5 years old. Childhood mortality, still calculated as a rate of such deaths per 1,000 children from birth to 5 years, is an important measure of a society's health. The World Health Organization (WHO) uses childhood mortality as part of a child survival index to make cross-national comparisons.

One can view the efforts of public health professionals over the past century as an effort to refine this broad health measure to assess infant health status better. As we have increasingly been able to affect the health of mothers and newborns, our ability to define and measure relevant components of infant health and morbidity has also improved. Measurement of MCH events is intended not only to enhance scientific understanding but also to facilitate effective interventions. By the 1870s, the present concept of infant mortality, the number of infant deaths per 1,000 live births, came into use. The turn of the 20th century brought into focus the role of infectious diseases and poor nutrition, which took a heavy toll on infants throughout their first year. The MCH community began to divide infant mortality into neonatal mortality (deaths in the first 27 days of life per 1,000 live births) and postneonatal mortality (deaths from 28 to 364 days per 1,000 live births minus neonatal deaths). Neonatal deaths were generally attributed to biological birth complications and postneonatal deaths to environmental conditions and infectious diseases.

International comparisons are troubled by different historical and cultural perspectives on the meaning of infants' lives and deaths. In China, newborns are counted as being 1 year old at the time of birth. In some societies, an infant is not considered to be alive (and age is not calculated) until the time of christening, circumcision, or naming. A baby that dies before achieving the required status would not be enumerated as an infant death, and classification of neonatal and postneonatal deaths would be skewed by varying definitions.

Birth weight has been universally recognized as an important predictor of infant mortality and morbidity. Historically, all societies have known that tiny babies were more likely to die and that small infants who survived were developmentally vulnerable. In industrialized countries, the growth of specialized services for newborns and neonatal intensive care units in the 1950s and 1960s increased the focus on low birth weight (LBW) and prematurity. Specific measures of newborn morbidity status arose in tandem with these developments. Differential categorizations of small size that became popularized included definitions based on birth weight, gestational age or prematurity, and growth (birth weight levels corresponding to gestational age).

In 1948, WHO established 2,500 g as the threshold for normal births. At first, LBW was the only criterion used to define infant size. With improved registration and the use of computerized databases, more detailed and sophisticated birth weight measures developed. Birth weight categories are generally defined as normal birth weight (NBW) (2,500 g or more or at least 5 lb., 8.5 oz.), LBW (less than 2,500 g), moderately LBW (1,500–2,499 g), very LBW (VLBW) (less than 1,500 g), and occasionally extra LBW (less than 750 g). Births at less than 500 g are sometimes considered marginally viable and may be excluded from live births, and infants weighing 4,000 g or greater are sometimes considered separately as a high-weight group with potential health risks. Birth weight rates (more properly called proportions) are defined as the percentages of births in a weight category (i.e., number of births in a given weight range per 100 live births).

LBW can be thought of as being caused by two possible causes, infants born too soon (prematurity) or infants born too small (intrauterine growth retardation). Interest in the measurement of prematurity is increasing with the recognition that most infant deaths are due to low gestational age and immaturity of the fetus, not size per se. Prematurity has been defined somewhat arbitrarily based on 40 weeks as the average length of pregnancy. Normal gestation is defined as 37–41 weeks. The criterion for premature gestation is 36 weeks or less, and for extremely premature, it is 32 weeks or less. Births at 42+ weeks of gestation are classified as postmature. Rates of prematurity are usually calculated as the number of premature births per total live births × 100.

Prematurity is more difficult to measure accurately than birth weight. Gestational age is usually defined as the difference between the last menstrual period and the birth date, minus 2 weeks; increasingly, ultrasonography and newborn observational criteria, such as the Dubowitz scoring system, are also used to estimate gestational age. The completeness and accuracy of birth certificate and medical record data on last menstrual period vary according to mothers' ability to recall menstrual information and the accuracy of clinical judgment and record keeping.

Growth measures, which define intrauterine growth retardation or small for gestational age (SGA), use percentages to rank infant birth weights for a given gestational age based on national norms (Alexander, Himes, Kaufman, Mor, & Kogan, 1996). For example, among all infants born at 39-weeks gestation in the United States, 50% weigh more than 3,400 g. Babies are usually defined as SGA if they rank in the lowest 10th percentile for a given gestational age. The distinction between prematurity and growth retardation has important implications for prevention efforts and for subsequent morbidity and treatment of the infant. Premature infants are more vulnerable to mortality, but if they survive, their life course may be quite normal. SGA infants have better survival rates but more subsequent developmental and health problems. Growth retardation often makes a greater contribution to LBW rates in developing countries compared with industrialized nations such as the United States. However, the utility of these growth measures is limited by the lack of international comparative norms as well as the need for fairly sophisticated data collection systems.

Public health analysts have attempted to capture the relationship between infant birth size and infant mortality by defining birth weight–specific mortality (BWSM), the number of infant deaths per 1,000 live births in a given weight category. For example, in the 2001 birth cohort in the United States, 58.6 infants died per every 1,000 born at LBW and 244.4 died for every 1,000 born at VLBW. These rates contrasted with only 6.8 deaths per 1,000 infants born at 2,500 g or more (Arias, MacDorman, Strobino, & Guyer, 2003). BWSM is a very effective measure of a society's capacity to keep small infants alive.

Technically, infant mortality can thus be defined as $IM = \Sigma(BWSM \times BW)$. That is, the total infant mortality in society is the sum of all the infant mortality within each birth weight group. The infant mortality within each birth weight group is influenced by the frequency or distribution of births and the rate of survival of those births within that birth weight category (BWSM). This formula is important because it suggests two approaches to improve infant mortality: reducing the number of small babies born through preventive public health interventions and improving the clinical neonatal health services to keep small babies alive. Both prevention and treatment approaches are critical to improving infant mortality rates in any society.

The timing of the loss of a product of pregnancy is also important, and there are a number of opportunities for loss along the embryogenic timeline (issues of conception are discussed in Chapter 4). It is not possible to estimate either the likelihood of fertilization or the rate of implantation of fertilized eggs. Once successful implantation of a fertilized egg is accomplished, research suggests that approximately 25% of implantations may fail before women are aware they are pregnant; spontaneous abortions or miscarriages then occur subsequently in approximately 15% of the clinically recognized pregnancies, although the measurement of any of these losses is imprecise. Thus, it appears that more than one third of all implanted pregnancies fail to result in a live birth. Spontaneous abortions frequently present a serious psychological loss for the mother and family. In spite of the high frequency of early loss, general inattention to this important topic in women's health has hindered the development of any standardized measurements. The MCH field has a very limited understanding of the causes, risk factors, and distribution of early fetal loss.

Deaths after 20 weeks, but before birth, are defined as fetal deaths and are also rather poorly understood. Fetal death rates are approximately equal to neonatal death rates but are much less frequently studied (Barfield, 2004). An arbitrary division is made between early (20–27 weeks) and late (28+ weeks) fetal deaths, often called stillbirths. Historically, these distinctions have become less clear with the increased potential for fetal surgery and life-saving interventions for infants born prematurely. In many European countries, the term perinatal mortality is used to refer to all deaths from 28 weeks gestation through 7 days of life (number of late fetal deaths plus early neonatal deaths per 1,000 live births). US studies occasionally use this term but with varying definitions.

As with indicators of infant health status, the definition of maternal outcomes has been evolving over time. Maternal mortality has traditionally been used as the sole women's health indicator, with measures estimating ratios of maternal deaths per 100,000 live births or women's average lifetime risks of dying from pregnancy-related causes. However, definitions and methods used for estimating maternal mortality have not been consistent. In 1974, a statistical working group in Geneva declared a maternal death to be "the death of a woman while pregnant or within 42 days of termination of pregnancy" (Royston & Armstrong, 1989, p. 12). By including "all known deaths of women known to be pregnant," this group recommended a definition based purely on the timing of death regardless of cause, similar to measures of infant mortality.

A limit of 42 days postpartum gives a narrow window for capturing fatalities related to the sequelae of pregnancy and childbearing. An important example is postpartum cardiomyopathy, a sometimes fatal condition that can manifest up to 6-months postpartum without previous signs. Studies that have extended the postpartum period to a full year have identified 6% to 11% additional deaths after 42 days (Atrash, Koonin, Lawson, Franks, & Smith, 1990; Rochat, Koonin, Atrash, & Jewett, 1988). The International Classification of Diseases, 10th ed., Clinical Modification (ICD-10-CM), which replaced ICD-9 on January 1, 1999, revised the time frame upward to 1 year after delivery.

ICD-10-CM, like the ICD-9 and earlier versions published by the WHO (1977), divides maternal deaths into two groups. The first category is made up of direct obstetric deaths, resulting from obstetric complications of the pregnant state (pregnancy, labor, and puerperium); from interventions, omissions, incorrect treatment; or from a chain of events resulting from any of the above. The second classification is indirect obstetric deaths resulting from previous existing disease or disease that developed during pregnancy, which was not caused by direct obstetric causes but was aggravated by the physiologic effects of pregnancy. Deaths from unintentional or incidental causes presumed to be independent of childbearing are excluded, an omission that ensures conservative estimates of maternal mortality.

Studies have shown that maternal mortality increases considerably with inclusion of deaths to pregnant and postpartum women caused by drugs, violence, and injury (Chavkin & Allen, 1993). Enhanced surveillance of maternal deaths in North Carolina found 119 pregnancy-related deaths from 1993 to 1997, only 65 (or 55%) of which were identified through underlying cause-of-death codes in death certificates (Buescher, Harper, & Meyer, 2002). Buescher et al. (2002) identified numerous sources of underreporting of maternal mortality. With their enhanced surveillance methods allowing for ascertainment of maternal deaths occurring within a year after childbirth, cardiomyopathy appeared as the leading cause of pregnancy-related death. Furthermore, the researchers identified 178 non–pregnancy-related maternal deaths during the 5-year study period.

As maternal deaths have become more rare in developed countries, a new measure has been developed: the reproductive mortality rate. The concept of reproductive mortality includes risks sustained by women trying to avoid pregnancy, or deaths related to contraceptive use. The rate consists of the number of reproductive deaths per 100,000 women in a given age group. In the United States, mortality risks sustained by women trying to avoid or delay pregnancy have become as important as pregnancy-associated risks. "Whereas in 1955, 99 percent of the reproductive deaths in the US were pregnancy-related, only slightly more than one-half (53 percent) were so in 1975" (Royston & Armstrong, 1989, p. 16). The concept of reproductive mortality highlights the need for careful monitoring of new contraceptive and reproductive technologies.

The decline of maternal mortality calls for more sensitive measures of maternal morbidity, an area that has been relatively understudied. Severe pregnancy complications have been measured by the ratio of pregnancy-related hospitalizations per 100 deliveries. The ratio of hospitalizations for pregnancy complications declined markedly between 1986–1987 and 1991–1992, but this apparent improvement may have been illusory (Bennett, Kotelchuck, Cox, Tucker, & Nadeau, 1998). More recent data suggest a continuing sharp decline in pregnancy-related hospitalizations (Bacak, Callaghan, Dietz, & Crouse, 2003). However, reductions in hospital admissions may reflect changes in hospital policy and standards of medical practice rather than a true decline in morbidity. Cost containment policies and shifts to outpatient management of many conditions could mask health problems while lowering hospitalization rates.

For these reasons, the one objective pertaining to maternal morbidity in the US Department of Health and Human Services' *Healthy People 2010: Understanding and Improving Health* (2000) was restricted to reduction of maternal complications during hospitalized labor and delivery. The vast majority of women in the United States deliver in hospitals, and thus, record review of delivery hospitalizations is less biased by nonmedical factors than predelivery hospitalizations during pregnancy. Recommendations were made in *Healthy People 2010* to monitor ectopic (i.e., nonuterine) pregnancies and postpartum complications, including postpartum depression, but adequate data were not available for these purposes.

## Epidemiologic Trends

### Infant Mortality

The reduction of the infant mortality rate from 150 deaths per 1,000 live births in 1900 to 7 per 1,000 today is one of the great public health success stories in the United States. Over the last century, infant mortality has gone from being a common family tragedy to a relatively rare event. Infant mortality rates did not, however, improve steadily in the 20th century in the United States. Infant mortality has had four periods of limited or no decline: during the Great Depression in the 1930s, the period from the 1950s to the mid-1960s, the early 1980s, and recently in 2002. In 1960, the United States ranked 11th worldwide; by 1999, the United States had slipped to 28th place (National Center for Health Statistics, 2003).

The 2001 US infant mortality rate of 6.8 deaths per 1,000 live births represented a decrease of 10.5% from 1995 (Arias et al., 2003; Mathews, Menacker, & MacDorman, 2003). Preliminary data for 2002 indicated an increase to 7.0 deaths per 1,000 births, attributable in part to a decline in survival during the first week of life (Kochanek & Martin, 2004). This increase would represent the first rise in infant mortality in the United States in over 45 years. The target in *Healthy People 2010* is 4.5 per 1,000. Modest declines occurred between 1995 and 2001 for infants of non-Hispanic white, African American, and Mexican American mothers (Mathews et al., 2003). The continued ranking of the United States at the bottom of developed countries is primarily due to its adverse birth weight distribution (i.e., higher proportion of LBW infants) (Arias et al., 2003).

With gains in technological control over environmental conditions and infectious diseases, the timing of infant mortality has historically shifted toward early deaths, suggesting stronger biological determinants. Currently, most infant deaths occur in the neonatal period (4.5 deaths per 1,000 births in 2001) rather than the postneonatal period (2.3 deaths per 1,000 births in 2001). In recent years, improvements in infant mortality have also been concentrated in the neonatal period, perhaps because of rapid gains in neonatology and enhanced regionalization of tertiary care. *Healthy People 2010* targets are 2.9 per 1,000 for neonatal deaths and 1.2 per 1,000 for postneonatal deaths.

Approximately half of all infant deaths in 2001 were attributed to four causes: congenital malformations, disorders related to prematurity and LBW, sudden infant death syndrome (SIDS), and newborn consequences of maternal pregnancy complications (Arias et al., 2003). The dramatic drop in SIDS deaths after the 1992 recommendation of the American Academy of Pediatrics to put infants to sleep on their backs or sides, rather than placing them on their stomachs, has continued at a slower pace. The use of surfactant treatment has made respiratory distress syndrome (RDS) less of a lethal threat to premature and underweight infants since 1990; only 3.7% of infant deaths were caused by RDS in 2001 (Arias et al., 2003).

Major racial disparities in infant mortality show no sign of diminishing. In 2001, infants of African American mothers were 2.3 times as likely to die in the first year as infants of white mothers (13.3 vs. 5.7 deaths per 1,000 live births). Racial comparisons in infant mortality usually focus on black/white differences because of the extreme gap in the outcomes for these groups. Overall mortality rates for Asian and Pacific Islander and Latino infants are similar or better than the white rate, although regional and subgroup variations underlie the appearance of homogeneity (see Chapter 9). For example, in 2001, the Hispanic/Latino infant mortality rate in the United States as a whole was 5.4 deaths per 1,000 births. In the same year, the infant morality rate in Puerto Rico was 9.9, and Latino rates in the United States varied by ethnicity, 4.2 for Cubans, 5.2 for Mexicans, and 8.5 for Puerto Ricans. Similarly, ethnic variations are noted for Asian and Pacific Islanders (4.7 births per 1,000 deaths overall) with rates of 3.2 for Chinese, 4.0 for Japanese, and 7.3 for Hawaiians. Native American rates are also elevated at 9.7 deaths per 1,000 births (Mathews et al., 2003).

Infant mortality rates in the United States tend to vary by geographic region and state. The highest rates tend to cluster among states in the South and Midwest. Both remote rural areas and metropolitan centers with large pockets of poverty and unemployment tend to have extremely high rates. Variations by state also exist for race-specific rates. African Americans consistently fare worse, but the racial gap is more severe in some states than in others. For example, black:white infant mortality ratios in 1991–2001 were as high as 2.9 in Wisconsin and 2.7 in Missouri but were only 1.3 in Oregon and 1.4 in West Virginia (Mathews et al., 2003).

## Low Birth Weight

Low birth weight is an intransigent problem in the United States. The lowest recorded percentage of births below 2,500 g was 6.7% in 1984, and the rate slowly but steadily increased over the next 2 decades. The percentage of LBW births for the whole population rose from 7.0% in 1990 to 7.8% in 2002, whereas the percentage of VLBW remained fairly stable (1.27% in 1990 and 1.46% in 2002) (Arias et al., 2003; Martin, Hamilton, Sutton, Ventura, Menacker, & Munson, 2003). These trends make achievement of 2010 objectives (5.0% LBW and 0.9% VLBW) seem unlikely.

The increase in LBW between 1990 and 1999 was specific to non-Hispanic white, Native American, and Asian/Pacific Islander infants

(Guyer, Freedman, Strobino, & Sondik, 2000). Among white women, the increase in LBW is primarily associated with a rise in multiple births caused by fertility drugs and other assisted reproductive technologies; LBW has also risen, although more modestly, among singleton infants (Martin et al., 2003). Rates of LBW (13.3%) and VLBW (3.1%) among African Americans remain substantially elevated compared with the rates for white infants (6.8% LBW and 1.2% VLBW). These persistent problems have presented a frustrating challenge to the MCH community in its efforts to improve birth outcomes and eliminate inequities. Buekens and Klebanoff (2001) have observed that high rates of LBW and preterm delivery may begin to seem inevitable to US observers because of public health failure, and thus, innovative research and intervention strategies are more critically important than ever.

### Gestational Age

In 2002, the proportion of babies delivered prematurely (before 37 full weeks of gestation) was 12.1% compared with 10.6% in 1990 and the target of 7.6% in *Healthy People 2010*. Preterm births declined from 18.8% to 17.5% for African Americans between 1990 and 2002 but rose from 8.5% to 11.1% for white women during that period, reducing the black:white prematurity ratio from 2.2 to 1.6. Similar to the birth weight trends, increasing prematurity among white women has been associated with a rise in assisted reproductive technologies–related multiple births. In 1999, 1.9% of all births occurred before 32 weeks of gestation, and 66% of all LBW births were premature (March of Dimes Birth Defects Foundation, 1999). Although decreases in preterm delivery are desirable for reduction of infant mortality, morbidity, and disability, improved prenatal screening and treatment sometimes contribute to iatrogenic prematurity when early intervention is judged to be beneficial. In other words, medically induced prematurity may sometimes be preferable to longer gestations in cases of maternal or fetal distress or a multiparous pregnancy. Postterm births at 42 weeks gestation or later, also considered an adverse health outcome, declined to 6.7% in 2002 from 11.3% of all births in 1990 (Martin et al., 2003).

### Birth Weight-Specific Mortality

Birth outcomes differ dramatically by birth weight. Thus, infant mortality trends are determined by changes in both the distribution of birth weights and the likelihood of death in each birth weight category. The majority of infants who die are both very premature and VLBW. Newborns weighing 3,500–4,499 g are least likely to die in the first year. Over two thirds (67%) of all infants who died in 2001 were LBW, and over half (53%) of infant deaths were VLBW. Infants of African American mothers died of causes associated with LBW at a rate 3.8 times the rate for white infants (Arias et al., 2003).

Although there is much debate over explanations for such differences, the BWSM survival rates of African Americans and whites of similar birth weight are not markedly different. The major source of the racial gap in infant mortality is clearly due to differences in birth weight distributions, specifically the substantially greater rates of LBW and prematurity among African Americans. An excess of LBW in the entire US population explains our low international ranking in infant mortality.

Although progress in reducing LBW has been forestalled, dramatic declines in BWSM occurred between 1960 and 2001. The reduction of infant mortality rates during that period averaged approximately 80% in every weight category. Odds of survival improved between 1995 and 2001 for all birth weight categories, except the highest birth weight infants (4,500 g or more).

Because of sophisticated neonatal intensive care technologies, the likelihood of survival is now approximately 95% at 1,250–1,499 g compared with only 52% in 1960. Such dramatic improvements explain the overall decline in infant mortality over the last several decades, but technology may be reaching its limit in saving tiny newborns. Death rates for VLBW infants less than 500 g dropped 5% between 1995 and 2001, but 86% still died. The smallest survivors "are at much greater risk of experiencing lifetime disabilities such as blindness, developmental delays, and neurologic disorders, necessitating increased levels of medical and parental care" (Arias et al., 2003, p. 1224). The dissemination of high technology in neonatal and infant health services in the United States rivals any other country, but our population-based prevention efforts lag behind.

At the time of this writing (July 2004), the US Congress was debating legislation intended to lower rates of prematurity. Senate Bill 1726, the "PREEMIE Act" (Prematurity Research Expansion and Education for Mothers Who Deliver Infants Early Act), was introduced with bipartisan support to increase research on causes of premature delivery at the National Institutes of Health and Centers for Disease Control and

Prevention (CDC), to improve the treatment and health of premature babies, and to create programs to support the emotional and informational needs of their families. It is hoped that this act will reduce the number of babies who are born below NBW and thereby reduce health care costs. In 2003, the March of Dimes initiated a major 5-year Prematurity Campaign, with the goals of increasing public awareness about the problems of prematurity and decreasing the rate of preterm births in the United States by at least 15%.

## Maternal Mortality and Morbidity

An estimated 500,000 women worldwide die of maternal causes each year; 99% of these deaths occur in developing countries. Regional and national variations are extreme, ranging from average estimates of 55 deaths per 100,000 live births in East Asia to 700/100,000 in West Africa. Leading causes of maternal death in developing countries are hemorrhage, sepsis or infection, toxemia and hypertensive disease, illegal and unsafe abortion, and obstructed labor/ruptured uterus. The vast majority of these deaths would be preventable with better health services and transportation systems, as well as additional societal resources to improve sanitation, nutrition, education, and the overall health status of women (Royston & Armstrong, 1989). These maternal deaths are the target of the WHO Safe Motherhood campaign.

In industrialized countries, the average maternal death rate is 30 deaths per 100,000 births (Royston & Armstrong, 1989). The ratio of maternal deaths per 100,000 live births in the United States was 7.1 in 1998, an incredible decline from 619 deaths per 100,000 births in 1933 (Enkin, 1994; *Health People 2010*, 2000). However, essentially no progress has been made in the last 2 decades (despite an ambitious target of 3.3 deaths per 100,000 births in the *Healthy People 2010* objectives). This indicator is characterized by an alarmingly high racial differential in the United States. In 1998, the non-Hispanic African American ratio was 17.4 compared with 4.9 for non-Hispanic whites. The black maternal death ratio has consistently been threefold to fourfold the risk for whites since the 1940s. Major causes for all US maternal deaths reported in 1997 were hemorrhage, ectopic pregnancy, pregnancy-induced hypertension, embolism, infection, and other complications of pregnancy and childbirth.

Maternal mortality is known to be underestimated in all countries' registration systems, including US statistics. According to studies of mortality surveillance, the actual US rate may be 25% higher than reported (Royston & Armstrong, 1989). Sachs, Brown, Driscoll, Schulman, Acker, Ransil, et al. (1992) examined maternal mortality in Massachusetts between 1954 and 1985 and noted a shift to trauma (suicide, homicide, motor vehicle injuries) and pulmonary embolus as leading causes of death. Inadequate prenatal care also assumed greater prominence as a risk factor in Massachusetts, and one third to one half of the deaths were judged to be preventable. Improvements in environmental and health care factors, including the legalization of abortion, have gone a long way toward protecting women's health during pregnancy and delivery. The United States has not optimized these advantages, however, because inequities persist and maternal deaths are still more likely to occur in the United States compared with many other developed countries.

A recent Safe Motherhood initiative led by CDC has helped to focus greater attention on women's health and maternal morbidity (Wilcox, 2002), but resources required for improved monitoring are not yet available. The *Healthy People 2010* target for maternal illness and complications caused by pregnancy would reduce the 1998 baseline of 31.2% labor and delivery hospitalizations with maternal complications to 24%. The objective is "better than the best," meaning that all population subgroups would achieve a proportion of 24% or lower. Special effort would be required to reduce the complication rates of African American women, however, who suffered complications in 37.7% of delivery hospitalizations in 1998 (compared with 30.3% for whites).

## REPRODUCTIVE RISK

Extensive research has established many associations between maternal characteristics and infant health outcomes. The listing of principal risk factors for LBW from the 1985 Institute of Medicine report, *Preventing Low Birthweight*, is reproduced in Table 5–1. This list is organized by type of risk—demographic factors, medical conditions preceding and arising during pregnancy, behavioral and environmental exposures, health care characteristics, and evolving concepts of risk, such as stress, that are still not well understood. Table 5–2 classifies risk factors for preterm birth according to the certainty of association demonstrated by current research (Berkowitz & Papiernik, 1993). According to Kramer (1987), less than a

**Table 5–1**  Principal Risk Factors for Low Birth Weight

I. Demographic risks
   A. Age (less than 17 years; over 34 years)
   B. Race (black)
   C. Low socioeconomic status
   D. Unmarried
   E. Low level of education

II. Medical risks predating pregnancy
   A. Parity (0 or more than 4)
   B. Low weight for height
   C. Genitourinary anomalies/surgery
   D. Selected diseases such as diabetes, chronic hypertension
   E. Nonimmune status for selected infections such as rubella
   F. Poor obstetric history, including previous low birth weight infant, multiple spontaneous abortions
   G. Maternal genetic factors (such as low maternal weight at own birth)

III. Medical risks in current pregnancy
   A. Multiple pregnancy
   B. Poor weight gain
   C. Short interpregnancy interval
   D. Hypotension
   E. Hypertension/preeclampsia/toxemia
   F. Selected infections such as symptomatic bacteriuria, rubella, and cytomegalovirus
   G. First- or second-trimester bleeding
   H. Placental problems such as placenta previa, abruptio placentae
   I. Hyperemesis
   J. Oligohydramnios/polyhydramnios
   K. Anemia/abnormal hemoglobin
   L. Isoimmunization
   M. Fetal anomalies
   N. Incompetent cervix
   O. Spontaneous premature rupture of membranes

IV. Behavioral and environmental risks
   A. Smoking
   B. Poor nutritional status
   C. Alcohol and other substance abuse
   D. DES exposure and other toxic exposures, including occupational hazards
   E. High altitude

*continues*

---

**Table 5-1** continued

V. Health care risks
   A. Absent or inadequate prenatal care
   B. Iatrogenic prematurity
VI. Evolving concepts of risk
   A. Stress, physical and psychosocial
   B. Uterine irritability
   C. Events triggering uterine contractions
   D. Cervical changes detected before onset of labor
   E. Selected infections such as mycoplasma and *Chlamydia trachomatis*
   F. Inadequate plasma volume expansion
   G. Progesterone deficiency

---

*Definition of abbreviation:* DES = diethylstilbestrol, a form of synthetic estrogen that was found to cause vaginal cancer in the female offspring of women who had been administered the drug during pregnancy.

Source: Committee to Study the Prevention of Low Birthweight (1985).

third of premature deliveries in developed countries can be predicted by these known risk factors.

Later in this chapter we discuss the strengths and limitations of risk assessments for clinical predictions based on known factors. First, we wish to examine the notion of risk in the MCH context. A close look at the items listed in Table 5–1 and Table 5–2 reveals a heterogeneous mixture of elements with unclear causal links to LBW and prematurity.

Krieger (1994) has traced the historical evolution of explanatory models in medical research from the mechanistic "doctrine of specific etiology" to a more complex understanding of "multiple causation" in epidemiology. Risk factors tend to be viewed as independent entities, although in reality they often cluster together and interact. For many of the listed risks, we know little about the casual mechanisms that contribute to outcomes. Some of these factors are actually "risk markers" that indicate certain problems may be present. For example, unmarried status is often accompanied by mothers' low incomes. Reliability of risk markers is variable, and the amenability of risk factors to interventions is changeable. We often use available information as imperfect proxies for missing data (e.g., marital status to represent income or race/ethnicity to substitute for socioeconomic status) but fail to measure relevant factors directly. Emanuel, Hale, & Berg (1989) noted that we seldom take into account significant aspects

## Table 5–2  Risk Factors for Preterm Birth

Established risk factors
    Black race
    Single marital status
    Low socioeconomic status
    Previous LBW or preterm delivery
    Multiple second-trimester spontaneous abortions
    In vitro fertilization pregnancy
    Placental abnormalities
    Gestational bleeding
    Cervical and uterine anomalies
    In utero diethylstilbestrol exposure
    Multiple gestations
    Cigarette smoking
Probable risk factors
    Urogenital infections
    Cocaine use
    No prenatal care or inadequate prenatal care
    Seasonality
Factors weakly associated or not associated with preterm birth
    Maternal age
    Infant sex
    Maternal weight gain
    Dietary intake
    Parity
    Short interpregnancy interval
    Prior first trimester induced abortion
    Alcohol consumption
    Caffeine intake
    Sexual activity during late pregnancy
Inconclusive risk factors
    Psychosocial stress
    Short stature
    Low prepregnancy weight/low body mass index
    Anemia
    Employment-related physical activity
Factors for which there are insufficient data
    Familial and intergenerational factors
    History of infertility
    Use of marijuana and other illicit drugs
    Leisure-time physical activity
    Occupational and environmental toxicants

Source: Berkowitz and Papiernik (1993).

of mothers' childhoods, such as nutritional adequacy, or of adult women's environments during pregnancy, such as domestic violence.

A potential problem with risk factor analysis is the narrow focus on single outcomes rather than a more holistic context. The search to explain LBW and prematurity is extremely important, but not to the exclusion of other concerns. For example, alcohol consumption may not be associated with preterm delivery, but fetal alcohol syndrome and fetal alcohol effect are serious problems for infant and child development. Alcohol or drug use may also be a marker for domestic violence or other problems. Conclusive evidence may not exist to implicate anemia in prematurity; however, as with alcohol abuse, anemia is not only a risk for LBW, it is also a danger to women's subsequent health.

Wise (1993) pointed out that the relevance of individual risks must be evaluated in terms of their prevalence in the larger population, not just the magnitude of risk in extreme cases. For example, women who use illicit drugs or receive no prenatal care are frequently cited as being central to the infant mortality dilemma; overall, a very small proportion of infant deaths are attributable to women in those situations. Although these serious problems need to be addressed, a distortion of their extent in the population often serves a moralistic or judgmental rather than a preventive purpose. It is also notable that the root causes of many health risks— social inequalities and discrimination—are missing from the usual lists of risk factors.

In an ethnographic study at a public teaching hospital, Handwerker (1994) concluded that the labeling of low-income pregnant women as "high risk" has a stigmatizing function, to the extent of blaming and even prosecuting women who suffer fetal or infant deaths after failure to follow medical advice. "While addiction or other 'high risk' behavior occurring in white middle class women is often considered a health problem, poor women of color are increasingly viewed as criminals" (Handwerker, 1994, p. 672). Health professionals' values and training may influence risk classification at least as much as scientific criteria do. For pregnant women, identification as "high risk" determines the nature of their prenatal care and delivery experience, exposure to technological interventions, relationship with health care providers, and even their ability to maintain custody of their infants. The recent focus on unintended pregnancy as a risk factor, although meant to be supportive of women's right to reproductive choice, can imply that women in high-risk populations should be discouraged from childbearing.

Ethical issues in prenatal care have proliferated with the growth of reproductive technologies and sophisticated maternal and fetal interventions. Enkin (1994) has critiqued the framework of risk in pregnancy because it suggests the need for control by professionals rather than women and families, and it interferes with birth as a natural process. "Objecting to the risk management approach to childbirth is difficult, because the idea of risk management is a product of the culture in which we live. . . . Perhaps it is time to look for alternatives. It is essentially a question of strengthening the woman to give birth and to take care of her own baby" (Enkin, 1994, pp. 133–134). Incorporating strategies for empowerment of women and respect for the natural processes of pregnancy and childbirth with judicious use of medical advances is a major challenge for MCH practitioners and advocates.

## INTERVENTIONS

The manifestation of a poor pregnancy outcome is a function both of the maternal risks and any intervention that ameliorates those risks. Interventions to improve pregnancy outcomes have probably existed since the earliest days of humanity, and folk traditions still abound. The histories of both public health and modern medicine are intimately tied to efforts to enhance the safety of mothers and newborns. The dramatic reduction of both maternal and infant mortality in the 20th century testifies to the cumulative effects of multiple interventions.

Today a wide range of interventions aims to ensure healthy and successful pregnancies. Some of these interventions are tied directly to specific risk amelioration, whereas others are more closely associated with general health promotion. We can divide interventions into four broad groups reflecting the developmental course of pregnancy and birth: preconception, antepartum or prenatal, intrapartum, and postpartum or internatal.

Optimal reproductive outcomes result from a continuous process of health promotion and disease prevention throughout the entire course of women's lives (Lu & Halfon, 2003) (see Chapter 10). Infant health is intimately related to a mother's well-being from the time of her own conception, and the lifetime effects of childbearing are influenced by the totality of self-care and health care that mothers receive. Continuity of primary preventive care and adequate access to family planning services are essential for women's well-being before pregnancy occurs.

## Preconceptional Health Care

We now recognize that critical stages of early fetal development are completed before many women enter prenatal care or even know with certainty that they are pregnant. "The period of greatest environmental sensitivity for [the] developing fetus is between 17 and 56 days after fertilization. Cell organization, cell differentiation, and organogenesis take place during this period, and any insult, whether nutritional, drug-related, or viral, can jeopardize fetal development. . . . By the end of the eighth week after conception and certainly by the end of the first trimester, any major structural anomalies in the fetus have already developed" (Cefalo & Moos, 1994, pp. 2–3). Congenital anomalies, such as LBW, represent a major cause of infant mortality and morbidity that has not improved in response to recent technological developments. Little change has occurred in the overall incidence of birth defects, and some increases have been observed in rates of specific anomalies.

A new model of preconceptional health care has been introduced in hopes of shifting medical care and counseling to an earlier period with greater potential for primary prevention of early fetal loss, birth defects, and other adverse pregnancy outcomes (Cefalo & Moos, 1994). Cefalo and Moos (1994), authors of a guide to preconceptional counseling, stress the importance of adequate information in assuring full reproductive choice. The goal of preconceptional counseling is to teach women the extent to which they can increase the chances of a healthy pregnancy and positive birth outcome. Women must also be helped to understand that some occurrences are beyond their control and that medical professionals have significant limitations in their capacity to predict and prevent problems. Skill and training are required to implement preconceptional health promotion successfully, but this approach offers multiple opportunities to empower parents and improve birth outcomes.

One example is the potential for nutrition counseling, specifically to convey the recent recommendation that women contemplating pregnancy take folic acid supplements to prevent neural tube defects. Folate is a B vitamin needed to make DNA, the building block of cells. In the fetus, folate has also been found to play a key role in the development of the neural tube. Folate must be present during the development of the neural tube and before it closes at 8 weeks gestation, a time when many women are not yet aware that they are pregnant. A deficiency of folate during this period may cause neural tube defects, for example, spina bifida, which can result in serious disability. A recommended daily supplement of 0.4 to 0.8 mg of folate for all women has been shown to reduce the risk of a first occurrence, and a 4-mg dose has been recommended for women who have had a neural defect occur in a previous pregnancy. In order to ensure adequate supplementation, women must be educated and encouraged to take folate before pregnancy and throughout the first trimester.

A preconceptional visit is increasingly being integrated into prenatal care and is now routinely recommended by the March of Dimes and encouraged by the American College of Obstetrics and Gynecologists. Unfortunately, however, most pregnancies are not planned; thus, a planned preconceptional visit is not always likely. The source of payment for preconceptional visits has not yet been fully established, although some states incorporate preconceptional care as part of family planning visits in their Medicaid programs.

The efficacy and content of preconceptional visits are not yet well established. Korenbrot et al. (2002) reviewed the published obstetric and MCH literature to examine the clinical domains in which evidence for the value of preconceptional interventions could be shown. Relatively few areas were noted, although evidence for effectiveness was found for screening women who are seeking family planning for risk conditions, having sexually active women of reproductive age take dietary folate supplements, and providing women affected by certain metabolic conditions (diabetes and hyperphenyalanemia) with nutritional services. Over the past decade, the concept of preconceptional health care has broadened to cover not just women's health immediately before pregnancy, but to address women's health across the lifespan and serve as a bridge to more continuous services for women's general health needs. This concept is captured by Moos (2002, p. 72):

> Rather than pursuing the "add a category of service" mentality, further fragmenting care, we should reframe our existing array of services to look at the total woman, first, and her reproductive status, second. There is, in fact, little that could be recommended in routine preconceptional

counseling that would not benefit the average woman's general health status, irrespective of eventual conceptions. For instance, whether the woman plans to become pregnant or not, her smoking habits should be determined at every visit and clear recommendations and strategies for cessation, if needed, offered. Nutrition counseling during preconception could have lifelong benefits for women. To do less is to give poor care relative to the woman's immediate needs; however, in providing this emphasis in each routine visit, not only is the woman's health addressed but also her preconceptional wellness. "Preconceptional wellness is women's wellness—healthy women are more likely to have healthy pregnancies and healthy offspring: It is that simple."

Preconceptional health can also be conceptually associated with longitudinal or life course perspectives on the causation of poor birth outcomes and racial disparities. Risk factors present only during the course of the pregnancy do not provide satisfactory explanations for the occurrence of these events (Lu & Halfon, 2003). Life-course perspectives derive from both a women's health orientation and a temporal expansion of the preconceptional health care model consistent with the aphorism that "one can't cure a lifetime of ills during 9 months of a pregnancy."

Three domains of research support a longitudinal women's health framework: cross-generational reproductive outcome studies, the Barker hypothesis that fetal experiences influence subsequent adult health, and the weathering hypothesis that cumulative negative life experiences influence subsequent birth outcomes. The conversion of the current preconceptional health care model into organized longitudinal MCH or public health programs is just beginning. Such programs would likely focus on general health promotion and health educational programs for growing young women, multisectoral health promotion programs, and family planning. Some recent programmatic efforts have been based on longitudinal women's health care models, although their impact on reproductive health has yet to be demonstrated.

### Prenatal Care

The American College of Obstetricians and Gynecologists (ACOG) described four functions of prenatal care: risk assessment, serial surveillance, health education, and psychosocial support (Brann & Cefalo, 1992). The goals of risk assessment are to screen women in order to detect specific pregnancy risks for poor birth outcomes and to determine the most appropriate level of prenatal care, for example, to determine which women are medically at high risk needing tertiary prenatal or obstetric care and which women have psychosocial needs requiring specialized social services. The task of comprehensive prenatal care programs is to provide treatment for women appropriate to their level of need. Formal risk assessment is usually conducted at the first prenatal care visit. Currently, there are several popular screening tools, such as the Problem-Oriented Risk Assessment System, that identify and weigh a variety of demographic, medical, psychosocial, and behavioral risks using a standardized protocol.

Currently, risk screening tools have relatively low predictive value. At best, existing prenatal instruments can identify 54% of women who go on to experience perinatal deaths. Screening systems have inherent problems and limitations (Selwyn, 1990). Risk assessments are limited by our relatively weak understanding of mechanisms explaining poor pregnancy outcomes. Currently, the strongest predictors of adverse pregnancy outcomes are prior poor obstetric history, use of substances (including cigarettes), multiple gestations (i.e., twins, triplets, etc.), and vaginal infections. Predictions are much stronger for multiparous than for primiparous women.

Selwyn (1990) has outlined several dilemmas associated with risk assessment instruments based on the trade-off between sensitivity (detection of true positives) and specificity (detection of true negatives). The greater the chance of identifying women who are actually at risk (i.e., those who have preterm birth), the lower the likelihood of accurately classifying low risk women (i.e., those with full-term deliveries). In other words, in selecting the cutoff points for measuring risks, providers must choose between overdiagnosis with unnecessary treatment of false positives as opposed to underdiagnosis and missed opportunities for preventive treatment of false negatives. Both of these possibilities carry the risk of medical complications and psychological distress. Repeated screening may be one way to improve the accuracy of risk assessment.

Serial surveillance is successive monitoring of the pregnant women and fetus to ensure that they are progressing properly through the normal developmental stages. The purpose of this screening is to detect deviations and then to make appropriate referrals or provide treatments for any identified problems of the pregnancy. For most women, this routine surveillance involves urinalysis, fundal (i.e., uterine) height measurement, weighing, and sometimes other tests such as alpha-fetoprotein screening and ultrasound to detect fetal abnormalities. Both ACOG and the US Public Health Service (PHS) Expert Panel on the Content of Prenatal Care have developed detailed protocols for the timing and content of prenatal surveillance (Brann & Cefalo, 1992; PHS, 1989).

Health education is the provision of health information about the impact of pregnancy on women's health and physical changes, advice on behaviors to promote a healthy pregnancy and healthy infant (including nutrition, weight gain, exercise, substance use), preparation for delivery, and knowledge of newborn care. Pregnancy provides a significant opportunity for instruction and advice to improve the health of the mother, her future offspring, and the entire family. Studies repeatedly show that pregnancy is a receptive period for health behavior change. Two thirds of women who have given birth have taken childbirth education classes, but disproportionately more white women (76%) than African American women (44%) receive this benefit (Lu, Prentice, Yu, Inkelas, Lange, & Halfon, 2003).

Psychosocial support recognizes that pregnancy does not simply involve maternal physiological changes and embryological growth, but is embedded in a social, cultural, and emotional context. For many women, pregnancy is a time of great emotional flux. Clinical prenatal care providers as well as family and friends can provide needed support, both instrumental and psychological. Maternal depression, social isolation, exposure to violence, and substance use are some of the many psychosocial issues that may arise during and after pregnancy. Beyond clinical care settings, a variety of support programs have been developed to address prenatal psychosocial needs, including case management, pregnancy support groups, home visitation programs, and fatherhood involvement programs. Historically, a women's mental health during pregnancy was thought to influence the health of her fetus; this concept continues into the 21st century and requires more attention.

Currently in the United States, ACOG recommends 13 prenatal visits during pregnancy for a normal low-risk woman: the initial visit in the first 6 weeks, one visit per month until the 28th week, one visit every 2 weeks until the 36th week, and one visit per week thereafter. This standardized universal visit schedule was developed in the early part of the century in order to prevent maternal mortality, especially from eclampsia, a hypertensive disorder generally manifesting toward the end of pregnancy. It is important to note that this prenatal care schedule was developed primarily to improve maternal, not infant, health.

There have been some suggestions to change the visitation pattern. The US PHS report, *Caring for Our Future: The Content of Prenatal Care*, suggested fewer but more intensive prenatal care visits (PHS, 1989). According to the report, the timing of care should be shifted to increase visits toward the beginning of the pregnancy, including a preconceptional visit, in order to focus more on maternal health promotion activities. The PHS also recommended the establishment of different visitation schedules for primiparous and multiparous women. This and other proposals to modify the standard schedule have met with strong opposition from the professional obstetric community, even though the United States recommends more prenatal care visits than most European countries.

Prenatal care can be conceptualized very broadly or very narrowly. Narrowly defined, prenatal care represents only the ACOG recommended visits to a medical provider, that is, the provision of medical care during pregnancy. Broadly conceptualized, prenatal care comprises any intervention during pregnancy that enhances the health and well-being of mothers and their offspring. A comprehensive definition of prenatal care would include nutrition counseling and food supplementation, childbirth preparation classes, mentoring and advice from a "resource mother," home visitation, and an array of other services.

In general, the MCH field takes a very broad view of prenatal care and encourages the inclusion of psychosocial, nutrition, health education, case management, and other services. Definitions of the scope of prenatal care reflect fundamental beliefs about what is truly needed to ensure a successful pregnancy. Surprisingly, inadequate evidence exists to assess conflicting beliefs about pregnancy care or to update guidelines for the content of prenatal care in the United States.

There is widespread agreement that prenatal care is important and positive, but little research is available that documents the efficacy of prenatal care use or specific interventions to enhance birth outcomes and maternal health. The linkage between prenatal care and birth outcomes is actually quite a difficult area to study, as it involves complex definitional, methodological, design, and ethical issues. Randomized clinical trials (RCTs) assigning some women to a no-PNC group are not possible or desirable for ethical reasons, although RCTs of added new components of PNC are possible.

Kotelchuck (1994) showed that the impact of prenatal care on birth outcomes is a U-shaped function; women with inadequate and intensive care have the poorest birth outcomes. Inadequate care is often a marker for psychosocial and socioeconomic difficulties that may result in medical conditions. A lack of preventive care or early treatment may exacerbate those problems. Women with intensive care are likely to have more severe medical needs and complications, although they may not necessarily be easily addressed by PNC interventions. Their outcomes, although not optimal, would undoubtedly be worse without the intensive treatment they receive.

In the late 1980s and early 1990s, a public health/MCH consensus emerged that access to comprehensive PNC was the solution to high rates of infant mortality and racial disparities. Numerous federal and state public health/MCH programs were developed and implemented in this period, including expansion of allowable Medicaid income eligibility for maternity care to 185% of the federal poverty level, Medicaid reimbursement for nonclinical services (including health education, social work, nutrition, home visitation, and case management services), development of the federal Healthy Futures/Healthy Generation Programs and the Healthy Start Initiatives, and the establishment of numerous State/National Infant Mortality Reduction Commissions. The MCH community has been very successful at addressing access to PNC via outreach efforts, telephone hotlines, simplified Medicaid enrollment forms and presumptive eligibility, cross-program referrals, and incentive programs. PNC has improved steadily in the United States since 1988, with 74.6% of women in 2002 receiving at least adequate PNC. The gap in adequate use of prenatal care between racial/ethnic groups has also narrowed substantially (in California in 2002, 75.9% for whites and 67.5% for African Americans) (Rittenhouse, Braveman, & Marchi, 2003).

Most recent RCTs of enhanced or comprehensive PNC programs have not conclusively shown any impact on prematurity, LBW, or infant mortality. Various review articles have now concluded that PNC has, at best, only a limited impact on birth outcomes (Fiscella, 1995; Goldenberg & Rouse, 1998). Moreover, despite the steadily improving PNC use rates in recent years, prematurity and LBW rates have worsened in the United States. These findings have cast doubt on the efficacy and cost-effectiveness of comprehensive public PNC programs as interventions for improving pregnancy outcomes. In contrast to psychosocial PNC models, biologic models—especially of infectious diseases—have been gaining scientific credibility and popularity as the etiologic explanation in the past decade.

Recent efforts to enhance the effectiveness of prenatal care have attempted to incorporate new clinical understandings of infectious diseases, including sexually transmitted infections and bacterial vaginosis, into the treatment and prevention of preterm labor. This has led to a growing number of clinical trials of antibiotic prophylaxis to reduce prematurity, either among symptomatic or "high-risk" populations. The results have been quite disappointing to date (Ugwumadu, 2002). There remains much debate in the clinical literature about the nature and timing of the prophylaxis and the recurrent nature of infectious diseases. There is also growing recognition that host factors (such as maternal nutritional status, douching, sexual practices, or drug usage) can influence disease susceptibility. To date, only one preventive RCT trial involving weekly progesterone treatments started before 20 weeks gestation in women with a prior history of recurrent miscarriages has shown a significant positive impact on prematurity (Meis, Klebanoff, Thom, Dombrowski, Sibai, Moawad, et al., 2003).

The current debates about whether public health-oriented comprehensive PNC programs or infectious disease prophylaxis are more effective interventions to improve pregnancy outcomes reflect debates over public health philosophy as well as the etiology of perinatal conditions. Prenatal care is and will likely remain the principal mode of health service delivery during pregnancy, as PNC provides primary health care for mothers. The MCH field, in this era of health care reorganization and cost containment, is being challenged to demonstrate the effectiveness of specific components of prenatal care, especially the psychosocial and other non-medical services. Yet researchers have only begun to examine the specific content or constellation of prenatal care, in order to refine their assessment of overall PNC use.

Research findings from national survey data (Kogan, Alexander, Kotelchuck, Nagey, & Jack, 1994) indicate that receipt of health advice from prenatal care providers is an important contributor to LBW prevention. Unfortunately, research suggests that the ACOG prenatal care recommendations, especially for risk assessment and health education, are not routinely followed (Peoples-Sheps, Hogan, & Ng'andu, 1996). For example, Kogan et al. (1994) found that African American women were more likely than white women to have the recommended prenatal medical procedures performed but less likely to receive advice about health behaviors.

The Special Supplemental Food Program for Women, Infants, and Children (WIC) has been consistently associated with reduced rates of LBW and infant mortality, as well as with more adequate prenatal care use (Kotelchuck, Schwartz, Anderka, & Finison, 1984; Rush, Kurzon, Seaver, & Shanklin, 1988). Women's use of comprehensive or enhanced services is often facilitated through WIC's care coordination or case management. Comprehensive prenatal care most often takes place in health departments or community health centers. Birth outcomes for low-income women appear to be better if care is provided in such community-based clinics rather than in private practice settings (Buescher, Smith, Holliday, & Levine, 1987). Private practitioners often lack the extensive referral and support networks necessary to implement models of comprehensive care.

Most of the prenatal care literature is restricted to outpatient or ambulatory care and focuses on "normal" pregnancies; nevertheless, many women experience complications, and the likelihood of hospitalization during pregnancy is relatively high. In 2002, over 31.9% of women received more than ACOG's recommended number of prenatal visits, and such women disproportionately account for LBW infants (Kotelchuck, 1994). Among North Carolina Medicaid participants, approximately 14% of women are hospitalized during the course of their pregnancies; 5% have more than one hospitalization. Among those with LBW infants, one third were hospitalized at least once while pregnant (Bennett & Kotelchuck, unpublished data). For women receiving inpatient and more intensive outpatient antenatal care, many opportunities exist to improve birth outcomes, monitor long-term health issues, and address psychosocial needs.

### Intrapartum Interventions

The delivery or intrapartum period is also an important time for interventions to improve birth outcomes for mothers and infants. Many of these interventions are pharmacological protocols and surgical procedures to augment the speed and safety of the birth process. Conflicting ideologies and values about childbirth have led to controversy about intercession in this period. Proponents of natural childbirth can cite evidence of the psychological and medical benefits of nonintervention, although most would recommend that women receive the highest quality of medical services at the first indication of need. In contrast, many clinical providers advocate for routine use of the latest medical technologies as an attempt to prevent any possible risk to the infant during delivery. Legal liability concerns, changing hospital practices, and trends in consumer demand influence the balance between these two orientations.

This chapter does not review the literature about obstetric delivery practices other than to note that there is much debate over the use of specific technologies during delivery. Electronic fetal monitoring is very widely used to assess fetal heart rate during delivery (85.2% of births in 2002), although it has not been recommended for universal use. Some argue for routine monitoring in order to alert providers to fetal distress; others are concerned about unnecessary C-sections resulting from misreadings. Induction and augmentation of labor are widespread (20.6% of births in 2002), but the use of drugs—no matter how benign—is controversial because of the potential impact on mothers and on the subsequent health and development of newborns. Yet pain control and length of delivery are important issues for most women. Forceps deliveries and vacuum extractions (5.9% of births in 2002) have declined in recent years as C-section rates have increased. The use of tocolytic drugs (e.g., ritodrine) to reduce the onset of early labor is now widespread, although major improvements in preterm delivery and LBW are not expected to result from tocolysis (Klein & Goldenberg, 1990).

Cesarean sections are very widely performed in the United States. The national objective for *Healthy People 2010* is to reduce the cesarean delivery rate for first-time mothers to no more than 15 per 100 deliveries. This will likely be difficult to achieve as C-section rates are once again increasing after having declined slightly in the mid-1990s. C-section deliveries accounted for 26.1% of all births in 2002, including 18.0% by primary C-section. There is very strong evidence that C-sections reduce maternal and infant mortality in specific delivery situations, such as obstructed labor and eclamptic conditions. However, the optimal level of C-sections is subject to much debate because C-sections entail major surgery that introduces new risk to both mothers and infants (e.g., anesthesia complications, infection, iatrogenic prematurity).

Most European countries have much lower rates of C-sections than the United States, although European rates are rising rapidly. C-section rates in some Latin American countries are even higher than in the United States. High cesarean rates have alarmed many obstetricians, prompting the initiation of a series of second-opinion programs that succeeded in reducing C-sections; however, others have implicitly encouraged elective C-sections by defining the issue as one of maternal choice. Many financial, convenience, and legal incentives still make C-section delivery a popular procedure for obstetricians. In 2004, the ACOG endorsed elective C-section on demand (in the absence of medical indications).

For a limited period of time, there was a growing willingness to allow trials of vaginal birth after cesarean section (VBAC) in the United States. The year 2010 objective for VBACs is to reduce the proportion of C-sections among women with prior cesarean births to 63% (from a 1998 baseline of 72%). The past decade has seen dramatic changes in the extent of VBACs in the United States. VBACs increased through 1996, reaching 28.3% of women with prior C-sections, but then declined very rapidly to only 12.6% in 2002 as concerns arose about very rare, but life threatening, intrauterine ruptures. ACOG has now mandated very stringent requirements for VBAC efforts, such as 24-hour anesthesiologist availability. These requirements present particular problems for smaller, rural, and suburban hospitals, many of which have now ceased performing VBACs.

Controversy over the desirability of obstetric interventions and hospital competition has led both to more midwifery-attended births and to marketing of more supportive, family-friendly birthing practices within hospitals. The vast majority of births (99%) take place in hospitals in the United States, and most deliveries are assisted by physicians (91.3%). With increasing professionalization of the midwifery field, including the ability to obtain third-party reimbursement, there has been a steady increase to 8.1% in midwifery-assisted births over the past decade (7.7% by certified nurse midwives and 0.4% by other midwives). Several European countries, including the Netherlands, have substantially more births assisted by midwives and home deliveries. There has also been growth in the use of doulas (labor support coaches) to further enhance the birthing process for women.

Debate continues, however, about optimal settings and attendants for deliveries. For low-risk women, tertiary centers have been shown to have better birth outcomes, but also more surgical interventions (Albers & Savitz, 1991). The National Birth Center Study examined outcomes of care in 84 US nonhospital birth centers that deliver "family-centered" maternity care to medically low-risk women. Nearly 80% of deliveries of the 12,000 women in the study were attended by nurse midwives. The rest of the women were cared for by obstetricians or other physicians, other midwives, or registered nurses. The total rate of C-sections was only 4.4% per 100 deliveries, and rates of LBW and infant mortality were extremely low. When surveyed, 99% of the women said they would recommend the birth center to a friend (Rooks, Weatherby, Ernst, Stapleton, Rosen, & Rosenfield, 1989).

For women at high risk—those whose conditions are recognized during crises in labor as well as those identified through early assessment—regionalization of obstetric and postpartum care has been very successful in improving birth outcomes. Regionalized care is a system of coordination among hospitals for the transfer of high-risk mothers or newborns to more intensive levels of care, including air transport for women in isolated rural areas. Hospitals are designated as Level I, Level II, or Level III. Level III hospitals are tertiary-care centers with specially trained obstetric staff and neonatal intensive care units. Ideally, all women deliver at the appropriate level hospital after having been screened throughout pregnancy for their risks and needs. Regionalization of obstetric services became widespread in the 1960s and 1970s and dramatically reduced infant mortality by making tertiary neonatal services available for most births. In North Carolina, for example, 70% of VLBW infants are now born in Level III hospitals, and in Massachusetts, 87% of higher order multiple births are born in Level III hospitals.

Favorable rates of BWSM in the United States reflect both the high level of technology and the regionalization of programs that give the entire population access to that technology. Regionalized perinatal care may be vulnerable to fiscal trends dictating multiple hospital mergers and closures, particularly in rural areas. Furthermore, Wise (1990) has cautioned that improvements in infant mortality may level off and even increase if we achieve the maximum benefits of neonatal technology without rectifying social risks to health and deficiencies in preventive health care. Indeed, another interpretation of the rise in infant mortality in 2002 is that the continued improvements in BWSM caused by enhanced neonatology and regionalization no longer outweigh the negative impact of the continuous rise of LBW and prematurity in the United States.

Two major advances in fetal medicine have had significant effects on fetal survivability. The use of antenatal corticosteroids to mature the lungs of the fetus has become widespread in anticipation of a premature delivery. This treatment, coupled with the use of tocolytic agents to delay labor for a limited time period, has lowered the incidence of RDS. The broad efficacy of important new treatments such as steroids and tocolytic agents depends on the regular involvement of all women in high-quality prenatal and obstetric care. Any inequities in access to new advances in maternal and fetal medicine will reinforce social injustices and impair the overall improvement of MCH outcomes.

### Postpartum or Internatal Care

A wide range of postpartum treatments can influence birth outcomes. The postpartum period, like the preconceptional period, is becoming a major focus for reproductive health initiatives. Traditionally, the postpartum period has addressed the quality of services and access to neonatal medicine as well as public health infant mortality and morbidity prevention programs. Today, a new focus is emerging on internatal care for maternal and infant health.

Access to regionalized neonatal intensive care units for high-risk infants and improvements in neonatal medicine have dramatically improved infant survival (BWSM rates). Recent advancements in intrapartum antibiotics, high-frequency ventilation, and surfactant, an agent that enhances the elasticity of the fetal lung surface, have dramatically improved birth outcomes and the quality of life for premature VLBW newborns. Surfactant has had a major impact on premature infants with RDS; it is estimated that 50% of the decrease in the US infant mortality rates in the 1990s was due to the introduction and use of this agent. There is some concern that the increasing frequency of VLBW infant survival may be associated with an increase in the incidence of cerebral palsy.

The past decade has seen a growth in postpartum public health-oriented programs. In particular, the American Academy of Pediatrics' successful "Back to Sleep" campaign encourages parents to place infants to sleep on their backs in order to reduce the incidence of SIDS. WIC is the largest postpartum program in the United States, providing nutritional supplementation and education to over 40% of all newborns and their breastfeeding mothers. WIC fosters continuity from prenatal to postpartum participation, a particularly valuable programmatic feature. Numerous public health programs foster the linkage of high-risk infants to early intervention programs. In contrast, very few prevention programs focus on resumption of maternal smoking in the postpartum period, despite the fact that half of women who stop smoking cigarettes during pregnancy resume smoking after delivery.

For routine uncomplicated deliveries, the postpartum period is also extremely important as the initiation into parenthood for new mothers, their partners, and their families. The postpartum hospitalization should offer opportunities for physical recovery and stabilization of the mother and newborn, psychological adaptation, maternal education, and observation of both the mother's and infant's health status. Current insurance and hospital policies allow little time for any of these functions, and the duration of hospitalization for delivery has become a major public health and policy issue. The average length of stay for a hospital delivery is approximately 2 days for a vaginal birth and 4 days for a C-section, much shorter than the time required for manifestation of many problems that require medical care and advice. Often women are discharged even more quickly. In an extensive review of early discharge published in 1995, Braveman, Egerter, Pearl, Marchi, & Miller (1995) noted that 12 to 24 hours was a typical stay in the Western states for a vaginal delivery without complications.

Initially, early discharge programs were offered only to low-risk women in order to free hospital beds and to meet consumer demand for a less medicalized birth experience. In such programs in the 1970s, women were carefully screened for participation and received extensive in-home follow-up services. As cost-containment pressures have become more dominant, early discharge has become routine and involuntary for almost all women without serious medical complications.

Margolis, Kotelchuck, & Chang (1997) showed that women discharged early are actually more likely to be those with risk characteristics, such as teenagers and women lacking private health insurance. The consequences of this fiscally driven policy for MCH are unknown. Braveman et al. (1995) concluded, "No adequately designed studies have examined discharge before 48 hours after delivery without additional post-discharge services. . . . Some studies suggested adverse outcomes associated with early discharge even with early follow-up" (p. 716). By the late 1990s, the US Congress and 43 states had passed legislation mandating insurers to cover postpartum hospital stays for a minimum of 48 hours after vaginal deliveries and 96 hours after C-sections. The impact of that legislation has generally been favorable, with decreases in rehospitalization for neonatal jaundice and fewer subsequent emergency department visits, especially for those newborns with early home follow-up visits (Meara, Kotagal, Atherton, & Lieu, 2004).

In the past decade, there has been a growth in the concept of internatal care, that is, in the development of an organized system care for maternal (and infant) health care in the postpartum period. The nursing literature sometimes refers to this as fourth-trimester care. Traditionally, the 6-week postpartum follow-up visit is the only formal health care visit recommended to address maternal health. This visit focuses primarily on delivery follow-up care and family planning resumption. Too many mothers in the United States have no further contact with the health care system for themselves until their next pregnancy; in most states, Medicaid reproductive health care coverage stops at 60 days postpartum. Traditional public health nurse postpartum home visits have long ceased (often for budgetary reasons), although a few states and local communities have reinstituted postpartum visitation programs for specialized high-risk populations. The current system of care for postpartum women is clearly inadequate for maternal health.

The postpartum period should be an important period for intervention. Pregnancy is a major life event, and several critical health risks may emerge that can have an impact on the woman's own subsequent health, her reproductive health for future pregnancies, and her optimal parenting capacity. These include diabetes, hypertension, overweight and obesity, injuries and violence, and mental health. Several other key health issues also emerge in this period, including subsequent family planning, breastfeeding, resumption of smoking or use of other substances, access to health care, and folic acid consumption. Much as preconceptional health care addresses women's health (and reproductive health before pregnancy), internatal care also addresses women's health but further on in the life course. Internatal care can also be a form of preconceptional care for a subsequent pregnancy.

Internatal care programs have some practical advantages over preconceptional care, as they do not depend on a planned pregnancy. Virtually all women who have a birth or late fetal loss can be located and contacted. Several current initiatives foster the development of internatal care. The Safe Motherhood Initiative of the CDC focuses on keeping women healthy before, during, and after pregnancy. The Healthy Start Initiative is a longstanding federal MCH Bureau community-based reproductive health initiative to address racial disparities in high-risk communities. Healthy Start has recently changed its mandate to include the period of pregnancy until 2-years postpartum, with a special mandate for internatal continuity of care. The MCH Bureau has also initiated a program on women's health within the MCH Title V programs. The broader women's health movement is beginning to expand the scope of reproductive health to examine the impact of pregnancy on women's health in addition to the influence of women's health on infant outcomes.

There has also been a new focus in the National Institute of Mental Health and the MCH Bureau on maternal depression and other mood disorders during and after pregnancy and their impact on subsequent women's and children's health and development. It is estimated that approximately 15% of women experience postpartum depression. Maternal depression is increasingly being viewed as a chronic illness, not solely as a postpartum episodic phenomenon. It has been linked to smoking, substance use, interpersonal violence, poor nutrition, and decreased access and use of health care and family planning services. New efforts in the Healthy Start Initiative and other federal programs are addressing the identification, referral, and treatment of women with chronic depression around the time of pregnancy and early motherhood. These initiatives include enhanced maternal depression screening and referral in pediatric care (a two-generational model of pediatric care) and in child development programs (including Head Start), as well as the development of community-based nonprofessional treatment programs and activities. The linkage of traditional MCH and reproductive clinical care with mental health services is a critical public health issue that deserves increased attention.

Formal internatal care programs are just now being organized with several large initiatives underway. These programs have not yet been evaluated for impacts on the health of mothers or infants. Internatal programs face numerous barriers, for example, who should be the provider, who will pay for the care, what content should be addressed, and what would motivate maternal attendance. In the future, internatal programs will be seen as routine and necessary primary care for postnatal women in the same way that prenatal care is viewed for pregnant women today. Internatal programs are part of the larger women's health and longitudinal agenda for reproductive health services.

## OUTSTANDING CONCERNS

### Racial Disparities in Birth Outcomes

What are the causes of racial disparities in birth outcomes between African Americans and whites in the United States, and how can these disparities be eliminated? The racial gap has confounded the MCH field for many decades. Historically, biological and eugenic explanations were offered but later shown to be scientifically invalid. Economic explanations became predominant in the 1960s, with the focus on high poverty rates in black communities. Race is often viewed as a proxy for socioeconomic status, as African Americans are less likely on average than whites to have private health insurance coverage or access to services and are more likely to be exposed to poverty and environmental hazards.

Recent analyses have suggested that race is not simply a marker of social class; for example, the racial gap in LBW rates is highest among college-educated women (Schoendorf, Hogue, Kleinman, & Rowley, 1992). The "Hispanic paradox" of good birth outcomes in relatively poor and under-insured Latino communities also challenges the assumption of a simple relationship between social class and birth outcomes. Recent attention has turned to the role of psychosocial stressors, including the experience of racist treatment, in determining adverse health outcomes such as prema-ture delivery among African Americans (McLean, 1993; Rowley, 2001). New research paradigms are being developed to determine the interactive and longitudinal effects of racism, sexism, and class discrimination on women's reproductive health (e.g., differential treatment by prenatal care providers, vulnerability to infections, neurophysiological expressions of stress), as well as the protective influence of cultural beliefs and responses (e.g., low rates of tobacco use, intergenerational supports) (Krieger, Rowley, Herman, Avery, & Phillips, 1993; Lu & Halfon, 2003). The con-tinued existence of severe disparities remains an unacceptable burden on the African American community, a stark reminder of societal inequities and injustice, and a compelling challenge to MCH (see Chapter 9).

## Intransigence of LBW and Prematurity Rates

Can any public health initiative reduce our unacceptable and rising LBW and prematurity rates? For the past 40 years, since the federal War on Poverty in the 1960s, wide-ranging public health programs have aimed to improve these birth outcomes. In spite of interventions to improve (1) nutrition (e.g., WIC), (2) access to medical care (via expanded income eligibility for Medicaid maternity coverage), and (3) content of prenatal care (e.g., home visitation, comprehensive services), birth weight distribu-tions have barely changed. Are birth outcomes impervious to public health interventions? The success of European experiences with comprehensive health and social benefits for mothers and families suggests otherwise. Identification of key factors that influence birth weight and are amenable to change still eludes us in the United States. Perhaps the impact of our interventions has been obscured by countervailing pressures such as overuse of C-section, increasing substance use, multiple births due to assisted reproductive technology, or new environmental assaults. LBW and prematurity, with their lifetime consequences for children and families, will hinder national progress until we can solve this puzzle and mobilize the political will to support necessary solutions. The new March of Dimes Prematurity Campaign and the PREEMIE Act perhaps signal a shift in our nation's attention to this critical topic.

### Prevention Versus Treatment

What is the wisest allocation of resources for improving reproductive health? Both prevention to reduce the number of LBW infants and treatment to lower BWSM rates are crucial in the fight against infant mortality. These aspects of prevention should not be seen as mutually exclusive, but the two domains are quite distinct and often competitive in the professional and political process of funding decisions. Almost all of our recent improvements in infant mortality have been due to developments in neonatal treatment and access to care. Pressures to abandon regionalized care networks that have made newborn tertiary care almost universally available could have devastating consequences, especially in poor and rural communities.

Should we continue to invest new funds in enhanced neonatal treatment, or have we maximized the effectiveness of this strategy? To what extent are we producing serious new morbidity by saving increasingly smaller infants? Should we assume that further technological expenses are justified, or should we spend money on uncertain experiments in hopes of preventing LBW and prematurity? Epidemiologic findings alone cannot provide a final answer to this dilemma, which rests on values as well as science.

### Location and Content of Preconceptional and Internatal Health Care

Preconceptional and internatal care address general health promotion for women, family planning needs, and preparation for subsequent pregnancies. In an integrated health system with comprehensive coverage, preconceptional and internatal care could fit easily into a continuum of services. In our current disciplinary-structured and underfunded public health care system, we face major policy decisions about the inclusion of preconceptional and internatal health care as part of Title X family planning or Title V prenatal care services in the public health sector, or as part of obstetrics, pediatrics, family practice, or internal medicine in the clinical sector. In the current health system, there is no guarantor of women's health outside of the maternal role. Tensions arise over whether preconceptional and internatal health must always be linked to a maternity focus, as well as over the question of who will pay for these new services. Family planning reaches a broader population but still addresses women's health in the context of reproduction. What should be the content of preconceptional and internatal health care? How can we transform these concepts and longitudinal models of women's health care into more formal public health programs?

## Timing and Number of Visits

Should the current ACOG recommendations on timing and number of prenatal care visits be modified? These recommendations were originally based on protection of the mother's health (especially mortality caused by pre-eclampsia) with an emphasis on frequency of visits in late pregnancy. Maternal mortality has been significantly reduced with largely effective management of hypertensive conditions. Should the recommendations be changed to encourage more visits early in pregnancy (as suggested by PHS) in order to promote infant health through maternal behavioral changes, social support, or earlier infectious disease detection? Is there a chance that women's health could be impaired by decreased surveillance near term?

## Balancing Visions and Risks of Childbirth

How should the MCH community balance the competing visions of birth as a natural process or a risky event requiring the most advanced medical techniques available? Both views on the birth process capture a truth and express concern for the health of mothers and newborns. Women who have been historically excluded from high-quality health services may rightfully perceive an equal entitlement to technology. To some, natural childbirth is seen as the most psychologically and physically healthy manner to have a child; to others, it represents unnecessary endangerment of both mother and child. The debate is shaped by strong ideologic views and personal experience, as well as strong professional identities and economic interests. How can we continue to reduce mortality and morbidity without disempowering women in the experience of pregnancy and birth?

## Early Pregnancy Loss

What is the epidemiology of miscarriage or early pregnancy loss? For all of our sophistication about infant morbidity and mortality, we still lack a full assessment of the outcomes of all conceptions. We do not really know how many early pregnancy losses occur, the nature of geographic and temporal trends, or the true impact on the subsequent physical, mental, and reproductive health of women. Do these deficiencies simply reflect technical measurement issues, or do they indicate a lack of attention to a major issue for women and families and the health of the entire population? The environmental disaster at Love Canal was detected, after all, by elevated miscarriage rates in the community. Measuring early fetal loss is another challenge for MCH research and an important topic for mothers and families.

## Who Will Survive?

Neonatal technology has allowed society to keep smaller and smaller babies alive. These tiny premature infants have the highest risks of dying, and those who survive often have significant health burdens. Many attempts to save 500- to 750-g or smaller infants are still very experimental and invasive. To what extent should we be striving to keep all premature infants alive? Is there a societal commitment to provide early intervention and special education services to the increasing number of children born with cerebral palsy and other developmental disabilities? Should research funding be allocated to extend fetal viability to younger ages? Who should decide when it is time to allow a child to die—the parents, the physicians, the federal government via the Baby Doe Law, the courts, or hospital committees? These complex ethical issues are part of the responsibility undertaken by MCH professionals.

## Measurement Issues

Some researchers do not believe that our nation's infant mortality ranking is an accurate indicator of our nation's health. Equivalent definitions of infant mortality become critical when making international comparisons. Japan, for example, defines infant deaths only as those occurring to babies born weighing at least 1,000 g. Because death rates are highest at low weights, some observers have questioned whether this definition introduces a conservative bias into Japanese estimates of infant mortality.

Cities and states in the United States vary widely in the extent to which they report infants born under 500 g as live births. These are problems of measurement, not biology or ethics. Should we adopt the European measure of perinatal mortality to avoid the distinction between live births and fetal deaths? Is there a risk of obscuring our infant mortality problem— or defining it away—by changing our measurement system?

Many measurement issues cloud our debates over MCH strategies. At what gestational age should pregnancy losses be considered fetal deaths? Should the definition of fetal deaths be tied to the age of viability? Should we collect MCH data by race, ethnicity, and/or social class? Do these categories highlight real population differences or only reinforce social stereotypes? As the number of infant deaths declines, classification decisions become more critical to the estimation and perception of infant mortality.

### Women's Health

Why do we study maternal health as a component of infant health rather than women's health? This chapter's analysis of MCH epidemiology indicated the relative paucity of information on maternal health and morbidity, particularly on the long-term impact of pregnancy on women's health. Maternal mortality is no longer sufficient to describe maternal health and pregnancy-related morbidity. What other universal measurements of maternal health are available? Hospitalization rates? Specific morbidity rates for conditions such as pregnancy-related hypertension or gestational diabetes? Rates of injury, either intentional or unintentional, during pregnancy? The MCH field needs to develop broad measures of women's health during pregnancy. Connecting maternal morbidity to subsequent issues in women's health, not simply infant outcomes, remains a challenge for the field (see Chapter 10).

### Multisectoral Collaboration for MCH Goals

How do we foster more far-reaching community-based strategies for infant mortality reduction transcending a predominantly medical focus? In some developing countries, the current approach to infant mortality involves multiple sectors of society in collective efforts. Women's organizations, community development groups, educators, religious leaders, and others join with the health sector to tackle the social roots of the problem. The challenge for MCH in the United States is to mobilize entire communities, including medical professionals, in initiatives that attack the full range of health risks and barriers to health care. One of the tasks of community coalitions is to work toward social policies to achieve their goals. In Europe, social welfare policies are integrated with health planning to reduce social inequities that manifest in health differentials. Women in most European countries have universal entitlements such as child allowances and paid maternity leave; single mothers and others with greater need often receive special benefits. Multisectoral collaboration, implicit in longitudinal models of women's health, is rarely attempted in the United States.

In 1996, the Personal Responsibility Work Opportunity Reconciliation Act (P.L. 104-193) restructured US social welfare policy to eliminate entitlements to income support for poor families. Temporary Assistance to Needy Families replaced Aid to Families with Dependent Children, a program with many limitations that nonetheless provided a basic safety net. Work requirements, lifetime time limits on benefits, and other provisions of Temporary Assistance to Needy Families have raised concerns about the potential health impact on low-income women, children, and families. The most recent version of the "New Federalism" reduces federal dollars and emphasizes variations among states. Particular concerns have been loss of benefits for immigrant families and lack of protection for children with disabilities as well as women coping with domestic violence, chronic disease, and mental illness. Monitoring of health and insurance effects has thus far produced mixed results (Ellwood & Ku, 1998; Korenbrot et al., 2000). Because positive program outcomes are linked closely to economic indicators and job availability, public health advocates need to monitor potential health effects on women and children with special care during economic downturns.

## Continued Improvements in Reproductive Health into the 21st Century

Major improvements in reproductive health were one of the great achievements of public health in the 20th century. Reductions in infant mortality (from 150 to 7 infant deaths per 1,000 births) and maternal mortality (from 750 to 10 maternal deaths per 100,000 births) have dramatically changed the lives and expectations of mothers, children, and families. These achievements were accomplished through a broad array of public health activities and struggles. There have been substantial changes in our understanding of the causes of poor birth outcomes, in clinical and public health practices to address reproductive health, in opportunities for women, and in the overall public health of our communities, as well as changes in the role and responsibility of government for the health of our newest citizens and their parents.

As this chapter has attempted to make clear, many ongoing professional and political challenges remain to further improving reproductive health in the United States and globally. Specifically, our scientific and epidemiologic knowledge base about reproductive outcomes remains inadequate. We need to strengthen our preconceptional, prenatal, delivery, postpartum, and internatal intervention programs. Finally, and perhaps most importantly, we must improve our reproductive health policies and funding support in order to implement necessary and successful public health and social welfare programs. The political and professional legacy of our MCH foremothers and forefathers should be a challenge, and an inspiration, to improve reproductive health care further for mothers and infants in the 21st century.

# REFERENCES

Albers, L.L., & Savitz, D.A. (1991). Hospital setting for birth and use of medical procedures in low-risk women. *Journal of Nurse-Midwifery, 36,* 327–333.

Alexander, G.R., Himes, J.H., Kaufman, R.B., Mor, J., & Kogan, M. (1996). A United States national reference for fetal growth. *Obstetrics Gynecology, 87,* 163–168.

Arias, E., MacDorman, M.F., Strobino, D.M., & Guyer, B. (2003). Annual summary of vital statistics: 2002. *Pediatrics, 112,* 1215–1230.

Atrash, H.K., Koonin, L.M., Lawson, H.W., Franks, A.L., & Smith, J.C. (1990). Maternal mortality in the United States, 1979–1986. *American Journal of Obstetrics and Gynecology, 76,* 1055–1060.

Bacak, S.J., Callaghan, W.M., Dietz, P.M., & Crouse, C. (2003, December). Pregnancy-associated hospitalizations in the United States, 1999–2000. Paper presented at the annual Maternal, Infant, and Child Health Epidemiology meetings, Tucson, Arizona.

Barfield, W. (2004). Racial/ethnic trends in fetal mortality: United States, 1990. *Morbidity and Mortality Weekly Report, 53,* 529–532.

Bennett, T.A., Kotelchuck, M., Cox, C.E., Tucker, M.J., & Nadeau, D.A. (1998). Pregnancy-associated hospitalizations in the United States in 1991 and 1992: A comprehensive view of maternal morbidity. *American Journal of Obstetrics and Gynecology, 178*, 346–354.

Berkowitz, G.S., & Papiernik, E. (1993). Epidemiology of preterm birth. *Epidemiologic Reviews, 15*, 414–443.

Brann, A.W., & Cefalo, R.C. (Eds.). (1992). *Guidelines for perinatal care* (3rd ed.). Evanston, IL, Washington, DC: American Academy of Pediatrics and American College of Obstetricians and Gynecologists.

Braveman, P., Egerter, S., Pearl, M., Marchi, K., & Miller, C. (1995). Early discharge of newborns and mothers: A critical review of the literature. *Pediatrics, 96*, 716–729.

Bremner, R.H. (Ed.). (1971). *Children and youth in America: A documentary history* (Vol. 2, Pt. 8). Cambridge, MA: Harvard University Press.

Buekens, P., & Klebanoff, M. (2001). Preterm birth research: From disillusion to the search for new mechanisms. *Pediatric and Perinatal Epidemiology, 15* (Suppl. 2), 159–161.

Buescher, P.A., Smith, C., Holliday, J.L., & Levine, R.H. (1987). Source of prenatal care and infant birth weight: The case of a North Carolina county. *American Journal of Obstetrics and Gynecology, 156*, 204–210.

Buescher, P.A., Harper, M., & Meyer, R.E. (2002). Enhanced surveillance of maternal mortality in North Carolina. *North Carolina Medical Journal, 63*, 76–79.

Cefalo, R.C., & Moos, M.K. (1994). *Preconceptional health care: A practical guide.* St. Louis, MO: Mosby.

Chavkin, W., & Allen, M. (1993). Questionable category of nonmaternal death [Letter]. *American Journal of Obstetrics and Gynecology, 168*, 1640–1641.

Committee to Study the Prevention of Low Birthweight, Division of Health Promotion and Disease Prevention, Institute of Medicine. (1985). *Preventing low birthweight* (p. 7). Washington, DC: National Academy Press.

Ellwood, M.R., & Ku, L. (1998). Welfare and immigration reform: Unintended side effects for Medicaid. *Health Affairs, 17*, 137–151.

Emanuel, I., Hale, C.B., & Berg, C.J. (1989). Poor birth outcomes of American black women: An alternative explanation. *Journal of Public Health Policy, 10*, 299–308.

Enkin, M.W. (1994). Risk in pregnancy: The reality, the perception, and the concept. *Birth, 21*, 131–134.

Fiscella, K. (1995). Does prenatal care improve birth outcomes? A critical review. *Obstetrics and Gynecology, 85*, 468–479.

Goldenberg, R.L., & Rouse, D.J. (1998). Prevention of premature birth. *New England Journal of Medicine, 339*, 313–320.

Guyer, B., Freedman, M.A., Strobino, D.M., & Sondik, E.J. (2000). Annual summary of vital statistics: Trends in the health of Americans during the 20th century. *Pediatrics, 106*, 1307–1317.

Handwerker, L. (1994). Medical risk: Implicating poor pregnant women. *Social Science and Medicine, 38*, 665–675.

*Healthy People 2010: Understanding and improving health.* (2000). Washington, DC: US Department of Health and Human Services, Public Health Service.

Klein, L., & Goldenberg, R.L. (1990). Prenatal care and its effect on preterm birth and low birth weight. In I.R. Merkatz & J.E. Thompson (Eds.), *New perspectives on prenatal care.* New York: Elsevier.

Kochanek, K.D., & Martin, J.A. (2004). Supplemental analysis of recent trends in infant mortality. Health E-Stats accessed June 28, 2004, at http://www.cdc.gov/nchs/products/pubs/pubd/hestats/infantmort/infantmort.htm

Kogan, M.D., Alexander, G.R., Kotelchuck, M., Nagey, D.A., & Jack, B.W. (1994). Comparing mothers' reports on the content of prenatal care received with recommended national guidelines for care. *Public Health Reports, 109,* 637–646.

Korenbrot, C.C., et al. (2000). Change in births to foreign-born women after welfare and immigration policy reforms in California. *Maternal and Child Health Journal 4(4),* 241–250.

Korenbrot, C.C. (2002). Preconception care: A systematic review. *Maternal and Child Health Journal, 6,* 75–88.

Kotelchuck, M. (1994). The adequacy of prenatal care utilization index: Its US distribution and association with low birthweight. *American Journal of Public Health, 74,* 1086–1092.

Kotelchuck, M., Schwartz, J.B., Anderka, M.T., & Finison, K.S. (1984). WIC participation and pregnancy outcomes: Massachusetts statewide evaluation study. *American Journal of Public Health, 74,* 1086–1092.

Kramer, M.S. (1987). Determinants of low birth weight: Methodological assessment and meta-analysis. *Bulletin of the World Health Organization, 65,* 663–737.

Krieger, N. (1994). Epidemiology and the web of causation. *Social Science and Medicine, 39,* 887–903.

Krieger, N., Rowley, D.L., Herman, A.A., Avery, B., & Phillips, M.T. (1993). Racism, sexism, and social class: Implications for studies of health, disease and well being. In D. Rowley & H. Tosteson, (Eds.), *Racial differences in preterm delivery: Developing a new research paradigm* (pp. 82–122). New York: Oxford University Press.

Lu, M.C., & Halfon, N. (2003). Racial and ethnic disparities in birth outcomes: A life-course perspective. *Maternal and Child Health Journal, 7,* 13–30.

Lu, M.C., Prentice, J., Yu, S.M., Inkelas, M., Lange, L.O., & Halfon, N. (2003). Childbirth education classes: Sociodemographic disparities in attendance and the association of attendance with breastfeeding initiation. *Maternal and Child Health Journal, 7,* 87–94.

March of Dimes Birth Defects Foundation. (1999). *March of Dimes StatBook: Statistics for healthier mothers and babies.* White Plains, NY: March of Dimes Birth Defects Foundation.

Margolis, L.H., Kotelchuck, M., & Chang, H.Y. (1997). Factors associated with early maternal postpartum discharge from hospital. *Archives of Pediatric and Adolescent Medicine, 151,* 466–472.

Martin, J.A., Hamilton, B.E., Sutton, P.D., Ventura, S.J., Menacker, F., & Munson, M.L. (2003). *Births: Final Data for 2002: National Vital Statistics Reports, 52*(10). Hyattsville, MD: National Center for Health Statistics.

Mathews, T.J., Menacker, F., & MacDorman, M.F. (2003). *Infant mortality statistics from the 2001 period linked birth/infant death data set: National Vital Statistics Reports, 52*(2). Hyattsville, MD: National Center for Health Statistics.

McLean, D.E. (1993). Psychosocial measurement: Implications for the study of preterm delivery in black women. In D. Rowley & H. Toteston (Eds.), *Racial differences in preterm delivery: Developing a new research paradigm* (pp. 39–81). New York: Oxford University Press.

Meara, E., Kotagal, U.R., Atherton, H.D., & Lieu, T.A. (2004). Impact of early newborn discharge legislation and early follow-up visits on infant outcomes in a state Medicaid population. *Pediatrics, 113*, 1619–1627.

Meis, P.J., Klebanoff, M., Thom, E., Dombrowski, M.P., Sibai, B., Moawad, A.H., Spong, C.Y., Hauth, J.C., Miodovnik, M., Varner, M.W., Leveno, K.J., Caritis, S.N., Iams, J.D., Wapner, R.J., Conway, D., O'Sullivan, M.J., Carpenter, M., Mercer, B., Ramin, S.M., Thorp, J.M., Peaceman, A.M., & Gabbe, S. (2003). Prevention of recurrent preterm delivery by 17 alpha-hydroxyprogesterone caproate. *New England Journal of Medicine, 348*, 2379–2385.

Moos, M.K. (2002). Preconceptional health promotion: Opportunities abound. *Maternal and Child Health Journal, 6*, 71–74.

Mrs. A-C-P to Julia Lathrop, Chief of the US Children's Bureau (1971, June 24). October 19, 1916, folder 634, Ethel S. Dummer Papers. Schlesinger Library, Radcliffe College. In R. H. Bremner (Ed.), *Children and youth in America: A documentary history*, 1971, p. 1071. Cambridge, MA: Harvard University Press, 1971.

National Center for Health Statistics. (2003). *Health, United States, 2003*. Hyattsville, MD: US Department of Health and Human Services, Centers for Disease Control and Prevention, National Center for Health Statistics.

Peoples-Sheps, M.D., Hogan, V.K., & Ng'andu, N. (1996). Content of prenatal care during the initial work-up. *American Journal of Obstetrics and Gynecology, 174*, 220–226.

Public Health Service Expert Panel on the Content of Prenatal Care. (1989). *Caring for our future: The content of prenatal care*. Washington, DC: US Public Health Service.

Rittenhouse, D.R., Braveman, P., & Marchi, K. (2003). Improvements in prenatal insurance coverage and utilization of care in California: An unsung public health victory. *Maternal and Child Health Journal, 7*, 75–86.

Rochat, R., Koonin, L.M., Atrash, H.K., & Jewett, J.F. (1988). Maternal mortality in the United States: Report from the Maternal Mortality Collaborative. *Obstetrics and Gynecology, 72*, 91–97.

Rooks, J.P., Weatherby, N.L., Ernst, E.K., Stapleton, S., Rosen, D., & Rosenfield, A. (1989). Outcomes of care in birth centers: The National Birth Center Study. *The New England Journal of Medicine, 321*, 1804–1811.

Rowley, D.L. (2001). Closing the gap, opening the process: Why study social contributors to preterm delivery among black women. *Maternal and Child Health Journal, 5,* 71–74.

Royston, E., & Armstrong, S. (Eds.). (1989). *Preventing maternal deaths.* Geneva: World Health Organization.

Rush, D., Kurzon, M.R., Seaver, W.B., & Shanklin, D.S. (1988). The national WIC evaluation: Evaluation of the Special Supplemental Food Program for Women, Infants and Children. VII. Study of food expenditures. *American Journal of Clinical Nutrition, 48* (2 Suppl), 512–519.

Sachs, B.P., Brown, D.A., Driscoll, S.G., Schulman, E., Acker, D., Ransil, B.J., & Jewett, J.F. (1992). Maternal mortality in Massachusetts: Trends and prevention. *The New England Journal of Medicine, 316,* 677–672.

Schoendorf, K., Hogue, C., Kleinman, J., & Rowley, D. (1992). Infant mortality in college educated families: Narrowing the racial gap. *The New England Journal of Medicine, 326,* 1522–1526.

Selwyn, B.J. (1990). The accuracy of obstetric risk assessment instruments for predicting mortality, low birth weight, and preterm birth. In I.R. Merkatz & J.E. Thompson (Eds.), *New perspectives on prenatal care.* New York: Elsevier.

Ugwumadu, A. (2002). Bacterial vaginosis in pregnancy. *Current Opinion in Obstetrics and Gynecology 14,* 115–118.

Wertz, R.W., & D.C. Wertz. (1982). *Lying-In: A history of childbirth in America.* New York: Schocken Books.

Wilcox, L.S. (2002). Pregnancy and women's lives in the twenty-first century: The United States Safe Motherhood movement. *Maternal and Child Health Journal, 6,* 215–220.

Wile, I.S. (1971). Do medical schools adequately train students for the prevention of infant mortality? Transactions of the American Association for Study and Prevention of Infant Mortality. In R. H. Bremner (Ed.), *Children and youth in America: A documentary history* (Vol. 2, Pt. 8, p. 965). Cambridge, MA: Harvard University Press.

Wise, P.H. (1990). Poverty, technology and recent trends in the United States infant mortality rate. *Paediatric and Perinatal Epidemiology, 4,* 390–401.

Wise, P.H. (1993). Confronting racial disparities in infant mortality: Reconciling science and politics. In R. Rowley & H. Tosteson (Eds.), *Racial differences in preterm delivery: Developing a new research paradigm* (pp. 7–16). New York: Oxford University Press.

World Health Organization. (1977). *International classification of diseases: Manual of the international statistical classification of diseases, injuries, and causes of death* (9th rev.). Geneva: World Health Organization.

# CHAPTER 6

# The Child from 1 to 4: The Toddler and Preschool Years

*Anita M. Farel and Jonathan B. Kotch*

*"A child is the greatest gift from Wakatanka,"* the Great Mystery, a tribesman explained years later, sent *"in response to many devout prayers, sacrifices, and promises."* As the tribe's future, children enjoyed outpourings of parental affection, indulgence, gentle but persistent instruction, and a complete absence of physical punishment. (Utley, 1993)

## INTRODUCTION

The preschool years witness growth rates not experienced again until adolescence. The importance of early childhood for future health cannot be overstated. During this period, the child, born totally helpless and dependent, develops language, locomotion, social relationships, and the knowledge and skills that make successful school entry possible. It is also a period of great risk, not only because inadequate nutrition or health care can predispose the preschool child to potential health problems that compromise future growth and development, but also because inadequate parenting or insufficient social and cognitive stimulation can jeopardize the successful transition to school and lead to subsequent academic and social problems.

According to Erikson (1950), the preschool child's developmental tasks are to achieve a sense of autonomy and to experience individual initiative. The successful completion of these tasks is a necessary prerequisite to the individuality and purposeful activity that will be called on when the child enters school. The interpersonal relationships that the child develops during this period will be long lasting, as in the case of family relationships and also models for future relationships. Poor health habits initiated during this period can lead to obesity, cardiovascular disease, and even interpersonal violence (Margolis, Sparrow, & Swanson, 1989).

Whereas preventive health services, exemplified by immunizations, play a prominent role at this age period, it is also true that, as children approach school age, the greatest threat to their lives becomes intentional and unintentional injury, which at best can only modestly be affected by personal health care. Similarly, many of the leading causes of morbidity in this period either seem resistant to medical intervention or are increasing in prevalence as a result of advances in medical technology and treatment. All of these circumstances suggest the need to consider community-based prevention strategies and social policy as interventions of choice in this age group. In this chapter, we describe the demographics, history, and health status of 1 to 4 year olds in the United States, their access to health services, and programs and policies relevant to this age group.

## DEMOGRAPHICS

Although birth rates and fertility rates have decreased steadily in this country since the late 1970s, the *number* of births started increasing in 1975 because of the increased number of women born during the baby boom having babies of their own (Guyer, Freedman, Strobino, & Sondik, 2000). That year there were 3,154,198 infants born alive in the United States. In 2000, that number was 4,058,814, declining slightly to 4,025,933 in 2001 and 4,021,726 in 2002, when the crude US birth rate, 13.9 per 1,000, was the lowest ever recorded (Martin et al., 2003). As a result of this trend, the total under 5 years population on July 1, 2003, is estimated to have been 19,769,279 (US Census Bureau, 2004) compared with 18,354,443 in April 1990 and 19,175,798 in April 2000, an increase of 4.5% (Meyer,

2001). There are slightly more boys born than girls, 51.2% of all births, but because boys have a higher mortality rate, females become the majority by the age of 30 years. Among the 19,175,798 were 1,817,543 female and 1,900,431 male children of Hispanic or Latino origin, who could have been of any race (US Census Bureau, 2000). The sex and race distribution of children less than 5 years in the United States as of April 2000 is shown in Table 6–1.

Demographic trends indicate that the ethnic composition of the preschool population, and consequently of all children in the United States, is shifting toward nonwhite. The percentage of children who are Hispanic or Asian increased from 11% in 1980 to 22% in 2001. These children are projected to comprise almost 30% of the child population by 2020. In contrast, the percentage of black, non-Hispanic children has remained at approximately 15% since 1980 and will decline slightly to 14% by 2020. The percentage of non-Hispanic White children fell from 74% in 1980 to 62% in 2001 and is expected to decline further to 55% by 2020 (Child Trends Data Bank, 2003).

Poverty is one of the most powerful determinants of a young child's health. From birth through infancy and childhood, poverty is associated with higher mortality and morbidity for a wide range of conditions, including behavioral and emotional disorders, spanning virtually every sphere of a child's life. Approximately one in five US children (and one in four minority children) lives in poverty—the highest child poverty rate in the world among developed countries (Dalaker, 2001). Six million children, representing 15% of poor children, live in families whose income is

**Table 6–1** US Under-5 Population by Sex and Race, April 2000

|  | Male | Female |
| --- | --- | --- |
| White | 6,597,764 | 6,262,128 |
| African American | 1,424,275 | 1,380,511 |
| American Indian/Alaska Native | 108,659 | 104,393 |
| Asian | 337,149 | 333,257 |
| Native Hawaiian/Pacific Islander | 17,254 | 16,137 |
| Other race | 843,478 | 802,578 |
| Two or more races | 482,154 | 466,061 |

Source: US Census Bureau, 2000.

less than 50% of the poverty level (Wood, 2003). Almost two million of these children are white, with the remainder roughly divided equally between Hispanic and non-Hispanic black. The duration of poverty also varies with race. Only 6% of white children who are poor were poor 5 years ago. In contrast, 29% of black children who are poor were poor 10 years ago (Wood, 2003). Poverty and the low educational level of the household combine to form an almost insurmountable culture of deprivation, which is difficult to overcome.

Several national trends over the past 35 years contributed to the rise in poverty: decreased real value of wages earned by workers with less education, reductions in real value of income transfer programs, increased numbers of single-parent, female-headed families, and adverse interactions between these factors and social and emotional problems of families, such as domestic violence. Twenty percent of female heads of households on Temporary Assistance for Needy Families (TANF) were abused compared with only 1.5% of a comparable group who were not on TANF. Sixty-five percent of children who are poor live in households without their biological father, whereas 25% of children who are not poor live in a single-parent household (Feeley, 2000). Regardless of whether the mother works, the low income level of mother-headed families is made worse by the persistent failure of fathers to meet child support obligations. Low-income single female parents have two to four times the rate of clinical depression as that found in the general population (Lennon, Blome, & English, 2001).

Poverty is an underlying cause of preventable illness in children in the United States. Beginning with the landmark study of infant deaths in 1913 by the Children's Bureau (US Department of Health, Education and Welfare, 1976), many studies, summarized by Gortmaker and Wise (1994), have repeatedly documented this association, not only for natural causes of mortality and morbidity (Starfield, 1982), but also for external causes (Nelson, 1992; Nersesian, Petit, Shaper, Lemieux, & Naor, 1985). Nevertheless, debate persists over the dynamics of the relationship between poverty and child illness. In Denmark, for example, child health statistics remained favorable even during economic hardship. Gortmaker and Wise (1994) attribute this stability to redistribution of resources in this very egalitarian society. Consistent with this finding is the observation that, rather than mean income, the magnitude of the gap between the highest and lowest income groups in the United States is closely correlated with infant mortality (Kawachi, Kennedy, Lochner, & Prothow-Stith, 1997).

Poverty is associated with many risks for poor health among young children. Adverse pregnancy outcomes among poor women include a greater likelihood of low birthweight and postnatal complications. Poor children are more likely to have inadequate or inappropriate nutrition. Malnutrition is associated with iron deficiency anemia, weakness, fatigue, growth retardation, impaired social development, slow learning, and increased susceptibility to infection (Oberg, 1987).

Approximately half of families that are poor live in neighborhoods with concentrated poverty (Casey, 2000). Poor communities suffer from a lack of public resources, economic investment, and political power, all of which exacerbate the disadvantages of poverty (Knitzer, 2002). For example, four to five million children, the vast majority of whom are poor, reside in older homes with lead levels exceeding the accepted threshold for safety (Brody et al., 1994). Poor communities offer few safe places for children to congregate and play. Consequently, children who live in neighborhoods that are poor are less likely to participate in sports or after-school activities. Economic, social, health, and other factors thus converge to stunt the intellectual, emotional, and physical development of poor children.

Child poverty also permeates need for special education services because it affects children's health, behavior, and as a consequence, cognitive development and academic achievement. One third of mothers of poor children with individualized education plans (IEPs) did not finish high school compared with 7% of mothers whose children with IEPs are not in poverty, reinforcing the conclusion that parental education is the best predictor of poverty. Poverty alone had a negative effect on teacher ratings of approaches to learning (US Department of Education, 2001).

The relationship between poverty and health status has ominous implications for the future of children's health and well-being. Assessments of health, cognitive development, school achievement, and emotional well-being are all related to the level of family affluence (Brooks-Gunn, Duncan, & Maritato, 1997). Despite the fact that between 1993 and 1997 the number of young children in poverty declined approximately 19%, the poverty rate for children less than 6 years of age remained higher than any other age group (Morgan & Kickham, 2001). Major adjustments in the economy, such as the replacement of skilled, unionized manufacturing jobs with lower paid, lesser skilled, nonunionized service sector jobs, coupled with increasing proportions of children living with one parent, usually the mother, and failure of social welfare programs to keep pace with inflation, conspire to keep approximately one in five children (and one in four minority children) in poverty.

# HEALTH STATUS

## Historical Changes

The improvement in the health status of preschool age children in the United States in the 20th century is the greatest of any infant or child age bracket. Using fatality as a proxy measure of health status, it may be said that preschool children in the United States are healthier now than ever before. Fatalities among 1 to 4 year olds fell 98% from 1900 to 1998 (Guyer et al., 2000). Indisputably, the story behind this modern public health miracle is the control of infectious diseases. Of the 97% decline in mortality that occurred between 1900 and 1985, 93% occurred before 1950, approximately the time of the introduction of antibiotics to the general public (Fingerhut, 1989). Therefore, the lives saved and morbidities prevented are attributable almost entirely to improved public health services such as sanitation, immunization, food safety, and the promotion of personal hygiene by public health workers on the one hand and to improved living standards resulting in reductions in family size, improved nutrition, improved housing conditions, and decreased crowding on the other. There is no credible basis for the claim that personal medical care made anything more than a marginal contribution to this "spectacular" (Guyer et al., 2000, p. 1313) improvement in health and life expectancy enjoyed by US children.

In her autobiography, Dr. Sara Josephine Baker (1873 to 1945), the first woman to receive a doctorate in public health and founder of New York City's Division of Child Hygiene, the first government-sponsored agency in the world dedicated to child health, described the activities contributing to the improvement of the health of children in her jurisdiction. These included training 30 public health nurses to teach recent immigrants preventive health practices such as proper ventilation, bathing, breastfeeding, and clothing for infants and young children. Baker's Division of Child Hygiene offered health education and advice, screening and referral, and pure milk in the "baby hygiene stations" that she set up. She trained midwives, introduced hygiene into New York City classrooms, isolated children with infectious diseases by keeping them out of school, and placed orphaned children from hospitals with loving foster mothers. By the time of her retirement in 1923, New York's child death rate was the lowest of any city in the United States or Europe (Grolier Library of North American Biographies, 1994).

In her comprehensive review of trends in childhood mortality in the United States, Fingerhut (1989) documented the precipitous drop in death rates for the 1- to 4-year-old age group, from 1980 per 100,000 (based on death registration states which included 26% of the US population) in 1900 to 50 per 100,000 in 1985. By 2000, this rate had declined still further to 32 per 100,000, rising to 33.3 in 2001 because of increases in deaths caused by congenital malformations, homicide, and diseases of the heart (Arias, MacDorman, Strobino, & Guyer, 2003). At the same time, preschool children in the United States experience higher mortality rates than their peers in other Western countries, primarily because of excess injury deaths. The success in reducing the death rate in this age group represents primarily the success in reducing natural causes of death. In 1900, natural causes accounted for the death of 93% of all 1 to 4 year olds in the United States. Diphtheria, diarrhea, enteritis, and pneumonia together caused the deaths of 10% of all 1 to 4 year olds. By 1985, however, all natural causes (including but not limited to infectious diseases) accounted for the deaths of 55% of all 1 to 4 year olds (Fingerhut, 1989). By 2001, the leading causes of death in this age group, in order, have become unintentional injury, congenital anomalies, malignant neoplasms, homicide, heart disease, and (finally) influenza and pneumonia, reflecting the relatively greater success in preventing natural causes of death compared with external causes (Centers for Disease Control and Prevention, 2001). The rate of every one of them decreased with the single exception of homicide. The 1- to 4-year homicide rate increased from 0.6 per 100,000 in 1950 to 2.9 in 1995, after which it resumed its decline, to 2.3 per 100,000 in 2000 (Health, US, 2003).

## Epidemiology of Major Health Problems

### Infectious Diseases

Excluding routine visits, the five leading reasons for visiting pediatricians are infectious diseases. In 1988, the Child Health Supplement of the National Health Interview Survey (still the most recent national survey of its kind as of this writing) asked questions about nine of the more common childhood infectious diseases (Hardy, 1991). Among preschool children, approximately half of all doctor visits are for infectious illness. The annual incidence of repeated ear infections for the 0- to 4-year-old age group, 16 per 100 per year, is the highest in all of childhood. Nearly 30% of all US preschoolers have had repeated ear infections, and they visited the doctor on average more than five times per year. Among infectious conditions, preschool children in the United States (including infants) visited the doctor next most often for repeated tonsillitis, followed by mononucleosis, frequent diarrhea or colic, pneumonia, and bladder or urinary tract infection (in descending order) (Hardy, 1991).

Infectious illness takes its toll in other ways. Preschool children who are ill because of infectious disease may miss preschool or child care or experience activity limitation and days in bed, requiring working parents to lose days at work. A high proportion of preschoolers with infectious disease take prescribed medications (over 90% of those with ear infections, tonsillitis, and pneumonia) (Hardy, 1991), although the proportion of children 0 to 4 years old who used prescription antibiotics has declined from 47.9% in 1996 to 38.1% in 2000 (Carroll & Miller, 2004). Hospitalization, although infrequent, does occur, most commonly for diseases of the respiratory system. Infectious and parasitic disease is the third leading discharge diagnosis for children 1 to 4 years old (US DHHS/HRSA/MCHB, Child Health USA, 2002). Infectious disease is still a killer, the underlying cause of over 8% of deaths among 1- to 4-year-old children in 2001 (Arias, Anderson, Kung, Murphy, & Kochanek, 2003).

### Congenital Conditions

Birth defects are the leading cause of infant mortality (Anderson & Smith, 2003). Although most children with birth defects do not die in infancy, many of the more serious congenital malformations contribute substantially to childhood morbidity and long-term disability and thus have health care, social, and economic implications for young children. Costs for care for children with birth defects include expenses associated with a range of services, including diagnosis and treatment, and possible hospitalization, special education, rehabilitation, and residential placement.

Waitzman, Scheffler, and Romano (1996) used data from the California Birth Defects Monitoring Program to estimate the lifetime economic consequences of birth defects. They estimate the societal costs associated with medical, educational, and developmental resources used by individuals born with at least 1 of 18 birth defects and provide evidence for how cost estimates for selected birth defects can be used to argue for preventive interventions, including folate supplementation of food to prevent neural tube defects. Direct medical costs include corrective surgery, treating infections associated with several birth defects, and special appliances and prostheses for severe cases. The high rates of activity limitations for chronic diseases such as cerebral palsy, Down syndrome, and spina bifida incur high nonmedical expenses for special education and developmental services. Similarly, costs related to long-term care for conditions such as these are higher than for other birth defects.

A study of hospital discharge and census data from South Carolina and California used to document the contribution of birth defects and genetic diseases to the high percentage of pediatric hospitalizations found that pediatric hospitalizations related to birth defects and genetic conditions were more costly than other types of pediatric hospitalizations. Hospitalizations were higher for black children compared with those for white or Hispanic children. For preschool-age children, the rates were 4 per 1,000 in South Carolina and 5 per 1,000 in California. Birth defects-related hospital charges accounted for 16% and 28% of all pediatric hospitalization charges in South Carolina and California. More hospitalizations related to birth defects, and genetic diseases were paid for by government sources than hospitalizations for other reasons. Similar patterns of hospitalization were found in the two states, despite ethnic and geographic differences (Yoon et al., 1997).

In both South Carolina and California, half of all hospitalizations for black children related to birth defects and genetic diseases could be attributed to sickle cell diseases.

Three percent of infants are diagnosed with birth defects during the first year of life. By the age of 2 years, 5% to 7% are diagnosed, and by the age of 5 years, 7% to 10% of all children have recognizable birth defects. The prevalence of birth defects is affected by diverse demographic and environmental factors, genetics, and type of defects. Birth defects include structural malformations, metabolic disorders, and other conditions that originate during the prenatal period. The etiology of only a small proportion of birth defects is understood (Nelson & Holmes, 1989). In addition to certain teratogens, risk factors such as gender, birth rank, and mother's age have been identified. Most defects are identified within codes

740.0–759.9 of the International Classification of Diseases, Ninth revision, Clinical Modification (US Public Health Service, 1991).

Increasing awareness of the relationship between the incidence of birth defects and teratogenic factors, such as use of thalidomide in the 1960s, and infectious diseases such as rubella in the 1950s, stimulated the development of surveillance programs. Organized in 1974, the International Clearinghouse for Birth Defects Monitoring Systems now includes 24 programs from around the world. Over half of all state health departments have also developed their own birth defects surveillance systems. Surveillance programs are important for documenting the incidence of birth defects, examining potential etiologic agents, and assessing the effectiveness of interventions. When risk factors are identified, preventive interventions can be implemented. Program managers can use data from surveillance programs to evaluate the success of programs in reaching populations targeted for services. Information collected by different monitoring programs is useful for tracking changes in the incidence of anomalies that are detected at birth and demographic variations among conditions. Although initially developed as a means for determining the etiology of certain birth defects, surveillance systems have evolved into a means for monitoring the effectiveness of interventions (Lynberg & Edmonds, 1992). Progress in understanding the etiology of some birth defects has led to campaigns such as that directed at the consumption of folic acid to prevent spina bifida (Centers for Disease Control and Prevention, 1992).

Significant measurement issues surround the reporting of birth defects. Birth defects that involve structural malformations are more easily identified than, for example, subtle metabolic disorders. Surveillance systems that use multiple ascertainment methods, such as the Metropolitan Atlanta Congenital Defects Program, will be more accurate than programs that use only newborn hospital discharge information. The Metropolitan Atlanta Congenital Defects Program is a population-based surveillance system for birth defects and other perinatal conditions that occur in infants born to women who live in the five-county metropolitan Atlanta area. The program has statutory authority to conduct program activities such as reviewing records from maternity units, newborn nurseries, and genetic counseling (Edmonds et al., 1981).

### Mental Health

Despite its seriousness, attention to the prevalence and distribution of mental health disorders among preschool-aged children is relatively new

(Knitzer, 2000). Studies conducted in London, Hong Kong, and rural and urban areas of the United States estimate the prevalence rates for mental health disorders at 22% to 24% of 3 year olds, with 5% to 7% having a moderate to severe disorder and 15% to 18% a mild disorder (Anderson & Werry, 1994). Commonly identified problems include overactivity, restlessness, attention-seeking and difficult-to-control behavior, bedwetting, daytime wetting, food fads, difficulty settling down at bedtime, and night waking. These problems are most frequently associated with maternal depression, poor family relationships, and marital disharmony.

A study of preschool children found that the prevalence of conditions in this population, was comparable to that of other age groups (Lavigne et al., 1996). Other studies have indicated that as many as two thirds of children with problems at the age of 3 years will still have them at the age of 9 years (Campbell & Ewing, 1990). Bricker, Davis, and Squires (2004) asserted that the prevalence of young children with evidence of mental health problems is rising, reporting that recent surveys suggest that 10% to 25% of young children have mild to serious disorders. One quarter of parents of children enrolled in Head Start reported that their children had problem behaviors the parents consider to be clinically significant (Webster-Stratton, 1997).

Early identification of mental health problems is urgent. Children whose conditions are identified early would likely benefit from earlier preventive interventions (Costello, Burns, Angold, & Leaf, 1993; Lavigne et al., 1996). Without such intervention, mental health problems in young children may limit the formation of strong and constructive relationships with peers and adults and impair the acquisition of adaptive, cognitive, and language skills.

However, Bricker, Davis, & Squires (2004) described five barriers to early identification.

1. The development of mental health screening programs is impeded by the intrinsic variability of behavior among young children (Squires, 2000).
2. Physicians and other providers are often not as attuned to mental health evaluation as they are to other health indicators. A survey conducted by the National Alliance for the Mentally Ill (2000) reported that less than half of the parents responding indicated that their child's primary care physician recognized serious mental illness in their children.

3. Poor recognition of mental health problems by providers may be confounded by uneasiness at labeling a child as well as awareness that many insurance plans provide only limited coverage.

4. Family members or other caregivers may not be sensitive to possible disturbances in a child's development. Guidelines for the identification of early mental health and behavior problems in 3- to 5-year-old children under the Individuals with Disabilities Education Act (IDEA) are limited. Vague eligibility guidelines under IDEA, in addition to limited community-based options for screening, diagnosing, and evaluating children in this age group, reduce opportunities for treating problems.

5. There are few low-cost, easily administered instruments for screening young children.

The authors identify three recently developed low-cost screening measures that can be administered by individuals who do not have professional training. These economical instruments hold great promise for involving parents and caregivers earlier in the identification process.

### Developmental Disabilities

Mental retardation is one among a group of diverse conditions termed developmental disabilities that are attributable to mental and/or physical impairments, manifest between birth to 21 years of age, and likely to continue indefinitely (Decoufle, Yeargin-Allsopp, Boyle, & Doernberg, 1994). Mental retardation is a broad classification, including conditions for which the etiologies are numerous and diverse. Legislative and social initiatives can reduce the incidence of some conditions associated with mental retardation such as preterm births and alcohol consumption during pregnancy, but most cases of mental retardation have no known cause. In addition to mental retardation, neuromuscular disorders such as muscular dystrophy, sensory impairments such as blindness and deafness, learning disabilities, and conditions such as epilepsy and autism all fall under the developmental disabilities classification.

In the 1960s, intelligence tests were used to identify children with mental retardation, and services were offered primarily in special schools or residential institutions. The current practice of mainstreaming children with mental retardation grew out of concern that the segregated environment of special classes or institutions deprived children with mental retardation of experiences necessary for effective socialization. The widespread use of IQ testing as the criterion for decisions about services was also criticized for having stigmatizing consequences that were difficult to overcome. Although there is not a consistent viewpoint about classifying children with mild mental retardation, severe mental retardation (defined as IQ < 50) is usually recognizable before children reach school age. The prevalence of preschool-age children with severe mental retardation ranges from 3 to 5 per 1,000 children. However, the definition of severe mental retardation as an IQ of less than 50 is problematic because IQ alone does not describe individual differences in adaptive skills or the presence of other conditions that may impede effective coping by a child whose IQ is above this cutoff.

Accurate prevalence rates for developmental disabilities are not available. Children with developmental disabilities, by definition, have functional limitations in at least three of the following seven areas: self-care, receptive or expressive language, learning, mobility, self-direction, capacity for independent living, and economic self-sufficiency (Crocker, 1989). Based on records from local special education programs, an estimated 8% to 16% of school-age children with developmental disabilities receive special education services. Because legislative mandates provide educational services to all school-age children with specific physical, emotional, or cognitive impairments, Decoufle et al. (1994) argued that school records provide the most comprehensive means of identifying school-age children with developmental disabilities. Consequently, recent mandates to provide preschool special education services may also generate useful data about children under 4 years with developmental disabilities.

Surveillance of developmental disabilities is difficult because case definitions often rely on clinical judgment, and there are no standard national or state-specific definitions for developmental disabilities. Furthermore, developmental disabilities may not be manifest at the age of 1 year and only become apparent as the child matures. In the United States, the Centers for Disease Control and Prevention has conducted the Metropolitan Atlanta Developmental Disabilities Surveillance Program, a population-based surveillance system for mental retardation, cerebral palsy, vision impairment, and hearing impairment among children aged 3 to 10 years whose parents are residents of the Atlanta metropolitan area. Educational, medical, and social services records are used to ascertain cases.

## External Causes

Injuries are the single leading cause of death among all children over the age of 6 months. In the 1- to 4-year-old age group, intentional and unintentional injuries combined account for over 40% of all deaths (Arias, MacDorman, Strobino, & Guyer, 2003). Motor vehicle injury, drowning, and fires and burns are the most common unintentional injury causes of death among preschoolers (US DHHS/HRSA/MCHB, Child Health USA, 2002). Whereas deaths caused by unintentional injury declined between 2000 and 2001, homicides increased 35%, from 356 to 415 (Arias, MacDorman, Strobino, & Guyer, 2003).

Among these increasing homicides, perhaps the most tragic is child abuse, defined here as physical harm deliberately inflicted by a caretaker. Although many parents whose use of corporal punishment may have led to the death of a child might not have "intended" to kill the child, the result is the same. The difference between the intention to teach the child a lesson by hurting him and deliberately intending to harm him is merely semantic. Unfortunately, many cases of child abuse fail to achieve the medical examiner's threshold for diagnosing child maltreatment as the cause of death, resulting in underreporting of the incidence of fatal child abuse (Herman-Giddens, 1991; Kotch, Chalmers, Fanslow, Marshall, & Langley, 1993). Despite the fact that child maltreatment reports appear to be declining in the United States, estimated child maltreatment fatalities are going up (US DHHS, ACYF, 2004). The proliferation of child fatality teams in the United States is evidence of the recognition that fatal child abuse is preventable if, by more accurate identification, we can learn who is at risk and when to intervene.

It is impossible to know the true incidence of child maltreatment in the United States. Official statistics reflect the activities of public agencies in response to reported cases, and child protection teams do not even investigate a third of referrals that come to their attention (US DHHS, ACYF, 2004). The most recent National Incidence Study (Sedlack & Broadhurst, 1996), a survey within a sample of counties in the United States to enumerate cases both known to child protective services (CPS) and known to other agencies and organizations, was last conducted in 1993.

Far more injuries are nonfatal than fatal, but the causes and incidence of nonfatal injury are less well documented than those of fatal injury. Leading causes of emergency room visits and hospitalizations for injury in this age group include falls, burns, motor vehicle injury, and poisoning. Although less serious medically, nonfatal injuries, the leading cause of disability after congenital and perinatal causes, actually cost the United States more in indirect costs than fatal injuries, given that the present value of total lost productivity caused by nonfatal injuries is greater than that caused by fatal injuries. In fact, of the over $4 billion lifetime cost of injury in the 0- to 4-year-old age group in 1985, 33% is the indirect cost of injury morbidity compared with 23% for injury mortality (Rice, MacKenzie and Associates, 1989).     •

# HEALTH CARE ACCESS

Despite the decreasing rate of children with no health insurance in the late 1990s, children most in need of health care continue to be those with the most limited access (Rhoades, Vistnes, & Cohen, 2002). In 2002, almost half of children with poor or fair health status were covered by public-only health insurance. The Medical Expenditure Panel Survey, an annual household survey sponsored by the Agency for Healthcare Research and Quality, provides data for evaluating trends in health insurance status that include estimates of health care use, expenditures, sources of payment, quality, and insurance coverage. According to a recent report, the percentage of uninsured children under the age of 18 years declined from 15.7% to 12.9% from 1996 to 2002. However, the percentage of children covered by public-only health insurance during the same period increased from 21.3% to 26.3%. Younger children were more likely to be enrolled in public-only health insurance. In 2002, 32.1% of children aged 0 to 3 years were covered by public-only health insurance. Black children had the highest rate of public-only health insurance (46.9% in 2002), and Hispanic children were the most likely to be uninsured (23.8% in 2002) (Rhoades & Cohen, 2003). Government, or public, health insurance for children consists primarily of Medicaid but also includes Medicare, the State Children's Health Insurance Program (see Chapter 2), and CHAMPUS/Tricare, the health benefit program for members of the armed forces and their dependents.

Simpson et al. (2004), also using the Medical Expenditure Panel Survey data set to examine changes in insurance coverage and health care use, reported that approximately 40% of all hospital stays (1995–2000) for 1 to 4 year olds were for respiratory conditions. Although hospital admission for asthma can be avoided by appropriate outpatient care, admissions increased between 1995 and 2000 (11.2% to 12.6%, respectively). However, the mean length of stay in a hospital for respiratory conditions decreased during this period, possibly the result of the impact of managed care arrangements on hospitalizations and strides in pharmacologic interventions.

As a result of the State Children's Health Insurance Program, eligibility expansions in state Medicaid programs, and expanded employer-based coverage, health insurance coverage for children of all ages has improved. However, there continue to be reports that a majority (at least 65%) of uninsured children are eligible but not enrolled in public programs. Holahan, Dubay, and Kenney (2003) argued that the key policy issue among children is the lack of participation among eligible families rather than inadequate eligibility levels. The reasons for lack of participation are complex. If a family's experience with public welfare was not positive or if information about Medicaid rules under welfare reform were not adequately communicated, families may not know that their children are eligible for public sources of health insurance. Cumbersome enrollment procedures, stigma associated with public programs, language barriers, and misunderstanding about the value of insurance all undermine enrollment. Gains in coverage during recent years are challenged by economic downturns. For example, in 2003, Oklahoma reduced eligibility for children less than 5 years of age from 185% to 133% poverty level. It also required more frequent reporting of eligibility and eliminated strategies, such as media outreach, that brought children into these programs.

# PROGRAMS

Several federal programs are of particular importance for this age group.

## Immunizations

Immunizations are the *sine qua non* of a personal preventive health intervention. Immunizations exemplify disease prevention, the delivery of a direct service to individuals for the purpose of preventing a specific disease. Immunizations have been proven to be cost beneficial and are the basis for the routine schedule of health maintenance services recommended for preschool children by the American Academy of Pediatrics and others. *Healthy People 2010* proposes an immunization goal of 80% coverage of 19 to 35 month olds. To achieve this goal, all the recommended doses of available vaccines for the prevention of polio, diphtheria/

pertussis/tetanus (DPT) or diphtheria and tetanus (DT), measles, and *Haemophilus influenzae* type B (Hib), a more organized child health services delivery system is necessary. Up-to-date immunization of 19 to 35 month olds in the United States went down from 1998 to 2001 for DPT/DT, measles-containing vaccine (MCV), Hib,[1] and polio, and up for the newer chicken pox and hepatitis B vaccines (Centers for Disease Control and Prevention, 2003). Children with family incomes below the poverty level had lower rates of coverage with the combined series than children with family incomes at or above the poverty line—72% of children below poverty compared with 79% of higher income children (Forum on Family and Child Statistics, 2003). As a result, in the year 2000, there were 10 cases of rubella, 37 cases of measles, 43 cases of hepatitis B, 57 cases of mumps, 294 cases of *H. influenzae*, and 2,878 cases of pertussis among US children less than 5 years. The numbers for *H. influenzae* increased over 1999 (US DHHS/HRSA/MCHB, 2002).

## IDEA

Many health programs address the needs of particular populations and target services to eligible groups. In contrast, all children are entitled to public education. For children with disabilities, significant amendments to the Education of the Handicapped Act in 1986 (P.L. 99-457) extended these entitlements to 3 to 5 year olds (Preschool Grants Program, Section 619 of Part B) and offered states funding to plan systems of services for infants and toddlers from birth to 2 years of age (Part C, Infant and Toddler Program).

### Part B Preschool Grants Programs

Compelling evidence over the past 50 years has affirmed that special interventions for young children with disabilities and their families during the preschool years increase the child's developmental and educational gains. In 1986, the federal government reinforced the importance of preschool services for children with developmental delays or disabilities by establishing the Preschool Grants Program (Section 619 of Part B) under amendments to the Education of the Handicapped Act, referred to as the IDEA since 1990. This legislation expanded earlier incentives to encour-

---

[1]Diphtheria, pertussis tetanus/diphtheria tetanus; measles, mumps, rubella; *H. influenza* type B, inactivated polio vaccine.

age states to entitle all 3- through 5-year-old children with disabilities to a free and appropriate public education. By 1993, every state and jurisdiction assured free and appropriate public education for all preschoolers with disabilities. The Preschool Grants Program is the only federal program exclusively serving preschool-age children with disabilities. State education agencies are awarded formula grants from the US Department of Education to implement the program through local education agencies and other community service agencies. The Preschool Grants Program is the second largest federal program focusing on 3- to 5-year-old children.

Services provided under Part B may include, but are not limited to, assistive technology devices and services, audiology, counseling services, early identification and assessment, medical services for diagnosis or evaluation, occupational therapy, parent counseling and training, physical therapy, psychological services, recreation, rehabilitation counseling services, school health services, social work services in schools, special education, speech pathology, and transportation. All children who are eligible for services under Part B must have an IEP developed by parents and providers to develop goals for a child's program of services and to determine which special education and related services are necessary to reach these goals and the setting(s) in which these services will be provided. Related services are provided when they are necessary to assist a child to benefit from special education. As a result of successful outreach and child find campaigns, the number of children being served under the Preschool Grants Program grew from 478,627 in 1994 to 647,420 in the 2002–2003 school year for the United States and outlying areas (Danaher, Kraus, Armijo, & Hipps, 2003). Innovations and increased interagency collaboration have promoted services that are comprehensive and cost-effective. The larger number of children served by Part B is likely a result of the availability of more accurate screening and assessment instruments, parental concern about the course of a child's development and behavior as children get older, and variable eligibility policies between the two programs (Harbin & Danaher, 1994).

However, some difficult issues persist. Translating the vision of inclusion is difficult in many communities where, historically, children with disabilities may have been placed in more segregated, distinct settings. Although local school systems may be integrating older children into the public school classrooms, childcare settings have traditionally been more autonomous. This situation is compounded by the dearth of preschool or childcare resources, particularly in rural areas. Furthermore, providing services for children with more rare conditions requires establishing channels of communication among diverse providers, resources in the public and private sector, and families. Communities in which child care rather than preschool services is the norm require special collaborative initiatives between health care and educational providers.

Capitalizing on possibilities for flexible use of Part B funds to translate the spirit of the legislation requires skills in collaboration and a comprehensive, less categorical vision of a child's and family's needs. Amendments to the law retracted the requirement that states report the numbers of 3- to 5-year-old children served by disability category and subsequently allowed states to incorporate an additional *preschool-specific category* for children experiencing developmental delays. Such amendments have made it possible for programs to use more flexible, noncategorical eligibility criteria. In 1997, 35 states and Guam now use developmental delay, and 19 extend it beyond the age of 5 years (Danaher, 2001).

## Part C Infant and Toddler Program

Part C, the infant/toddler section of IDEA, is a mechanism for developing systems of family-centered services for infants and toddlers, with or at risk for disabilities, and their families. The 1986 legislation required states that chose to participate in the Part C (previously, Part H) program to develop state and local infrastructures to respond to the requirement for service delivery systems. Over the course of the 5-year planning period, states were required to apply for continued funding from the US Department of Education and to document their progress in developing the different elements of the system required by the legislation. At the end of the 5-year program implementation process, it was expected that all eligible infants, toddlers, and their families would be entitled to a gamut of comprehensive, coordinated services. By 1992, the complicated process of developing appropriate policies, including interagency agreements, at the state and local levels slowed progress toward full implementation of the law. Furthermore, budget constraints experienced by many federal and state programs forced states to narrow their conceptualization of appropriate populations to serve. In fact, only nine states and jurisdictions opted ultimately to serve infants and toddlers "at risk" for developmental problems (Shackelford, 2004).

All states are required to address 16 minimum requirements in their state plans. States are required to identify a "lead agency" for the Part H program. In more than half of the states, the health department is the lead agency. An Individualized Family Service Plan (IFSP) for each eligible child must be developed with families in order to assure its responsiveness to families' unique concerns, priorities, and needs. Extensive regulations direct state early intervention programs to improve community awareness and identification of children with or at risk for developmental disabilities. For example, under IDEA, the child find system requires each state to ensure that all children with disabilities or suspected of having disabilities are located, identified, and evaluated. The child find system must be coordinated with all other child find initiatives, including Supplemental Security Income (SSI), Title V, and Early and Periodic Screening, Diagnosis, and Treatment (EPSDT). Explicit regulations for community outreach, participation of diverse early childhood personnel, and development and monitoring of IFSP have shaped the implementation and evaluation of early intervention programs. The IFSP has several components related to health care. For example, the IFSP must describe the child's physical development, including vision and hearing. Health care services and nursing services that would enable the child to benefit from other early intervention services must be provided. Medical services, in so far as they are necessary for diagnostic and assessment purposes, are also included in early intervention services. Other services that the child needs such as well-child care or surgery must also be documented in the IFSP, although not paid for by Part C. Such information helps provide a more complete picture of the child and family's needs for services and for tracking a child's health status, particularly when the child does not have a primary care physician.

## Early Intervention

Early intervention refers to the provision of services to young children between birth and school age with or at risk for developmental disabilities and their families. Educational, health care, supportive, social, and therapeutic services are among those provided. Rather than a specific program model, early intervention has been referred to as a concept that addresses the developmental needs of young children with a wide range of disabilities (Guralnick, 1998; Shonkoff & Meisels, 2000).

Early intervention services can be delivered in a center or the child's home. Teams of specialized professionals (teachers, social workers, allied health therapists) as well as community workers, who may provide very personal support even if they lack formal training or education, staff early intervention programs.

The health care system historically has been the first point of professional contact for families with young children with developmental problems. Initially, services for young children with disabilities were primarily rehabilitative and emphasized functional and cognitive development (Hutt & Gibby, 1976). In the 1960s, the importance of the interaction between the child and caregiver was considered the single most important factor in developmental achievement. As a result, children with mental retardation were no longer segregated in separate preschool programs, nor were children considered to be at risk for poor development because of social disadvantage.

Assessing a child's needs and resources in the context of the family shifted the orientation of the relationship between caregivers and interventionists and fostered the development of more refined identification and assessment procedures for infants and preschool children. The importance of the family is emphasized. Families and children develop unique mechanisms to compensate for the child's special needs. Consequently, the family must be the context where assessment and intervention take place.

Under federal law, states are given considerable discretion in establishing eligibility criteria for early intervention services among the following three groups: infants with established conditions that are likely to lead to delay, infants with developmental delay, or infants who are at risk for developmental delay. However, identifying accurate, culturally sensitive risk factors has been difficult.

Although there is agreement that early intervention programs should be provided for infants with disabilities and those at some level of identifiable risk for developmental problems (Guralnick, 1998), identifying less easily defined potential risk factors in order to determine who should be served by an early intervention program has proved elusive (Upshur, 1990). The use of perinatal factors, such as low birthweight or preterm birth, to estimate number of children at risk proved to be relatively insensitive (Scott & Masi, 1979).

Most recent early intervention initiatives address the child's needs in the context of the family. Bronfenbrenner, Moen, and Garbarino (1984) focused attention on the complex interaction among risk factors for developmental problems by emphasizing that the family is embedded in neighborhoods and communities that have broad social and cultural influences. Precursors of developmental delay have been identified more accurately by including the impact of multiple family risk factors, such as stressful life events, mother's educational level, mother's mental health status, and father's presence in the home.

The child's relationships within the larger context of family and community are central to understanding the likelihood of success in school. No single variable—health, socioeconomic, environmental—can encompass the potential adverse influences that can affect a child's development. Gorman and Pollitt (1996) examined the relationship among several environmental, medical, and developmental risk factors and children's risk for academic problems and concluded that a good school has some protective value for those most at risk. Other research has confirmed that psychosocial factors such as maternal depression and substance abuse affect children's health and development regardless of whether they have socioeconomic risk factors.

There is considerable evidence that properly designed programs with well-defined goals can affect parenting behavior that, in turn, can facilitate favorable outcomes. By this means, children with developmental disabilities and socioeconomic disruption are given the greatest opportunity to pursue a life course in which the consequences of these risk factors are kept to a minimum.

### Special Supplemental Food Program for Women, Infants, and Children

The Special Supplemental Food Program for Women, Infants, and Children (WIC) began as a demonstration in 1972. The goal was to improve the health of pregnant and lactating women, infants, and children by combining nutrition supplements, nutrition education, and access to health services. From its inception, WIC was conceived of as a food and nutrition program with a necessary connection to health services. Congress deliberately chose to avoid any stigma associated with welfare programs by administratively placing WIC in the Food and Nutrition Service of the Department of Agriculture. As Senator Hubert H. Humphrey (1972), one of the architects of the new program, said at the time, such placement would ensure that the program would "not be mismanaged in terms of some other programs."

Since 1972, thanks in part to a series of lawsuits to overcome the Nixon administration's deliberate impounding of WIC funds, the program has expanded rapidly. Today it serves nearly 7.5 million clients in an average month, including 3.74 million children 1 to 4 years old, at an annual cost of $4.5 billion (USDA, 2004). A beneficiary of the combined forces of agricultural interests, retail stores, child health and nutrition advocates, and drug companies that produce infant formula, WIC has survived major policy challenges, including threats of budget cuts in 1995. The success of WIC is undoubtedly attributable also to the fact that it is the most evaluated program of all federal social programs, and most of those evaluations have demonstrated the health benefits and the cost-effectiveness of WIC.

The overwhelming majority of these evaluations have focused on pregnancy outcome. During pregnancy, WIC services include vouchers for milk, cheese, eggs, fruit juice, dried peas, beans or peanut butter, and iron-fortified grain products. In addition, WIC services are offered as an adjunct to health care, and thus, women attracted by free food also receive prenatal care, as well as group and individual nutrition education. The evaluations of WIC have not attempted to disaggregate the separate contributions of health care, nutrition supplements, and nutrition education, but as a package, WIC has been shown to increase the mean birthweight and mean gestational age of newborns (Kennedy & Kotelchuck, 1984; Rush et al., 1988). WIC also has been shown to reduce Medicaid expenses for newborns in the first year of life (Schramm, 1986), hence the assertion that, in addition to providing a net health benefit, WIC also saves money.

There is less evidence about the benefits of WIC for the preschool child. As with the pregnant woman, an eligible child who has a nutritional risk and who is income eligible ($<$ 185% of the Federal Poverty Income Guidelines in most states) is entitled to food vouchers for milk and milk products, eggs, peanut butter, iron-fortified cereals, and vitamin C–rich juices. In addition, the parent or guardian (and in some cases the child) participates in nutrition education, and the child must have access to medical care. One study demonstrated that the requirement for access to medical care increased immunization rates for children in a local health department (Kotch & Whiteman, 1982). Rush's National WIC Evaluation included the tantalizing suggestion that children's head circumferences were 0.5 cm larger if they were on WIC in utero, and he attempted to link that finding with the observation that older children on WIC performed better on some cognitive tests such as digit memory (Rush et al.,

1988). However, because of issues of confidentiality and cost, these findings were never followed, and in 1989, the Congress refused to fund studies of the WIC impact on children that had been solicited by the Food and Nutrition Service.

More recent studies of WIC have documented its positive effect on the nutrition intake and access to health care of preschool children. For example, Rose, Habicht, and Devaney (1998) demonstrated that WIC benefits positively influenced ($p < 0.05$) the intakes of 10 of 15 nutrients studied. For iron and zinc, the average increase because of WIC represented 16.6% and 10.6%, respectively, of the preschooler recommended dietary allowance for these nutrients. Buescher et al. (2003) used linked birth, Medicaid, and WIC records to show that WIC children used more health services, both preventive and curative, than matched children on Medicaid but not on WIC. Finally, Lee, Rozier, Kotch, Norton, and Vann (2004) used the same data set to look specifically at the use of dental services. Not only did WIC increase the use of preventive and restorative dental care for children 0 to 5 years old compared with Medicaid children not on WIC, those on WIC also used fewer emergency dental care services.

## Head Start

The federal Head Start program was launched in 1965 as part of President Johnson's War on Poverty. The program was a response to sobering statistics about the number of young children who were very poor. The Head Start program was a national initiative to help improve the odds that poor young children would succeed in life. From the beginning, Head Start was envisioned as a comprehensive program that would provide child care and parent education, evaluate enrolled children's health systematically, monitor children's nutritional and emotional status, screen for hearing and vision, and provide a climate that would nurture social and behavioral competence among enrolled children to ensure that they enter school with a foundation similar to that of their more economically advantaged peers.

Access to health services was a fundamental theme in Head Start programming. These services include (1) a comprehensive health services program that encompasses a broad range of medical, dental, nutrition, and mental health services; (2) preventive health services and early intervention; and (3) service coordination to link the child's family to an ongoing health care system to insure that the child continues to receive comprehensive health care even after leaving Head Start (Zigler, Piotrkowski, & Collins, 1994). Ten percent of Head Start enrollment is reserved for children with disabilities, most of whom have hearing or speech/language impairments. Children with low-incidence, severe disabilities such as blindness, deafness, and mental retardation are enrolled in the Head Start population in approximately the same proportion as in the IDEA, Part B program for 3 and 4 year olds. Head Start also enrolls children with feeding tubes and children served by full-time aids. For low-income areas and neighborhoods, Head Start is often the only program serving families who have children with severe disabilities (US DHHS, 2004).

The importance of starting positive child development experiences at birth was reinforced by a new component included in the reauthorization of the Head Start Act in 1994, Early Head Start. The concept for Early Head Start was similar to that of the initial Head Start program, but support and education for the parents of these very young children were reinforced. By 2000, 6% of the overall Head Start enrollment was served in Early Head Start (US DHHS, 2000). As many low-income parents with young children shifted from public assistance to regular employment and hours away from home, the need for the unique family supports provided by Head Start programs grew. However, the parent involvement component, with the goal of engaging parents as classroom volunteers or as recipients of home visits, cannot be effective when parents are expected to be employed full-time or enrolled in job training. Changes in the economic and political environment will continue to have a powerful effect on the demand for Head Start programs.

Challenges for Head Start include the demand for expanding the program and ensuring the quality of Head Start services, particularly training teachers. The low wages typically paid to Head Start staff precipitate turnover and jeopardize program quality. Economic uncertainty and the vulnerability of young children form the crucible within which child development services are designed. These services consequently are heavily weighted toward ameliorating existing situations rather than improving outcomes in the long term. Nonetheless, evaluations of Head Start emphasize the positive outcomes for most of the children and families who have been enrolled in these services. Not surprisingly, Head Start programs enjoy bipartisan support.

## Home Visiting

Over the past 10 years, home visiting programs, funded by private and public sources, have flourished. Once a strategy for addressing the special needs of immigrant populations, current models build on evidence about the critical early years in a child's life and positive reports from specific home visiting models. All home visiting programs emphasize the delivery of services to young children and their families in their homes and parents' vital role in guiding their child's development. The overarching home visiting model asserts that by seeing the young child in the environment in which the family lives, the home visitor can tailor services to meet the unique needs of the family. In addition, the personal relationship between parents and home visitors bridges the loneliness and isolation between families and their communities. Similar to early intervention programs, home visiting describes a strategy for delivering services rather than a homogeneous or unalterable program. By providing social support and practical assistance, home visitors attempt to stimulate and nurture changes in parents' attitudes, knowledge, and behavior (Gomby, Culross, & Behrman, 1999).

The implementation of home visiting programs varies widely. For example, most programs attempt to prevent child abuse and neglect by improving parenting skills and promoting healthy child development. Some programs also work to improve mothers' lives by supporting their efforts to return to school, to postpone subsequent pregnancies, and to earn a living. Some programs begin during pregnancy, whereas others begin when a child is born or even later. The length of most programs is 2 to 4 years. The background for home visitors ranges from individuals with bachelor's, master's, or nursing degrees to paraprofessionals who live in the communities being served (Gomby, Culross, & Behrman, 1999).

Almost unique among evaluation protocols in the field of maternal and child health, several home visiting programs have attempted to provide evidence for a causal connection between their programs and outcomes by using experimental designs that randomly assign families either to receive home visiting services or to be in control groups that receive other services or no services beyond periodic screenings.

In a review of recent home visiting program evaluations, Gomby Culross, & Behrman, (1999) concluded that results from evaluations are mixed. Furthermore, even evaluations showing a positive effect indicate that improvement is modest. Program evaluators used an array of approaches to assess whether parents' knowledge of child development and parents' perceptions of their effectiveness changed. In some cases, parent self-report scales and observations of mother–children interaction were used. Results from six program evaluations (Gomby, Culross, & Behrman,

1999) document some change in parents' attitudes as a result of the home visiting program, but not necessarily in their behaviors (e.g., Daro, McCurdy, & Harding, 1998). Similarly, despite promoting the importance of prenatal care and the use of preventive health visits, none of the six evaluation studies found improvements in immunization rates or number of well-child visits. Results for assessments of children's development and behavior similarly suggested only modest, if any, improvement. The Nurse Home Visitation Program (Olds et al., 1999) has documented significant benefits to unmarried (largely teenage) women. The young mothers who received home visits had fewer subsequent pregnancies, were more likely to defer second births, spent fewer months on welfare or receiving food stamps, and had fewer problems with arrests and substance abuse than mothers who did not receive home visits. Olds et al. (1999) argued that altering a mother's life course has important implications for her children. A mother's ability to assume responsibilities associated with a steady job and postpone a second pregnancy may make it possible for her to emerge from poverty and focus the efforts on her child.

All home visiting programs depend on changes in parents' behavior to nurture children's health and development. However, the complexity and variety of the family situations affect the consistency with which a home visiting program can be implemented. The results from evaluations of home visiting programs to date suggest that expectations for home visiting programs can only be modest and, most importantly, that home visiting cannot be the only strategy for serving families with young children at risk for poor health and development.

## OUTSTANDING ISSUES

### Child Abuse and Neglect

Public involvement in child protection in the United States can be traced to the case of Mary Ellen, a beaten, emaciated New York City child who was found chained to a bed in her tenement apartment. The New York Society for the Prevention of Cruelty to Animals, in the absence of any analogous agency, public or private, dedicated to the prevention of cruelty to children, took the case to court and won. Subsequently, the N.Y. Society for the Prevention of Cruelty to Children emerged, later becoming the American Humane Association (American Humane Association, 2004).

Child protection remained primarily a responsibility of voluntary agencies until the outcry, prompted by the publication of Kempe's seminal article, "The Battered Child Syndrome," resulted in local and state social service involvement (Kempe, Silverman, Steele, Droegemueller, & Silver, 1962).

The federal government has been directly involved in child abuse and neglect services since 1973, when model Child Abuse and Neglect legislation was first passed (US Congress, 1973). Because social services are under state jurisdiction, the federal government is limited to providing child maltreatment services through grants-in-aid. In the model legislation, the Congress provided funds for state CPS, which defined child maltreatment more or less the same way that the model legislation does, and included mandatory reporting in state legislation. As a result, every state now has a mandatory reporting law, and federal support for child maltreatment services is channeled to states through the social services block grant (Title XX of the Social Security Act).

Overworked and understaffed CPS agencies are constrained to investigate every legitimate report and provide services to the substantiated cases (approximately 30% of all reports), leaving little time, money, or energy for prevention. Public health has been in the forefront of prevention services for families at risk of abuse and neglect (Barber-Madden, Cohn, & Schloesser, 1988), but identifying such families remains a crude science at best. Although there is some evidence that home visiting services can reduce reporting rates among at-risk families, there is no evidence that, short of removing the child from the home, CPS interventions actually reduce the risk of subsequent abuse. Approximately one third of CPS cases are re-reported, and because there is little interest and no funding for rigorous evaluation of CPS, there is no way of knowing if this recidivism rate is higher or lower than would be the case without CPS. The National Study of Child and Adolescent Well-being, a longitudinal study of a representative sample of CPS cases funded by the Administration on Children and Families under Congressional mandate that is following a representative sample of CPS cases, is still in progress as of this writing.

## Child Care

Increasing numbers of preschool children are being cared for outside the home. In 2001, 61% of children from birth through 6 years of age (not yet in kindergarten) received some form of child care on a regular basis from persons other than their parents (Forum on Child and Family Statistics, 2003). This is a consequence of mothers with young children entering the labor force, 57.6% of mothers in married-couple families and 63.8% in families maintained by women (US Department of Labor, 2001). Children from birth through the age of 2 years were more likely to be in home-based care, either with a relative or nonrelative than to be in center-based care. Children ages 3 to 6 years who were not yet in kindergarten were more likely to be in a center-based child care arrangement.

The use of child daycare is not without risk. Strong evidence shows that group child care increases the frequency of infectious diseases among young children. For example, a typical toddler raised at home in the United States may have two episodes of diarrhea a year, whereas a daycare–reared child may have four or more (Haskins & Kotch, 1986). Similarly, the risk of upper respiratory infection is increased among children attending child care. Most of the illnesses that children are exposed to in daycare are annoying but benign. However, the same mode of transmission that increases the risk of diarrhea also increases the risk of hepatitis A. The same mode of transmission that increases the risk of upper respiratory infection also increases the risk of otitis media and meningitis.

The means to prevent the most common form of meningitis in preschoolers, *H. influenza* meningitis, is straightforward—immunization. There is no immunization for diarrhea, however, which may be caused by any of a number of parasites, viruses, and bacteria. Most prevention strategies rely on scrupulous handwashing, which was shown in one study (Black et al., 1981) to reduce diarrhea in child care 50%. However, when Bartlett et al. (1988) replicated their own similar study, they discovered that training child daycare workers to monitor diarrhea episodes in their classrooms resulted in the same reduction in diarrhea that the classrooms whose workers had been trained to wash their hands enjoyed. In the only randomized, controlled trial of handwashing, Kotch et al. (1994) demonstrated a small but significant decrease in severe diarrhea, but no effect on mild diarrhea. More recent studies have corroborated these results (Roberts, 2000; Uhari & Mottonen, 1999) and added reduced parents' days absent from work and reduced prescriptions to the reduction in diarrheal illness outcome.

The picture with respect to injuries among children in out of home care is even less clear, given the absence of any US studies based on community-wide samples of children. Of 156,040 injuries sustained in 1999 playground equipment designed for public use, 13% occurred in child care (US Consumer Product Safety Commission, 2002).

Early studies of injury risk in child care centers that do exist (Rivara, DiGuiseppi, Thompson, & Calonge, 1989; Sachs et al., 1989) identify the playground and particularly playground equipment as potentially hazardous, but rates of injury requiring medical attention or bed rest in center-based care may be no greater than the injury rates reported for similarly aged children reared at home or cared for in family home child care (Kotch et al., 1997). The challenge is to make child care even safer. Adult supervision, safer playground equipment and impact-absorbing playground surfaces, scheduled activities, barriers to exposure to household hazards such as poisonous cleaning substances and medications, and less time spent in the car all contribute to reduced injury risk for children in organized child care centers.

## Homelessness

Congress passed the Stewart B. McKinney Homeless Assistance Act (42 USC 11301, et seq., 1994) in response to the growing crisis of homelessness, particularly the large numbers of homeless families with children (Shinn & Weitzman, 1996). The National Resource Center on Homelessness and Mental Illness refers to individuals who are homeless as "the poorest of the poor" (National Resource Center on Homelessness and Mental Illness, 2003). Homelessness among American families is increasing, and families with children are one of the fastest growing segments of the homeless population. Families with children accounted for 36% of the homeless population (US Conference of Mayors, 2000). Forty-two percent of homeless children are under 5 years of age (National Resource Center on Homelessness and Mental Illness, 2003). The increasing number of homeless families can be attributed in large part to the growth of American families headed by women and economic hardship incurred by single-parent households. According to the National Coalition for the Homeless, poverty and the lack of affordable housing are the principal causes of homelessness (National Coalition for the Homeless, 2001). However, the National Center on Homelessness and Mental Illness identified high rates of other background characteristics: 25% were physically or sexually abused as children, 27% were in foster care or institutions as children, and 21% were homeless as children.

Separation from their families is one of the devastating consequences of homelessness for children. Many women who live in shelters for single adults have children in foster care or other living arrangements. More than half of the cities surveyed by the US Conference of Mayors in 1994 reported that 15% to 30% of children in foster care were removed from their families or remained in foster care primarily because of housing problems. The shift of parents from welfare rolls to low-wage positions exacerbates the situation. Subsidized housing is in such short supply that fewer than one in four TANF families lives in public housing or receives a housing voucher to help them rent a private unit. In addition, housing subsidies are not an option for most families (National Coalition for the Homeless, 2001). In 1998, the gap between the number of affordable housing units and the number of people needing them was the largest on record (Daskal, 1998).

Among the myriad problems they face, homeless children have more severe health problems and less chance of being immunized than other poor children. Although the height-for-age and weight-for-age measurements of homeless children in this study were comparable to those of a national sample of low-income children, 9% of children living in emergency shelters were below the fifth percentile for height and weight.

Homeless children are in fair or poor health at twice the frequency of other children. Homeless children have higher rates of asthma, ear infections, stomach problems, and speech problems (Better Homes Fund, 1999). Mental health problems such as anxiety, depression, and withdrawal are found in 12% of homeless preschool children, and 16% of homeless preschoolers have behavior problems, including severe aggression and hostility. Homeless children are twice as likely to experience hunger and four times as likely to have delayed development. Acts of violence, particularly against their mother, are witnessed by almost 25% of homeless children. The rate of physical and sexual abuse against homeless children occurs at two to three times the rate of other children (National Resource Center on Homelessness and Mental Illness, 2003).

## Foster Care

Broadly, *foster care* refers to out-of-home placements for children who cannot remain with their birth parents largely as a result of maltreatment (The Future of Children, 2004). Over the past 20 years, the number of children who require foster care has grown substantially. Preschool-age children are the largest group of children entering care and the cohort remaining the longest in care. Over the past decade, the number of infants and toddlers coming into foster care has increased by 110% (Dicker, Gordon, & Knitzer, 2002). Concomitantly, the rate of reunification has been declining. Approximately half the children in foster care will be reunited with their parents, but children who entered the foster care system in 1997 had a 13% slower rate of reunification than children who entered in 1990. This trend may be attributable to the 1997 Adoption and Safe Family Act, which encouraged states to promote adoptions and reduced the time parents had to reunify with their children (The Future of Children, 2004). The Child and Family Services Reviews, originally passed in 1994, was the first attempt by the federal government to assess the ability of state child welfare agencies to meet national goals of promoting safety, permanency, and well-being described in established national standards.

Most of the children in foster care have health and/or developmental problems. Rosenfeld et al. (1997) estimated that children in foster care have more acute and chronic health conditions, developmental delay, and emotional maladjustment than children not in foster care. Halfon, Mendonca, and Berkowitz (1995) identified developmental or emotional problems in 83% of foster children 13 to 36 months of age and 92% of foster children 37 to 60 months of age. Approximately 40% of the children in foster care had been born preterm, experienced hearing and vision problems, failure to thrive, and had developmental delay. Parental stress underlying foster home placement may have been generated by the financial and emotional demands of raising a child with a disability (Lessenberry & Rehfeldt, 2004). Children with chronic health conditions and developmental disability are more likely to be the objects of mistreatment than healthy children. Unfortunately, disabilities not only affect the child's development and planning for care (Leslie, Gordon, Ganger, & Gist, 2002) but also stability of foster placement and reunification. The Committee on Early Childhood, Adoption, and Foster Care (American Academy of Pediatrics, 2000) recommended assessment of children within 30 days of placement. However, a national study of child welfare policies in 36 states found that over 40% of the sampling units did not have policies for identifying foster children with emotional or developmental disorders (Leslie et al., 2003).

## Obesity

Childhood obesity is associated with a range of complications that affect a child's risk for poor physical and mental health. Obese children are more likely to develop type II diabetes, cardiovascular disease, orthopedic problems, hypertension, and many other medical and psychological conditions including social rejection and low self-esteem (Strauss, 2000). Although certain individuals may have a greater genetic predisposition to obesity, the prevalence of obesity has occurred far too rapidly for increased prevalence of these genes to account for the epidemic.

The Pediatric Nutrition Surveillance System (PedNSS) monitors the nutritional status of low-income children who participate in federal maternal and child health programs for routine care, nutrition education, and supplemental food. The 2002 PedNSS, which summarized 2001 data, reported that the prevalence of overweight was 13.5% for children aged birth to 5 years old and 14.3% for children 2 to 5 years old. The highest rates were among American Indian or Alaska Native (17.7%) and Hispanic (19.0%) children, and the lowest rates were among black and white children (11.8%). The prevalence of overweight in children 2 to 5 years old has increased steadily from 10.7% in 1992 to 14.3% in 2002. Overweight has increased among all racial and ethnic groups, with the greatest increase occurring among white children. An increase was seen in all racial and ethnic groups except American Indian and Alaska Native children, whose prevalence has remained stable, although consistently higher than all other groups. Findings from PedNSS are consistent with trends found for the increase overweight in children in the US population (Polhamus et al., 2004).

Early recognition and prevention are essential for addressing obesity. Research into conditions that precipitate early childhood obesity has focused on different issues. For example, several studies of the role of breastfeeding and introduction of solid foods during infancy concluded that an infant's dietary patterns alone do not explain the development of overweight in early childhood (Parsons, Power, Logan, & Summerbell, 1999). Other studies have investigated feeding practices among mothers of children 2 to 5 years of age. Baughcum et al. (2001) argued that a mother's feeding practices and her beliefs about a child's desirable weight affect the growing child's ability to regulate his or her own appetite. Although there was not a specific style of feeding that was associated with obesity in young children, low-income mothers had significantly different feeding behaviors from high-income mothers, as measured by the Preschooler Feeding Questionnaire. The impact of having a television in the bedroom on a child's risk of obesity was examined in children ($n = 2,761$) between 1 and 5 years of age. Based on a survey conducted among families enrolled in one of New York State's WIC programs and specific information about the child's height, weight, and body mass index, a television in the child's bedroom was a strong marker of increased risk for being overweight (Dennison, Erb, & Jenkins, 2002). Another survey of participants in the New York City Neighborhood WIC Program was attached to demographic information collected as part of certification for WIC. Nelson, Chiasson, and Ford (2004) concluded that 40% of the children 2 to 4 years of age were or were at risk for overweight.

## CONCLUSION

A social problem becomes a part of a nation's policy agenda when a particular issue catches public attention or when a group with a special interest advocates for its own particular cause. We do not have a national agenda with a child health focus. Rather than being an end to be valued in itself, child health is more often considered a means to some other end, such as literacy. Despite rhetoric to the contrary, the United States, alone among developed countries, has not committed the resources necessary to assure access to an appropriate level of health services nor committed itself to achievable health status standards for its youngest citizens. Rather, it has chosen a categorical approach to child health, ignoring opportunities to address the underlying causes of suboptimal child health. The current legislative process, through US House and Senate committee structures, perpetuates the practice of addressing pervasive social problems from the fragmented perspectives of the many different health and developmental outcomes occurring at the furthest ends of the chain of causality. In fact, the broad array of public programs supported by the federal government is symptomatic of the fact that health status for growing subpopulations of preschool children in the United States has been deteriorating relative to that observed in other developed countries. Perhaps the most serious criticism leveled against the US child health system is that it is neither equitable nor efficient. That is, children who need comprehensive health services the most do not have access to them because of varied program eligibility requirements and inconsistent benefits, and those who do have access pay more than any other children in the developed world. However, even before committing itself to achieving reasonable child health goals, the United States must make a national commitment to children themselves. As of this writing, the country is moving away from such a commitment.

# REFERENCES

American Academy of Pediatrics. (2000). Committee on early childhood and adoption and dependent care: Developmental issues for young children in foster care. *Pediatrics, 106,* 1145–1150.

American Humane Association. (2004). *The story of Mary Ellen.* Available from: http://www.americanhumane.org/site/PageServer?pagename=wh_mission_maryellen [cited] November 24, 2004.

Anderson, J., & Werry, J.S. (1994). Emotional and behavioral disorders. In I.B. Pless (Ed.), *The epidemiology of childhood disorders* (pp. 304–338). New York: Oxford University Press.

Anderson, R.N., & Smith, B.L. (2003). Deaths: Leading causes for 2001. National Vital Statistics Reports; Vol 52, No 9. Hyattsville, Maryland: National Center for Health Statistics, 86 pp.

Arias, E., Anderson, R.A., Kung, H.-C., Murphy, S.L., & Kochanek, K.D. (2003). Deaths: Final data for 2001 (Table 10). *National Vital Statistics Reports, 52*(3), 30–33. Available May 16, 2004, from: http://www.cdc.gov/nchs/data/nvsr/nvsr52/nvsr52_03.pdf

Arias, E., MacDorman, M.F., Strobino, D.M., & Guyer, B. (2003). Annual Summary of Vital Statistics: 2002. *Pediatrics, 112,* 1215–1250.

Barber-Madden, R., Cohn, A., & Schloesser, P. (1988). Prevention of child abuse: A public health agenda. *Journal of Public Health Policy, 9,* 167–176.

Bartlett, A.V., Jarvis, B.A., Ross, V., Katz, T.M., Dalia, M.A., Englender, S.J., & Anderson, L.J. (1988). Diarrheal illness among infants and toddlers in day care centers: Effects of active surveillance and staff training without subsequent monitoring. *American Journal of Epidemiology, 127,* 808–817.

Baughcum, A.D., Powers, S.W., Johnson, S.B., Chamberlin, L.A., Deeks, C.M., Jain, A., & Whitaker, R.C. (2001). Maternal feeding practices and beliefs and their relationships to overweight in early childhood. *Journal of Developmental and Behavioral Pediatrics, 22,* 391–408.

Better Homes Fund. (1999). Homeless children: America's new outcasts. National Center on Family Homelessness. Newton, MA. Available March 28, 2004, from: www.familyhomelessness.org

Black, R.E., Dykes, A.C., Anderson, K.E., Wells, J.G., Sinclair, S.P., Gary, G.W., Jr., Hatch, M.H., & Gangarosa, E.A. (1981). Hand washing to prevent diarrhea in day care centers. *American Journal of Epidemiology, 113,* 445–451.

Brenner, M.H. (1973). Fetal, infant and maternal mortality during periods of economic stress. *International Journal of Health Services, 3,* 145–159.

Bricker, D., Davis, M.S., & Squires, J. (2004, April–June). Mental health screening in young children. *Infants and Young Children, 17,* 129–144.

Brody, D.J., Pirkle, J.L., Kramer, R.A., Flegal, K.M., Matte, T.D., Gunter, E.W., & Paschal, D.C. (1994). Blood lead levels in the US population: Phase 1 of the Third National Health and Nutrition Examination Survey (NHANES III, 1988 to 1991). *Journal of the American Medical Association, 272,* 277–283.

Bronfenbrenner, U., Moen, P., & Garbarino, J. (1984). Child, family, and community. In R.D. Parke (Ed.), *Review of child development research (Vol. 7): Handbook of Early Childhood Intervention.* Chicago, IL: University of Chicago Press, 283–328.

Brooks-Gunn, J., Duncan, G., & Maritato, N. (1997). Poor families, poor outcomes: The well-being of children and youth. In G.J. Duncan & J. Brooks-Gunn (Eds.), *Consequences of growing up poor* (pp. 1–17). New York: Russell Sage Foundation.

Buescher, P., Horton, S., Devaney, B., Roholt, S., Lenihan, A., Whitmire, T., & Kotch, J.B. (2003). Child participation in WIC: Medicaid costs and use of health care services. *American Journal of Public Health, 93,* 145–150.

Campbell, S.B., & Ewing, L.J. (1990). Follow-up of hard-to-manage preschoolers: Adjustment at age 9 and predictors of continuing symptoms. *Journal of Child Psychology and Psychiatry, 31,* 871–889.

Carroll, W.A., & Miller, G.E. (2004). Trends in antibiotic use among US children aged 0 to 4 years, 1996–2000. Agency for Health Research and Quality Statistical Brief #35. Available May 16, 2004, from: http://www.meps.ahrq.gov/papers/st35/stat35.pdf

Casey, A.E. (2000). *Kids count data book 2000: State profiles of child well-being.* Baltimore, MD: Anne E. Casey Foundation.

Centers for Disease Control and Prevention. (1992). Recommendations for the use of folic acid to reduce the number of cases of spina bifida and other neural tube defects. *Morbidity and Mortality Weekly Report, 41,* 1–7.

Centers for Disease Control and Prevention. (1995). Monthly immunization table. *Morbidity and Mortality Weekly Report, 44,* 903.

Centers for Disease Control and Prevention. (2001). Table 32. *Leading causes of death and numbers of deaths, according to age: United States, 1980 and 2001* (Vol. II, Mortality, Part A, 1980). National Center for Health Statistics, National Vital Statistics System, Vital statistics of the United States. Available June 11, 2004, from: http://www.cdc.gov/nchs/data/hus/tables/2003/03hus032.pdf

Centers for Disease Control and Prevention. (2003). *National, state, and urban area vaccination levels among children aged 19–35 months: United States, 2002. MMWR Morbidity and Mortality Weekly Report, 52*(31), 728–732.

Centers for Disease Control and Prevention. (2004). Fatal injuries: Mortality reports. National Center for Injury Prevention and Control. Available March 28, 2004, from:http://webappa.cdc.gov/sasweb/ncipc/output_options_9.htm

Child Trends Data Bank. (2003). Racial and ethnic composition of the child population, Figure 1. Available June 11, 2004, from: www.childtrendsdatabank.org/indicators/60RaceandEthnicComposition.cfm

Costello, E.J., Burns, B.J., Angold, A., & Leaf, P.J. (1993). How can epidemiology improve mental health services for children and adolescents? *Journal of American Academy of Child and Adolescent Psychiatry, 32,* 1106–1114.

Crocker, A. (1989). The spectrum of medical care for developmental disabilities. In I.L. Rubin & A.C. Crocker (Eds.), *Developmental disabilities: Delivery of medical care for children and adults* (pp. 10–29). London: Lea and Feiber.

Dalaker, J. (2001). *Poverty in the United States 2000, Current Population Reports. Series P60-214.* Washington, DC: US Census Bureau, US Government Printing Office.

Danaher, J. (2001). Eligibility policies and practices for young children under Part B of IDEA. *NECTAC Notes,* Issue No 9, 1–17.

Danaher, J., Kraus, R., Armijo, C., & Hipps, C. (Eds.). (2003). Section 619 profile (12th ed.). Chapel Hill: The University of North Carolina, FPG Child Development Institute, National Early Childhood Technical Assistance Center.

Daro, D., McCurdy, K., & Harding, K. (1998). *The role of home visiting in preventing child abuse: An evaluation of the Hawaii Healthy Start Program.* Chicago: National Committee to Prevent Child Abuse.

Daskal, J. (1998). *In search of shelter: The growing shortage of affordable rental housing.* Washington, DC: Center on Budget and Policy Priorities.

Decoufle, P., Yeargin-Allsopp, M., Boyle, C.A., & Doernberg, N.S. (1994). Developmental disabilities. In L.S. Wilcox & J.S. Marks (Eds.), *From data to action* (pp. 335–350). Atlanta, GA: Centers for Disease Control and Prevention.

Dennison, B.A., Erb, T.A., & Jenkins, P.L. (2002). Television viewing and television in bedroom associated with overweight risk among low-income preschool children. *Pediatrics, 109,* 1028–1035.

Dicker, W.L., Gordon, E., & Knitzer, J. (2002). *Improving the odds for the healthy development of young children in foster care* (Policy Paper No. 2). New York: National Center for Children in Poverty, Promoting the Emotional Well-Being of Children and Families Series.

Edmonds, L.D., Layde, P.M., James, L.M., Plynt, J.W., Erickson, J.D., & Oakley, G.P., Jr. (1981). Congenital malformations surveillance: Two American systems. *International Journal of Epidemiology, 10,* 247–252.

Erikson, E.H. (1950). *Childhood and society* (2nd ed.). New York: W.W. Norton and Co.

Feeley, T.J. (2000). *Low income non-custodial fathers: A child advocates' guide to helping them contribute to the support of their children.* Washington, DC: National Association of Child Advocates, Issue Brief, National Association of Child Advocates. Available November 7, 2002, from http://www.childadvocacy.org/

Fingerhut, L.A. (1989). *Trends and current status in childhood mortality, United States, 1900–1985* (Series 3, No. 26. DHHS Pub. No. [PHS] 89-1410). Washington, DC: US Department of Health and Human Services, Public Health Service, Centers for Disease Control, National Center for Health Statistics.

Forum on Child and Family Statistics. (2003). "Childhood immunization" in *America's Children: Key National Indicators of Well-Being.* [available] May 16, 2004, from: http://www.childstats.gov/ac2003/indicators.asp?IID=123&id=4

Gomby, D.S., Culross, P.L., & Behrman, R.E. (1999, Spring/Summer). Home visiting: Recent program evaluations—analysis and recommendations. *The Future of Children, Vol. 9*(1), 4–26.

Gorman, K.S., & Pollitt, E. (1996). Does schooling buffer the effects of early risk? *Child Development, 67,* 314–326.

Gortmaker, S., & Wise, P. (1994). *The first economic injustice: Socioeconomic disparities in infant mortality in the United States: Theoretical and policy perspectives* (Society and Health Working Paper Series No. 94-4). Boston, MA: Society and Health Working Group, The Health Institute, New England Medical Center and Harvard School of Public Health.

Grolier Library of North American Biographies. (1994). *Activists* (Vol. 1, pp. 15–16). Danbury, CT: Grolier Educational Corporation.

Guralnick, M.J. (1998). Effectiveness of early intervention for vulnerable children: A developmental perspective. *American Journal on Mental Retardation, 102,* 319–345.

Guyer, B., Freedman, M.A., Strobino, D.M., & Sondik, E.J. (2000). Annual summary of vital statistics: Trends in the health of Americans during the 20th century. *Pediatrics, 106,* 1307–1317.

Halfon, J.S., Mendonca, A., & Berkowitz, G. (1995). Health status of children in foster care. *Archives of Pediatric and Adolescent Medicine, 149,* 386–392.

Harbin, G., & Danaher, J. (1994). Comparison of eligibility policies for infant/toddler programs and preschool special education programs. *Topics in Early Childhood Special Education, 14,* 455–471.

Hardy, A.M. (1991). *Incidence and impact of selected infectious diseases in childhood.* National Center for Health Statistics. Vital Health Stat, 10(180) DHHS Pub. No. (PHS) 91-1508).

Harvey, B. (1991). Why we need a national child health policy. *Pediatrics, 87,* 1–6.

Haskins, R., & Kotch, J.B. (1986). Day care and illness: Evidence, costs, and public policy. *Pediatrics, 77*(6 Suppl), 951–982.

Health, US. (2003). National Center for Health Statistics (Table 45). Available June 17, 2004, from: http://www.cdc.gov/nchs/data/hus/tables/2003/03hus045.pdf.

Herman-Giddens, M.E. (1991). Underreporting of child abuse and neglect fatalities in North Carolina. *North Carolina Medical Journal, 52,* 634–639.

Holahan, J., Dubay, L., & Kenney, G. (2003). Which children are still uninsured and why. *Health Insurance for Children, The Future of Children, 13*(1), 55–79.

Humphrey, H.H. (1972, August 16). *Congressional record.* US Congress, 92d congress, 2d session, S28588. Government Printing Office, Washington, DC.

Hutt, M.L., & Gibby, R.G. (1976). *The mentally retarded child: Development, education and treatment* (3rd ed.). Boston, MA: Allyn and Bacon.

Kawachi, I., Kennedy, B.P., Lochner, K., & Prothow-Stith, D. (1997). Social capital, income inequality, and mortality. *American Journal of Public Health, 87*(9), 1491–1498.

Kempe, C.H., Silverman, F.N., Steele, B.F., Droegemueller, W., & Silver, H.K. (1962). The battered child syndrome. *Journal of the American Medical Association, 181,* 17–24.

Kennedy, E.T., & Kotelchuck, M. (1984). The effect of WIC supplemental feeding birth weight: A case-control analysis. *American Journal of Clinical Nutrition, 40,* 579–585.

Knitzer, J. (2000). Early childhood mental health programs. In J. Shonkoff & S. Meisels (Eds.), *Handbook of early childhood intervention* (2nd ed., pp. 906–956). New York: Cambridge University Press.

Knitzer, J. (2002). *Promoting resilience: Helping young children and parents affected by substance abuse, domestic violence, and depression in the context of welfare reform* (Children and welfare reform Issue Brief 8). New York: National Center for Children in Poverty, Columbia University.

Kotch, J.B., & Whiteman, D. (1982). Effect of a WIC program on children's clinic activity in a local health department. *Medical Care, 20,* 691–698.

Kotch, J.B., Chalmers, D.J., Fanslow, J.L., Marshall, S., & Langley, J.D. (1993). Morbidity and death due to child abuse in New Zealand. *Child Abuse and Neglect, 17,* 233–247.

Kotch, J.B., Dufort, V.M., Stewart, P., Fieberg, J., McMurray, M., O'Brien S., Ngui, E.M., & Brennan, M. (1997). Injuries among children in home and out-of-home care. *Injury Prevention, 3,* 267–271.

Kotch, J.B., Weigle, K.A., Weber, D.J., Clifford R.M., Harms, T.O., Loda, F.A., Gallagher, P.N., Jr., Edwards, R.W., LaBorde, D., McMurray, M.P., Rolandelli, P.S., & Faircloth, A.H. (1994). Evaluation of an hygienic intervention in child day-care centers. *Pediatrics, 94*(6 Suppl), 991–994.

Lavigne, J.V., Gibbons, R.D., Christoffel, K.K., Arend, R., Rosenbaum, D., Binns, H., Dawson, N., Sobel, H., & Isaacs, C. (1996). Prevalence rates and correlates of psychiatric disorders among preschool children. *Journal of the American Academy of Child and Adolescent Psychiatry, 35*(2), 204–214.

Lee, J.Y., Rozier, R.G., Kotch, J.B., Norton, E.C., & Vann, W.F., Jr. (2004). The effects of child WIC participation on use of oral health services. *American Journal of Public Health, 94*(5), 772–777.

Lennon, M.C., Blome, J., & English, K. (Eds.). (2001). *Depression and low-income women: Challenges for TANF and welfare-to-work policies and programs.* New York: National Center for Poverty, Columbia University.

Leslie, L.K., Gordon, J.N., Ganger, W., & Gist, K. (2002). Developmental delay in young children in child welfare by initial placement type. *Infant Mental Health Journal, 23,* 496–516.

Leslie, L.K., Hurlburt, M.S., Landsverk, J., Rolls, J.A., Wood, P.A., & Kelleher, K.J. (2003). Comprehensive assessments for children entering foster care: A national perspective. *Pediatrics, 112,* 134–141.

Lessenberry, B.M., & Rehfeldt, R.A. (2004). Evaluating stress levels of parents of children with disabilities. *Exceptional Children, 70,* 231–244.

Lynberg, M.C., & Edmonds, L.D. (1992). Surveillance of birth defects. In W. Halperin & E. Baker (Eds.), *Public health surveillance.* New York: Van Nostrand Reinhold.

Margolis, L.H., Sparrow, A.W., & Swanson, G.M. (1989). *Growing into healthy adults: Pediatric antecedents of adult disease.* Lansing, MI: Michigan Department of Public Health.

Martin, J.A., Hamilton, B.E., Sutton, P.D., Ventura, S.J., Menaker, F., & Munson, M.L. (2003). *Births: Final data for 2002* (Vol 52, no. 10): *National vital statistics reports.* Hyattsville, MD: National Center for Health Statistics.

Meyer, J. (2001). *Age 2000: Census 2000 brief.* Washington, DC: US Department of Commerce, Economics and Statistics Administration, US Census Bureau.

Morgan, D.R., & Kickham, K. (2001). Children in poverty: Do state policies matter? *Social Science Quarterly, 82*(3), 478–493.

National Alliance for the Mentally Ill. (2000, October 30). *Families on the brink: Executive summary: The impact of ignoring children with serious mental illness.* Available May 10, 2004, from: http://www.nami.org/youth/brink3/html

National Center for Health Statistics. (1995). *Health, United States, 1994.* Hyattsville, MD: US Public Health Service.

National Center for Injury Prevention and Control, Office of Programming and Statistics. (2001). *10 Leading causes of death by age group—2001.* Centers for Disease Control and Prevention. Available March 28, 2004, from: http://www.cdc.gov/ncipc/osp/charts.htm

National Coalition for the Homeless. (2001). *Homeless families with children: NCH Fact Sheet #7.* Available March 18, 2004, from: http://www.national homelessness.org/families.html

National Resource Center on Homelessness and Mental Illness. (2003, June 6). *Substance Abuse and Mental Health Services Administration, US Department of Health and Human Services.* Available March 18, 2004, from: http://www. nrchmi.samhsa.gov/facts/default.asp

Nelson, J.A., Chiasson, M.A., & Ford, V. (2004). Childhood overweight in a New York City WIC population. *American Journal of Public Health, 94,* 458–462.

Nelson, K., & Holmes, L.B. (1989). Malformation due to presumed spontaneous mutations in newborn infants. *New England J Medicine, 320,* 19–23.

Nelson, M.D. (1992). Socioeconomic status and childhood mortality in North Carolina. *American Journal of Public Health, 82,* 1131–1133.

Nersesian, W.S., Petit, M.R., Shaper, R., Lemieux, D., & Naor, E. (1985). Childhood death and poverty: A study of childhood deaths in Maine, 1976–1980. *Pediatrics, 75,* 41–50.

Oberg, C.N. (1987). Pediatrics and poverty. *Pediatrics, 79,* 567–569.

Olds, D.I., & Kitzman, H. (1993). Review of research on home visiting for pregnant women and parents of young children. *The Future of Children, 3,* 53–90.

Olds, D.L., Henderson, C.R., Kitzman, H.J., Eckenrode, J.J., Cole, R.E., & Tatelbaum, R.C. (1999). Prenatal and infancy home visiting by nurses: Recent findings. *The Future of Children Home Visiting: Recent Program Evaluations, 9,* 44–65.

Parsons, T.J., Power, C., Logan, S., & Summerbell, C.D. (1999). Childhood predictors of adult obesity: A systematic review. *International Journal of Obesity Related Metabolism Disorders, 23*(Suppl 8), S1–S107.

Polhamus, B., Dalenius, K., Thompson, D., Scanlon, K., Borland, E., Smith, B., & Grummer-Strawn, L. (2004). *Pediatric nutrition surveillance 2002 report.* Atlanta: US Department of Health and Human Services, Centers for Disease Control and Prevention.

Rhoades, J.A., & Cohen, J.W. (2003). *AHRQ statistical brief #28 health insurance status of children in America: 1996–2002: Estimates for the non-institutionalized population under age 18.* Available from: http://www.meps.ahrq.gov/papers/st28/stat28.pdf

Rhoades, J.A., Vistnes, J.P., & Cohen, J.W. (2002). *The uninsured in America: 1996–2000.* Rockville, MD: Agency for Healthcare Research and Quality.

Rice, D.P., MacKenzie, E.J., & Associates. (1989). *Cost of injury in the United States: A report to Congress.* San Francisco, CA: Institute for Health and Aging, University of California and Injury Prevention Center, The Johns Hopkins University.

Rivara, F.P., DiGuiseppi, C., Thomson R.S., & Calonge, N. (1989). Risk of injury to children less than five years of age in day care versus home care settings. *Pediatrics, 84,* 1011–1016.

Roberts, S. (1994). *Who we are.* New York: *The New York Times.*

Roberts, L., Jorm, L., Patel, M., Smith, W., Douglas, R.M., & McGilchrist, C. (2000). Effect of infection control measures on the frequency of diarrheal episodes in child care: A randomized, controlled trial. *Pediatrics, 105*(4 Pt 1), 743–746.

Rose, D., Habicht, J.P., & Devaney, B. (1998). Household participation in the Food Stamp and WIC programs increase the nutrient intakes of preschool children. *The Journal of Nutrition, 128,* 548–555.

Rosenfeld, A., Pilowsky, D., Fine, P., Thorpe, M., Fein, E., Simms, M., Halfon, N., Irwin, M., Alfaro, J., Saletsky, R., & Nickman, S. (1997). Foster care: An update. *Journal of the American Academy of Child and Adolescent Psychiatry, 36*(4), 448–456.

Rush, D., Alvir, J.M., Horvitz, D.G., Seaver, W.B., Garbowski, C.G., Johnson S.S., Kulka, R.A., & Devore, J.W. (1988). The national WIC evaluation: Evaluation of the special supplemental food program for women, infants and children. *American Journal of Clinical Nutrition, 48,* 389–519.

Sachs, J.J., Smith, J.D., Kaplan, K.M., Lambert, D.A., Sattin, R.W., & Sikes, R.K. (1989). The epidemiology of injuries in Atlanta day care centers. *Journal of the American Medical Association, 262,* 1641–1645.

Schramm, W.F. (1986). Prenatal participation in WIC related to Medicaid costs for Missouri newborns: 1982 Update. *Public Health Reports, 101,* 607–615.

Scott, K.G., & Masi, W. (1979). The outcome from and utility of registers of risk. In T.M. Field, A.M. Sostek, S. Goldberg, & H.H. Shuman (Eds.), *Infants born at risk.* New York: Spectrum Publications.

Sedlack, A.J., & Broadhurst, D.D. (1996). Third national incidence study of child abuse and neglect. Washington, DC: US Department of Health and Human Services.

Shackelford, J. (2004). *State and jurisdictional eligibility definitions for infants and toddlers with disabilities under IDEA* (NECTAC Notes No. 14). Chapel Hill: The University of North Carolina, FPG Child Development Institute, National Early Childhood Technical Assistance Center.

Shinn, M., & Weitzman, B. (1996). Homeless families are different. In J. Baumohl (Ed.), *Homelessness in America*. Phoenix, AZ: Oryx Press.

Shonkoff, J.P., & Meisels, S.J. (Eds.). (2000). *Handbook of early childhood intervention*. New York: Cambridge University Press.

Simpson, L., Zodet, M.S., Chevarley, F.M., Owens, P.L., Dougherty, D., & McCormick, M. (2004). Health care for children and youth in the United States: 2002: Report on trends in access, utilization, quality, and expenditures. *Ambulatory Pediatrics, 4,* 131–153.

Squires, J.K. (2000). Identifying social/emotional and behavioral problems in infants and toddlers. *Infant-Toddler Intervention, 10*(2), 107–119.

Starfield, B. (1982). Family income, ill health, and medial care of US children. *J Public Health Policy, 3,* 244–259.

Strauss, R.S. (2000). Childhood obesity and self-esteem. *Pediatrics, 105*(1), e15.

Taylor, M.L., & Koblinsky, S.A. (1993). Dietary intake and growth status of young homeless children. *Journal of the American Dietetic Association, 93,* 464–466.

The Future of Children. (2004, Winter). Children, families, and foster care. *14*(1).

Uhari, M., & Mottonen, M. (1999). An open randomized controlled trial of infection prevention in child day-care centers. *Pediatric Infectious Disease Journal, 18*(8), 672–677.

Upshur, C.C. (1990). Early intervention as preventive intervention. In S.J. Meisels & J.P. Shonkoff (Eds.), *Handbook of early childhood intervention*. New York: Cambridge University Press.

US Census Bureau. (2000). *Population division: Population by age, sex, race, and Hispanic or Latino Origin for the United States: 2000 (PHC-T-9)*. Available July 28, 2004, from: http://www.census.gov/population/www/cen2000/phc-t9.html

US Census Bureau. (2004). *Population division: Population estimates*. Available March 29, 2004, from: http://eire.census.gov/popest/data/states/ST-EST2003-01.php

US Conference of Mayors. (2000). *A status report on hunger and homelessness in America's cities: 2000*. Washington, DC.

US Congress. (1973). Child Abuse Prevention and Treatment Act, PL 93-247.

US Consumer Product Safety Commission. (2002). *Playground-related statistics*. Available July 8, 2004, from: http://www.uni.edu/playground/resources/statistics.html

USDA, Food and Nutrition Service, Nutrition Program Facts (2004). *WIC. The Special Supplemental Nutrition Program for Women, Infants and Children*. [available] November, 2004, from: http://www.fns.usda.gov/wic/WIC-FactSheet.pdf [cited] November 24, 2004.

US Department of Health and Human Services, Administration on Children, Youth and Families. *Child Maltreatment 2002*. Washington DC: US Government Printing Office, 2004.

US Department of Education. (2001). *24th Annual report to Congress on the implementation of the Individuals with Disabilities Education Act.* Washington, DC: US Government Printing Office.

US Department of Health, Education and Welfare, Public Health Service, Health Services Administration, Bureau of Community Health Services. (1976). *Child health in America* (DHEW Publication No. [HSA] 76-5015). Government Printing Office, Rockville, MD.

US Department of Labor. (2001). *Employment characteristics of families in 2001.* Bureau of Labor Statistics. Washington, DC.

US DHHS. (2000). Head Start Bureau. Administration for Children and Families. Washington, DC.

US DHHS. (2004). Head Start Bureau. *Head start program performance standards and other regulations.* Administration for Children and Families, Administration on Children, Youth and Families. Washington, DC.

US DHHS, ACYF. (2004). *Child maltreatment 2002: Reports from the states to the national child abuse and neglect data systems.* National statistics on child abuse and neglect. Washington, DC: USGPO.

US DHHS/HRSA/MCHB, *Child Health USA.* (2002). Available May 16, 2004, from: http://www.mchb.hrsa.gov/chusa02/main_pages/page_03.htm

US Public Health Service. (1991). International Classification of Disease, Ninth Revision, Clinical Modification. US Department of Health and Human Services, Health Care Financing Administration. DHHS Publication No. (PHS) 91-1260.

Utley, R.M. (1993). *The lance and the shield* (p. 7). New York: Ballentine.

Waitzman, N.J., Scheffler, R.M., & Romano, P.S. (1996). *The cost of birth defects.* New York: University Press of America.

Webster-Stratton, C. (1997). Early intervention for families of preschool children with conduct problems. In M. Guralnick (Ed.), *The effectiveness of early intervention* (pp. 429–453). Baltimore, MD: Brookes.

Wood, D. (2003). Effect of child and family poverty on child health in the United States. *Pediatrics, 112*(3), 707–711.

Woodruff, G., & Sterzin, E.D. (1993). Family support services for drug- and AIDS-affected families. In R.P. Barth, J. Pietrzak, & M. Ramler (Eds.), *Families living with drugs and HIV* (pp. 219–237). New York: Guilford Press.

Yoon, P.W., Olney, R.S., Khoury, M.J., Sappenfield, W.M., Chavez, G.F., & Taylor, D. (1997). Contribution of birth defects and genetic diseases to pediatric hospitalizations. *Archives of Pediatric and Adolescent Medicine, 151.*

Zigler, E., Piotrkowski, C.S., & Collins, R. (1994). Health services in Head Start. *Annual Review of Public Health, 15,* 511–534.

CHAPTER 7

# The School-Age Child

*Joseph Telfair and Jonathan B. Kotch*

> *"When I was born in 1920, if you wanted to visit your family on Sundays you . . . went to the graveyard . . . My brother and sister died when I was seven. Half of my family was gone! Tell me, dear children, how many of your friends died while you were growing up?"*
> *"None," said Rodney at last.*
> *"None! You hear that? . . . Six of my best friends died by the time I was ten!"* (Bradbury, 1994, pp. 133, 135)

## INTRODUCTION

The transition to school for any child, whether reared primarily at home or with significant experience in out-of-home care, is the most profound transition for most children until the transition to work or residential college. Upon school entry, the child becomes a worker, responsible for "producing things" (Erikson, 1950, p. 259). Although success in making this transition does not guarantee future health and happiness, in the developed world these days, it is a rare individual who can become a healthy and productive adult after a failed career in school. Indeed, years of completed education are a powerful predictor of health status. Applying regression techniques to data from the National Vital Statistics System, the National Longitudinal Mortality Study, and the Area Resource File, Singh and Yu (1996) concluded, "The lower the level of educational attainment and the greater the poverty, the higher the childhood mortality rates" (p. 512).

The child entering the realm of formal education moves from a learning style based mostly on personal contacts to one based on symbols. The child's world expands from the familiar, circumscribed environment of direct experience to one whose history extends back over centuries and forward infinitely in time and space (Dewey, 1956). As his or her physical and intellectual worlds expand, so do physical risks. It is in the early school years that injury becomes the cause of nearly half (46%) of all childhood deaths (Anderson & Smith, 2003). In this chapter, we review the demography, health status, health services, and health programs affecting US children who are 5 to 9 years of age.

# DEMOGRAPHICS

Currently, children who are 5 to 9 years old constitute 7.3% of the American population (US Census Bureau, 2000). The US population of children who are 5 to 9 years old declined from 1970 to 1980 and then increased in 1990. By 2000, US children 5 to 9 years old numbered approximately 20,549,505. There were 10,523,277 boys and 10,026,228 girls (US Census Bureau, 2000). The racial composition of the population is as follows: there were 13,944,882 white children, 3,205,512 African American children, 239,007 American Indian and Alaska Native children, 2,464,999 Asian children, 127,179 Native Hawaiian and other Pacific Islander children, and 3,623,680 Hispanic children (US Census Bureau, 2000).

## Family Structure

Within the last decade, the percentage of families with children has increased slightly. In 2000, 52.2% of all families had related children who were less than 18 years of age present (US Census Bureau, 2000). The decline in the proportion of households with children less than the age of 18 years is an important component in the overall decline in household and family size over the last 30 years. Households with their own children decreased from 45% of all households in 1970 to 35% in 1990 and 33% in 2000 (US Census Bureau, 2000).

In 1970, there were only 3 million single-mother families and 393,000 single-father families (Fields & Casper, 2001). By 2000, the number of one-parent families had increased to 12 million, of which 10 million were maintained by the mother. The percentage of families maintained by a single-parent varies greatly by race, with 19.8% for whites, 58.1% for African Americans, 38.8% for American Indian/Alaska Native, 17.1% for Asians, and 28.7% for Hispanics (US Census Bureau, 2000).

### Children and Poverty

In 2000, 8.4% of married couple families with children under 18 years old were below the poverty line compared with 40.6% of families of female householders with children less than 18 years old (US Census Bureau, 2000). This contrast by family structure is especially pronounced among certain racial and ethnic groups. For example, in 2000, 8% of black children in married-couple families lived in poverty compared with 49% of black children in female-householder families. Twenty-one percent of Hispanic children in married-couple families lived in poverty compared with 48% in female-householder families (see Table 7–1) (US Census Bureau, 2000).

## HEALTH STATUS

The years from 5 to 9 are the healthiest of any age bracket in the United States if judged by the mortality rate, 15.3 per 100,000 in 2001 (Anderson & Smith, 2003). Between 1980 and 1999, the death rate declined by almost one third, from 31 to 19 deaths per 100,000 children ages 5 to 14 years old. Major concerns in child health have shifted from "natural causes" (infectious diseases primarily) to so-called new morbidities (injury-related mortality and morbidity; psychological, emotional, and learning disorders; and chronic physical and developmental condi-

**Table 7–1** Percentage of Poverty by Household Type and Race for US Children, 2000

| Household Type | All (%) | White (%) | Hispanic (%) | Black (%) |
|---|---|---|---|---|
| All | 16.2 | 6.9 | 18.5 | 19.1 |
| Married | 8.2 | 4.4 | 14.1 | 6.1 |
| Female-headed household | 39.8 | 20.0 | 34.2 | 34.6 |

Source: US Census Bureau, 2000.

tions) (Maternal and Child Health Bureau, 1991). Improved living standards, community-based health promotion and disease prevention, and effective immunization against infectious diseases have all made major contributions in reducing childhood mortality and morbidity in this century. Nevertheless, the United States is still behind other industrialized nations in childhood mortality, primarily because if excess deaths attributable to injury (Williams & Kotch, 1990). The majority of unintentional injury deaths among children 5 to 14 years old resulted from motor vehicle traffic crashes. In 1999, more than 65% of children 5 to 14 years old who died in traffic crashes were not wearing a seatbelt or other restraint (Health Resources and Services Administration, 2001b). Although seat belt use and other safety measures (such as child proof safety caps, smoke detectors, bicycle helmets, flame-retardant clothing) have reduced mortality rates caused by unintentional injury, rates of death because of violence rose among children until about 1991 in the case of homicide (Fox & Zawitz, 2003) and 1994 in the case of suicide (Snyder & Swahn, 2003). Both declined somewhat since then without reaching the levels of the 1960s.

# EPIDEMIOLOGY OF MAJOR HEALTH PROBLEMS

## Natural Causes

Death rates in this age group declined 66% from 1900 to 1933, 62.5% between 1933 and 1950, 33.3% from 1950 to 1970, and 50% from 1970 to 1985 (Fingerhut, 1989). That 50% decline was the highest of any age bracket among all people in the United States. Deaths among US 5- to 9-year-old children declined another 19.2% between 1985 and 1998 (CDC Wonder, 2004). Over the course of the 20th century, from 1900 and 1998, the death rate for 5–9 year olds in the United States declined 96%. Because natural causes were declining faster than external causes (e.g., 69% between 1933 and 1950 for natural causes compared with 35% for external causes) (Fingerhut, 1989), the proportion of all deaths attributable to external causes has been increasing. In 1900, an estimated 89.9% of child deaths were due to natural causes. Sometime between 1970 and 1971, natural causes resulted in fewer than 50% of deaths among US 5- to 9-year-old children for the first time in history (Fingerhut, 1989).

## Infectious Diseases

In 1900, diphtheria alone caused 10% of all deaths in US school-aged children (Fingerhut, 1989). By 1992, there was no infectious disease among the top five killers of such children (Maternal and Child Health Bureau, 1995; Guyer, Freedman, Strobino, & Sondik, 2000). On the other hand, infectious disease is the leading cause of visits to the doctor for sick care (Hardy, 1991) and a major cause of hospitalization in this age group (Maternal and Child Health Bureau, 1995).

The 1988 Child Health Supplement to the National Health Interview Survey (NHIS-CHS) (National Center for Health Statistics, 1989) asked respondents about nine of the most common childhood infectious diseases. Using a 7-year age bracket (5 to 11), the survey discovered that repeated ear infections were the most common complaint in the past year (8.8%), followed by repeated tonsillitis (5.5%). Half of school-age children who had either condition had to limit their activity. Pneumonia was the leading infectious disease cause of hospitalization, but children with mononucleosis were hospitalized longer. Children in the 5- to 11-year-old bracket were the most likely to have surgery for repeated tonsillitis or repeated ear infections, to lose the most school days and spend more time in bed because of mononucleosis, and to see the doctor for repeated tonsillitis and bladder or urinary infections (Hardy, 1991).

## Chronic Illness

In 1998, the Maternal and Child Health Bureau defined children with special health needs or chronic conditions as "children with special health care needs are those who have or are at increased risk for a chronic physical, developmental, behavioral, or emotional condition and who also require health and related services of a type or amount beyond that required by children generally" (McPherson et al., 1998, p. 138). Approximately 14 million children have mild to moderate chronic problems such as persistent ear infections, respiratory allergies, asthma, eczema and skin allergies, and speech defects. Another, 10%, approximately 7 million children, have one or more severe chronic conditions, such as congenital heart defects, neural tube defects, juvenile diabetes mellitus, sickle cell disease, or HIV infections (Institute of Medicine, 1998). Expenditures for this group account for 70% to 80% of all medical expenditures for all children (Institute of Medicine, 1998). Data from the new National Health Interview Survey on Disability (NHIS-D) (1994) survey suggest that 16% to 18% of US children under age of 18 years have chronic physical, developmental, behavioral, or emotional conditions having some degree of functional impact or requiring services (Newacheck & Halfon, 1998). The most recent prevalence reports from 1992 indicate that for children under the age of 18 years, the most prevalent conditions included respiratory allergies (9.7%), asthma (4.2%), eczema and skin allergies (3.3%), frequent or severe headaches (2.5%), and speech defects (2.6%). Diabetes (0.1%), sickle cell disease (0.1%), and cerebral palsy (0.2%) were among the less prevalent conditions (Newacheck & Taylor, 1992). However, the prevalence of these conditions is higher in certain populations (e.g., the prevalence of sickle cell disease for blacks is 1 in 400). Furthermore, the severity of chronic conditions for children less than 18 years of age varies. For example, 20% were mildly affected. Nine percent of children experienced more than occasional bother or limitation of activity, but not both, and 2% were severely affected (Newacheck & Taylor, 1992).

The absolute numbers of children with chronic illness are not expected to change dramatically in the coming decades (Newacheck & Taylor, 1992). Although more children with chronic conditions will survive because of improvements in medical technology and practice, these increases will be offset by demographic trends leading to fewer births (National Center for Health Statistics, 1995). Nonetheless, the prevalence of children with chronic conditions continues to increase. Growing populations of children with special health care needs include those with HIV infection and the population of children who are dependent on advanced medical technology such as ventilators, gastrostomies, and tracheostomies (Palfrey et al., 1991). However, improvements in diagnosis (e.g., asthma, hearing impairments) and longer survival because of medical advances (e.g., cystic fibrosis) are credited in the increasing prevalence of certain diseases (Richardson, 1989; Schidlow & Fiel, 1990). A fuller discussion of chronic illness in children by A. Farel is in Chapter 11 of this volume.

## Mental Health

In previous decades, emotional and behavioral problems among children were treated because they were seen as precursors of adult disorders. More recently, these problems have come to be seen as also important in their own right (Drotar & Bush, 1985). The President's New Freedom Commission on Mental Health reports that between 5% and 9% of school-age children suffer from serious emotional disorders, manifesting in impairments that range from behavioral problems to depression. Findings from the 1992 to 1994 NHIS-D and related studies suggest that between 17% to 22% of children birth to 17 years old suffer from some form of diagnosable mental illness, indicating that the use of psychologic assistance for children had increased by more than 7% to 12% since results of the 1988 NHIS-CHS results were published (Halfon & Newacheck, 1998).

Data from the 1988 NHIS-CHS indicate that the cumulative proportion of children who have ever had emotional or behavioral problems should increase fairly steadily with age. The proportion of children who had ever had an emotional or behavioral problem rose from 5.3% at the age of 3–5 years, to 12.7% at ages 6–11 years, to 18.5% at ages 12–17 years. One quarter emerged during the preschool years (3–5) and another quarter during the early elementary years (6–8). Twenty-two percent became evident during the adolescent years (12–17). Increases in childhood psychological disorders have been attributed to the growing proportions of children who experience parental divorce, were born outside of marriage, or are raised in conflict-filled families or low-income, low-education, single-parent households (Zill & Schoenborn, 1990).

NHIS-CHS data also indicate that the prevalence of childhood emotional and behavioral problems showed significant variation across family income groups, with children from less advantaged backgrounds standing a somewhat greater chance of exhibiting such problems (Zill & Schoenborn, 1990). The prevalence declined from 15.8% among children from families with incomes less than $10,000 per year or 12.8% among those with family incomes of $40,000 or more (Zill & Schoenborn, 1990). Income-related differences were more pronounced among elementary school children and adolescents than among preschoolers.

Furthermore, the 1988 NHIS-CHS indicates that the prevalence of childhood emotional and behavioral problems varied by differences in family structure. The prevalence of emotional and behavioral problems was 8.3% in mother–father families, 19.1% in mother-only families, 23.6% in mother–stepfather families, and 22.2% in other family situations (Zill & Schoenborn, 1990). However, the frequency of problems among children in mother-only families may have been understated because of the large proportions of black and Hispanic persons in this group (Zill & Schoenborn, 1990). Although mental health problems are relatively common among children, especially among those with health problems (Drotar, 1981; Goldberg et al., 1979), most cases are mild and resolve without treatment. Nonetheless, there is a core of persistent, disabling disorders—notably conduct disorder, multiple disorders, autism, and child schizophrenia—that require focused and sustained treatment. Data from the 1988 NHIS-CHS indicate that the overall prevalence of emotional or behavioral problems was 13.4% of all children 3–17 years old. By 1996, the 6-month prevalence of any mental or additive disorders among 9–17 year olds was reported by the Surgeon General to be 20% (Children and Mental Health, 2004). Yet just 10% of these had ever received counseling or treatment (Zill & Schoenborn, 1990). This fact should be of great concern to Maternal and Child Health practitioners in that (1) the etiology of most childhood emotional and behavioral problems is not well understood, (2) many providers have not been adequately trained to recognize and deal with these types of problems, and (3) procedures for referring children for psychological diagnosis and treatment are not standardized. Thus, there is believed to be a substantial group of young people with developmental or behavioral disorders whose problems go untreated and perhaps even unrecognized (Silverman & Koretz, 1989). Because of the significant life stresses faced by children with emotional and behavioral difficulties, untreated mental health problems can often lead to further difficulties in adolescence and adulthood. There is growing recognition that prevention and early intervention work to reduce the prevalence of, or the consequences of, mental health problems in children (Children and Mental Health, 2004).

### Developmental Disabilities

In 1984, The Developmental Disabilities Act (PL 98-527) referred to a developmental disability as a "severe, chronic condition attributable to a mental or physical impairment, manifest before the age of 22 and likely to continue indefinitely." More recently, the Developmental Disabilities Assistance and Bill of Rights Act Amendments of 1999 define the concept of developmental concerns of young children "to include both substantial developmental delays or specific congenital or acquired conditions that will likely result in substantial functional limitations in three or more major life activities, including self-care, receptive and expressive language, learning, mobility, self-direction, capacity for independent living, and economic self-sufficiency if services are not provided." Developmental concerns experienced by children can challenge typical development in the key domains: cognition, social and emotional growth, language and communication, and physical growth and skill (Hogan, Rogers & Msall, 2000). These concerns may be due to inherited genetic influences or environmental influences (or a combination of genetic and environmental factors) and may have their genesis during the prenatal, perinatal, or postnatal periods. Examples of genetically based concerns include Down syndrome, Fragile X syndrome, phenylketonuria, and Tay-Sachs disease. Environmentally based concerns may include the consequences of encephalitis, meningitis, rubella (German measles), fetal alcohol syndrome, lead poisoning, poor nutrition, unintentional injury, and child abuse. A host of individual and cultural–familial factors is associated with environmentally based concerns such as parental educational level, family history, and patterns of parent–child interaction. The prevalence estimate data from the 1994 and 1995 NHIS-D indicate that 13% in 1994 and 13.6% in 1995 of US children 17 years old and less have had a delay in their development (National Center for Health Statistics, 1999).

Finally, in the 1988 and 1994 NHIS-CHS, between 2% to 5% of all children 17 years old and less had ever received treatment or counseling for a delay in growth or development. That is, less than half (49%) of those reported to have had such a delay received some form of treatment, with half of this group (25%) receiving treatment in the previous 12 months. As with mental health problems, this low rate of treatment for these problems should be of concern to MCH practitioners.

## Learning Disabilities

The proportion of children who were reported in 1988 NHIS-CHS to have learning disabilities (LDs) (speech or language disorder, an academic skill disorder, or other diagnoses affecting children's ability to learn) was higher than the proportion known to be receiving special educational services according to school record data. Of total public school children, 4.8% were recorded as receiving special educational services for LDs in 1987, more than double the 1.8% recorded in 1977. However, 6.5% of all children 3 to 17 years old (or 3.4 million) were reported in the 1988 NHIS-CHS to have LDs, and 5.5% of those 6 to 17 years old were reported to have attended special classes or a special school because of such disabilities (Zill & Schoenborn, 1990). By 1997 to 1998, National Center for Health Statistics reported that 7% of all 6- to 11-year-old children had a learning disorder (including 4% of the 7% who also had attention deficit disorder [ADD]); another 3% had ADD, but only 54% of children with LD were receiving special education services (Pastor & Reuben, 2002). The prevalence of LD did not change significantly by 2002 (Child Trends Data Bank, Learning Disabilities, 2003). Furthermore, in contrast to developmental delays, most LDs are not fully apparent until the child gets to school and starts trying to read, write, and calculate. Therefore, there is a substantial rise in the prevalence of LDs as children reached school age, as was expected. The proportion of children with LDs jumped from 1% at 3 to 5 years old to 11% among 12 to 17 year olds (Child Trends Data Bank, Learning Disabilities, 2003).

The prevalence of LDs also varied by family structure, income, parental education, and gender. Low-income, single mother as parent, male gender, and low parental educational achievement are all associated with an increased prevalence of LD (Pastor & Reuben, 2002). The situation for race/ethnicity is more complicated, however. White non-Hispanics are more likely to have a diagnosis of ADD, whereas there were no significant racial/ethnic differences for LD or LD plus ADD.

Moreover, Zill and Schoenborn pointed out that there is evidence that LDs were underidentified in populations of different race in 1988. The reason for this is that blacks and Hispanics have higher rates than whites of the risk factors for LDs—low parental education and income levels, low birth weight, single parenthood, etc. However, significant racial/ethnic differences in prevalence of LD were not reported. Explanations of this paradox have included a lack of familiarity with the terms used to describe LDs and differential recall of past events between whites and peoples of different races (Zill & Schoenborn, 1990). However, it is important to keep in mind the different cultural perceptions and mores of whites and persons of difference race regarding what constitutes a learning deficiency (how it is both perceived and defined) and how much and what type of information should be shared with strangers (Jackson, 1981; Jones & Roberts, 1994; Nettles, 1994; Telfair & Nash, 1996). Finally, private health insurance coverage is associated with a higher prevalence of ADD only (Pastor & Reuben, 2002). Given more limited access to medical care (discussed later here), black children may be less likely to have had a LD diagnosed as such than white children.

Finally, in the 1988 NHIS-CHS, approximately 5% of all children 3 to 17 years old, or more than three quarters of those with LDs, had received treatment or counseling for their disabilities, and most of these children (three fifths) had received treatment or counseling in the previous 12 months (Zill & Schoenborn, 1990).

## External Causes

External causes (including both intentional and unintentional injury) are the leading causes of death of children 1 to 14 years old. Unintentional injury causes the most deaths between ages 5 and 14 years. Homicide is the fourth leading injury cause of death for 5 to 9 year olds (after congenital anomalies and malignant neoplasms), and suicide is the third leading cause of death in 10 to 14 year olds (after malignant neoplasms) (Centers for Disease Control and Prevention, 2004). The majority of unintentional injury deaths among children 5 to 14 years old result from motor vehicle traffic crashes. More than 65% of children 5 to 14 years old that died in traffic crashes in 1999 were not wearing a seatbelt or other restraint. Injury disproportionately affects poor children and children of different races. Similar to mortality patterns for children under the age of 5 years, among children 5 to 14 years old, black children had the highest death rates in 1999, at 29 deaths per 100,000 compared with 19 per 100,000 overall (Maternal and Child Health Bureau, 1995).

Community-based strategies to prevent injury death have largely been successful in reducing death rates. Examples of such successes include seat belt use and other safety measures, which have lowered traffic fatalities, smoke detectors to reduce deaths caused by house fires, childproof caps on medications, and bicycle helmets (Singh & Yu, 1996). Rates of death caused by homicide rose among children 5 to 14 years old by a factor of two to three between the mid 1980s and the mid 1990s, after which date homicide rates have been decreasing (Fox & Zawitz, 2003).

Injuries more often are not fatal. In the 5- to 9-year-old age, injury is the second leading cause of hospitalization, resulting in 60,000 hospital discharges a year (Maternal and Child Health Bureau, 1995). Unfortunately, not all of these children are discharged well. Injury is the leading cause of acquired disability among school-aged children. In addition to hospitalization, injury may result in an emergency room or doctor visit, activity limitation, days lost from school, bed-disability days, etc.

# HEALTH CARE ACCESS AND USE

The use of health services by children is qualitatively different from that of adults. Children use proportionately more ambulatory and preventive care and less hospital care than adults (Keane, Lave, Ricci, & LaVallee, 1999). As a direct result, annual healthcare costs for children (excluding infants) are less than those of adults, even of adults less than 65 years old. For the majority of children 6 to 17 years old (85%), between 1996 and 1998, medical care expenditures averaged $1,019 (McCormick et al., 2001). Nevertheless, 21% of that expense was paid out of pocket (McCormick et al., 2001).

The need for immunizations and indeed for routine well-child visits in general declines in the school years. This explains why older school-age children (8 to 11 years) were the least likely age group among all children less than 18 years old to have had a routine doctor visit during the years of 1993 to 1996 (Newacheck, Hughes, Hung, Wong, & Stoddard, 2000). Another reason for lack of a doctor visit for routine medical care or for not having a regular source of routine health care in the first place is uninsuredness (Kenney, Dubay, & Haley, 2000; Newacheck, Hughes, Hung, Wong, & Stoddard, 2000; Schoen & Dezroches, 2000). Children constitute a significant proportion of the growing uninsured population. In 1999, 11 million children under 18 years of age lacked health insurance. In actual numbers, this corresponded to an increase of nearly 1 million over the levels of uninsured children reported 2 years previously (Kaiser Commission and Medicaid and the Uninsured, 2001). According to the Survey of Income and Program Participation, the percentage of children less than 17 years old who had health insurance coverage for the entire year went down from 74.9% in 1999 to 71.4% in 2002, a significant decline at the 5% level (Boushey & Wright, 2004). Not surprisingly, privately insured children were more likely to use health care than either the uninsured or the publicly insured (predominantly those on Medicaid), despite the fact that privately insured children are reported to experience more favorable health status (McCormick et al., 2001).

This inequity seems to characterize the nation's approach to children's health care needs in general. Children are disproportionately uninsured. There is a big drop in Medicaid coverage between the children less than 5 years old (25% coverage) and the children 5 to 14 years old (15.6%), which is not made up for by a proportionate increase in either private insurance coverage (National Center for Health Statistics, 1995) or the State Child Health Insurance Program (Boushey & Wright, 2004). In fact, private insurance coverage of all children less than 18 years old, particularly employer-based health insurance coverage, is decreasing steadily. Private health insurance coverage of all children under 18 years declined from 73.5% in 1988 to 69.3% in 1992 (Newacheck, Hughes, & Cisternas,

1995). Although Medicaid and other public insurance has been able to compensate so far, policy initiatives at the national level to cut Medicaid funding and eliminate federal entitlements to Medicaid are ominous.

The Medicaid program is associated with substantial improvement in, access to, and use of health care services for low-income children. However, numerous barriers to Medicaid enrollment have prevented many eligible children from enrolling in the program; hence, they remain uninsured. This problem has been further exacerbated by welfare reform (welfare-to-work initiatives), which dismantled previous policies that automatically conferred Medicaid eligibility to children in families receiving Aid to Families with Dependent Children or welfare (Garrett & Holahan, 2000; Sochalski & Villarruel, 1999). Sochalski and Villarruel (1999) reported that many children in families leaving welfare are still eligible for Medicaid based on income eligibility criteria. However, several reasons are given for many of these children becoming uninsured. First, welfare administrators fail to inform families of their continuing eligibility. Second, families may not understand the eligibility rules. Third, a stigma is frequently attached to receiving Medicaid, and finally, many administrative challenges exist for states and families (Garrett & Holahan, 2000; Sochalski & Villarruel, 1999).

The fate of children who are eligible for Medicaid but who remain unenrolled mirrors that of children who are uninsured. Davidoff et al. (2000) pooled Medicaid-eligible children (<17 years old) from the 1994 and 1995 National Health Interview Survey and classified them according to insurance status (Medicaid enrollee; eligible but unenrolled and without insurance, and eligible but unenrolled with private insurance). Comparative analyses were completed examining measures of access (having a particular physician at a usual source of care, clinic waiting time, having an unmet health need) and use of health care services (adequacy of immunizations, having visited a doctor's office in the past two weeks, amount of money spent on medical care). Uninsured Medicaid-eligible children fared least well on all the access to care indicators studied. With respect to use, uninsured Medicaid eligible children had the lowest levels of immunization adequacy and tended to be less likely to have visited the doctor's office in the past 2 weeks. They were more likely to have used nonhospital outpatient, hospital outpatient, and the hospital emergency room than Medicaid enrollees. Although privately insured Medicaid-eligible children generally had better health care access and use profiles than Medicaid enrollees, they were significantly more likely to spend more than $500 per year for out-of-pocket health care expenses.

In view of the evidence that having some form of insurance, whether private or public, improves access to health care for children, attempts to provide health insurance coverage to other uninsured low-income non-Medicaid eligible children are warranted. The State Children's Health Insurance Program was created in response to the growing problem of these uninsured children. The program was enacted as Title XXI of the Social Security Act and appropriates funds through the Balanced Budget Act of 1997 for states to provide health insurance to children from birth through 18 years old (Halfon et al., 1999; Sochalski & Villarruel, 1999). The program is funded for 10 years, and states have the option to use the funds to expand their Medicaid programs, to establish new or expand existing child health insurance programs apart from the Medicaid program, or to use a combination plan with Medicaid expansion and a state plan available. The State Children's Health Insurance Program offers tremendous potential for improving access to care for children in the target population.

In 2000, 88% of children had health insurance coverage at some point during the year. That number has ranged from 85% to 88% for each year since 1987 (Health Resources and Services Administration, 2001a). The number of children who had no health insurance at any time during 2000 was 8.4 million (12% of all children). This was significantly lower than the 1999 number of 9.1 million (13% of all children). The proportion of children covered by private health insurance decreased from 74% in 1987 to 66% in 1994 and then increased to 71% in 2000 (Health Resources and Services Administration, 2001c). During the same time period, the proportion of children covered by government health insurance grew from 19% in 1987 to a high of 27% in 1993; it has since decreased to 23% in 1997 and has been fairly stable (Bloom & Tonthat, 2002). Hispanic children are less likely to have health insurance than white, non-Hispanic, or black children. In 2000, 75% of Hispanic children were covered by health insurance compared with 93% of white, non-Hispanic children and 87% of black children (Health Resources and Services Administration, 2001a). Overall rates of coverage did not differ by the child's age. However, the type of insurance does vary by the age of the child: government-provided insurance decreased but private health insurance increased with age. Nearly, 7% of children had no usual source of health care between 1993 and 2000. This overall percentage remained relatively stable. Children with public insurance, such as Medicaid, were more likely to have no usual source of care than were children with private insurance (5% and 3%, respectively) (Health Resources and Services Administration, 2001a). Children who were uninsured were nearly nine times as likely as those with private insurance to have no usual source of care. In 2000, 12% of children in families below the poverty line had no usual source of care compared with 6% of children in higher income families (Health Resources and Services Administration, 2001a).

## Community-Based Services for Children and Families

Community-based services are those provided to children and families outside of traditional institutional settings and in proximity to where clients live. These services include those provided by local health departments, community clinics, social service satellite programs, specialized umbrella programs, etc. Community-based services for children and their families are best exemplified by the model of the Family Resource Center (FRC). FRCs (depending on size and range of services), like most community-based programs, attempt to encompass a holistic or ecological approach to serving children and families that includes both health and human services. Precursors of FRCs were the community family service agencies that had as their primary mission to assist families after they have experienced a crisis. The primary goal was to provide whatever services the family needed that would enable them to stay together after the crisis experience (Weiss & Halpern, 1990; Weissbourd & Patrick, 1988).

In the mid 1960s, as the war on poverty heated up and the concept of empowerment entered the human services repertoire (Kadushin, 1980), there was a recognition of the need for a broad range of programs that should be available to families on a continuum from prevention through early intervention to crisis management and long-term supportive measures. This recognition led to the current emphasis of prevention and building on the strengths of families. The first of the programs on the continuum, preventive programs, are designed to help families before they are in crisis by attempting to reach all families (program access) and to reflect the strengths, needs, and culture of the families whom they serve (cultural access). An overall goal of these programs is to assess families' competencies and strengths and empower them (through the provision of support services) to function adeptly within their existing environments.

The focus is on the building, preserving, reinforcing, and maintaining of family strengths, sense of worth, and competence. Current family resource programs, like other community-based services programs, may take a variety of forms or service emphases. These include (1) comprehensive drop-in centers, (2) parent education, (3) crisis intervention services, (4) support groups services, (5) home visitors services, (6) information and referral services, (7) parent advocacy services, (8) other family-center service delivery models, and (9) any combination of these emphases. Given the range of program or service emphases, FRCs and other community-based service programs having a family-centered and public health focus rely on a number of basic principles. These principles are as follows.

### Focus on Prevention

Family resource programs clearly emphasize prevention over treatment. Such programs seek to assist families to meet their needs and head off problems before they develop. They also go one step further and embrace the concept of optimalism, which means "providing an environment conducive to the optimal development of children through the support of the family and maintenance of a viable community" (Weiss & Halpern, 1990; Weissbourd & Patrick, 1988). This definition does not specify a target population, as it implies that all children have the right to an optimal environment in which they can grow into healthy adults. Thus, family resource programs serve all families regardless of economic status, race ethnicity, composition, or capabilities.

### Recognition of the Importance of the Early Years

Research has demonstrated that strong, healthy attachments and positive experiences in the early years provide a solid foundation for further positive social, cognitive, and emotional development. As a result, family resource programs often provide support programs and services for extended periods of time, primarily during pregnancy, through the preschool years, so as to help establish an optimal reciprocal relationship between parents and their young children.

### Ecological Approach

Children do not exist in a vacuum but are embedded in families and communities. If a child is to develop in a truly healthy manner, attention must be paid to the family and community where that child lives. Such attention takes two forms in the context of family resource programs. First, family resource programs respect the cultural and social traditions of the many diverse groups that currently reside in the United States. Second, family resource programs seek to build communities by strengthening the bonds between people and the services in the community in which they live, thereby strengthening the informal support system of communities.

### Holistic View of Parents

Family resource programs take a holistic view of parents. Parents have their own needs, desires, and interests aside from those of their children, and they are more than vessels into which to pour information. They learn from experience as well as from facts and tend to assimilate information as it relates to their lives. Adults who have positive self-esteem and express confidence in their child-rearing skills in turn enhance their children's social and cognitive development.

### Value of Support

Family support services help reduce social isolation, provide information, and enhance coping abilities. They seek to build on family strengths rather than emphasize deficits. The ability of a family to develop friendships, to make linkages with other groups, and to seek advice and information is considered a strength. Parents may become empowered to take control of their lives from the neighborhood to the national level through their experiences with a family resource program.

Finally, because of the advantages of access (physical and cultural) and emphasis on prevention, empowerment, and support, community-based programs play an important role in the provision of needed services to school-age children and their families.

## School Health

School health activities were one of the earliest public health interventions targeted specifically at children. Leading the way were Dr. Sarah Josephine Baker (see Chapter 1) and Lillian Wald, who based in New York's Henry Street Settlement, organized in 1893 the first visiting nurse service and subsequently the first school health nursing program in the country. These early efforts both used the school setting to shortcut infectious disease surveillance strategies in an effort to identify and quarantine children who were a threat to others and directed health education, screening, and disease prevention activities for the benefit of the children served and their families.

Public school entry is the first time since birth that essentially all children in the United States are within the purview of an institutional setting. This creates an opportunity for proactive health intervention that has only partly been taken advantage of in this country. Traditional school health activities, such as screening tests and routine medical history and examination, are of "low effectiveness" (p. 112) and "limited value" (p. 123), respectively (American Academy of Pediatrics, 1981). On the other hand, a comprehensive school health program cannot only promote a child's achievement of health literacy, "the capacity to obtain, interpret, and understand basic health information and services and the competence to use such information and services in ways which enhance health" (Joint Committee on National Health Education Standards, 1995, p. 5). It can also make a direct contribution to the general education of the child. According to J. Michael McGinnis, former Director of Disease Prevention and Health Promotion of the US Public Health Service, a child who is not healthy will not "profit optimally from the educational process" (American School Health Association, 1994).

The goals of a comprehensive school health program are to promote health, prevent injury and disease, prevent high-risk behavior, intervene to help children in need or at risk, help those with special needs, and promote positive health and safety behaviors. The program has eight separate components: school environment; health education; health services; physical education; counseling, guidance, and mental health; food service and nutrition; worksite health promotion; and integration of school and community activities. The school environment addresses not only the safety of the physical environment but a supportive psychosocial environment as well. Health education is to be integrated into the academic curriculum and to result in changes in students' knowledge, attitudes, behaviors, and skills (American School Health Association, 1994).

Physical education should devote at least 60% the time to instruction that can translate into a program of lifetime, health-related physical activity. Counseling, guidance, and mental health address direct services to students with psychosocial needs, in conjunction with other community-based resources. School food service and nutrition includes both nutritionally appropriate meals at a reasonable price and education in making responsible, healthy food choices. Worksite health promotion is directed at school district employees. Integration of school and community health activities seeks to maximize health and health-related services for school-age children through coordination, integration, and communication with existing health resources, including parents (American School Health Association, 1994).

Health services in school are a special case. These may vary from the minimum required by law (such as dental, hearing, vision and spinal screening, and sports physicals) to the delivery of hands-on personal health services on school grounds. School-based and school-linked health centers, totaling approximately 30 in the early 1980s, now number in the hundreds (US General Accounting Office, 1994). Although more common in middle and high schools, school-based health centers are not unknown at the elementary level. Approximately 9% of all school-based and school-linked health centers serve primary school children, and another 12% serve both primary and secondary school students (US General Accounting Office, 1994).

Many different school-based and school-linked health center models exist. They may be staffed by school district employees or local health department employees, may be available to a specific subpopulation of the student body or to all (with parental consent), may be limited to screening and referral for initial complaints, or may provide comprehensive primary and preventive care. In most cases, midlevel providers, primarily nurse practitioners and physician assistants, provide the bulk of the services. The most controversial issue that has to be confronted in establishing a school-based health center at the secondary school level, the provision of reproductive health services, is less of an issue at the elementary school level. Financing, staffing, third-party reimbursement, and responding to dental and mental health needs are continuing problems. Nevertheless, the school-based health centers are low cost, convenient, and "can improve children's access to health care . . . especially those who are poor or uninsured" (US General Accounting Office, 1994, p. 5).

# OUTSTANDING ISSUES

## Child Abuse and Neglect

After declining somewhat in the 1990s, official reports of child abuse and neglect went up somewhat in 2000 from 1.18% to 1.22% of all US children (USDHHS, 2002). The increase does not reflect an increased awareness and willingness to report alone (National Center for Health Statistics, 1995). In her reanalysis of the 1986 national incidence study, Sedlak (1991) concluded that the increased incidence of child maltreatment between 1980 and 1986 "reflected increases in the incidence of occurrence of moderate injury cases" (Sedlak, 1991, p. 3–15). Subsequent to Sedlak's analysis, a Gallup poll reported that a survey of parents revealed a rate of abuse 16 times that estimated by official statistics (Lewin, 1995).

An estimated 879,000 children were victims of abuse and neglect in 2000 (USDHHS, 2002). There was a slight difference in percentages of the victims based on gender; the male victimization rate was 11.2 male children per 1,000 in the population compared with a rate of 12.8 female children per 1,000 in the population. Children in the age group of birth to 3 years had the highest victimization rate. Overall, the rate of victimization is inversely related to the age of the child (USDHHS, 2002). The victimization rates ranged from 15.7 children per 1,000 children aged birth to 3 years to 5.7 children per 1,000 aged 16 to 17 years. More than 34% of maltreatment deaths were associated with neglect, making this the single leading cause of maltreatment death in 1999. The second leading cause of maltreatment death was physical abuse alone (28%), followed by physical abuse and neglect combined (22%) (USDHHS, 2002). In 2000, 63% of child maltreatment victims suffered neglect (including medical neglect). Nineteen percent were physically abused. Ten percent were sexually abused, and 8% were emotionally or psychologically maltreated (USDHHS, 2002).

Children who have experienced abuse and neglect are at increased risk for experiencing adverse health effects and behaviors as adults, including smoking, alcoholism, drug abuse, physical inactivity, severe obesity, depression, suicide, sexual promiscuity, and certain chronic diseases (USDHHS, 2002). The role of the child protective services (CPS) agency is to respond to the needs of children who are alleged to have been maltreated and to ensure that they remain safe. In 2000, almost 3 million children were the subjects of a CPS investigation or assessment, but this represents only two thirds of the referrals received by child protective agencies. The rest were not accepted for investigation (USDHHS, 2002).

Different patterns of abuse exist among school-age children compared with infants and preschoolers. Older children are significantly more likely to experience physical abuse than those in younger age groups, but the youngest children are more likely to be fatally abused and the older more likely to experience moderate injury (Sedlak, 1991). Overall, there were no age differences for neglect, but two subcategories, emotional and educational neglect, were higher for older children. Finally, sexual abuse rates also increased with age (Sedlak, 1991).

In order to qualify for federal CPS funding, states must implement child abuse and neglect legislation that mandates reporting, conforms with federal definitions of abuse and neglect, and provides prevention and treatment services within the guidelines of the law (US Congress, 1973). Unfortunately, CPS agencies as currently constituted are inadequate to the task. Problems include underfunding; inadequate and inadequately trained staff; lack of coordination among the legal, criminal justice, health, social service, and education communities; inadequate or conflicting laws and policies; and a lack of responsibility among the general public (US Advisory Board, 1995). Most cases reported to CPS and accepted for investigation are not substantiated, and according to McCurdy and Daro (1992), hundreds of thousands of substantiated cases do not even receive basic services.

The answer to child maltreatment is prevention, but prevention requires knowing the underlying causes. As of yet, few resources have been expended to understand the etiology of abuse and neglect. Not only are the funds available for child abuse and neglect research inadequate, but the very agency designated by Congress to lead the national effort to investigate the phenomenon of child maltreatment, the National Center on Child Abuse and Neglect, was abolished by the welfare reform legislation that emerged from the 1996 Congress and replaced by a lower level Office on Child Abuse and Neglect. Nevertheless, it is clear that child abuse and neglect cannot be overcome without attention to social and economic conditions (poverty, substandard housing, inadequate education, broken families, unwanted pregnancy, unemployment, substance abuse, and low-quality child care) that put children and families at risk of a myriad of health problems. In addition, stressful life events and lack of social support have been shown to contribute to the risk of reported abuse and neglect (Kotch et al., 1995).

## AIDS/HIV

Pediatric acquired immunodeficiency syndrome (AIDS) is defined as clinical AIDS in children less than 13 years of age. AIDS was not recognized in children until well after its initial description in adults (Work Group on

HIV/AIDS, 1988). Initially, it was difficult to distinguish AIDS from other rare congenital immunodeficiency diseases in children, but several researchers convincingly demonstrated that the human immunodeficiency virus (HIV) affects the pediatric as well as the adult population (Work Group on HIV/AIDS, 1988). The face of pediatric AIDS has changed. When first recognized in children, HIV infections were seen primarily among hemophiliacs and neonatal intensive care unit graduates, as these were children who had multiple exposures to blood products. Effective screening and processing of the blood supply have largely eliminated this vector of transmission (Stuber, 1989). It is now well understood that HIV in children is transmitted by three routes: (1) from mothers to infants during the perinatal period, (2) through parenteral exposure to infected body fluids, primarily blood, and (3) through sexual contact (Rogers, 1987). Recent reports indicate that perinatal transmission remains the primary form of transmission of HIV in children. Evidence suggests that HIV is transmitted from infected mothers to their infants in utero by transplacental passage of the virus, during labor and delivery through exposure to infected maternal blood and/or vaginal secretions, and postnatally through breastfeeding. The risk of transmitting HIV from mother to infant in the absence of treatment ranges from 15 to 35%. It is lowest in Europe and highest in Africa (Peckham & Gibb, 1995). New HIV infections among newborns have dropped significantly since the introduction of AZT-based regimens in 1995. Perinatal transmission continues to occur because of HIV-positive pregnant women who have not received appropriate care. With proper maternal treatment, the risk of passing HIV from mother to child is 1.5% compared with over 20% without treatment (National Institute of Allergy and Infectious Disease, 2002). Despite what we know about preventing perinatal HIV transmission, 216 infants were born with HIV infection in 2001. HIV infection is often difficult to diagnose in very young children. Infected babies, especially in the first few months of life, often appear very normal, with no telltale signs that would allow a definitive diagnosis of HIV infection (National Institute of Allergy and Infectious Diseases, 2002). In recent years, researchers have used a highly accurate blood test in diagnosing HIV in children 6 months of age and younger (National Institute of Allergy and Infectious Diseases, 2002).

   The United States has a relatively small percentage of the world's children living with HIV/AIDS. At the end of 2000, 3,787 infants and children from birth through the age of 13 years were believed to be living with

AIDS in the United States (Centers for Disease Control and Prevention, 2001, p. 33). The number of new pediatric AIDS cases fell from 952 in 1992 to 92 in 2002 (Centers for Disease Control and Prevention, 2002). Since 1998, the US cities with the highest rates of pediatric AIDS were New York City; Miami, Florida; Newark, New Jersey; Washington, DC; and San Juan, Puerto Rico. The disease disproportionately affects children in minority groups, especially African Americans.

Pediatric HIV disease, including AIDS, differs from the disease in adults in a variety of ways. Children with AIDS often develop severe bacterial infections, and a large proportion have mental or motor retardation (National Institute of Allergy and Infectious Diseases, 2002). The natural history of the disease is not only different in children; it is less well understood than in adults. Moreover, AIDS progresses very differently in different children. Most of the children reported with perinatally acquired AIDS (87%) had met the Centers for Disease Control case definition for AIDS before their third birthday, whereas 3% were diagnosed after their sixth birthday.

The pediatric AIDS crisis is one small part of the overall crisis of AIDS, and it is also distinct from it. Today, most children with AIDS were born with HIV infection—born into families often living in poverty in which one or both parents may be HIV infected and drug dependent (Oleske, 1989). Minority children, many of whom face urban poverty, poor health, a lack of access to adequate health care, and educational disadvantages, comprise the majority of pediatric AIDS cases (Work Group on HIV/AIDS, 1988). At the end of 2001, black children accounted for 66% of AIDS cases reported in children under the age of 13 years; 18% of AIDS cases were among Hispanic children (Centers for Disease Control and Prevention, 2001, p. 22). The AIDS rate (per 100,000) among children under the age of 13 years by race are the following: black (1.7), Hispanic (0.3), American Indian/Alaska native (0.2), white (0.1), and Asian/Pacific Islander (0.1). These counts reflect only those children with AIDS who have been reported to Centers for Disease Control. They do not include other infected children who are either asymptomatic or symptomatic at any of the earlier stages of disease. It is likely that for every child who meets the definition of AIDS another 2 to 10 are infected with HIV (Work Group on HIV/AIDS, 1988).

Researchers have observed two patterns of illness in HIV-infected children. Approximately 20% of children develop serious disease in the first few years of life, and most of these children die by the age of 4 years (National Institute of Allergy and Infectious Disease, 2000). The remaining 80% of infected children have a slower rate of disease progression, many not developing the most serious symptoms of AIDS until school entry or even adolescence (National Institute of Allergy and Infectious Disease, 2000). Many children with HIV infection do not gain weight or grow normally. HIV-infected children frequently are slow to reach milestones in motor skills and mental development such as crawling, walking, and speaking. As the disease progresses, many children develop neurologic problems such as difficulty walking, poor school performance, seizures, and other symptoms of HIV (National Institute of Allergy and Infectious Disease, 2000). Children with AIDS become sicker and die faster than do adults. Like adults with HIV infection, children with HIV develop life-threatening opportunistic infections. Serious bacterial infections occur in children more frequently than adults, and they are more likely to suffer from chronic diarrhea. *Pneumocystis carinii* pneumonias the leading cause of death in HIV-infected children with AIDS. In addition, a lung disease called lymphocytic interstitial pneumonitis, rarely seen in adults, occurs more frequently in HIV-infected children. This condition, like *Pneumocystis carinii* pneumonia, can make breathing more progressively difficult and often results in hospitalization (National Institute of Allergy and Infectious Disease, 2000). Infected infants and children who receive comprehensive health care have markedly fewer hospitalizations and experience an improved quality of life. However, this care comes at a price. Oleske (1989), Osterholm and MacDonald (1987), and Boland et al. (1992) pointed out that on average the lengths of hospital stay for children with AIDS are longer and their bills are higher than comparable children with acute or other chronic conditions. However, the Work Group on HIV/AIDS (1988) pointed out that comprehensive ambulatory care and community-based services could considerably reduce in-hospital occupancy and its attendant costs.

The Pediatric Section of the Work Group on HIV/AIDS (1988) and others (Boland et al., 1992; Osterholm & MacDonald, 1987; Stuber, 1989) pointed out that coordination of care for these children and mothers is complicated by the precautions necessary to protect confidentiality and by the sheer enormity and complexity of the problems encountered. In addition, Stuber (1989) stated that there is an enormous emotional cost of dealing with the problems involved in the treatment of HIV-infected patients as a group, especially children in families. These authors all believe that the expertise of many disciplines is needed to provide optimal care, including (but not limited to) nursing, social work, nutrition, psychiatry, psychology, child development, law, ethics, immunology, infectious disease, and obstetrics. Stuber (1989) argued that a multidisciplinary team can provide the mutual education, support, and understanding needed to overcome the fear and exhaustion reported by many health care professionals when they work with HIV infection or AIDS in these groups who are less than 13 years old.

Families raising children with HIV/AIDS differ from families living with other chronic illnesses in important ways. Most children with HIV infection acquire it perinatally from their mothers. Sometimes fathers and siblings also may be infected. Thus, several family members may require medical treatment, and the family may have experienced the death of one or more of its members. Moreover, HIV/AIDS is a stigmatized condition that can isolate individuals or families from usual supports, which is often compounded by stigma associated with drug use, poverty, and minority ethnic status (Rehm & Franck, 2000).

MCH practitioners must keep in mind that children with AIDS have a particular dependency—in many cases, virtually total dependency—on the community and on government. This unique dependency arises from the complexity of their health care needs and the high costs of treatment, the stigma that they often face, the fragility of their families, and the poverty into which they are so often born. Furthermore, as paraphrased from Osterholm and MacDonald (1987), MCH practitioners must first realize in a straightforward but compassionate manner that the great weight of pediatric AIDS will continue to fall on our communities of different races, particularly in the inner city. It will be important for those working with these communities and the communities themselves to take ownership in developing creative solutions to addressing the complex problems associated with pediatric HIV/AIDS. In other words, individuals, communities, public health agencies, MCH practitioners, and government all need to respond.

## Homelessness

One of the fastest growing segments of the homeless population is families with children. A survey of 25 US cities found that in 2000 families with children accounted for 36% of the homeless population (US Conference of Mayors, 2001). These proportions are likely to be higher in rural areas; research indicates that families, single mothers, and children make up the largest group of people who are homeless in rural areas (Vissing, 1996).

Recent evidence confirms that homelessness among families is increasing. Requests for emergency shelter by families with children in 25 US cities increased by an average of 17% between 1999 and 2000 (US Conference of Mayors, 2001). The same study found that 27% of requests for shelter by homeless families were denied in 2000 because of a lack of resources. Moreover, 79% of the cities surveyed expected an increase in the number of requests for emergency shelter by families with children in 2001. There are several national estimates of homelessness. Unfortunately, many are dated or are based on dated information. However, the best approximation is provided by the Urban Institute and the National Survey of Homeless Assistance Providers, which findings indicate that there are 3.5 million homeless persons in the United States (Urban Institute, 2000). Recent attention to this problem has revealed a changing composition of the homeless population. What once consisted largely of older males now consists of increasing numbers of young men, women, and children. In the United States, approximately 1.35 million children are homeless every year. Children represent an estimated 39% of the homeless population (Urban Institute, 2000). It is important to note that the figures from this study are based on a national survey of service providers, and not all homeless persons use services. The number of persons experiencing homelessness is likely higher. In addition, it is acknowledged that the latter statistic may be a gross undercount because it does not account for children and families living in rural areas, abandoned shacks, bus terminals, and street shanties or for runaway or "throwaway" adolescent youth (Reyes & Waxman, 1987; Children's Defense Fund, 1988).

The fastest growing segment of the homeless is families, most commonly single mothers with two or three children. Research indicates that a worker earning minimum wage would have to work 97 hours a week to pay the rent of an average two-bedroom apartment (US Department of Housing and Urban Development, 1999). The largest number of homeless families resides in the major urban areas that include New York City, Denver, Philadelphia, San Francisco, St. Paul, Salt Lake City, San Antonio, Seattle, and Washington, DC (Alperstein & Arnstein, 1988). For example, according to Alperstein and Arnstein (1988), in New York State, it is estimated that there are 50,000 homeless, of whom 85% are in New York

City. Of these, the fastest growing segment of the homeless are families, most commonly single mothers with two or three children, who now comprise 40% to 45% of that city's homeless population. In addition, Edelman and Mihaly (1989) reported that in Washington, DC, the number of families seeking shelter jumped 500% during 1986. A more recent study of 27 US cities found that in 2001 37% of all requests for emergency shelter for an individual went unmet because of a lack of resources; this was a 13% increase from 2000. In these urban areas, there is a significant lack of appropriate shelters for families with children; in 2001, 52% of emergency shelter requests from families were denied, a 22% increase from 2000 (US Conference of Mayors, 2001).

It has only been within the last decade that "welfare hotels" (those willing to take government subsidies to house homeless persons) and homeless shelters have had to make accommodation for women and children. These facilities are generally dilapidated, are overcrowded, lack privacy or cooking facilities, and are breeding grounds for unsafe behaviors like substance abuse, violence, and prostitution. Many of these facilities provide day-to-day temporary sheltering; that is (for a number of reasons, including encouraging children to attend school and parent to search for jobs), families must stay outside of the shelters during the daytime (Alperstein & Arnstein, 1988; Edelman & Mihaly, 1989). On average, most of these facilities have an upper time limit for how long a family can stay (e.g., 14 months). However, in cities such as New York, families have stayed for as long as 5 years (Alperstein & Arnstein, 1988).

The experience of unstable housing, however long, has a significant impact on the health, education, and emotional development of children. Homeless children, compared with domiciled children of poor families, are generally less healthy and experience greater psychosocial stress as a result in living under more adverse conditions (Acker, Fierman, & Deyer, 1987; Alperstein & Arnstein, 1988; Edelman & Mihaly, 1989; Redlender, 1994). Very little is known, and even less has been published, on the health status of children who are also homeless. Alperstein and Arnstein (1989) and Redlender (1994) reported that, from what little is known, a disturbing pattern describing the health conditions of these young homeless children has emerged. These children have limited access to primary care. As a result, chronic health problems that include delayed immunizations, poor hygiene, anemia, poor diet and nutrition, and undetected and untreated emotional difficulties are much more likely in this population than in their domiciled, poor, same-age peers (Edelman & Mihaly, 1989). In addition, because of overcrowding, inadequate toilet facilities, and lack of knowledge of good hygiene, homeless children are also at high risk for various contagious diseases such as enteric illness, childhood exanthemas, and possibly tuberculosis (Alperstein & Arnstein, 1988). Consequently, homeless children get sick four times as often as children in domiciled families. In addition, they tend to suffer from more mental health problems than other children yet less than half receive treatment (Better Homes Fund, 1999).

Alperstein and Arnstein (1988) pointed out that if care is obtained these children are more likely to use emergency health care providers than are domiciled poor families. Furthermore, the difficulties of access to health care for the poor are exacerbated by their homelessness. Homeless families also have to deal with the difficulties of finding their way around unfamiliar neighborhoods to reach health providers. Thus, already overburdened by frequent changes in abode, the daily searches for affordable food, and the periodic attempts to find housing, parents are unlikely to be able to manage the health care system except for emergency care. Finally, emotional difficulties experienced by all family members can threaten not only the well-being of the child but also can lead to temporary or permanent family dissolution. Like most problems experienced by children in general, homelessness affects the "whole health" of the child, his/her physical, psychological, spiritual, and social health.

Housing instability often interferes with a child's opportunity for education. At least 12% of homeless school-age children are not enrolled in school while they are homeless, and 45% of homeless children do not attend school on a regular basis when they are homeless (Better Homes Fund, 1999). Often homeless children are prevented from going to school because of lack of transportation, frequent moving, no permanent address, and no medical or school records (Better Homes Fund, 1999). Frequent moving does not allow a child to establish a base of relationships with teachers or peers, nor does it allow the school to put in place the necessary supports needed to allow the child to "catch up" academically with his or her peers. Unfortunately, as Edelman and Mihaly (1989) stated, many school systems may be indifferent to homeless children and, with some exceptions, are not equipped to help these children continue their education. Even for homeless children who are able to continue their education, their poor living conditions and poor health, hygiene, and nutrition make it difficult for them to keep up with the required work. In addition, emotional difficulties (e.g., depression) resulting from living under adverse conditions and exacerbated by stigmatization and teasing from peers only make a focus on learning much more difficult. Homeless children are likely to repeat a grade twice as often as other children. In addition, 41% of homeless children attend two schools in 1 year, and 28% go to three or more schools in 1 year (Better Homes Fund, 1999). Children who are homeless have significant health and human service needs related to a number of factors including profound poverty, the stress of unstable housing, lack of a peer system, interrupted schooling, and living in a generally unsafe environment.

In 1987, the US Congress passed the Stewart B. McKinney Act, the first federal legislation that specifically addressed the issue of homelessness. Nearly 14 years later, the McKinney-Vento Act of 2001 was signed into law, as Title X, Part C, of the No Child Left Behind Act. The McKinney-Vento Homeless Assistance Act requires the Secretary of Education to develop, issue, and publish the Federal school enrollment guidelines that describe (1) successful ways that a State can assist local educational agencies in immediately enrolling homeless children and youth in school and (2) how a state can review its requirements regarding immunization and medical or school records and make whatever revisions are appropriate and necessary to immediately enroll homeless children and youth in school (US Department of Education, 2002). Under the McKinney-Vento Homeless Children and Youths Program, state educational agencies must ensure that homeless children and youth have equal access to the same free public education, including a public preschool education, as is provided to other children and youth. States must review and undertake steps to revise any laws, regulations, practices, or policies that may act as barriers to the enrollment, attendance, or success in school of homeless children and youth (US Department of Education, 2002). School districts and schools may not separate homeless students from the mainstream school environment on the basis of their homelessness. Homeless students must also have access to the education and other services that they need to have an opportunity to meet the same challenging state academic achievement standards to which all students are held (US Department of Education, 2002).

MCH practitioners should take a holistic approach to addressing the needs of these children and families. This approach must include efforts to insure that health, welfare, and education systems are sensitive to the egregious circumstances of family homelessness. Interventions that attempt to create a welcoming environment also should provide advocacy for the empowerment of families and the amelioration of their problems.

## Immigrant Children

A subgroup of the school-aged population that has grown exponentially over the last decade is the offspring of immigrants to the United States. Children of immigrants are expected to account for more than half of the growth in the school-aged population between 1990 and 2010 (Nord & Griffin, 2000). Research indicates that from 1990 to 1997 the number of children in immigrant families grew by 47% compared with only 7% for the children of native-born parents, and by 1997, nearly one of every five children (14 million) was the child of an immigrant (Hernandez, 2000). It is estimated that most of the growth over the next 30 years will occur through immigration and births to immigrants and there children. The majority of children in immigrant families are of Hispanic or Asian origin, the proportion of children in the United States who are non-Hispanic whites is projected to drop from 69% in 1990 to only 50% in 2030 (Hernandez, 2000).

Several federal agencies are dedicated to collecting data and monitoring and understanding the mental and physical health needs of immigrant children in the United States. However, very limited research is available on the circumstances, health status, and overall development of children of immigrant families. The children of immigrants experience the overwhelming issues involved with growing up in a way that is unique to most children. Several factors are believed to elevate a child's risk for negative health, developmental, and educational outcomes, including family incomes below the poverty threshold, parents who have low educational attainments, only one parent or many siblings in the home, or living in overcrowded housing (Hernandez, 2000). In 2001, immigrant children with foreign-born parents were more likely than native-born children with foreign-born parents to live below the poverty level—28% and 20%, respectively (Health Resources and Services Administration, 2001a). The percentage of children whose parents have less than a high school diploma is much higher (42%) among children with at least one foreign-born parent than among native children with native-born parents (11%) (Health Resources and Services Administration, 2001c).

## Current Trends in Education for School-Age Children

The current state of public education in the United States is often an issue debated by many parents, administrators, teachers, and policy makers. Several factors have helped to shape the recent trends of the educational system and how it is perceived by the American public. Some of these factors include inconsistent performance on standardized testing, low reading scores, school accountability, and overwhelming diversity in student body population.

The No Child Left Behind Act of 2001 is a landmark in education reform designed to improve student achievement and change the culture of America's schools. President George W. Bush described this law as the "cornerstone of my administration." Clearly, our children are our future and, as President Bush has expressed, "Too many of our neediest children are being left behind." With passage of No Child Left Behind, Congress reauthorized the Elementary and Secondary Education Act, the principal federal law affecting education from kindergarten through high school. In amending the Elementary and Secondary Education Act, the new law represents efforts to support elementary and secondary education in the United States (US Department of Education, 2002). In addition, this legislation reauthorizes the McKinney-Vento Homeless Assistance Act's Education for Homeless Children and Youth program, along with most other federal elementary and secondary education programs. The McKinney-Vento Act is a federal law that entitles children who are homeless to a free, appropriate public education and requires schools to remove barriers to their enrollment, attendance, and success in school. Today, more than $7,000 on average is spent per pupil by local, state, and federal taxpayers. States and local school districts are now receiving more federal funding than ever before for all programs under No Child Left Behind: $23.7 billion, most of which will be used during the 2003–2004 school year. This represents an increase of 59.8% from 2000 to 2003. It is built on four major ideas: accountability for results, an emphasis on doing what works based on scientific research, expanded parental options, and expanded local control and flexibility. Each state must measure every public school student's progress in reading and math in each of grades 3 through 8 and at least once during grades 10 through 12. These assessments must be aligned with state academic content and achievement standards. They will provide parents with objective data on where their child stands academically. No Child Left Behind requires states and school districts to give parents easy-to-read, detailed report cards on schools and districts, telling them which ones are succeeding and why. Included in the report cards are student achievement data broken out by race, ethnicity, gender, English language proficiency, migrant status, disability status, and low-income status, as well as important information about the professional qualifications of teachers. With these provisions, parents have important, timely information about the schools their children attend—whether they are performing well or not for *all* children, regardless of their background.

In 1999, the National Center for Educational Statistics administered the Parent Survey of the National Household Education Surveys Program. This was the first study conducted to provide a comprehensive set of information that may be used to estimate the number and characteristics of homeschoolers in the United States (US Department of Education, 1999). This report, *Homeschooling in the United States: 1999*, presents an estimate of the number of homeschooled students, characteristics of homeschooled children and their families, parents' reasons for homeschooling, and public school support for homeschoolers. Students were considered to be homeschooled if their parents reported them being schooled at home instead of a public or private school, if their enrollment in public or private schools did not exceed 25 hours a week, and if they were not being homeschooled solely because of a temporary illness. In the spring of 1999, an estimated 850,000 students nationwide were being homeschooled, thus, 1.7% of US students, 5 to 17 years old, with a grade equivalent of kindergarten through grade 12. The study concluded that a greater percentage of homeschoolers (75%) compared with non-homeschoolers (65%) were white. At the same time, a smaller percentage of homeschoolers were black, non-Hispanic students, and an even smaller percentage were Hispanic students. There appeared to be no difference in the household income of homeschoolers than non-homeschoolers. However, parents of homeschoolers had higher levels of educational attainment than did parents of non-homeschoolers. Parents gave a wide variety of reasons for homeschooling their children. The top three reasons included being able to give their child a better education at home (48.9%), having religious reasons (38.4%), and having a poor learning environment at school (25.6%).

# CONCLUSION

Although on average school-age children may be the healthiest population group in the United States, they are also among the most vulnerable. Although benefiting from an unprecedented extent from public health advances in the areas of infectious disease and other natural causes of morbidity and mortality, children are threatened by injuries, both intentional and unintentional. Chronic and handicapping conditions, behavioral morbidities, including social and emotional problems, LDs, and social problems such as hunger, homelessness, abuse, and exploitation demand attention. Nevertheless, it is during the school-age years that enormous potential exists for reaching vast numbers of children with services and health-promoting strategies; it is in this age group, for the first time since birth, that children in the United States are nearly universally accessible through a helping institution. Using the schools to enforce immunization requirements demonstrates how reaching children and their families at this stage of their development can be successful. Recognizing this, Freedman, Klepper, Duncan, and Bell (1988) proposed that public schools be used to define insurable groups for the purpose of obtaining health care coverage for uninsured and underinsured children and their families. Initiatives like this could be expanded to include setting the stage for healthier adolescence and adulthood by emphasizing injury prevention, physical activity, oral health, good nutrition, and healthful, prosocial interpersonal relationships. Teachers and others in schools see children every day and would be appropriate sources for early referral for health, developmental, social, and emotional problems, if resources were available to respond. Inadequate funding and preoccupation with so-called family rights has prevented the United States from maximizing the potential of generations of children.

## Acknowledgments

The authors thank Kai Stewart and Savannah Weaver for their help in the preparation of this chapter.

# REFERENCES

Acker, R.J., Fierman, A.H., & Dreyer, B.P. (1987). An assessment of parameters of health care and nutrition in homeless children. *American Journal of Diseases in Children, 141*, 388.

Alperstein, G., & Arnstein, E. (1988). Homeless children: A challenge for pediatricians. *Pediatric Clinics of North America, 35,* 1413–1425.

American Academy of Pediatrics. (1981). *School health: A guide for health professionals.* Evanston, IL: Author.

American School Health Association. (1994). *Guidelines for comprehensive school health programs* (2nd ed., ASHA publication #G011). Kent, OH: American School Health Association.

Anderson, R.N., & Smith, B.L. (2003). Deaths: Leading causes for 2001. *National Vital Statistics Reports* (Vol. 52, No. 9). Hyattsville, MD: National Center for Health Statistics.

Better Homes Fund. (1999). *Homeless children: America's new outcasts.* Available from: http://www.nationalhomeless.org/

Bloom, B., & Tonthat, L. (2002). Summary statistics for U.S. children: National Health Interview Survey, 1997. *Vital and Health Statistics, 10*(203).

Boland, M., Conviser, R., Kelly, M., Connor, E., Rapkin, R., & Oleske, J. (1992). Care needs of HIV-infected children at New Jersey Children's Hospital. *Aids & Public Policy Journal, 7,* 7–17.

Boushey, H, & Wright, J. (2004). *Health insurance coverage in the United States: Health insurance data brief #2.* Washington, DC: Center for Economic and Policy Research.

Bradbury, R. (1994). No news, or what killed the dog? *American Way, 27,* 133, 135.

CDC Wonder. (2004). *Compressed mortality data request screen for the years 1979–1998 with ICD-9 codes.* Available April 7, 2004, from: http://wonder.cdc.gov/mortICD9J.html

Centers for Disease Control and Prevention. (2001). U.S. HIV and AIDS cases reported through June 2001. *HIV/AIDS Surveillance Report.* Midyear edition Vol. 13, No. 1. Atlanta, GA: U.S. Department of Health and Human Services.

Centers for Disease Control and Prevention. (2002). Cases of HIV infection and AIDS in the United States, 2002. *HIV/AIDS Surveillance Report,* Vol. 14, pp. 1–40.

Centers for Disease Control and Prevention. National Center for Injury Prevention and Control. (2004). *Leading causes of death, US, 2001.* Available March 27, 2004, from: http://webappa.cdc.gov/sasweb/ncipc/leadcaus10.html

Children and Mental Health. *Mental health: A report of the Surgeon General 1999.* Available April 25, 2004, from: http://www.surgeongeneral.gov/library/mentalhealth/chapter3/sec1.html

Children's Defense Fund. (1988). *The children's defense budget: An analysis of our nation's investment in children.* Washington, DC: Author.

Child Trends Data Bank, Learning Disabilities. (2003). Available April 25, 2004, from: http://www.childtrendsdatabank.org/indicators/65learningdisabilities.cfm.

Davidoff, A.J., Garrett, A.B., Makuc, D.M., & Schirmer, M. (2000). Medicaid-eligible children who don't enroll: health status, access to care, and implications for Medicaid enrollment. *Inquiry. 37*(2):203–18.

Dewey, J. (1956). *The child and the curriculum.* Chicago: University of Chicago Press.

Drotar, D. (1981). Psychological perspectives in chronic childhood illness. *Journal of Pediatric Psychology, 6,* 211–228.

Drotar, D., & Bush, M. (1985). Mental health issues and services. In N. Hobbs & J.M. Perrin (Eds.), *Issues in the care of children with chronic illness.* San Francisco: Jossey-Bass.

Edelman, M.W., & Mihaly, L. (1989). Homeless families and the housing crisis in the United States. *Children and Youth Services Review, 11,* 99–108.

Erikson, E.H. (1950). *Childhood and society* (2nd ed.). New York: W.W. Norton and Co.

Fields, J., & Casper, L.M. (2001). *America's Families and Living Arrangements: March 2000.* Current Population Reports P20-537. Washington, D.C.: U.S. Census Bureau.

Fingerhut, L.A., National Center for Health Statistics. (1989). *Trends and current status in childhood mortality, United States, 1900–1985.* Vital and health statistics, Series 3 (No. 26. DHHS Pub. No. [PHS] 89-1410).

Fox, J.A., & Zawitz, M.W. (2003, January). *Homicide trends in the US: 2000 update.* NCJ 197471. BJS Crime Data Brief, Washington, DC.

Freedman, S.A., Klepper, B.R., Duncan, R.P., & Bell, S.P., Jr. (1988). Coverage of the uninsured and underinsured: A proposal for school enrollment-based family health insurance. *New England J Medicine, 318,* 843–847.

Garrett, B., & Holahan, J. (2000). Welfare leavers, Medicaid coverage, and private health insurance. *Assessing the New Federalism Brief B-13.* Washington, DC: The Urban Institute.

Goldberg, R.T., Isralsky, M. & Shwachman, H. (1979). Vocational development and adjustment of adolescent with cystic fibrosis. *Arch Phys Med Rehabil, 60,* 369–374.

Guyer, B., Freedman, M.A., Strobino, D.M., & Sondik, E.J. (2000). Annual summary of vital statistics: Trends in the health of Americans during the 20th century. *Pediatrics, 106,* 1307–1317.

Halfon, N., & Newacheck, P.W. (1998). Prevalence and impact of parent reported disabling mental health conditions among U.S. children. *Child & Adolescent Psychiatry, 38,* 600–609.

Halfon, N., Inkelas, M., & Newacheck, P.W. (1999). Enrollment in the State Child Health Insurance Program: A conceptual framework for evaluation and continuous quality improvement. *Milbank Q. 77*(2):181–204, 173.

Hardy, A.M., National Center for Health Statistics. (1991). *Incidence and impact of selected infectious diseases in childhood.* Vital and health statistics, Series 10, No. 180 (DHHS Pub. No. [PHS] 91-1508).

Health Resources and Services Administration. (2001a). America's children report 2001. *Indicators of children's well-being: Population and family characteristics.* Available from: http://www.childstats.gov

Health Resources and Services Administration. (2001b). America's children report 2001. *Indicators of children's well-being: Economic security.* Available from: http://www.childstats.gov

Health Resources and Services Administration. (2001c). America's children report 2001. *Indicators of children's well-being: Health indicators.* Available from: http://www.childstats.gov

Hernandez, D. (2000). *Children of immigrants: Health, adjustment and public assistance.* Available from: http://www.nap.edu/openbook/0309065453/html

Hogan, D.P., Rogers, M.L., & Msall, M.E. (2000). Functional limitation and key indicators of well-being in children with disability. *Archives of Pediatric and Adolescent Medicine, 154,* 1042–1048.

Institute of Medicine. (1998). The Future of Public Health. Washington, DC: National Academy Press.

Jackson, J.J. (1981). Urban black Americans. In A. Harwood (Ed.), *Ethnicity and medical care.* Cambridge, MA: Harvard University Press.

Joint Committee on National Health Education Standards. (1995). *National Health Education Standards: Achieving Health Literacy.* New York: American Cancer Society.

Jones, D.J., & Roberts, V.A. (1994). Black children: Growth, development, and health. In L. Livingston (Ed.), *Handbook of black American health: The mosaic of conditions, issues, policies, and prospects.* Westport, CT: Greenwood Press.

Kadushin, A. (1980). *Child welfare services* (3rd ed.). New York: McMillan Publishing Co.

Kaiser Commission on Medicaid and the Uninsured. (2001). *Final Report.* San Francisco: Kaiser Family Foundation.

Keane, C.R., Lave, J.R., Ricci, E.M., & LaVallee, C.P., (1999). The impact of a children's health insurance program by age. *Pediatrics, 104,* 1051–1058.

Kenney, G., Dubay, L., & Haley, J. (2000). Health insurance, access, and health status of children: Findings from the nation survey of America's families, in Urban Institute, *SNAPSHOTS of America's Families II* (1–8), Washington, DC: Urban Institute.

Kotch, J.B., Browne, D., Ringwalt, C.L., Stewart, P.W., Ruina, E., Holt, K., Lowman, B., & Jung, J.-W. (1995). Risk of child abuse or neglect among a cohort of low income infants. *Child Abuse and Neglect, 19,* 1115–1130.

Lewin, T. (1995, December 7). Parents poll finds child abuse to be more common. *The New York Times.*

Maternal and Child Health Bureau, Health Resources and Services Administration, Public Health Service, US Department of Health and Human Services. (1991). *Healthy children 2000* (DHHS Pub. No. HRSA-M-CH-91-2). Washington, DC: US Government Printing Office.

Maternal and Child Health Bureau, Health Resources and Services Administration, Public Health Service, US Department of Health and Human Services. (1995). *Child Health USA '94* (DHHS Pub. No. HRSA-MCH-95-1). Washington, DC: US Government Printing Office.

McCormick, M.C., Weinick, R.M, Elixhauser, A., Stagnitti, M.N., Thompson, J., & Simpson, L. (2001). Annual report on access to and utilization of health care for children and youth in the United States: 2000. *Ambulatory Pediatrics, 1,* 3–15.

McCurdy, K., & Daro, D. (1992). *Current trends in child abuse reporting and fatalities: The results of the 1991 annual fifty state survey.* Chicago: National Center on Child Abuse Prevention Research.

McPherson, M., Arango, P., Fox, H., Lauver, C., McManus, M., Newacheck, P.W., Perrin, J.M., Shonkoff, J.P., & Strickland, B. (1998). A new definition of children with special health care needs. *Pediatrics, 102,* 137–140.

National Center for Health Statistics. (1989). Current estimates from the national health interview survey: United States, 1988. *Vital and Health Statistics,* Series 10, No. 173.

National Center for Health Statistics. (1995). *Health, United States, 1994.* Hyattsville, MD: US Public Health Service.

National Center for Health Statistics. (1999). *National health interview survey on disability (NHIS-D)* (database on CD-ROM) (CD-ROM Series, Vol. 10, No. 8). Hyattsville, MD: National Center for Health Statistics.

*National Health Interview Survey-Disability Supplement.* (1994). Rockville, MD: National Center for Health Statistics.

National Institute of Allergy and Infectious Disease. (2002). *Mother-to-infant HIV transmission rate less than 2% in Phase III perinatal trial (PACTG 316).* Bethesda, MD: Author [available] http://www.niaid.nih.gov/daids/therapeutics/geninfo/PACTG316Statement.pdf [cited] December 28, 2004.

Nettles, A. (1994). Scholastic performance of children with sickle cell disease. *Journal of Health and Social Policy, 5,* 123–140.

Newacheck, P.W., & Halfon, N. (1998). Prevalence and impact of disabling chronic condition in childhood. *American Journal of Public Health, 88,* 610–617.

Newacheck, P.W., & Taylor, W.R. (1992). Childhood chronic illness: Prevalence, severity, and impact. *American Journal of Public Health, 82,* 364–370.

Newacheck, P.W., Hughes, D.C., & Cisternas, M. (1995, Spring). Children and health insurance: an overview of recent trends. *Health policy and child health.* Washington, DC: Center for Health Policy Research, The George Washington University.

Newacheck, P.W., Hughes, D.C., Hung, Y., Wong, S., & Stoddard, J.J. (2000). The unmet needs of America's children. *Pediatrics, 105,* 989–997.

Nord, C.W., & Griffin, J.A. (2000). *Children of immigrants: Health, adjustment, and public assistance: Educational profile of 3 to 8 year old children of immigrants.* Available from: http://www.nap.edu/openbook/0309065453/html

Oleske, J.M. (1989). Children with HIV infection: Dilemmas in management. *Caring, VIII,* 32–35.

Osterholm, M.T., & MacDonald, K.L. (1987). Facing the complex issues of pediatric AIDS: A public health perspective. *Journal of the American Medical Association, 258,* 2736–2737.

Palfrey, J.S., Walker, D.K., Haynie, H., Singer, J.D., Porter, S., Bushey, B., & Cooperman, P. (1991). Technology's children: Report of a statewide census of children dependent on medical supports. *Pediatrics, 87,* 611–618.

Pastor, P.N., & Reuben, C.A. (2002). Attention deficit disorder and learning disability: United States, 1997–98. National Center for Health Statistics. *Vital Health Statistics, 10*(206).

Peckham, C., & Gibb, D. (1995). Mother-to-child transmission of the human immunodeficiency virus. *New England J Medicine, 333,* 298–302.

Redlender, I. (1994). Health care of homeless women and children. In H.M. Wallace, R.P. Nelson, & P.J. Sweeny (Eds.), *Maternal and child health practices* (4th ed.). Oakland, CA: Third Party Publishing Company.

Rehm, R.S., & Franck, L.S. (2000). Long-term goals and normalization strategies of children and families affected by HIV/AIDS. *Advance Nursing Science, 23,* 69–82.

Reyes, L.M., & Waxman, L.D. (1987). *The continuing growth of hunger, homelessness, and poverty in American cities: 1986.* Washington, DC: US Conference of Mayors.

Richardson, S.A. (1989). Transition to adulthood. In R.E.K. Stein (Ed.), *Caring for children with chronic illness: Issues and strategies.* New York: Springer Publishing Company.

Rogers, M.F. (1987). Transmission of human immunodeficiency virus infection in the US. In DHHS *Report of the Surgeon General's workshop on children with HIV infection and their families.* Rockville, MD: US Department of Health and Human Services, Public Health Service, Health Resources and Services Administration, Bureau of Health Care Delivery and Assistance, Division of Maternal and Child Health.

Schidlow, D., & Fiel, S. (1990). Life beyond pediatrics: transition of chronically ill adolescents from pediatric to adult care systems. *Medical Clinics of North America, 74,* 1113.

Schoen, C., & Dezroches, C. (2000). Uninsured and unstably insured: The importance of continuous insurance coverage. *Health Services Research, 35,* 187–206.

Sedlak, A. (1991, September 5). *National incidence and prevalence of child abuse and neglect: 1988* (revised report). Rockville, MD: Westat.

Silverman, M.M., & Koretz, D.S. (1989). Preventing mental health problems. In R.E.K. Stein (Ed.). *Caring for Children with Chronic Illness, Issues, and Strategies.* New York: Springer Publishing Co., 213–229.

Simpson, G. (1993, Winter). *Determining childhood disability and special needs children in the 1994–95 NHIS on disability.* Paper presented at the ASA annual meeting.

Singh, G.K., & Yu, S.M. (1996). US childhood mortality, 1950–1993: Trends and socioeconomic differentials. *American Journal of Public Health, 86,* 505–512.

Snyder, H.N., & Swahn, M.H. (2003, March). Juvenile suicides, 1981–98. *Youth Violence Research Bull.* OJJDP and CDC, NCJ 196978.

Sochalski, J.A., & Villarruel, A.M. (1999). Improving access to healthcare for children. *Journal of the Society of Pediatric Nursing, 4,* 147–154.

Stuber, M.L. (1989). Coordination of care for pediatric AIDS: The development of a maternal-child HIV task force. *Developmental and Behavioral Pediatrics, 10,* 201–204.

Telfair, J., & Nash, K.B. (1996). Delivery of genetic services to African Americans. In N.L. Fisher (Ed.), *Ethnic and cultural diversity and its impact on the delivery of genetic services.* Baltimore, MD: The Johns Hopkins University Press.

Urban Institute. (2000). *A new look at homeless in America.* Washington, DC: Urban Institute. Available from: http://www.urban.org

US Advisory Board on Child Abuse and Neglect. (1995). *A nation's shame: Fatal child abuse and neglect in the US.* Executive Summary. Washington, DC: US Advisory Board on Child Abuse and Neglect.

US Census Bureau. (2000). Profile of general demographic statistics: 2000. *2000 Census of Population and Housing.* Washington, DC: US Department of Commerce.

US Conference of Mayors. (2001). *A status report on hunger and homelessness in America's cities: 1998.* Washington, DC: Author.

US Congress. (1973). Child Abuse Prevention and Treatment Act, PL 93-247.

US Department of Education. (1999). *Parent survey of national household education surveys program.* Washington, DC: National Center of Educational Statistics.

US Department of Education. (2002). McKinney-Vento Act Education for Homeless Children and Youths Program, Office of Elementary and Secondary Education. Federal Register: Volume 67, Number 46. Available from: http://www.ed.gov/legislation/FedRegister/other/2002-1/030802a.html

USDHHS, ACYF. (2002). *Child Maltreatment, 2000.* Washington, DC: USGPO.

US Department of Housing and Urban Development (1999). Annual Housing and American Housing Survey. Washington, DC: Author.

US General Accounting Office. (1994). *Health care reform: School-based health centers can promote access to care* (GAO/HEHS-94-166). Washington, DC: Author.

Vissing, Y. (1996). *Out of sight, out of mind: Homeless children and families in small-town America.* Lexington, KY: The University Press of Kentucky.

Weiss, H., & Halpern, R. (1990). Family support and educational programs: Something old or something new? New York: National Center for Children in Poverty.

Weissbourd, B., & Patrick, M. (1988). In the best interest of the family: The emergence of the family resource programs. *Infants and Young Children, 1,* 46–54.

Williams, B., & Kotch, J.B. (1990). Excess injury mortality among children in the US: Comparison of recent international statistics. *Pediatrics, 86*(Suppl), 1067–1073.

Work Group on HIV/AIDS. (1988). Pediatric AIDS. *Public Health Reports, 103*(Suppl 1), 94–98.

Zill, N., & Schoenborn, C.A. (1990). Developmental, learning, and emotional problems: Health of our nation's children, US, 1988. *Advance data from vital and health statistics* (No. 190). Hyattsville, MD: National Center for Health Statistics.

# CHAPTER 8

# Improving Adolescent Health

*David Knopf*

*I would there were no age between ten and three-and-twenty, or that youth would sleep out the rest; for there is nothing in between but getting wenches with child, wronging the ancientry, stealing, fighting.* (Shakespeare, 1925)

*Adolescence is a new birth, for the higher and completely human traits are now born. . . . These years are the best decade of life. No age is so responsive to all the best and wisest adult endeavor.* (Hall, 1904, pp. xiii and xviii)

## INTRODUCTION

No age group is more maligned or idealized than adolescence. This cultural ambivalence has profound implications for the health of adolescents, resulting in sometimes dismissing adolescent problems as inevitable, sometimes minimizing adolescent concerns and issues as trivial, and sometimes developing anxiety-driven, ideologically based policies. Adolescent health is often injected into the core political/cultural debates regarding justice and the range and role of government in such areas as abortion, sexuality, family values, poverty, and social opportunity. Clearly, adolescents have significant problems as a population, and these problems have significant repercussions for young people and society now and in the future. Public health professionals and advocates have long sought to improve the health of adolescents, increase concern for their needs, and apply public health principles to efforts to improve their health, both now and in the future.

Compared with other age groups, adolescents are generally healthy, but they should be of high public health concern for several reasons. Certain populations of adolescents have poor health status, and many of these are in the direct care of public agencies, such as the incarcerated, those in foster care, and Native Americans. Many of the major health problems of adolescents are psychosocially based and thus should be amenable to prevention efforts. Because many health-related behaviors that cause significant adult morbidity and mortality begin in adolescence and may be less well embedded in younger people, changes in these behaviors during adolescence may pay long dividends for the public's health (Burt, 2002). Another important reason to attend closely to adolescent health is that adolescents are the immediate next pool of parents, workers, and citizens, and thus, their health will very soon affect the health of succeeding generations, the economy, and the body politic. Adolescent problems such as juvenile crime, motor vehicle injuries, pregnancy, and sexually transmitted diseases often affect other generations directly. Finally, just as parents feel some urgency to complete the unfinished business of socialization as the opportunity to influence the development of their offspring draws to a close in adolescence (Smetana, 1989) so too should society.

This chapter considers the importance, nature, and context of adolescent development. The epidemiology of adolescent health problems illustrates the pervasiveness of psychosocial factors in mortality, morbidity, and risk behavior. A consideration of the state of current health care for adolescents will show the lack of access and underuse of relevant health care and illustrate the need for broadly conceived, comprehensive, youth-oriented approaches that address youth development, health promotion, prevention, primary care, and treatment services. Recent public health efforts have been developed at the local, state, and federal levels to address some of these needs. Major problem areas of providing quality health care; preventing fatal injury, suicide, pregnancy, and obesity; and serving stigmatized populations are considered in light of evaluation research.

First, who are adolescents? Some use biological markers such as the beginning and completion of puberty. Others would use social definitions such as leaving the family of origin, becoming economically independent, or becoming a legally responsible adult (usually at 21 years old). Some would even combine in the adolescent group both teenagers and youth and thus include those up to their mid 20s, reflecting the continued lack of true independence of many in their mid 20s. For public health purposes, age-based definitions, although crude, are easiest to apply, but even age definitions vary. Some resources such as the Centers for Disease Control and Prevention (CDC) typically report health data in varying age blocks such as less than 18, 5–14, 15–24, or even 15–64, thus confusing and obscuring much data with issues of other ages. For the purposes here, adolescence usually refers to those who are in the second decade of life.

# ADOLESCENCE IN THE 21ST CENTURY

## Historical Perspectives on Adolescence

Some have argued that adolescence is a recent invention (Kett, 1993), but historical reviews illustrate a long awareness of unique issues in the second decade of life and some important differences over time. The term *adolescent* was not in common use until G. Stanley Hall's (1904) publication in 1904 of a two-volume text, *Adolescence: Its Psychology, and its Relations to Anthropology, Sex, Crime, Religion, and Education*. Before this time, the age group was more often referred to as *Youth*, which had a connotation of semi-independent participation in economic activities and typically ranged from age 12 to the early to mid 20s (Modell & Goodman, 1990).

Industrialization changed the ways youth become adults, and this distressed many. The transition by youth to full adulthood before industrialization often included fostering out of the family to apprenticeships for working class youth and to boarding school for the elite, both of which were seen as semiautonomous phases still monitored by adults. With industrialization, urbanization, and the expansion of the middle class in the late 19th century, such transitions faded, and youth became increasingly dependent on their family and marginalized economically. Age-segregated training became the norm for the second decade of life, and the mixed social class American public high school emerged as the uniquely American means to foster upward social mobility for the working and middle classes. Hall's publication became an important part of the movement that focused on the character development of an age group, which was seen as vulnerable and malleable (but when working class youth did not respond to these bourgeois reformers' attempts, they were again seen as troublesome, and the label of juvenile delinquent developed). Hall believed adolescents should be protected from precocity—adult experiences and responsibilities that come too early. This view fit well with the changing needs of the economy for fewer unskilled laborers and the changing view of the family as less an economic unit and more an emotional refuge to protect children. In contrast to the popular imagination, protected child development, family stability, and multigenerational relationships have only become a possible norm within the last century. This changing view of adolescence as a protected transition time may not be universally accepted and may be particularly difficult for non-European immigrants, who come from different historical, economic, and cultural traditions.

## Demographics of Adolescence

In the last decade, the total adolescent population between 10 and 19 years increased from 34 million in 1990 to 40 million in 2000. The adolescent population will be increasingly heterogeneous, with the percentage of those who do not consider their heritage primarily European going from 18.5% in 1980 to 45% by 2025 according to Census Bureau projections (National Adolescent Health Information Center [NAHIC], 2003a). This change may result in adolescents being seen as even more alien and becoming more marginalized. Hispanic youth are expected to be 22% of the total in 2025, African American 14%, and Asian/Pacific Islander 8%. Although two thirds of all young people less than 18 years lived with two parents in 2000, this percentage is down considerably since 1970, when 87.1% lived with two parents. In 2002, one of six adolescents lived in poverty, the lowest rate since measurement began. There continue to be large racial differences, with 46% of African American adolescents living with two parents, and nearly a third of all African American youth living in poverty in 2000 (NAHIC, 2003a). Most adolescents now live in suburbs (54%) rather than central cities (27%) or rural areas (19%), and more live in the South than any other region.

## The Context of Adolescent Development

Part of the difficulty in approaching adolescence has been in understanding the nature of adolescence. Many still think of adolescents not as people but as monstrosities to be avoided at best and endured and controlled at worst. Population-based studies do not confirm this negative view of normal adolescence. Most adolescents do not describe extreme moodiness but rather describe positive relationships with their parents; most parents describe their own adolescents in mostly positive terms. Numerous studies find that 80% of adolescents are growing up and becoming responsible adults without major difficulty (Offer & Schonert-Reichl, 1992). The consequence of the view that adolescence is inevitably a time of "storm and stress" for most youth is that problems may be dismissed as inherent to adolescence rather than seen as signs of significant social problems that can be modified. A more rounded view has developed in the social psychological literature of adolescence as a time of transitions with occasional perturbation (Steinberg, 2000) needing a "prolonged supportive environment with graded steps toward autonomy" (Irwin, 1987, p. 2). Indeed, some research suggests adolescence is more problematic for parents than for teenagers because of the parent's own developmental and relationship issues (Steinberg, 2000).

## Biological Development

Biological changes, particularly the development of the reproductive and endocrine systems, are often considered the engine for the train of many issues related to adolescent development. For females, the normal process may begin as early as age 8 years with the first stages of breast development. Height spurts commonly occur between the ages of 9.5 to 14.5 years and menarche between 10.5 and 15.5 years of age. Males are usually a little later, with testicular enlargement between 10.5 and 13.5 years of age and rapid growth in height and other dimensions approximately a year after that (US Congress, 1991b). Although the process takes a predictable course, there is much variation in timing between individuals such that normal puberty may be considered anywhere from years 8 to 18.

There are also significant historical and environmental variations in the timing of puberty. At the beginning of the 20th century, menarche averaged 14.5 years in the United States, and thus puberty was often not completed until near the end of high school. Currently, the average age of menarche is 12.5 years, and thus, the process is now often completed before high school. The exact causes of this change are unknown but are usually attributed to reductions in infectious disease and improvement in overall nutrition. Most researchers now believe the declining age of menarche has reached a plateau but that girl's breast development is happening somewhat earlier, although this may be because of more accurate assessment (Coleman & Coleman, 2002).

### Psychological Development and Social Health

Because so much of public health work regarding adolescence is focused on the behavioral changes of adolescents, it is necessary for public health workers to have an understanding of adolescent psychological and social development. Although the growth and development of the reproductive system are widely recognized, few appreciate the increasing complexity of mental operations made possible by neurologic and cognitive maturation in adolescence, a process that facilitates the transformations during adolescence in identity, personal relationships, and social roles. Until the last decade, most thinking about young people's cognitive ability has followed Piaget's developmental stage theories of a necessary and inevitable sequence from concrete thinking through simple abstractions, cognitive comparisons, perspective taking, and empathy to formal operations and synthesis using self-awareness, experience, judgment about the thinking process, and multiple strategies for making logical inferences. It is now recognized that the processes are much more environmentally supported or hindered than previously thought and much more specific to content areas of interest (Keating, 1990). "Rampant relativism," questioning everything, intolerance of inconsistency, literalism, and difficulty with understanding inferences and consequences, all common to earlier adolescents, may be seen as expected signs of incomplete cognitive maturity. Those attempting to influence adolescent risky behavior will need to take particular notice of adolescent cognitive development and perceptions of risk and vulnerability (Millstein & Halpern-Felsher, 2002).

Much psychologic research and theorizing have described normal adolescence during three phases. In the early adolescence phase, the central tasks are described as coming to terms with physical changes, the accompanying need for a changing body image, and increased cognitive abilities. Ego development is described as frequently impulsive and self-focused (Sayer, Hauser, Jacobson, Willett, & Cole, 1995). In the middle adolescence phase, the central tasks are developing independent relationships with peers and establishing a sexual identity while balancing continuing relationships with family. Ego development is described as conformist because it is usually group and peer centered and thus externally imposed. The late adolescence phase is often described as having the central tasks of completing the establishment of autonomy by determining vocational orientations and planning to exit the family of origin. The ego in late adolescence is described as postconformist in that there is increased internal control, greater reliance on internalized principles, appreciation of more subtle differences in motivation, and awareness of multiple causation. Developmental maturation usually results in an adequate resolution and integration of the various tasks, but as Hauser, Powers, and Noam (1991) noted, severe trauma, stress, emotional deprivation, and severely restricted environments can result in *arrested, foreclosed,* or *regressive* ego development, which can lead to more problems in functioning.

Developmental theory suggests that the goal of maturity is an independent identity, a suggestion that has several implications challenged by recent developmental and feminist theorists. Gilligan (1987) suggested that maturity is more related to the development of *inter*dependence, the ability to care and be connected, and thus, the excessive attention to independence as a goal of development reflects an excessively individualistic approach based on building theories looking only at middle-class male development. Others approaching youth from a life development perspective echo this theme by emphasizing that youth development should be thought about more as moving toward having productive and satisfying adulthoods, which encompass five important ingredients (Lerner & Castellino, 2002). These elements include *connections* to family, peers, and community; *competence* in academic, social, and vocational activities; *confidence* or a positive self-identity; *character*, or positive values and integrity; and *compassion*.

During adolescence, there is a significant increase in human sexual interest, arousal, and behavior. In 2003, nearly half (46.7%) of all high school students reported having had sexual intercourse during their lifetime, which is down slightly from 54.1% in 1991 (Grunbaum et al., 2004). Adolescents are exposed to considerable sexually oriented advertisements and entertainment; nevertheless, adolescents receive inconsistent messages from adults about the acceptability of sexual expression. This American cultural contradiction between a sexualized environment and the unacceptability of sexual behavior places youth in a double bind, tends to drive sexual decision making away from adult influence, and makes accessing contraceptives psychologically difficult for many. One research study found that those who pledged virginity until marriage had about the same age of sexual initiation and fewer partners but more sexually transmitted infections because they were less likely to use a condom (Straziuso, 2004). Developmental challenges related to the sexual unfolding of adolescents have been defined as (1) developing positive feelings about one's body, (2) learning to manage feelings of sexual arousal and desire, (3) developing new forms of autonomy and intimacy, and (4) developing skills to control the consequences of sexual behavior (Brooks-Gunn & Paikoff, 1993).

National studies on the sexual behaviors of adolescents have assumed that all adolescent respondents are heterosexual. Although seldom considered unless as pariahs, a significant number of youth are struggling with issues of sexual orientation, identity, and behavior without identifying themselves as homosexual (Savin-Williams, 2001). A large survey of high school students in Minnesota found that 4.5% considered themselves "predominantly homosexual," and 10.7% "weren't sure" of their sexual orientation (Remafedi, Resnick, Blum, & Harris, 1992). The concept of normal, healthy homosexual behavior is rarely discussed, but a few attempts have noted issues in parallel with those of heterosexuals, including coming to terms with one's self-identity, being able to achieve intimacy, and planning for the consequences of sexual activity. The massive stigmatization, alienation from supportive adults, and violence toward those with different sexual orientations result in greater difficulty achieving a healthy sexual identity and lead to distinctive subcultures offering different forms of community supports (Remafedi, 1989).

Social relationships also go through changes in adolescence. Families continue to be important, and as noted previously here, relationships are generally positive; however, significant changes still exist. Boundaries become more permeable such that adolescents and their families often have to find ways to accommodate new relationships. Conflict increases somewhat during early adolescence, particularly between mothers and daughters, usually about household chores. The adolescent defines the conflict as about issues of personal choice, but parents perceive the conflict as about issues of social propriety. Parent–adolescent conflict usually subsides by middle adolescence and is seldom threatening to family cohesion (Smetana, 1995). A substantial amount of research has attempted to define parenting correlates of adolescent competency, usually defined in terms of school achievement, psychological health, and healthy behavior (Baumrind, 1987; Darling & Steinberg, 1993; Lamborn, Mounts, Steinberg, & Dornbusch, 1991). Using both longitudinal convenience samples and large-scale school population-based samples, these studies analyzed parenting on two dimensions: amount of control or demandingness and amount of nurturance or warmth. This approach identified four basic types of parenting: *authoritative* (sometimes called democratic) parents who are demanding but warm and nurturing, *authoritarian* families who may be demanding but are not seen by the adolescent as warm or nurturing, *permissive* parents who are nurturing but not demanding, and *neglectful* or inattentive parents who are neither demanding nor warm toward the adolescent. Adolescents with authoritarian or authoritative parents generally achieve better than the other two groups, but young people with authoritative parents score higher on measures of psychological health and healthy behavior. The youth who fared the worst were those with neglectful parents. The degree of effect in most studies is rather low, and the distinctions between types somewhat imprecise, as most parents fall toward the middle on the two dimensions. This has been replicated among other cultural groups with similar results, but the positive impact of authoritative parenting is even more modest among African American families (Steinberg, Mounts, Lamborn, & Dornbusch, 1991).

## Environmental Context of Adolescent Health and Development

The context of adolescent lives is also affected by the larger society. Legal structures, schools, neighborhoods, the economy, and the media all have influence on the health and well-being of young people.

### Legal structure

The legal structure affects adolescent development by establishing a series of regulatory steps designed to reduce risky behavior until the young person is deemed by virtue of age to be capable. Statutes related to tobacco, alcohol, driving, sexual consent, medical consent, and financial responsibility are all based on judgments about adolescent developmental abilities and needs for protection. Although states differ, generally beginning about age 12 years, adolescents begin to have more legal rights (such as the ability to get confidential treatment for sexually transmitted diseases), and they progress in the direction of increasing legal autonomy in the areas of driving privileges (usually 16–18 years), consent for medical treatment (14–18 years), sexual consent (13–18 years), confidentiality (14–18 years), contracts (18 years), purchase of controlled substances such tobacco (18 years), and the last legal right in most states, buying alcohol (21 years). On the surface, such variation seems inconsistent, which can be quite irritating to some youth, but such inconsistency reflects attempts at accommodation between the reality of increasing adolescent autonomy and the need for continued adult involvement and responsibility. Most important, state laws do recognize the need for minors to have confidentiality regarding sexual health issues to encourage treatment of sexually transmitted infections and to allow access to contraception (English & Kenney, 2003). The trend in the law has been to increase legal rights for young people. Nevertheless, the legal right for young people to seek medical treatment, especially regarding sexuality and abortion, continues to be highly controversial (English, 2002). The important issue of legal obligation to pay for services and the ability of minors to qualify for state-funded health care also varies widely. Some states allow minors to become eligible for Medicaid for reproductive health care services ("sensitive services") based on their own income and assets rather than their family's income. Without such eligibility, confidentiality provisions are rather hollow because the medical bill may be sent home.

### Schools

Schools have a major influence on adolescent health and development and are often a major site for public health interventions. Poor school adaptation as shown through dropping out, grade retention, and a lack of participation in school activities has been associated with pregnancy, delinquency, substance use, unemployment, and reduced earnings (US Congress, 1991b), and poor engagement in school has been associated with high-risk behavior (Resnick et al., 1997).

Although the problems of poor school adaptation may be most related to social class issues, some factors of school structure and environment have been associated with poorer adaptation and engagement, as reviewed by the Office of Technology Assessment (US Congress, 1991b). Efforts to increase academic standards by using standardized testing, requiring more courses, and tracking by ability have increased academic performance for a few but have also increased grade retention, school dropout, and alienation among more marginal students. Larger schools are problematic. Somewhat smaller schools, 500–1000 students, generally have more social cohesion and participation in school activities than larger schools and have proportionately fewer behavior problems, delinquency, dropping out, or health problems. Policies that facilitate participation by teachers, students, and parents in decision making have shown similar benefits. Schools that have more transitions—between classes, teachers, subjects, and/or grade level—tend to have worse behavior and less achievement, particularly among early adolescent girls and among poorer students. Studies of the effects of class size in adolescence have shown mixed results, but the negative impact of larger class size is worse again on the more marginal students.

Disparities based on ethnic and racial identity continue to plague schools. Seldom recognized has been the significant improvement in educational performance of minorities. Although African American and Hispanic youth still lag behind their white counterparts, the gap in standardized testing scores for 17 year olds has been reduced 45% for African American students from 1971 to 1996 and 27% for Hispanic students since 1975, the first year that results of Hispanics were separately reported (Ferguson, 2001). This improvement may reflect the tremendous discrepancy between whites and blacks under mostly officially segregated conditions until the 1970s, changes in family structure, and improvement in parental education (Grissmer, Kirby, Berends, & Williamson, 1995). Nevertheless, African American and Hispanic youth continue to do less well on standardized tests and in graduation rates (US Department of Education, 2003).

### Neighborhood and community

Neighborhood and community effects on adolescent development are most studied in terms of the consequences of concentrations of poverty in urban environments. Seldom studied are rural/urban differences. Poor urban neighborhoods have more single mothers, more unemployed men, more substance abuse, and fewer positive role models (National Research Council, Commission on Behavioral and Social Sciences and Education, 1993). The consequences on adolescents of living in a high poverty-concentration neighborhood include more risky behavior, poorer educational achievement, and high rates of pregnancy, delinquency, and violent crime. The effects are particularly strong on males (Katz, King, & Liebman, 2001). The negative effects have been attributed to (1) a lack of institutional resources, (2) impaired relationships and social connections, and (3) neighborhood norms that do not encourage collective efficacy and do not support social control over inappropriate behavior (Leventhal & Brooks-Gunn, 2003). The concentration of poverty in neighborhoods, which had been increasing for decades, declined substantially in the 1990s (Jargowsky, 2003).

Neighborhoods vary by more than poverty concentration. A study of small cities in the Midwest found important differences between communities independent of poverty. Community assets may be defined as policies and practices that support families, facilitate positive interactions with and between youth, and endorse more prosocial values (Blyth, 1993). Communities that had more of these assets tended to have adolescents who had lower frequency of risk behaviors, substance abuse, pregnancy, antisocial behavior, depression, and vandalism.

### Economic influences

Economic influences on adolescent health and development are poorly understood because researchers seldom obtain income data directly and instead use proxy measures such as parental education or race. Nevertheless, the influence on health and development is considerable. The poorer the adolescent, the more likely the youth will be disabled, have a chronic condition, have emotional or behavioral problems, lack health insurance, not see a health care provider, not see a dentist, or have unmet medical needs (Newacheck, Hung, Park, Brindis, & Irwin, 2003a). Poorer adolescents are more likely to have school problems, get pregnant, or be arrested (US Congress, 1991c). Economic changes affect family behavior. Because of declining wage structure, increasing single parenthood, and sky-rocketing housing prices in many areas, more family caretakers need to be employed outside of the home. Single-parent families have increased from 10% of the population in 1965 to 27% in 2001 (Ellwood & Jencks, 2002). Adolescents at home without adult supervision are engaged in more risk behavior, regardless of economic status (Richardson, Radziszewska, Dent, & Flay, 1993). Economic problems also affect parenting behavior. Studies of middle-class Iowa families who had major decreases in income found increased parental depression and hostility, particularly among the men, which resulted in greater negativity by the father toward the adolescent children in the family, which in turn was associated with more antisocial behavior and depression among the adolescents (Elder, Conger, Foster, & Ardelt, 1992). Other studies have associated poverty with fewer positive role models for adolescents, restricted geographic mobility resulting in exposure to riskier neighborhoods, greater disengagement from society (particularly among African American males), and greater difficulty with becoming employed (Sum & Fogg, 1991). Although poverty increases the risks of poor transitions, it should be recognized that two thirds of poor adolescents are not poor as adults (Edelman & Ladner, 1991).

### The media

The media, particularly television, is often seen as a major influence on adolescent development, usually in terms of stimulating desire, fostering violence, socializing adolescents into the market economy, and supporting passivity. American 11 to 13 year olds watch 23.6 hours per week, and 14 to 18 year olds average 17 hours per week (Roberts, 2000). For many parents, particularly those in middle school, the television has become the after-school plan to "keep kids out of trouble." A variety of studies using a variety of methods have established a relationship between TV watching and fearfulness, desensitization, and violent behavior (Brown & Witherspoon, 2002). Researchers have also identified negative effects of television on academic performance, weight, and increased risk behavior, including substance use and earlier sexual activity (Villani, 2001). Others have linked increases in gender stereotyping, consumerism, and aggressiveness to television watching (Strasburger, 2004). Research on other forms of electronic media such as the Internet or video games may have similar results but have not been comprehensively researched.

# ADOLESCENT HEALTH STATUS

Although adolescents are generally healthy, there are important exceptions, disparities, and unhealthy patterns. Adolescent mortality increased during the mid 1990s but is now at an all-time low. The causes of death have changed over the decades from mostly infectious disease-related causes in 1950 to mostly injury, both intentional and unintentional, today. Epidemiologic analysis of adolescent health problems indicates the pervasiveness of behavioral factors in the morbidity and mortality of adolescents, and many of these same behaviors initiated during adolescence contribute to the morbidities and mortalities experienced in adulthood.

## Data Sources for Adolescent Health

Data about adolescent health have increased over the last decade. The most widely used assessment of adolescent health behaviors has been the CDC's Youth Risk Behavior Surveillance System (YRBSS). The YRBSS uses national, state, and local samples of high school students throughout the United States to measure the incidence and prevalence of the specific behaviors among adolescents that lead to their most important health problems. The YRBSS is also used by schools, communities, and states to assess health risk status and to target interventions. An important limitation of the YRBSS has been that it does not include higher risk, out-of-school youth who may be incarcerated, homeless, or working. Another important national data source is the National Health Interview Survey carried out at regular intervals by the National Center for Health Statistics. This survey obtains baseline health data and information on varying topics. The federal governmental sponsors several more surveys, which include the National Survey of Family Growth, the National Survey of Drug Use and Health, and the University of Michigan's Monitoring the Future project, which evaluates substance use trends yearly. Information about data sources for adolescent health is readily available on the Internet (Ozer, Park, Paul, Brindis, & Irwin, 2003).

These surveys have limitations. Many continue to use differing age categories. Some do not include nonstudents; few surveys include information on the socioeconomic status of respondents. Although some have questioned whether responses on a survey vary by school or home setting, a comprehensive analysis found that such differences do not affect the validity of results (Brenner, Billy, & Grady, 2003). Some have noted that cultural controversy has emerged over whether surveys of youth are a violation of parental confidentiality and should require active parental consent. As a result, some surveys, particularly those regarding sexual behavior, have been withdrawn from the field.

## Mortality

Adolescent and young adult death rates have declined slowly over the last 20 years (Figure 8–1). There are important subgroups with much worse

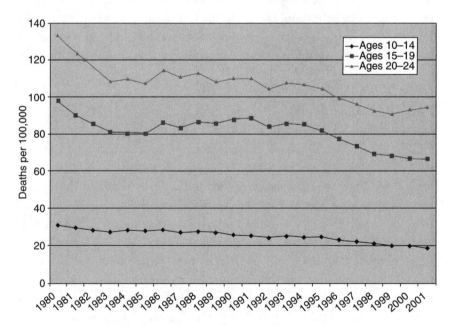

FIGURE 8–1 Adolescent mortality trends 1980–2001.

mortality. Mortality rates for males ages 10 to 14 years are 1.5 times female mortality rates, and males ages 15 to 19 years have a mortality rate that is 2.4 times that of females. There is also large variation by ethnicity, with Native American/Alaskan Natives and African Americans having much higher death rates. The differences among males and ethnic groups is largely accounted for by differences in injury mortality.

## Specific Adolescent Health Problems and Health-Related Behaviors

### Injuries

Injuries, both intentional and unintentional, are the major cause of death to adolescents. Among youth ages 15 to 19 years, injuries accounted for 75% of the 13,555 deaths in 2001, and among youth ages 10 to 14 years, injuries were 51% of the 4,002 deaths in the same year (CDC, 2004a). Motor vehicle injuries are the leading cause of death for both age groups (Figure 8–2). Males are more likely than females to die from injury, particularly among 15 to 19 year olds. American Indians/Alaskan Natives and Whites are more likely to die from motor vehicle injuries and suicide

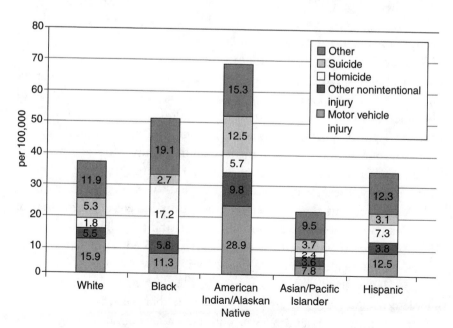

FIGURE 8–2  Mortality rates by ethnicity ages 10–19, 2001.

than others. African Americans have much higher rates of homicide, although these have declined dramatically since 1993 from a high of 140 per 100,000 to 60 per 100,000 in 2000 among 15 to 19 year olds (Ozer et al., 2003). Injuries cause much morbidity. It is estimated that for every fatal injury there are 41 adolescents hospitalized for a nonfatal injury (Runyan & Gerken, 1991).

### Unintentional injuries

The most common causes of death from unintentional injuries are motor vehicle crashes (73% of all unintentional injuries), drowning (6%), unintentional firearm injuries (2%), and other land transportation injuries (2.5%) (CDC, 2004a). Since 1980, there has been a steady reduction in motor vehicle fatalities (32% mortality rate reduction among 15 to 19 year olds) that has been attributed to increased seat belt use and reductions in alcohol-related fatalities (Sells & Blum, 1996).

### Intentional injuries and violence

Intentional injuries are defined as injuries resulting from interpersonal violence, including homicide and the self-directed violence of suicide. In 2002 there were 3,971 intentional deaths of 10 to 19 year olds, most of which were among the 15 to 19 year olds. Although homicide deaths to youth have decreased more than 50% since 1983, the US rate is still 10 to 15 times the rate of most European countries (Krug, Dahlberg, Mercy, Zwi, & Lozano, 2002). Males are much more likely to be victims, particularly black 15- to 19-year-old males, who were 17 times more likely to be killed as white youth the same age in 2000 (Ozer et al., 2003). Guns are involved in approximately three of four adolescent homicides, and three of four firearm deaths are with small handguns. Most victims knew their assailant; 60% of the shooting deaths were after an argument. Interestingly, the rate of *assaults* in Denmark is similar to that of the United States, but the *homicide* rate is approximately one fifth that of Ohio, a comparable size population, suggesting that the availability of guns rather than violent behavior per se is the predominant factor for increased homicide (Cohall & Cohall, 1995).

Suicide has been identified as the third leading cause of death among adolescents. Suicide rates are higher for males than for females, more frequent in rural areas and Western states, much higher among Native Americans, and somewhat higher among Hispanics and whites than among African American adolescents. Attempted suicide is even more common, with 8.5% of all adolescent students surveyed as part of the 2003 YRBSS reporting a suicide attempt (Grunbaum et al., 2004) (Table 8–1). Twice as many females as males made an attempt, Hispanic females more than white or African American females. Prior history of suicide attempt, substance abuse, presence of firearms in the home, family history of suicide, antisocial behavior, and psychiatric disorders have all been associated with increased risk for completed suicide (US Public Health Service, 1999).

### Chronic Illness and Disabilities

Chronic conditions include a wide spectrum of physical and mental health problems, including hay fever, asthma, cancer, cardiovascular disease, learning disabilities, epilepsy, juvenile-onset diabetes, hearing and visual impairments, leukemia, chronic kidney disease, and cystic fibrosis. Many of these disabilities result in a substantially reduced quality of life for the adolescent. Additionally, chronically ill adolescents may need more significant health and social services.

According to the National Child Health Interview Survey, 20.1% of all 12 to 17 year olds had an activity limitation in 2002 (Child Trends, 2004). The condition most frequently identified as a cause of functional limitation among all children aged 17 years was asthma, affecting 15% of all adolescents ages 12 to 17 years (Dey, Schiller, & Tai, 2004). Learning disability was the next highest at 10.5%. The percentage with activity limitation, emotional and behavioral problems, or being in only fair to poor health varied by income: the poorer the family background, the higher the rate of chronic symptoms (Newacheck et al., 2003a).

### Mental Health

No national prevalence studies have been conducted to assess specific diagnosable mental disorders in adolescents. In one national study, 23% of parents of 6 to 16 year olds reported on a standardized checklist that their youth had a symptom of emotional or psychiatric distress (Achenbach, Dumenci, & Rescorla, 2003). Another national study found that 8.8% of parents of 12 to 17 year olds reported that their adolescents had a high level of emotional or psychiatric distress (Vandivere, Gallagher, & Moore, 2004). Learning disabilities are among the most common mental health problems of young people, affecting 9.6% of adolescents,

**Table 8–1** Health Risk Behaviors, US 9th and 12th Grades, Youth Risk Behavior Surveillance Survey, 2003.

| Behavior | Total | Male | Female | 9th Grade | 12th Grade | White | Black | Hispanic |
|---|---|---|---|---|---|---|---|---|
| Injury-related behaviors | | | | | | | | |
| -Rarely or never uses a seat belt | 18% | 22% | 15% | 20% | 16% | 17% | 21% | 20% |
| -Rode within last 30 days with a driver who had been drinking alcohol | 30 | 29 | 31 | 28 | 33 | 28 | 31 | 36 |
| -Carried a weapon last month | 17 | 27 | 7 | 18 | 16 | 17 | 17 | 16 |
| -Made a suicide attempt within last year | 8.5 | 5.4 | 11 | 10 | 6.1 | 6.9 | 8.4 | 11 |
| Substance use related behaviors in last 30 days | | | | | | | | |
| -Smoked cigarettes | 22 | 22 | 22 | 17 | 26 | 25 | 15 | 18 |
| -Drank alcohol | 45 | 44 | 46 | 36 | 56 | 47 | 37 | 46 |
| -Had five or more drinks at a time | 28 | 29 | 28 | 20 | 37 | 32 | 15 | 29 |
| -Smoked marijuana | 22 | 25 | 19 | 18 | 26 | 22 | 24 | 24 |
| -Used cocaine | 4.1 | 4.6 | 3.5 | 3.6 | 4.7 | 3.8 | 2.2 | 5.7 |
| Sexual behaviors | | | | | | | | |
| -Had intercourse in the last 3 months | 34 | 34 | 35 | 21 | 49 | 31 | 49 | 37 |
| -Used a condom at last intercourse | 63 | 69 | 57 | 69 | 57 | 62 | 73 | 57 |
| Nutrition and exercise-related behaviors | | | | | | | | |
| -Trying to lose weight | 44 | 29 | 59 | 42 | 45 | 45 | 35 | 49 |
| -Engages in sufficient vigorous physical activity | 63 | 70 | 55 | 68 | 55 | 66 | 55 | 59 |

Totals that are more than 10% are rounded to nearest whole number.
Source: Grunbaum et al. (2004).

which includes 7.7% of all adolescent who have been diagnosed with attention deficit disorder (Blackwell, Vickerie, & Wondimu, 2003). Prolonged depressed mood within the last 6 months has been estimated to affect between 10% to 20% of adolescents, and 9.2% of adolescents meet formal diagnostic criteria for major depressive disorder (Rushton, Forcier, & Schecktman, 2002). Eating restriction is common in adolescence, with 56.2% of high school girls saying that they have dieted, 18.3% having fasted to lose weight, 11.3% having used diet pills, and 8.4% taking laxatives or vomiting for weight-related reasons (Grunbaum et al., 2004). Approximately 0.3% to 1% of high school girls meet psychiatric criteria for the diagnosis of anorexia nervosa, and approximately 4% to 10% struggle with bulimia (Whitaker, 1992).

## Sexual Behavior and its Health Consequences

There has been a small decrease in sexual intercourse among adolescents over the last several years, but sexual activity is still quite common. In 2003, nearly one third of ninth graders reported that they had had sexual intercourse, and nearly two thirds of seniors reported they had had intercourse (Grunbaum et al, 2004). These rates are substantially similar to other comparable countries (Darroch, Singh, & Frost, 2001). In addition to the decline in sexual activity among teens, there has been an increase in condom use. Among sexually active teens, 63% said that they used a condom at last intercourse in 2003 compared with 46% in 1991, with African American youth reporting the highest rate of condom use (72.8%) (Grunbaum et al., 2004). Nevertheless, youth in the United States continue to have much more negative consequences of sexual activity than their peers in comparable countries in spite of substantial improvement.

Approximately 846,000 adolescents became pregnant in 1999, which is a decrease from nearly a million in 1990 (NAHIC, 2003b). The rates of pregnancy, birth, abortion, and miscarriage among 15 to 19 year olds are approximately twice those of most European countries. The total *number* of pregnancies to non-Hispanic whites exceeds African American and Latina pregnancies, but the pregnancy *rates* of these two groups is twice the white rate. Being poor increases the birthrate among teens, with 83% of births to teens in families with incomes less $25,000, and half of all births to teens occur in families with income less than $12,000. Approximately one half of pregnancies result in a live birth. Approximately 21% result in an abortion, and the rest miscarry. Substantial risks have been associated with adolescent childbearing, including lower birthweight, higher mortality rates, poorer school performance, and less adequate parenting (National Campaign to Prevent Teen Pregnancy, 2004), although many of these effects may be more related to poverty than early child bearing (Geronimus, 1987; Luker, 1996).

Another important health consequence of adolescent sexual activity is sexually transmitted infection, including HIV. Adolescents account for approximately one fourth of the 15 million reported cases of sexually transmitted infections every year. Chlamydia, the most common of these diseases, has increased dramatically over the last decade, but this may be related to increased screening and less invasive testing (Ozer et al., 2003). Gonorrhea rates have generally declined but still are much more prevalent among African Americans (11 times the rate among Hispanic youth and 23 times that of white, non-Hispanic youth). Although AIDS is relatively uncommon among adolescents, the long incubation period of development from HIV infection to AIDS implies that many of those diagnosed with AIDS in their 20s contracted the disease as teens. Among teenagers, HIV is more often diagnosed among young women (CDC, 2002).

### Tobacco, Alcohol, and Other Drug Use

Prevalences of tobacco, alcohol, and other substance use by adolescents have long been identified as serious threats to the health of youth (Blum, 1987). Alcohol and other drug use frequently contribute to the causes of unintentional and intentional injuries, including motor vehicle-related injuries, homicide, and suicide, and may be a factor in unintended pregnancy and lead to a variety of medical, psychological, and social morbidities. The trend in substance use has been generally down since the 1980s, but there were increases in cigarette smoking and marijuana use until the late 1990s (CDC, 2004a).

Existing data on the incidence and prevalence of tobacco, alcohol, and other drugs used by adolescents are based on self-reports. Self-reported data may not be entirely accurate because of adolescents' attempts to provide socially desirable responses. Adolescents may also report engaging in behaviors that challenge what is socially desirable.

The most frequently used drugs by adolescents are those that eventually will be legal for them to use. Although nearly three fifths of students have tried cigarettes and almost four fifths have drunk alcohol at least once, regular and current use is less (Grunbaum et al., 2004). Students who have smoked within the last month are 21.9% of the high school population, and 15.8% have smoked nearly every day. Nearly half of all high school students have drunk alcohol within the last month, and nearly 30% have drunk five or more drinks on at least one occasion within the last 30 days. Out of school, adolescents were significantly more likely than in-school adolescents to have reported ever having smoked cigarettes (CDC, 1994). White and Hispanic students, older students, and out-of-school adolescents were significantly more likely than African American students to be current users of cigarettes (Table 8–1).

Illicit substance use is not as prevalent as use of alcohol and tobacco, but a significant number of adolescents reported use of marijuana and/or cocaine. In 2003 two fifths of students surveyed had used marijuana during their lifetime, and 22.4% used marijuana within the last month. Older, male, and out-of-school youth are more likely than others to report ever having used marijuana. Overall, 8.7% of students surveyed had used cocaine during their lifetime, and 4.1% were current cocaine users. Hispanic male and female students were significantly more likely than white or African American students to have tried cocaine. Despite the stereotype of cocaine as only an urban black problem, white youth were significantly more likely than African American young people to report ever having used cocaine (Grunbaum et al., 2004). Out-of-school adolescents were three times more likely than in-school adolescents to have reported ever having used cocaine (7.1% vs. 2.1%) (CDC, 1994). Rural substance abuse is as high or higher than other areas, particularly tobacco use and binge drinking (Atav & Spencer, 2002; Fahs et al., 1999).

## Obesity, Nutrition, and Physical Activity

The nutritional and activity statuses of adolescents are important for several reasons. First, adolescent growth and development require an increase in energy and an increase in nutrients, particularly iron, calcium, and certain other minerals. Second, as adolescents make more independent food choices, patterns are developing that could play important roles in several chronic diseases in adulthood. Third, eating habits may have even more direct effects on health during adolescence, such as obesity or deficits during pregnancy. Fourth, nutrition and physical activity patterns are changing for the worse.

Chronic diseases begin to develop during childhood and adolescence. Autopsies of young men in their early 20s, taken during the wars in Korea and Vietnam, showed fatty streaks indicative of atherosclerosis, thus confirming that this chronic disease starts early. Certain types of cancer, stroke, diabetes mellitus, and osteoporosis have been associated with long-term dietary behaviors. Certain chronic diseases, particularly diabetes, need careful attention to nutritional issues. Good bone development related to physical activity and calcium-rich diets in adolescence results in less osteoporosis in adult life (National Research Council, 1989).

Eating patterns, which relate to the development of obesity, are often established in adolescence and earlier. An ongoing national study of nutrition found that 15.5% of adolescents were overweight in 1999 to 2000 compared with 4.6% in the first survey period of 1966 to 1970 (Ogden, Flegal, Carroll, & Johnson, 2002). Again, there is much variation by ethnicity, with 12.4% of white teens, 26.6% of black teens, and 19.4% of Mexican-American teens being overweight in 1999–2000. Television watching, maternal inactivity, and irregular eating patterns have been associated with obesity. Among irregular eating patterns are three behaviors that are common during adolescence—skipping meals, snacking, and eating high-fat food, particularly "fast food." During pregnancy, nutritional needs for women increase, particularly for folic acid, but the general adolescent diet is low in this and other important nutrients. This is particularly important during the first several months when many do not know (or do not wish to know) that they are pregnant.

Although approximately two thirds of adolescents are vigorously physically active, the percentage declines with each age group (Grunbaum et al., 2004). The percentage of vigorously active adolescents has not changed since monitoring through the YRBSS began in 1993.

## Data on Well-Being of Adolescents

Traditionally, health care data have focused on mortality, morbidity, and related risk behaviors. Recently, researchers have noted that positive factors about adolescents prevent and moderate harm from risky behavior. These positive aspects of youth development may in fact be more critical to the successful transition to healthy and productive adulthood than most specific risk behaviors. Many indicators, from percentage volunteering to proportion attending religious services, have been considered, but two constructs have been particularly identified as linked to better health and less risky behavior: parental connectedness and school engagement (Resnick et al., 1997).

## Parental Connectedness

Adolescents who report feeling closer to their parents emotionally tend to do better in school, engage in fewer risk behaviors, and show more signs of psychological health, and thus, the degree of parental closeness reported by adolescents is one potential positive marker of adolescent well-being. Most adolescents describe feeling very close to their parents. In a study using a national database, of those adolescents living with their biological parents, 70% said they felt very close to their mothers, and 58% felt very close to their fathers (Resnick et al., 1997). Ethnic minority youth, less educated, and younger adolescents all reported more parental connectedness.

## School Connectedness

The degree of being engaged in school also shows an effect on school performance, risk behaviors, and psychological health, which is similar to that of parental connectedness. In 2002, 30.9% of parents reported indicators suggesting that their adolescent had a high degree of high engagement in school. Parents who were better educated and who had younger adolescents reported more school engagement (Vandivere et al., 2004). The parents perceived their youth as less highly engaged in school in 2002 than parents did in a previous study in 1997; adolescents from families with higher incomes had a bigger decrease in the percentage who indicated that they were highly engaged in school.

## *Health Care Use*

Adolescents use health care services for the treatment of acute (sore throat, injury, etc.) and chronic (hypertension, asthma, diabetes, etc.) conditions as well as for preventive services, including dental services, mental health services, substance abuse services, and reproductive health services. Although adolescents use health services less than any other age group, nearly three fourths do see a health care provider each year (Newacheck, Brindis, Cart, Marchi, & Irwin, 1999). Despite having worse health status, poor and minority youth have more time elapsed between visits to health care and fewer hospitalizations than white and non-poor youth. Rural and Southern youth also are less likely to receive such health services. Most health care is paid for by private insurance, but 30% is paid for out of pocket by families. Twelve percent of adolescents were uninsured in 2002. This decline in uninsured adolescents since

1995, even though private insurance coverage declined, is due to an expansion of Medicaid and the implementation of the State Child Health Insurance Program (Newacheck, Park, Brindis, Biehl, & Irwin, 2004).

Adolescents seek health services in a variety of places, including physicians' offices, emergency rooms, neighborhood and community health centers, public health departments, and school-based clinics. Of those seeing private physicians, early adolescents tend to see pediatricians rather than family practice doctors (41% vs. 25%). Middle adolescents 15 to 17 years old tend to see family practice physicians more than pediatricians (35% vs. 21%), but obstetricians/gynecologists see 19% of all females in this age group. Among late adolescents 19 to 21 years old, most medical visits are with family practice doctors (26.8%) rather than pediatricians (4%) or internal medicine physicians (7%), but obstetricians/gynecologists doctors see 37% of all female visits (Ziv, Boulet, & Slap, 1999).

Care is generally episodic rather than preventive. The most common health concerns and conditions prompting adolescent visits to a physician's office vary by age. Respiratory illnesses are the most common diagnoses, but the "V" code diagnostic category, which includes yearly general exams and preventive care, including immunizations, are the next most common diagnostic category in private office visits (14.7% of early adolescent visits, 23.5% of middle adolescent, and 29.4% of late adolescent visits). Despite this, important preventive opportunities are often missed. Only 2% of all visits include discussions about smoking cessation, weight control, nutrition, or HIV transmission (Igra & Millstein, 1993).

## THEMES FOR IMPROVING ADOLESCENT HEALTH

Analysis of adolescent health status and adolescent developmental issues has guided public health researchers, policy makers, and advocates to develop a few basic themes for improving the health of adolescents (Brindis et al., 1996). In addition to the US Congress's Office of Technology Assistance report in 1991, numerous foundations (e.g., Carnegie Council on Adolescent Development, 1989, 1995; William T. Grant Foundation, 1988) and government-sponsored collaborations (Health Futures of Youth, 1988; Irwin & Duncan, 2002; National Commission on Children, 1991) have concluded primarily the following:

1. Adolescent risk behaviors need to be addressed because of their tremendous impact on adolescent health now and throughout the life cycle.
2. Risk behavior may best be reduced by focusing on positive youth development and enhancing resilience.
3. Youth need better access to appropriate health care.
4. Research can guide our understanding of adolescent development, health status, and program effectiveness.

Undergirding all of these has been an increasing recognition that social and economic disparities are major factors in poorer health and that stigma about adolescents in general and about many adolescent subpopulations in particular inhibits adolescent growth and development.

## Ubiquitousness of Adolescent Risk

Although most adolescents are on track, doing their homework, arguing about their chores, and being generally responsible, most also engage in varying degrees of risky behavior. Most concerning are those who initiate multiple risk behaviors in early adolescence (Irwin, 1990; Jessor & Jessor, 1977). Although young people are often unfairly labeled by their problems (drug users, dropouts, gangsters), research confirms what youth service providers, parents, and teenagers have long known—youth who engage in one troubling behavior often engage in other risky behaviors. The adolescent who is initially identified with one problem likely has problems in other domains. The youth with drug problems, for example, has probably had school problems, tumultuous relationships with parents, and legal troubles and is more likely to have health problems from high-risk sexual behavior. Antecedents of high-risk behavior include early school failure and behavioral problems in elementary school, smoking tobacco in late childhood and early adolescence, and early puberty in girls. All of these suggest potential for earlier interventions and for evaluations of programs for younger children that monitor behavioral outcomes well into adolescence.

Risk taking may be particularly important for adolescent development in that it may assist with expectations regarding familial emancipation and help develop autonomy, mastery, and intimacy. Along these lines, Donovan and Jessor (1985) have argued that "problem behavior" should be seen as a functional aspect of development in that these behaviors may be means of achieving otherwise blocked goal obtainment, may be ways of expressing opposition to adult authority, may be ways of gaining access to peers and youth culture, and may be means of confirming self-identity. From this perspective, interventions aimed at reducing risk behaviors will need to address more dramatically the developmental needs of adolescents for mastery, peer relationships, and identity (Millstein & Igra, 1996).

## Resilience and Youth Development

Important concepts related to risk behavior emerging from longitudinal research are resilience and positive youth development. It has been noted that even among high-risk youth in high-risk environments, some young people succeed. One such study of high-risk children in Hawaii identified one third of the youth as high risk because they have four or more situations thought to be unfavorable to development—family situations such as poverty, conflict, alcoholism, or mental illness. These children showed signs of emotional distress in childhood, but at 18 years old, one third were doing well, and at 32 years old, nearly one half "loved well, worked well, played well, and expected well" (Werner, 1992, p. 263). The successful children connected to caring and supportive adults, had positive temperament and skills, and got second chances in late adolescence through military or adult education programs. Others have noted that communities and youth who have many assets such as those that encourage connectedness tend to have less risky behavior and less damage from risky behaviors (Blyth, 1993; Murphey, Lamonda, Carney, & Duncan, 2004).

Healthy development of youth involves more than being risk free. Programs and policies that aim to improve adolescent health need to focus more on youth development, which has been defined as

> . . . the ongoing growth process in which all youth are engaged in attempting (1) to meet their basic personal and social needs to be safe, feel cared for, be valued, be useful, and be spiritually grounded, and (2) to build skills and competencies that allow them to function and contribute in their daily lives. (Pittman, O'Brien, & Kimball, 1993, p. 8)

This leads to a view of youth as a resource who can be actively engaged in communities with caring adults rather than youth as just "at risk." Youth who are ". . . problem free are not fully prepared . . . but need skills, knowledge, and a variety of personal and social assets to function well during adolescence and adulthood" (Eccles & Gootman, 2002, p. 2–3). Such an orientation shifts the view of adolescence to focus more on healthy development and the institutions that support development rather than the individual undesirable behavior and the institutions which respond only to the isolated individual behavior. This also leads to more focus on building assets in the community context of adolescence (Lerner & .Castellino, 2002).

A wide variety of programs such as 4-H, mentoring, recreation, and civic action groups have been built on these principles. Increasingly, the research suggests that such programs, by and large, are effective in producing positive outcomes and less negative outcomes (Catalano, Hawkins, Berglund, Pollard, & Arthur, 2002; Eccles & Gootman, 2002; Roth & Brooks-Gunn, 2003).

## Access to Quality Health Care

Because young people and their families trust physicians and want guidance on development, sexuality, and health, these health care visits could be an opportunity for preventive health care and health promotion (Park et al., 2001). However, numerous financial and nonfinancial barriers to health care exist (Brindis, Morreale, & English, 2001).

Among financial barriers is a lack of insurance coverage and/or inadequate coverage. In addition to the uninsured, health insurance is often inadequate to the needs of adolescents. Approximately 30% of all adolescent health costs are paid by families out of pocket in the form of premiums, co-payments, uncovered prescriptions, and uncovered services (Newacheck, Wong, Galbraith, & Hung, 2003b). Although public and private insurance may generally both provide good coverage for traditional services, coverage for preventive services, confidential health care, mental health, and substance abuse treatment services is particularly inadequate (Fox, McManus, & Reichman, 2003). Inadequate reimbursement rates in fee-for-service systems or time pressures in managed-care environments discourage many physicians from screening and treating adolescents who require services that are more time intensive.

Many nonfinancial factors often make quality health care services difficult for adolescents. Adolescents who do not feel that their health concerns will remain confidential may be hesitant to seek medical care. In one survey of patients from 33 Wisconsin family planning clinics, one half of the adolescents reported that they would stop using health care services if their parent's permission were required for prescriptions for oral contraceptives (Reddy, Fleming, & Swain, 2002). Earlier studies have found even greater health care avoidance rates because of concerns about confidentiality (Council of Scientific Affairs, 1993). Only a third of the students in a Massachusetts study knew that they could get confidential care for sexually transmitted infections. Interestingly, an even higher percentage of youth said they did not want their friends to know their health concerns, a finding that needs to be considered in the development of school-based and school-linked health services and peer education programs (Cheng, Savageau, Sattler, & DeWitt, 1993).

Other nonfinancial impediments to quality health care are related to the complex biopsychosocial nature of adolescents' health problems. Youth and health care providers are often frustrated with the fragmentation of services across several different institutions—education, child welfare, juvenile justice, community mental health—each with its own priorities, cultures, and financing. Health care providers who work with adolescents often report that their training did not prepare them to manage these complexities. The focus on acute care within the health care system often makes difficult the screening, anticipatory guidance, relationship building, and problem solving that health promotion needs.

## Growing Research on Program Effectiveness

Research on adolescents and health has mushroomed. There are at least 12 academic journals on adolescent issues, meta-analyses, and syntheses on numerous topics and research issues (Millstein et al., 2000). One particular area of research has been on program evaluation, with several summaries and synthesis available outlining "Best Practices" (Child Trends, 2002; Hawkins, Catalano, & Arthur, 2002; Komro & Stigler, 2000; Nation et al., 2003; Schinke, Brounstein, & Gardner, 2002; Wandersman & Florin, 2003; Weissberg, Kumpfer, & Seligman, 2003).

Most of these reviews identified degrees of evidence (i.e., "effective," "noneffective," "unproven," and "promising") for evaluating programs and established criteria for program inclusion based on the quality of evaluation and program design. One review found that effective programs were comprehensive, had multiple intervention strategies, often were implemented in multiple settings, had explicit theoretical grounding, developed positive relationships, varied in teaching methods, paid attention to timing, were socioculturally relevant, had sufficient dosage, and hired well-trained staff (Wandersman & Florin, 2003). Another review of positive youth development programs found tremendous variety but that most worked in multiple social domains, particularly school involvement, included families and community, had a series of positive youth constructs in the program planning such as promoting bonding, self-efficacy, prosocial norms, and competency. These programs also made a point of measuring positive and negative behaviors (Catalano et al., 2002). The Substance Abuse and Mental Health Services administration has created a registry of programs judged to be effective by 15 criteria and has concluded similarly that programs are most effective when they create webs of influence in multiple domains, target positive and negative behaviors, include families and community, and pay close attention to program design, fidelity of implementation, and evaluation (Schinke et al., 2002).

Most evaluated programs depend on community-based efforts. Reviewers have found that although community-based programs have often had positive impacts, the results have been inconsistent (Wandersman & Florin, 2003). This has been particularly so when programs expand or replicate. One difficulty has been having valid, reliable, and ethical evaluations, as random assignment or using comparison sites can create suspiciousness in many communities. Another difficulty is that getting an adequate dose or amount of intervention may make difficult achieving significant results. Creating, maintaining, and sustaining a coalition are time consuming and often problematic because of the different agenda and cultural backgrounds of the various coalition members and researchers. As the Anne E. Casey Foundation (2001) learned through its *Making Connections* effort, communities change during the process; such initiatives take a long time, and issues of race, power, and equity are too often ignored but always present.

# PUBLIC HEALTH PROGRAMS FOR ADOLESCENTS

Reflecting the dilemmas of the American political structure (Brindis & Ott, 2001), public health efforts to improve adolescent health have been an interaction of federal, state, and local community efforts and a mix of public and private organizational involvement. This sometimes creates a multiplicity of efforts, some duplication, much organizational complexity, diversity of opinion, difficulty reaching consensus, some contradictory efforts, and perhaps some creativity.

## Federal Programs

A sometimes bewildering number of federal agencies, ranging from the Department of Agriculture to the Department of Transportation, have programs related to adolescent health. Within the Department of Health and Human Services are programs that fund direct health care services for poor youth through Medicaid and for low-income youth through the State Child Health Insurance Program. Also within the Department of Health and Human Services are programs that address specific issues related to youth health and development, including the Substance Abuse and Mental Health Administration, the CDC's Division of Adolescent and School Health, and the Health Resources and Services Administration. Particularly important for youth are programs linked to the Maternal and Child Health Bureau (MCHB).

### MCHB

The MCHB administers Title V of the Social Security Act, which underwrites most public health work for adolescents in the United States. Using both block grants to the states and Special Projects of Regional and National Significance (SPRANS) grants for infrastructure development and demonstration projects, MCHB has been the key federal agency for developing adolescent health as an area of concern. One of the major projects within the Office of Adolescent Health has been establishing State Adolescent Health Coordinators in each state to develop plans for meeting adolescent health care needs. The Office of Adolescent Health has also established national centers on adolescent health policy (NAHIC in San Francisco, the State Adolescent Health Resource Center in Minneapolis, and the School Mental Health Policy Centers in Los Angeles and Baltimore). The SPRANS program has modeled a wide variety of MCH programs such as reducing teen pregnancy and decreasing school bullying. SPRANS grants also attempt to reduce health disparity problems for high-risk populations such as homeless youth, African American males, and the physically disabled.

One important part of the federal role has been to support health professional training. The epidemiology of adolescent health presented in this chapter underscores the importance of addressing the complex psychosocial mortalities and morbidities with more broadly based training than traditional medically based models. Because of this, MCHB sponsors several programs to increase interdisciplinary training. One of the prime examples is the Leadership Education in Adolescent Health at university-based sites (Birmingham, Boston, Houston, Indianapolis, Minneapolis, Rochester, and San Francisco). Begun in 1978, the Leadership Education in Adolescent Health programs train graduate and postgraduate nurses, nutritionists, physicians, psychologists, and social workers to provide leadership for interdisciplinary work in adolescent health care. The MCHB also funds programs at 13 schools of public health. The Partners in Program Planning in Adolescent Health is a collaboration of several professional organizations sponsored by MCHB that aims to improve professional practice related to adolescent health.

MCHB also administers several other programs related to adolescent health, such as transition support for special health care needs youth, and collaborates with other federal agencies on projects such as the National Initiative to Improve Adolescent Health (discussed later here).

### Other Federal Efforts to Improve Adolescent Health

Other federal efforts to improve access to appropriate adolescent health care have included the Early Prevention, Screening, Diagnosis, and Treatment program, school-based and school-linked health services, and funding for reproductive health services.

The Early Prevention, Screening, Diagnosis, and Treatment program was supposed to increase access to screening and follow-up services for children and youth with some services of particular relevance to adolescents including reproductive health and mental health (English, 1993). Unfortunately, even with improved funding, the program has reached only a small percentage of eligible adolescents enrolled, and few states have established mental health screening protocols.

Another area of federal initiative has been to support school-based/ linked health care services. After initial reports suggesting that such services may reduce sexual activity and pregnancy, the federal government joined private foundations, state governments, and local school districts in funding sites such that by 2002 there were nearly 1,500 schools with school-based health centers (Center for Health and Health Care in Schools, 2003). These clinics vary in the amount of services provided and have often proven quite controversial because of concern from some that they would provide reproductive health care services and thus increase adolescent sexual activity. Subsequent evaluations have found for some time that school health clinics do achieve accessible, acceptable, comprehensive health care for adolescents, do not increase sexual activity among the students, and may decrease pregnancy rates (US Congress, 1991c).

Family Planning and Adolescent Family Life programs are other federal efforts to reduce teen pregnancy. Title X of the Public Health Service Act began in 1970 to fund family planning clinics, and Title XX of the Public Health Services Act of 1981 created the Adolescent Family Life Program, which funds both prevention programs and services for adolescents who are pregnant or parenting. Block grants to the states for MCH services and for social services are often used for adolescent pregnancy prevention efforts, as are SPRANS grants. The federal government also has created special initiatives that include teen pregnancy reduction efforts, often as part of other projects such as "Healthy Start," "Healthy Schools," "Healthy Communities," and in 1995 the Community Coalition Partnership Program.

### National Initiative to Improve Adolescent Health

One of the important projects of the Division of Adolescent and School Health and the Office of Adolescent Health within MCHB has been the National Initiative to Improve Adolescent Health by the year 2010. This initiative attempts to organize public health efforts to achieve the 21 Critical Objectives for Adolescents and Young Adults of the 2010 National Health Objectives (NAHIC, 2003c). To attain these objectives, the National Initiative aims to shift the focus of adolescent public health efforts from a primary focus on individual risk behaviors to a more broad-based, comprehensive youth development orientation that can be implemented by national, state, and local community efforts (Table 8–2).

Part of the National Initiative is to develop guidance for state and local community efforts to improve adolescent health through a companion document to the 21 Critical Objectives (CDC, 2004b). It describes a collaborative community process of building a coalition, assessing needs through using local sources of data, prioritizing, developing a logic model to conceptualize the change process, and finally leading to create an action plan. Difficulties of implementing, sustaining, and evaluating the interventions are also addressed.

## Collaborations to Improve Adolescent Health

Several public and private collaborations involving national organizations as well as local and state affiliates have been developed to improve adolescent health. The National Campaign to Prevent Teen Pregnancy is perhaps

**Table 8-2** Healthy People 2010–2021 Critical Health Objectives for Adolescents and Young Adults.

| Objective # | Objective | Baseline (1998 Unless Noted) | 2010 Target |
|---|---|---|---|
| *16-03 (a,b,c)* | *Reduce deaths of adolescent and young adults* | | |
| | 10–14 year olds | 21.5/100,000 | 16.8/100,000 |
| | 15–19 year olds | 69.5/ | 39.8/ |
| | 20–24 year olds | 92.7/ | 49.0/ |
| **Unintentional Injury** | | | |
| *15-15 (a)* | *Reduce deaths caused by motor vehicle crashes. 15–24 year olds* | 25,6/100,000 (1999) | Not established for age group |
| *26-01 (a)* | *Reduce deaths and injuries caused by alcohol and drug related motor vehicle crashes. 15–24 year olds* | 13.5/ | Not established for age group |
| 15-19 | Increase use of safety belts; 9th to 12th grade student | 84% (1999) | 92% |
| 26-06 | Reduce the proportion of high school students who report that during the previous 30 days, they rode with a driver who had been drinking | 33% (1999) | 30% |
| **Violence** | | | |
| 18-01 | *Reduce the suicide rate* | (1999) | Not established for age group |
| | 10–14 year olds | 1.2/100,000 | |
| | 15–19 year olds | 8.0/ | |
| 18-02 | Reduce the rate of suicide attempts by high school students that require medical attention | 2.6% (1999) | 1% |
| 15-32 | *Reduce the rate of homicide* | (1999) | Not established for age group |
| | 10–14 year olds | 1.2/100,000 | |
| | 15–19 year olds | 10.4/ | |
| 15-38 | Reduce physical fighting among high school students | 36% (1999) | 32% |
| 15-39 | Reduce weapon carrying on school property by high school students | 6.9% | 4.9% |
| **Substance Abuse and Mental Health** | | | |
| 26-11 (d) | Reduce the proportion of 12–17 year olds who binge drink alcohol regularly | 7.7% | 2% |
| 26-10 (b) | Reduce the proportion of 4–17 year olds with disabilities who are reported to be sad, unhappy, or depressed | 8.3% | 0.07% |

*continues*

**Table 8-2** Healthy People 2010–2021 Critical Health Objectives for Adolescents and Young Adults (continued).

| Objective # | Objective | Baseline (1998 Unless Noted) | 2010 Target |
|---|---|---|---|
| 06-02 | (Developmental) Increase the proportion of children with mental health problems who receive treatment | Age grouping beyond adolescent | Age grouping beyond adolescent |
| 18-07 | (Developmental) Increase the proportion of children with mental health problems who receive treatment | Baseline data not yet available | Target not yet available |
| **Reproductive Health** | | | |
| 09-07 | *Reduce pregnancies among 15–17 year olds* | 68 per 1,000 (1996) | 43 per 1,000 |
| 13-05 | (Developmental) Reduce new HIV diagnoses among 13–24 year olds | 16,479 | Target not yet available |
| 25-01 (a,b,c) | *Reduce the proportion of 15–24 year olds with chlamydia trachomatis* Females at family planning clinics Females at STD clinics Males at STD clinics | 5% (1997) 12.2% (1997) 15.7% (1997) | 3% 3% 3% |
| 25-11 | Increase the proportiion of high school students who abstain from sexual intercourse or use a condom if currently sexually active | 85% | 95% |
| **Chronic Diseases** | | | |
| 27-02 (a) | Reduce tobacco use by 9th to 12th graders | 40% | 21% |
| 19-03 (b) | *Reduce the proportion of 12–19 year olds who are overweight or obese* | 11% (1988–1994) | 5% |
| 22-07 | Increase the proportion of 9–12 graders who engage in vigorous physical activity 3 or more times a week for 20 or more minutes | 65.5% | 85% |

Source: adapted from National Adolescent Health Information Center (2004).
*Critical health outcomes are in italic;* behaviors that substantially contribute to important health outcomes are in normal font.

one of the best examples. It considers national and local collaborative efforts aimed at (1) improving the quality of clinical services through professional organizations, (2) preventing fatal injuries using the Haddon matrix, (3) reducing teen suicide through local and national initiatives, (4) decreasing teen pregnancy and the continuum of care, and (5) overcoming unhealthy behaviors linked to obesity through health promotion.

## Improving the Quality of Adolescent Health Services—Professional Partnerships

Although expansions of Medicaid and enactment of the State Child Health Insurance Program have more than offset declines in private health insurance coverage, adolescents still experience difficulty getting adequate health care. One set of efforts to improve adolescent health care has been to improve the skills of primary care providers to screen and respond to adolescent health issues through professional initiatives. The American Academy of Pediatrics, in cooperation with funding agencies of the federal government such as MCHB and others, has created a set of guidelines and materials regarding primary care for all of pediatrics, including adolescents, called *Bright Futures* (www.brightfutures.org). The American Academy of Pediatrics is also developing a program emphasizing the pediatrician as a "medical home" for children and youth with special health care needs, including those with mental health needs. The American Medical Association is the lead agency for a coalition that has worked toward defining, educating, and implementing preventive services within primary care called Guidelines for Adolescent Preventive Services (Elster & Kuznets, 1994). The Society of Adolescent Medicine has outlined a comprehensive view of the key elements in access to primary care (Klein, Slap, Elster, & Schonberg, 1992). Each of these projects emphasizes the physician's role as providing screening, health education, anticipatory guidance for common problems, basic problem solving, and referral for more complicated problems. These guidelines assume thorough links with health education and social services that are often unavailable or not well coordinated with health care delivery.

Proving the health effectiveness or the cost benefit of this type of clinic-based preventive care could be difficult. The cost benefits of interest to those who finance health care are usually shorter term benefits. Many adolescent health behaviors, however, do not have health consequences for many years (smoking, unhealthy eating, unsafe sexual behavior). Given the high long-term costs of many of these behaviors from cancer, obesity, or HIV, even a small effect of an intervention of 5% to 7% would be very effective for society as a whole in the long term (Downs & Klein, 1995).

### Preventing Fatal Injuries: Using the Haddon Matrix

As noted previously here, injuries account for more than 75% of all adolescent deaths. Injuries include both *unintentional* events such as motor vehicle and bicycle crashes, drowning, and occupational safety failures, as well as *intentional* injuries such as homicide, suicide, and abuse. Because the frequency and severity of injury in the population are predictable, public health workers focused on primary prevention avoid use of the word "accident," preferring the term "injury event." By intersecting the three time phases of the injury event, pre-event, event, and postevent, with the agent, host, and environment factors from the epidemiologic model, the Haddon matrix has been a successful public health tool for identifying strategies for injury prevention. It has been used in a wide variety of situations such as playground falls, handgun injury, and cancer deaths from smoking (Runyan, 2003). Here we focus on the leading cause of adolescent death, motor vehicle crashes (Table 8–3).

Partially as a result of interventions suggested by a public health approach such as the Haddon matrix and collaborations among police, parents, engineers, media, youth, regulators, legislators, and victims, unintentional motor vehicle fatalities in the 15- to 19-year-old age group have declined by nearly a third since 1980. Population-based strategies of benefit to all ages such as (1) improvements in highway design (e.g., interstate highways have one third the fatality rate of rural highways), (2) automobile crash-safety design, (3) seat belt use and passive restraint systems (40% to 50% less fatality), and (4) enhanced emergency medical services can be derived from this type of analysis. Efforts to reduce drunk driving by raising the drinking age, lowering the permissible blood alcohol levels, making the identification of a "designated driver" the social norm, sponsoring alcohol-free events, and even restricting automobile travel time are ways to improve the human pre-event factors related to injury. Efforts to increase the human factor of seat belt use during the event are only minimally successful unless they are also accompanied by a pre-event social environmental intervention with legal sanctions. Interestingly, driver education classes have not been shown to improve safety and in fact may decrease safety by enabling adolescents to drive at an earlier age (Mayhew & Simpson, 2002). Many states are finding graduated licensing to teenagers with restricted hour and limited numbers of passengers to be effective (McKnight, Peck, & Foss, 2002). The federal requirement of passive restraints and airbags is based on considering the rapid exchange of energy

**Table 8–3** Modified Haddon Matrix of Factors Related to Motor Vehicle Injury and Its Outcomes.

| | Human Factors | Agent or Vehicle Factors | Physical Environment Factors | Sociocultural Environment Factors |
|---|---|---|---|---|
| Before event | Driver vision<br>Alcohol<br>Experience<br>Amount of travel<br>Night/weekend<br>Traffic violations | Brakes, tires<br>Center of gravity<br>Jack-knife tendency<br>Speed capability<br>Ease of control | Visibility of hazards<br>Road curve and grade surface<br>Divided highway<br>Signals<br>Intersection access control | Attitudes about alcohol<br>Enforcement of speeding laws<br>Laws about teen driving |
| Event | Safety belt use<br>Age<br>Sex | Speed on impact<br>Vehicle size<br>Automatic restraints<br>Airbags<br>Type of contact<br>Rollover | Recovery areas<br>Guard rails<br>Median barriers<br>Roadside embankments<br>Speed limits | Attitudes about safety belt use<br>Laws about safety belt use<br>Enforcement of safety belt use |
| After event | Age<br>Physical condition<br>Severity of injury<br>Body region injured | Fuel system integrity | Emergency transport system (EMS)<br>Quality of EMS<br>Distance to trauma center<br>Rehabilitation programs | Support for trauma care Systems<br>Skill of EMS personnel<br>Laws and attitudes re disability<br>School integration |

Source: adapted from Lescohier and Gallagher (1996).

as the "agent" of injury at the time of the crash and may be one of the most significant factors for harm reduction (Table 8–3).

There have also been effective efforts to increase parent limit-setting and communication regarding driving behavior (Simons-Morton, Hartos, & Leaf, 2002). The importance of transportation in conflict with parents has a long history, as illustrated by the story told of Socrates, who asked a youth named Lysis whether his parents gratify all of his wishes. In response, Lysis complained that even though his parents seemed to want him to be happy his father would not let him ride the family's horses (quoted in Hall, 1904, p. 514).

## Reducing Teen Suicide: The Surgeon General's Initiative

Another form of injury that claims many lives and is an important challenge to community collaboration and mental health services is adolescent suicide. In 1999, Surgeon General Satcher called for a national response to suicide among all ages, which resulted in the development of a national strategy in 2000 (US Public Health Service, 2001). This strategy calls for action in three areas: *awareness, intervention*, and *methodology*. To improve *awareness*, the strategy calls for efforts to increase the recognition that suicide is a preventable public health problem and to increase support for broad based suicide prevention. It also aims to develop strategies to reduce the stigma that often prevents people from using mental health services. In the area of *intervention*, the strategy calls for developing local suicide prevention programs and reducing access to lethal means such as guns. An important part of intervention relates to clinical work by increasing training in recognition of risk behaviors, improving treatment, and enhancing community links with mental health and substance abuse services. Clustering of suicides has been noted, and thus, the strategy aims to reduce the contagion by improving the media's handling of suicidal behavior. In *methodology*, like any good public health recommendation, the strategy calls for increased research and surveillance.

Although the national strategy does not focus on adolescents, many of the recommendations have been researched regarding youth, and some studies have shown reductions in suicidal behaviors (Gould, Greenberg, Velting, & Shaffer, 2003). Several schools have developed suicide awareness curricula for students encouraging identification and help seeking. Although evaluators have generally been unable to show benefits and some have increased maladaptive coping, one multisite program has shown reduction in suicide attempts (Aseltine & DeMartino, 2004). Skills training to teach cognitive skills and problem-solving coping, particularly focusing on students in danger of school failure, have produced positive results. Likewise, teaching screening skills to gatekeepers such as teachers and primary care doctors has increased the referral rate to mental health services. Crisis response "postvention" usually includes planned small group discussions by trained staff and links to mental health services. Such postventions have had few evaluations, with one study reporting no improvements, but another 4-year follow-up showing significant reduction in suicidal behavior (cited in Gould et al., 2003).

Several community-based efforts to reduce adolescent suicide have been evaluated (Gould et al., 2003). Crisis hotlines have been developed and used by teens, but evaluators have generally been unable to show an impact on suicidal behavior. Firearm restriction has seemed a promising strategy, particularly because legal restrictions have a greater impact on adolescents and young adults, but the evaluations have been mixed. Because suicides often cluster, with one suicide apparently stimulating another, attempts to reduce this contagion have focused on educating media. Not dramatizing suicidal news excessively, not glorifying the victims, and including coping and treatment information have been urged. Austria and Switzerland both have reported significant reductions in suicides when following this approach. Other strategies have been to improve coordination of services for those who have attempted suicide and to enhance the availability and acceptability of mental health services to at-risk populations such as Native American youth, gay and lesbian youth, incarcerated youth, and homeless youth.

### Decreasing Adolescent Pregnancy: The Continuum of Care

Adolescent pregnancy is another public health problem that has become politicized, with much misinformation and distortion related to political expressions of concern. Because American sexual activity rates are similar to European rates yet US pregnancy rates are substantially higher, American adolescent pregnancy rates can hardly be attributed to the nature of adolescence, to the supposed generosity of the American welfare system compared with European welfare systems, or to greater promiscuity and related immoralities. Instead, the higher rates should be attributed to factors more unique to the American experience. In addition to widespread poverty, inequality, and a lack of universally available and accessible health care services, the high US teen pregnancy rate should be seen as related to American attitudes about sexuality and sexual behavior of adolescents, including family planning. Despite the controversies regarding sex education, the National Research Council notes that most adolescent pregnancy prevention programs enjoy wide support from the majority of Americans and that even those who did not initially support these programs can often find common ground with the idea that every child should be born to a welcoming family that is ready and able to care for it (Brown & Eisenberg, 1995).

Numerous major reviews have reached general agreement on best ways to prevent adolescent pregnancies (Kirby, 2002; Manlove et al., 2002; National Research Council, 1987). Each has affirmed that there is not one strategy, but that multiple, community-wide approaches are needed based on the classic public health service continuum of health promotion, prevention, treatment, and secondary prevention.

First, echoing Marion Wright Edelman's often repeated comment that the best contraception is hope, adolescent pregnancy prevention strategies need to promote life options for at-risk adolescents by increasing employment and educational opportunities, training in specific skills, and providing support for youth in transition. One such program in 30 states, the Teen Outreach Program, emphasized small discussion groups and community service. Participants in this program had reduced pregnancy rates, school failure, and school dropout by 30% to 50% compared with participants in comparison groups (Allen, Philliber, Herding, & Rupermine, 1997).

Second, prevention programs based on comprehensive education are needed. Most current sex education programs are too short, too late, and too cognitively based. Effective programs include clear messages about sexual activity as well as training in social skills, assertiveness, and peer pressure resistance and accurate, specific information on condom or contraceptive use, and access. Typically, programs such as "Reducing the Risk" aimed at grades 9–12 in Arkansas and California include didactic information, role playing, and small group discussions. Replication of this program has delayed onset of sexual activity and increased condom use in other states as well (Kirby, 2002). One preventive education approach that has received significant funding over the last several years has been the encouragement of abstinence. Traditionally, public health efforts have advised young people to avoid sexual activity but have focused more on encouraging contraception and improving service delivery. Advocates for abstinence programs believe preventing sexual activity outside of marriage would be more effective and that prevention efforts that also provide information on contraception give mixed messages that undermine the abstinence message. One study found an abstinence program aimed at 9th graders effective (Howard & McCabe, 1990), but further evaluation efforts to date have not been able to replicate this study (Kirby, 2002).

The third approach is to increase access to contraceptives for those sizable numbers of adolescents who are already sexually active. Education about their use, confidentiality in obtaining health care services, readily available services such as those through school-based/linked clinics, and payment mechanisms are critical to achieve this. In a model program that integrated school educational programs and contraceptive services at a nearby clinic, 3-year pregnancy rates declined by 30% among enrolled students compared with a 58% increase among nonenrolled students (Zabin & Hayward, 1993).

The fourth approach, secondary prevention, aims to improve outcomes for teen parents, usually by providing comprehensive medical, educational, and social services to teen parents. Such programs have had a variety of goals. Some have aimed to reduce low birth weight, some to prevent repeated childbearing, some to improve child outcomes, and some to speed entry to the job market to avoid welfare dependency. Results have been quite positive for some programs but not all. Effective programs, according to one review, shared several key characteristics (Seitz & Apfel, 1999). They have goals endorsed by the participants, such as maternal and child health and well-being rather than just job entry. They provide personalized care and attention. They use schools, and they pay close attention to the timing of involvement when the mothers are most open to assistance, which is earlier in pregnancy and parenting. Follow-up studies as long as 20 years later have indicated improved outcomes compared with controls (Seitz & Apfel, 1993).

## Promoting Healthy Lifestyles: Enhancing Nutrition and Physical Activity

Many unhealthy behaviors such as substance abuse, poor eating practices, and physical inactivity problems follow similar pathways to chronic illness requiring expensive secondary level medical and social treatments, often much later in life. The pervasiveness of these psychosocial problems means interventions based solely on individual treatment approaches will require extensive and thus expensive use of professional time in systems that are frequently plagued by coordination problems, difficulties in equality of access, and a frequent lack of sensitivity to adolescent concerns. Too much focus on individual behaviors, psychopathologies, and addictions misses the opportunities, skills, and internal strengths that adolescents need to resist so much in their toxic social environments. Broadly based activities based on learning skills interactively for promoting health offer a paradigm for programs that have led to significant improvements in a variety of areas, particularly when such programs are integrated and reinforced by schools, communities, homes, medical settings, and public policy to create "webs of influence" (Elster, Panzarine, & Holt, 1993; Price, Cioci, Penner, & Trautlein, 1993; Schinke et al., 2002).

Obesity effects health throughout the life course. Efforts to restrict food intake or encourage dieting as an individual behavior seldom work and may in fact increase obesity (Dietz & Gortmaker, 2001). Collaborative public health interventions are just being developed and evaluations reported. Initial results from interventions on multiple dimensions, including family, school, neighborhood, primary care, and policy, have shown promising results. Programs that help families reduce the use of food as reward, establish family meal time, improve parental modeling, and structure more physical activity can reduce obesity (Ritchie et al., 2001). The most important physical activity is turning off the television (Dietz & Gortmaker, 2001), which is implemented at the family level but reinforced by school and primary care. School-based curricula such as the multiple subject Planet Health program have been effective at improving diet, decreasing television viewing, and increasing physical activity. Such curricula need supportive policy. The decline in participation in daily physical education classes from 42% in 1991 to 28.4% in 2003 (Grunbaum et al., 2004) reflects a lack of supportive policy. Other policy-linked efforts have focused on reducing access to unhealthy food such as vending machines or fast food restaurants during school hours and increasing access to healthier food. Creating physical education programs that emphasize fitness and life-long lifestyle activities rather than just competitive sports is also an important education policy with public health consequences. Neighborhood interventions, which enhance activity by creating safe places for outdoor play, are important avenues of health promotion. Primary care health care providers can reinforce these activities through anticipatory guidance, teaching, and advocacy (American Academy of Pediatrics, 2003).

## Special Populations and the Core Responsibilities of Public Health

Although public health uses population-based approaches, the population is heterogeneous, and certain groups of the population have worse health status, often based on being excluded from social resources, stigmatized, and blamed for their conditions. These special populations include groups such as ethnic and racial minorities, immigrants and migrants, the poor, the learning disabled, the incarcerated, pregnant and parenting youth, the mentally ill, foster youth, maltreated youth, and youth with different sexual orientations. For youth, the multiplicity of special population identities is probably the most significant factor in risk. For example, the Native American learning-disabled youth in the foster care system who is pregnant would be considered at "multiple jeopardy." Because of the alienated and/or outcast nature of many of these groups, public health work is particularly concerned with assessing the needs of these populations, assuring that appropriate, quality services are provided and creating policies that attempt to create a link with the larger society. Sometimes the assurance function leads public health agencies to provide direct services to some of these groups to demonstrate that provision of services to these groups is feasible, to establish a beginning point for wider collaboration, or to serve groups that are considered "too difficult" for traditional health care providers.

Furthermore, because of the degree of social alienation experienced by many of these groups, special efforts need to be made to establish collaborative relationships for health. The population of homeless youth, for instance, is difficult to assess because many avoid contact with adults for fear of being turned over to the police and returned to their homes. Efforts to understand their health problems will need significant street outreach and work with peers. Likewise, assuring quality may be more difficult with certain ethnic groups with traditions of alternative views of health and with traditions of not appearing to disagree with authority. Policy development regarding some particularly stigmatized groups such as the incarcerated creates many controversies beyond their immediate health care needs. Working with key people trusted by those within the group, recognizing existing community networks and supports, and engaging in collaborative processes around jointly identified problems have been ways that public health workers have tried to develop epidemiologic analysis, a continuum of care, and health promotion activities for special populations.

# FUTURE DIRECTIONS

Despite the widespread call for increased access to health care and improved environments for adolescents, the continuing cultural conflict about the role of government, the degree of individual versus social causation for problems, and adolescent sexual behavior will likely continue and make access for adolescents to health care difficult. Public health initiatives have had the most success when they deliberately and systematically build a wide base at the local, state, or national level. This may be time consuming and unpredictable, but it may also lead to stronger continuing support. Another future direction of public health work with adolescents will be efforts to include adolescent needs in any future system of health care reform—managed care, national health insurance, or whatever combination emerges. Particularly important is establishing systems of confidentiality for adolescents, enabling and training providers to have a working knowledge of adolescents' needs, abilities, and limitations, and establishing primary care with risk screening, health guidance, and coordination with appropriate ameliorative programs. Identifying adolescent health indicators and adolescent-specific evaluations will be important avenues to pursue in efforts to keep health care systems accountable to serving adolescents. Because these problems and solutions often cross institutional boundaries, creating partnerships and a broader view of social costs will be important for implementing "best practice" programs in communities on a broader scale.

Ultimately, adolescent health status may be affected more by broader social issues than by direct contact with the health care system. Factors that seem to increase health among adolescents have been described as not just the absence of maltreatment, infection, stress, or social oppression but also the presence of adults who maintain caring and connectedness with them within the community. Those wanting to improve the health of adolescents will need to find ways to institutionalize these traits and to enhance resilience, reduce the harm, secure the environment, and establish a sense of engagement in the lives of adolescents. This truly is the "best and wisest adult endeavor," which makes the "age between ten and three and twenty" a time to celebrate rather than bemoan.

## Acknowledgments

David Knopf is from the Pediatric Social Work Department, Children's Hospital at University of California, San Francisco, and from the Division of Adolescent Medicine and the NAHIC, School of Medicine, University of California, San Francisco. This work was supported in part by the Murdoch Endowment, Department of Pediatric Social Work, University of California, San Francisco and the United States Bureau of Maternal and Child Health grants 2U45-MC00002-11-00 and T71 MC00003.

## REFERENCES

Achenbach, T.M., Dumenci, L., & Rescorla, L.A. (2003). LA: Are American Children's problems still getting worse? A 23 year comparison. *Journal of Abnormal Child Psychology, 31,* 1–11.

Allen, J.P., Philliber, S., Herding, S., & Rupermine, G.P. (1997). Preventing teen pregnancy and academic failure. Experimental evaluation of a developmentally-base approach. *Child Development, 64,* 729–742.

American Academy of Pediatrics, Committee on Nutrition. (2003). Prevention of pediatric overweight and obesity. *Pediatrics, 112,* 424–430.

Anne E. Casey Foundation. (2001). *Change that abides: A retrospective look at community and family strengthening projects and their enduring results.* Boston: Anne E. Casey Foundation. Available from: http://www.aecf.org/publications/data/change_abides.pdf

Aseltine, R.H., & DeMartino, R. (2004). An outcome evaluation of the SOS Suicide Prevention Program. *American Journal of Public Health, 94,* 446–451.

Atav, S., & Spencer, G.A. (2002). Health risk behaviors among adolescents attending rural, suburban, and urban schools. *Family Community Health, 25,* 53–64.

Baumrind, D. (1987). Rearing competent children. In C.E. Irwin, Jr. (Ed.), *Adolescent social behavior and health: New directions for child development* (Vol. 37). San Francisco: Jossey Bass.

Blackwell, D.L., Vickerie, J.L., & Wondimu, E.A. (2003). Summary health statistics for U.S. children: National Health Interview Survey, 2000. National Center for Health Statistics. *Vital Health Stat, 10213,* 11.

Blum, R. (1987). Contemporary threats to adolescent health in the United States. *Journal of the American Medical Association, 257,* 3390–3395.

Blyth, D.A. (1993). *Healthy communities, healthy youth: How communities contribute to positive youth development.* Minneapolis, MN: Search Institute.

Brenner, N.D., Billy, J.O., & Grady, W.R. (2003). Assessment of factors affecting the validity of self-reported health-risk behavior among adolescents: Evidence from the scientific literature. *Journal of Adolescent Health, 33,* 436–457.

Brindis, C.D., & Ott, M.A. (2001). Adolescents, health policy, and the American political process. *Journal of Adolescent Health, 30,* 9–16.

Brindis, C.B., Handley, M., Millstein, S., Irwin, C.E., Knopf, D., & Ozer, E. (1996). *Improving adolescent lives: A synthesis of health policy recommendations.* San Francisco: National Adolescent Health Information Center.

Brindis, C.D., Morreale, M.C., & English, A. (2001). The unique health care needs of adolescents. *Future of Children, 13,* 117–136.

Brooks-Gunn, J., & Paikoff, R.L. (1993). "Sex is a gamble, kissing is a game": Adolescent sexuality and health promotion. In S.G. Millstein, A.C. Peterson, & E.O. Nightingale (Eds.), *Promoting the health of adolescents: New directions for the twenty-first century.* New York: Oxford University Press.

Brown, S.S., & Eisenberg, L. (1995). *The best intentions: Unintended pregnancy and the well-being of children and families.* Washington, DC: National Academy Press.

Brown, J.D., & Witherspoon, E.M. (2002). The mass media and American adolescents' health. *Journal of Adolescent Health, 31* (6, Suppl. 1), 153–170.

Burt, M.R. (2002). Reasons to invest in adolescents. *Journal of Adolescent Health, 31,* 136–152.

Carnegie Council on Adolescent Development. (1989). *Turning points: Preparing American youth for the twenty-first century: The report of the Task Force on Education of Young Adolescents.* Washington, DC: Author.

Carnegie Council on Adolescent Development. (1995). *Great transitions: Preparing adolescents for a new century/concluding report of the Carnegie Council on Adolescent Development.* New York: Carnegie Corporation of New York.

Catalano, R.F., Hawkins, J.D., Berglund, M.L., Pollard, J.A., & Arthur, M.W. (2002). Prevention science and positive youth development: Competitive or cooperative frameworks? *Journal of Adolescent Health, 31*(Suppl.), 230–239.

Centers for Disease Control and Prevention. (1994). Health risk behaviors among adolescents who do and do not attend school: US, 1992. *Morbidity and Mortality Weekly Report, 43,* 8.

Centers for Disease Control and Prevention. (2002). *Young people at risk: HIV/ AIDS among America's youth.* Available from: http://www.cdc.gov/hiv/pubs/ facts/youth.pdf

Centers for Disease Control and Prevention. (2004a). *Trends in the prevalence of selected risk behaviors: Youth risk behavior surveillance system: Fact sheet.* Available from: http://www.cdc.gov/nccdphp/dash/yrbs/pdf-factsheets/trends.pdf

Centers for Disease Control and Prevention, National Center for Chronic Disease Prevention and Health Promotion, Division of Adolescent and School Health; Health Resources and Services Administration, Maternal and Child Health Bureau, Office of Adolescent Health; National Adolescent Health Information

Center, University of California at San Francisco. (2004b). *Improving the health of adolescents and young adults: A guide for states and communities.* Atlanta, GA: Centers for Disease Control and Prevention. Available from: http://nahic.ucsf.edu.

Center for Health and Health Care in Schools. (2003). 2002 State survey of school-based health center initiatives. George Washington University. Available from: www.healthinschools.org/sbhcs/narrative02.asp.

Cheng, T.L., Savageau, J.A., Sattler, A.L., & DeWitt, T.G. (1993). Confidentiality in health care: A survey of knowledge, perceptions, and attitudes among high school students. *Journal of the American Medical Association, 269,* 1404–1407.

Child Trends. (2002). Building a better teenager: A summary of "what works" in adolescent development. *Child trends research briefs publication* (#2002-57). Washington, DC: Author. Available from: www.childtrends.org

Child Trends. (2004). *Children with limitations.* Washington, DC: Child Trends Data Bank. Available from: www.childtrendsdatabank.org

Cohall, A.T., & Cohall, R.M. (1995). Number one with a bullet. In K.K. Christoffel & C.W. Runyan (Eds.), Adolescent injury: epidemiology and prevention. *Adolescent Medicine State of the Art Reviews, 6,* 183–198.

Coleman, L, & Coleman, J. (2002). The measurement of puberty: A review. *Journal of Adolescence, 25,* 535–550.

Council of Scientific Affairs. (1993). Confidential health care services for adolescents. *Journal of the American Medical Association, 269,* 1420–1424.

Darling, N., & Steinberg, L. (1993). Parenting style as context: An integrative model. *Psychological Bulletin, 113,* 487–496.

Darroch, J.E., Singh, S., & Frost, S.J. (2001). Differences in teenage pregnancy rates among five developed countries: The roles of sexual activity and contraceptive use. *Family Planning Perspectives, 33,* 6.

Dey, A.N., Schiller, J.S., & Tai, D.A. (2004). Summary health statistics for U.S. children: National health interview survey, 2002. National Center for Health Statistics. *Vital Health Statistics, 10,* 221.

Dietz, W.H., & Gortmaker, S.L. (2001). Preventing obesity in children and adolescents. *Annual Review of Public Health, 22,* 337–355.

Donovan, J.E., & Jessor, R. (1985). Structure of problem behavior in adolescent and young adulthood. *Journal of Consulting and Clinical Psychology, 53,* 890–904.

Downs, S.M., & Klein, J.D. (1995). Clinical preventive services efficacy and adolescent risk behaviors. *Archives of Pediatric and Adolescent Medicine, 149,* 374–379.

Eccles, J., & Gootman, J.A. (Eds.). (2002). *Community programs to promote youth development.* Washington, DC: National Academy Press.

Edelman, P., & Ladner, J. (Eds.). (1991). *Adolescence and poverty.* Washington, DC: Center for National Policy Press.

Elder, G.H., Conger, R.D., Foster, E.M., & Ardelt, M. (1992). Families under economic pressure. *Journal of Family Issues, 13,* 5–37.

Ellwood, D.T., & Jencks, C. (2002). *The spread of single-parent families in the United States since 1960*. Working paper, John F. Kennedy School of Government, Harvard University, Cambridge, MA.

Elster, A.B., & Kuznets, N.J. (Eds.). (1994). *AMA guidelines for adolescent preventive services: Recommendations and rationale*. Baltimore, MD: Williams and Williams.

Elster, A., Panzarine, S., & Holt, K. (Eds.). (1993). *American Medical Association state-of-the-art conference on adolescent health promotion: Proceedings*. Arlington, VA: National Center of Education in Maternal and Child Health.

English, A. (1993). Early and periodic screening, diagnosis and treatment: A model for improving adolescents' access to health care. *Journal of Adolescent Health, 14*, 524–527.

English, A. (2002). Financing adolescent health care: Legal and policy issues for the coming decade. *Journal of Adolescent Health, 31*, 334–346.

English, A., & Kenney, K.E. (2003). *State minor consent laws: A summary* (2nd ed.). Chapel Hill, NC: Center for Adolescent Health & the Law.

Fahs, P.S., Smith, B.E., Atav, A.S., Britten, M.X., Collins, M.S., Morgan, L.C., & Spencer, G.A. (1999). Integrative research review of risk behaviors among adolescents in rural, suburban, and urban areas. *Journal of Adolescent Health, 24*, 230–243.

Ferguson, R.F. (2001). Test-score trends along racial lines, 1971–1996: Popular culture and community academic standards. In N.J. Smelser, W.J. Wilson, & F. Mitchell (Eds.), *America becoming: Racial trends and their consequences* (Vol. 1). Commission on Behavioral and Social Sciences and Education. Washington, DC: National Academy Press.

Fox, H.B., McManus, M.A., & Reichman, M.B. (2003). Private health insurance for adolescents: Is it adequate? *Journal of Adolescent Health, 32S*, 12–24.

Geronimus, A.T. (1987). On teenage childbearing in the United States. *Population and Development Review, 13*, 54–61.

Gilligan, C. (1987). Adolescent development reconsidered. In C.E. Irwin, Jr. (Ed.), *Adolescent social behavior and health: New directions in child development* (Vol. 37). San Francisco: Jossey-Bass.

Gould, M.S., Greenberg, T., Velting, D.M., & Shaffer, D. (2003). Youth suicide risk and preventive interventions: A review of the past 10 years. *Journal of the American Academy of Child and Adolescent Psychiatry, 42*, 386–405.

Grissmer, D.W., Kirby, S.N., Berends, M., & Williamson, S. (1995). *Student achievement and the changing American family* (RAND MR-488). Santa Monica, CA: Rand Corporation.

Grunbaum, J.A., Kann, L., Kinchen, S., Ross, J., Hawkins, J., Lowry, R., Harris, W.A., McManus, T., Chyen, D., & Collins, J. (2004). Youth risk behavior surveillance: United States, 2003. *Morbidity Mortality Weekly Report, 53* (SS-02), 1–96.

Hall, G.S. (1904). *Adolescence: Its psychology, and its relations to anthropology, sex, crime, religion, and education*. New York: Appleton and Company.

Hauser, S.T., Powers, S.I., & Noam, G.G. (1991). *Adolescents and their families: Paths of ego development.* New York: Free Press.

Hawkins, J.D., Catalano, R.F., & Arthur, M.W. (2002). Promoting science-based prevention in communities. *Addiction Behavior, 27,* 951–976.

Health Futures of Youth: Proceedings of a Conference. (1988, April). *Journal of Adolescent Health Care, 9,* 1–69.

Howard, M., & McCabe, J.B. (1990). Helping teenagers postpone sexual involvement. *Family Planning Perspectives, 2,* 21–26.

Igra, V., & Millstein, S.G. (1993). Current status and approaches to improving preventive services for adolescents. *Journal of the American Medical Association, 269,* 1408–1412.

Irwin, C.E., Jr. (1987). Editor's notes: Adolescent health and behavior. In C.E. Irwin, Jr. (Ed.), *New directions for child development* (Vol. 37). San Francisco: Jossey Bass.

Irwin, C.E., Jr. (1990). The theoretical concept of at-risk adolescents. *Adolescent Medicine: State of the Art Reviews, 1,* 1–14.

Irwin, C.E., Jr., & Duncan, P.M. (2002). Health futures of youth II: Pathways to adolescent health, executive summary and overview. *Journal of Adolescent Health, 31,* (Suppl. 1), 82–89.

Jargowsky, P.A. (2003). *Stunning progress, hidden problems: The dramatic decline of concentrated poverty in the 1990s.* Living Cities Census Series. Brookings Institution. Available from: http://www.brook.edu/es/urban/publications/ jargowskypoverty.htm

Jessor, R., & Jessor, S. (1977). *Problem behavior and psycho-social development: A longitudinal study of youth.* New York: Academic Press.

Katz, L.F., King, J.R., & Liebman, J.B. (2001). Moving to opportunity: Early results of a randomized mobility experiment. *Quarterly Journal of Economics, 116,* 607–654.

Keating, D.P. (1990). Adolescent thinking. In S.S. Feldman & G.R. Elliot (Eds.), *At the threshold: The developing adolescent.* Cambridge, MA: Harvard University Press.

Kett, J.F. (1993). Discovery and invention in the history of adolescence. *Journal of Adolescent Health, 14,* 605–612.

Kirby, D. (2002). Effective approaches to reducing adolescent unprotected sex, pregnancy, and child-bearing. *Journal of Sex Research, 39,* 51–57.

Klein, J.D., Slap, G.B., Elster, A.B., & Schonberg, S.K. (1992). Access to health care for adolescents: A position paper of the Society for Adolescent Medicine. *Journal of Adolescent Health, 13,* 162–170.

Komro, K.A., & Stigler, M.H. (2000). *Growing absolutely fantastic youth a review of the research on "best practices."* University of Minnesota, Minneapolis, MN: Konopka Institute for Best Practices in Adolescent Health. Available from: http://www.allaboutkids.umn.edu/cfahad/GAFY_Science.PDF

Krug, E.G., Dahlberg, L.L., Mercy, J.A., Zwi, A.B., Lozano, R. (Eds.). (2002). *World report on violence and health.* Geneva: World Health Organization.

Lamborn, S.D., Mounts, N.S., Steinberg, L., & Dornbusch, S.M. (1991). Patterns of competence and adjustment among adolescents from authoritative, authoritarian, indulgent, and neglectful families. *Child Development, 62,* 1049–1065.

Lerner, R.M., & Castellino, D.R. (2002). Contemporary developmental theory and adolescence: Developmental systems and applied developmental science. *Journal of Adolescent Health, 31,* 122–135.

Lescohier, D., & Gallagher, S.S. (1996). Unintentional injury. In R.J. Diclemente, W.B. Hansen, & L.E. Ponton (Eds.), *Handbook of adolescent risk behavior.* New York: Plenum Press.

Leventhal, T., & Brooks-Gunn, J. (2003). Children and youth in neighborhood contexts. *Current Directions in Psychological Science, 12,* 27–31.

Luker, K. (1996). *Dubious conceptions: The politics of teenage pregnancy.* Cambridge, MA: Harvard University Press.

Manlove, J., Terry-Humen, E., Papillor, A.G., Franzetta, K., Williams, S., & Ryan, S. (2002). *Preventing teenage pregnancy, childbearing, and sexually transmitted diseases: What research shows us?* Child Trends Research Brief, Washington, DC: Child Trends. Available from: http://www.childtrends.org/Files/K1Brief.pdf.

Mayhew, D.R., & Simpson, H.M. (2002). The safety value of driver education and training. *Injury Prevention, 8* (Suppl. 2), ii3–ii8.

McKnight, A.J., Peck, R.C., & Foss, R.D. (2002).Graduated driver licensing: What works? *Injury Prevention, 8* (Suppl. 2), ii32–ii38.

Millstein, S.G., & Halpern-Felsher, B.L. (2002). Perceptions of risk and vulnerability. *Journal of Adolescent Health, 31S,* 10–37.

Millstein, S.G., & Igra, V. (1996). Theoretical models of adolescent risk-behavior. In J.L. Wallander & L.J. Siegal (Eds.), *Adolescent health problems: Behavioral perspectives.* New York: Guilford Press.

Millstein, S.G., Ozer, E.J., Ozer, E.M., Brindis, C.D., Knopf, D.K., & Irwin, C.E. (2000). *Research priorities in adolescent health: An analysis and synthesis of research recommendations.* San Francisco: University of California, San Francisco, National Adolescent Health Information Center.

Modell, J., & Goodman, M. (1990). Historical perspective. In S.S. Feldman & G.R. Elliot (Eds.), *At the threshold: The developing adolescent.* Cambridge, MA: Harvard University Press.

Murphey, D.A., Lamonda, K.H., Carney, J.K., & Duncan, P. (2004). Relationships of a brief measure of youth assets to health-promoting and risk behaviors. *Journal of Adolescent Health, 34,* 184–191.

Nation, M., Crusto, C., Wandersman, A., Kumpfer, K.L., Seybolt, D., Morrissey-Kane, E., & Davino, K. (2003). What works in prevention: Principles of effective prevention programs. *American Psychologist, 58,* 449–456.

National Adolescent Health Information Center. (2003a). *Fact sheet on demographics.* San Francisco: University of California, San Francisco. Available from: http://nahic.ucsf.edu.

National Adolescent Health Information Center. (2003b). *Fact sheet on reproductive health.* San Francisco: University of California. Available from: http://nahic. ucsf.edu.

National Adolescent Health Information Center. (2003c). *21 Critical objectives for improving the health of adolescents by the year 2010.* San Francisco: University of California. Available from: http://nahic.ucsf.edu

National Adolescent Health Information Center. (2004). *Companion document to the National Initiative to Improve Adolescent Health by the year 2010.* San Francisco: University of California. Available from: http://youth/ucsf.edu/ nahic.

National Campaign to Prevent Teen Pregnancy. (2004). *Teen pregnancy: So what?* Washington, DC. Available from: http://www.teenpregnancy.org/whycare/pdf/ sowhat.pdf

National Commission on Children. (1991). *Beyond rhetoric: A new American agenda for children and families: Final report.* Washington, DC: US Government Printing Office.

National Research Council. (1989). *Diet and health: Implications for reducing chronic disease risk.* Washington, DC: National Academy Press.

National Research Council, Commission on Behavioral and Social Sciences and Education. (1993). *Losing generations.* Washington, DC: National Academy Press.

National Research Council, Panel on Adolescent Pregnancy and Childbearing, Committee on Child Development and Research, Commission on Behavioral and Social Sciences. (1987). *Risking the future: Adolescent sexuality, pregnancy, and childbearing.* Washington, DC: National Academy Press.

Newacheck, P.W., Brindis, C.D., Cart, C.U., Marchi, K., & Irwin, C.E. (1999). Adolescent health insurance coverage: Recent changes and access to care. *Pediatrics, 102*(2 Pt 1), 195–202.

Newacheck, P.W., Hung, Y.Y., Park, M.J., Brindis, C.D., & Irwin, C. E. (2003a). Disparities in adolescent health and health care: Does socio-economic status matter? *Health Services Research, 38,* 1235–1252.

Newacheck, P.W., Wong, S.T., Galbraith, A.A., & Hung, Y.Y. (2003b). Adolescent health care expenditures: A descriptive profile. *Journal of Adolescent Health, 32S,* 3–11.

Newacheck, P.W., Park, M.J., Brindis, C.D., Biehl, M., & Irwin, C.E. (2004). Trends in private and public health insurance for adolescents. *Journal of the American Medical Association, 291,* 1231–1237.

Offer, D., & Schonert-Reichl, K.A. (1992). Debunking the myths of adolescence: Findings from recent research. *Journal of the American Academy of Child and Adolescent Psychiatry, 31,* 1003–1014.

Ogden, C.L., Flegal, K.M., Carroll, M.D., Johnson, C.L. (2002). Prevalence and trends in overweight among US children and adolescents, 1999–2000. *Journal of the American Medical Association, 288,* 1728–1732.

Ozer, E.M., Park, M.J., Paul, T., Brindis, C.D., & Irwin, C.E. (2003). *America's adolescents: Are they healthy?* San Francisco: University of California, San Francisco, National Adolescent Health Information Center.

Park, M.J., MacDonald, T.M., Ozer, E.M., Burg, S.J., Millstein, S.G., Brindis, C.D., & Irwin C.E. (2001). *Investing in clinical preventive services for adolescents.* San Francisco: University of California, San Francisco, Policy Information and Analysis Center for Middle Childhood and Adolescence & the National Adolescent Health Information Center.

Pittman, K.J., O'Brien, R., & Kimball, M. (1993). *Youth development and resiliency research: Making connections to substance abuse prevention.* Washington, DC: Academy for Educational Development.

Price, R.H., Cioci, M., Penner, W., & Trautlein, B. (1993). Webs of influence: School and community programs that enhance adolescent health and education. *Teacher's College Record, 94,* 487–520.

Reddy, D.M., Fleming, R., & Swain, C. (2002). Effect of mandatory parental notification on adolescent girl's use of sexual health care services. *Journal of the American Medical Association, 288,* 710–714.

Remafedi, G. (1989). The healthy sexual development of gay and lesbian adolescents. *SIECUS Report, 17,* 7–8.

Remafedi, G., Resnick, M., Blum, R., & Harris, K.M. (1992). Demography of sexual orientation in adolescences. *Pediatrics, 89*(4 Pt. 2), 714–721.

Resnick, M.D., Bearman, P.S., Blum, R.W., Bauman, K.E., Harris, K.M., Jones, J., Tabor, J., Beuhring, T., Sieving, R.E., Shew, M., Ireland, M., Bearinger, L.H., & Udry, J.R. (1997). Protecting adolescents from harm: Findings from the National Longitudinal Study of Adolescent Health. *Journal of the American Medical Association, 278,* 823–832.

Richardson, J.L., Radziszewska, B., Dent, C.W., & Flay, B.R. (1993). Relationship between after-school care of adolescents and substance use, risk taking, depressed mood and academic achievement. *Pediatrics, 92,* 32–38.

Ritchie, L., Crawford, P., Woodward-Lopez, G., Ivey, S., Masch, M., & Ikeda, J. (2001). *Prevention of childhood overweight: What should be done.* Center for Weight and Health. University of California, Berkeley. Available from: http://www.cnr.berkeley.edu/cwh/

Roberts, D.F. (2000). Media and youth: Access, exposure, and privatization. *Journal of Adolescent Health, 27* (2 Suppl.), 8–14.

Roth, J.L., & Brooks-Gunn, J. (2003). Youth development program: Risk, prevention and policy. *Journal of Adolescent Health, 32,* 170–182.

Runyan, C.W. (2003). Introduction: Back to the future: Revisiting Haddon's conceptualization of injury epidemiology and prevention. *Epidemiological Reviews, 25,* 60–64.

Runyan, C.W., & Gerken, E.A. (1991). Injuries. In W.R. Hendee (Ed.), *The Health of Adolescents.* San Francisco: Jossey-Bass.

Rushton, J.L., Forcier, M., & Schecktman, R.M. (2002). Epidemiology of depressive symptoms in the National Longitudinal Study of Adolescent Health.

*Journal of the American Academy of Child and Adolescent Psychiatry, 41,* 199–205.

Savin-Williams, R.C. (2001). A critique of research on sexual-minority youth. *Journal of Adolescence, 42,* 5–13.

Sayer, A.G., Hauser, S.T., Jacobson, A.M., Willett, A.B., & Cole, C.F. (1995). Developmental influences on adolescent health. In J.L. Wallander & L.J. Siegel (Eds.), *Adolescent health problems: Behavioral perspectives.* New York: Guilford Press.

Schinke, S., Brounstein, P., & Gardner, S. (2002). *Science-based prevention programs and principles* (DHHS Pub. No. [SMA] 03-3764). Rockville, MD: Center for Substance Abuse Prevention, Substance Abuse and Mental Health Services Administration.

Seitz, V., & Apfel, N.H. (1993). Adolescent mothers and repeated childbearing: Effects of a school-based intervention program. *American Journal of Orthopsychiatry, 63,* 572–581.

Seitz, V., & Apfel, N.H. (1999). Effective interventions for adolescent mothers. *Clinical Psychology: Science and Practice, 6,* 50–66.

Sells, C.W., & Blum, R.W. (1996). Morbidity and mortality among US adolescents: An overview of data and trends. *American Journal of Public Health, 86,* 513–519.

Shakespeare, W. (1925). A winter's tale. *Complete works.* New York: P.F. Collier and Son Company. Act III, Scene iii.

Simons-Morton, B.D., Hartos, J.L., & Leaf, W.A. (2002). Promoting parental management of teen driving. *Injury Control, 8* (Suppl. 2), ii24–ii31.

Smetana, J.G. (1989). Adolescents' and parents' reasoning about actual family conflict. *Child Development, 60,* 1052–1067.

Smetana, J.G. (1995). Parenting styles and conceptions of parental authority during adolescence. *Child Development, 66,* 299–316.

Steinberg, L. (2000). The family at adolescence: transition and transformation. *Journal of Adolescent Health, 27,* 170–179.

Steinberg, L., Mounts, N.S., Lamborn, S.D., & Dornbusch, S.M. (1991). Authoritative parenting and adolescent adjustment across varied ecological niches. *Journal of Research on Adolescence, 1,* 19–36.

Strasburger, V.C. (2004). Children, adolescents, and the media. *Current Problems Pediatric Adolescent Health Care, 34,* 54–113.

Straziuso, J. (2004, March 9). Study examines STD rates of teen virgins. *Associated Press.* Reporting presentation by Peter Bearman and Hannah Bruckner at the National STD Prevention Conference, Philadelphia, March 9, 2004.

Sum, A.M., & Fogg, W.N. (1991). The adolescent poor and the transition to early adulthood. In P. Edelman & J. Ladner (Eds.), *Adolescence and poverty: Challenge for the 1990s.* Washington, DC: Center for National Policy Press.

US Congress, Office of Technology Assessment. (1991a). *Adolescent health: Volume I: Summary and Policy Options* (OTA-H-468). Washington, DC: US Government Printing Office.

US Congress, Office of Technology Assessment. (1991b). *Adolescent health: Volume II: Background and the effectiveness of selected prevention and treatment services* (OTA-H-468). Washington, DC: US Government Printing Office.

US Congress, Office of Technology Assessment. (1991c). *Adolescent health: Volume III: Crosscutting issues in the delivery of health and related services* (OTA-H-468). Washington, DC: US Government Printing Office.

US Department of Education, National Center for Education Statistics. (2003). *Digest of education statistics, 2002* (NCES 2003-060). Washington, DC: US Department of Education.

US Public Health Service. (1999). *The Surgeon General's call to action to prevent suicide.* Washington, DC: Author.

US Public Health Service. (2001). *National Strategy for Suicide Prevention: Goals and Objectives for Action.* Rockville, MD: US Department of Health and Human Services.

Vandivere, S., Gallagher, M., & Moore, K.A. (2004). Changes in children's well-being and family environments. *Snapshots of America's families III.* Washington, DC: The Urban Institute. Available from: www.urban.org

Villani, S. (2001). Impact of media on children and adolescents: A 10-year review of the research. *Journal of the American Academy of Child Adolescent Psychiatry, 40,* 392–401.

Wandersman, A., & Florin, P. (2003). Community interventions and effective prevention. *American Psychologist, 58,* 441–448.

Weissberg, R.P., Kumpfer, K.L., & Seligman, M.E. (2003). Prevention that works for children and youth: An introduction. *American Psychologist, 58,* 425–432.

Werner, E.E. (1992). The children of Kauai: Resiliency and recovery in adolescence and adulthood. *Journal of Adolescent Health, 22,* 262–268.

Whitaker, A.H. (1992). An epidemiological study of anorectic and bulimia symptoms in adolescent girls: Implications for pediatricians. *Pediatric Annals, 21,* 752–759.

William T. Grant Foundation, Commission on Work, Family, and Citizenship. (1988). *The forgotten half: Pathways to success for America's youth and young families.* Washington, DC: Author.

Zabin, L.S., & Hayward, S.C. (1993). *Adolescent sexual behavior and childbearing.* Newbury Park, CA: Sage Publications.

Ziv, A., Boulet, J.R., & Slap, G.B. (1999). Utilization of physician offices by adolescents in the United States. *Pediatrics, 104,* 38.

# SECTION III

# Crosscutting Issues

# CHAPTER 9

# Disparities in Maternal and Child Health in the United States

*Larry Crum, Vijaya Hogan, Theresa Chapple, Dorothy Browne, and Jody Greene*

*The demographic changes that are anticipated over the next decade magnify the importance of addressing disparities in health status. Groups currently experiencing poorer health status are expected to grow as a proportion of the total US population; therefore, the future health of America as a whole will be influenced substantially by our success in improving the health status of our racial and ethnic minorities.* (Former Surgeon General David Satcher, 2000)

## INTRODUCTION

The premiere challenge faced by public health today is the elimination of the inequitable health disparities that exist for African American, Native American, and certain Hispanic and Asian subpopulations in the United States. Inequities in health exist across the spectrum of maternal and child health (MCH) indicators, with little evidence of progress toward eliminating these disparities, even in cases where the ethnicity-specific rates are in decline (England, Martin, & Hogan, 1991; Iyasu, Becerra, Rowley, & Hogue, 1992; Kington & Nickens, 2001; Parker et al., 2000; Williams, 2001).

The fact that these inequities exist is not new. In 1899, DuBois, Anderson, and Eaton (1899) published a book called *The Philadelphia Negro* and documented the existence of higher rates of morbidity and mortality across many health outcomes in the black community compared with other populations. Similarly, in 1928, Meriam (1928) observed higher rates of disease among Native Americans compared with the general population.

Although improvement is seen over time in many overall health indicators, such as life expectancy among all groups, the picture for specific mortality indicators has not been as encouraging. The likelihood of reaching the national goal of eliminating health disparities is small. For example, among African Americans, rates of heart disease, HIV, and infant mortality have decreased between the years 1950 to 1995, but the black/white mortality ratio increased. Rates of mortality caused by cancer, diabetes, and cirrhosis have declined, but also with increases in the black/white risk ratio (Williams, 2001).

Part of the reason for this dire prognosis is the relatively short history of national action to eliminate disparities and the underdevelopment of the science focused on acknowledging, understanding, and acting on the complexities of eliminating disparities. Despite the early studies documenting the existence of disparities, it was not until 1980 that a British national report on inequalities in health was published. This report documented disparities in the United Kingdom by residential area, social class, and ethnic group. This report quite possibly stimulated similar surveillance in the United States to assess the extent of disparities among subgroups of the population. *Health 1983, United States*, (NCHS, 1983) first documented disparities across several health outcomes using national surveillance data. In response to this report, then Department of Health and Human Services (DHHS) Secretary Margaret Heckler commissioned the Minority Health Task Force in 1984. This task force published its groundbreaking report in 1985. The report, *The Secretary's Task Force Report on Black and Minority Health* (US Department of Health and Human Services, 1985), introduced the concept of *excess deaths* to denote the difference between the actual number of deaths in a subgroup and the number of deaths that would have occurred if the mortality rate of that group were the same as that for the white population (Figure 9–1).

For ethnic subpopulations compared with the white majority, the task force calculated excess deaths for those younger than 70 years to be 42.3% among blacks, 14% for the Spanish surnamed, 2% among Cuban-born

**White Infant Mortality Rate**

521 deaths / 73,815 live births = 7.1 per 1,000 live births

**Black Infant Mortality Rate**

416 deaths / 27,129 live births = 15.3 per 1,000 live births

*How many black deaths would there be if there was no racial disparity? For example,*

X black deaths / 27,129 live births = 7.1 per 1,000 live births

X = 0.0071 × 27,129

X = 193

Actual number of deaths (416) − expected number of deaths (193) = **223 excess deaths**

**Excess Death Rate = Expected / Actual × 100**

**FIGURE 9–1** Calculating excess deaths: example, North Carolina, 1996.

persons, 7.2% for those Mexican born, and 25% for Native Americans. The rate of excess deaths was particularly high (i.e., 43%) for Native Americans who were younger than 45 years. There were no excess deaths for the Asian/Pacific Islander population, suggesting that this group possesses a healthier mortality profile than all other racial or ethnic subgroups. However, the aggregation of data to obtain these large ethnic population groups masks the heterogeneity within these groupings. That is, when the data for the Asian ethnic population are disaggregated into its component ethnic/nationality groupings, the within-group excess morbidity and mortality, masked by the aggregation, becomes apparent. For example, data from the National Center for Health Statistics (Centers for Disease Control, 2003) reveal that the infant mortality rate of Asians/Pacific Islanders is variable depending on the national group. As indicated in Table 9–1, the infant mortality rate for all Asians/Pacific Islanders combined was 4.7 per 1,000 live births compared with 13.3 for African Americans. However, an examination of each of the subgroups represented in the overall category indicates that the infant mortality rates for Hawaiians (7.3) is considerably higher than that of Chinese (3.2). The aggregate statistics for the total category masks the diversity within each ethnic subgroup. More detailed data about infant mortality are presented in the infant mortality section of this chapter.

The Secretary's Task Force report also identified the six diseases that explained 80% of the excess mortality among blacks: cancer, diabetes,

**Table 9-1** Infant, Neonatal, and Postneonatal Mortality Rates by Specified Race or National Origin of Mother: United States, 2001 Linked File

| Race of Mother | Mortality Rate per 1,000 Births | | |
|---|---|---|---|
| | Infant | Neonatal | Postneonatal |
| All Races | 6.8 | 4.5 | 2.3 |
| White | 5.7 | 3.8 | 1.9 |
| Black | 13.3 | 8.9 | 4.4 |
| American Indian* | 9.7 | 4.2 | 5.4 |
| Asian/Pacific Islander | 4.7 | 3.1 | 1.6 |
| Chinese | 3.2 | 1.9 | 1.3 |
| Japanese | 4.0 | 2.5 | † |
| Hawaiian | 7.3 | 3.6 | 3.7 |
| Filipino | 5.5 | 4.0 | 1.5 |
| Other Asian/Pacific Islander | 4.8 | 3.2 | 1.6 |

*Includes Aleuts and Eskimos.
†The figure does not meet standard of reliability or precision; based on fewer than 20 deaths in the numerator.
Neonatal is less than 28 days, and postneonatal is 28 days to under 1 year.
Source: CDC (2003).

cardiovascular disease/stroke, accidents and homicide, liver disease, and infant mortality. This task force report stimulated the establishment of the Office of Minority Health, whose stated purpose was to influence policy, promote data collection, develop strategic communications, and conduct service demonstrations and policy assessments for the improvement of minority health.

In 1991, with the publication of *Healthy People 2000: National Health Promotion and Disease Prevention Objectives* (US Department of Health and Human Services, 1991), a number of objectives designed to reduce the disparities in risk factors, morbidity, mortality, and disability for ethnic and racial populations were set. As noted in *Healthy People 2000* and in subsequent publications (Centers for Disease Control and Prevention [CDC], 1993a, 1993b; US Department of Health and Human Services, 1992), a number of diseases continued to disproportionately strike racial and ethnic minorities, including AIDS, tuberculosis, high blood pressure, and cardiovascular disease. Furthermore, the mortality rates for diseases and conditions such as cancer, cardiovascular diseases, substance use, homicide, diabetes, suicide, and unintentional injuries and the low birthweight rate were higher for many of the ethnic and racial groups. *Healthy People 2000* established for the first time that one of the goals of the nation would be the reduction of the disparities in health for subgroups of the US population, including ethnic and racial minorities. *Healthy People 2000* set group-specific targets for reduction in disease rates among populations, with separate targets for African Americans and whites. The existence of separate targets stimulated national debate on whether it was more appropriate to set "attainable" 10-year goals for subgroups or whether the nation needed to focus on achieving total equity between subpopulations. The focus on health equity won the debate using human rights arguments and the subsequent version of the national health objectives, *Healthy People 2010* (US Department of Health and Human Services, 1991), focused on *eliminating* the group-specific targets in favor of eliminating all health inequities in all vulnerable populations.

In this chapter, we present data to illustrate the extent of the disparity in key MCH indicators across ethnic and racial subpopulations. The tables and discussions represent a variety of approaches to analysis and presentation of race and ethnic data. In addition, changing demographics are discussed, given their implications for the health of the nation. Although it is important to understand the extent of the disparity, it is also critical to understand the *causes* of disparities. It is ultimately this knowledge that will move us closer to addressing and ultimately eliminating health inequities. As such, we provide an overview of what are known to be factors that contribute to disparities. Finally, some of the methodologic, political, and conceptual challenges affecting the understanding of the health disparities among minorities are enumerated. The chapter concludes with recommendations for policy, programs, research, and training and for educating MCH professionals in an effort to increase knowledge of and improve the ability to effectively reduce and ultimately eliminate disparities.

# CHANGING DEMOGRAPHICS

## Population Projections

Health inequities take on even more significance in public health when one considers the projected changes in the demographics of the United States. The changing demographics of the US population play a huge role in the ability to totally eliminate health disparities. According to the US Census Bureau, in 2000 African Americans comprised 12.3% of the US population or 34.6 million. Hispanics represented almost 12.5% of the mainland US population or 35.3 million. Asians and Pacific Islanders comprise 3.7% and Native Americans 1% of the US population (US Department of Commerce, 2000).

Population projections to the year 2050 indicate changes in the size of ethnic and racial subpopulations. By 2050, the non-Hispanic white population is projected to decrease from the current figure of 73% to 53% of the US population (Sandefur, Eggerling-Boeck, Mannon, & Meier, 2001). Projections for 2050 for racial and ethnic populations are as follows: Hispanics, 32%; African Americans, 12%; Asian and Pacific Islanders, 12%; American Indians and Alaska Natives, 1% (Sandefur et al., 2001). This change in demographics is compounded by the fact that the US white population is becoming older, whereas the racial and ethnic minority populations have larger proportions of younger children and adolescents. Minority children comprised approximately 30% of the population under 19 years of age in 1990 (National Center for Health Statistics, 1991). It is estimated that by year 2020, children of racial and ethnic subpopulations will constitute 40% of the child population in the United States (US Department of Commerce, 1992).

The elementary and middle school population of children, ages 5 to 13 years, is expected to rise from approximately 32 million in 1990 to over 38 million in 2020 and to over 45 million in 2050. The high school age population, that is, children 14 to 17 years of age, is likely also to face increases by 2050. In fact, data indicate that this age group is estimated to reach almost 21 million by the year 2050. Again, it has been noted that the child population between the ages of 5 and 17 years will be increasingly composed of racial and ethnic groups other than non-Hispanic whites. Demographically, the racial and ethnic groups will have a higher proportion of individuals who are less than 15 years of age. In addition, these groups are projected to grow faster than the white population during the next 5 decades (US Department of Commerce, 1992). The rate of increase is such that in a matter of years the population groups characterized as minorities will no longer be minorities but as a group will constitute a majority of the population.

In addition, the foreign-born population of the United States, those citizens who were not US citizens at birth, grew from 10 million in 1970 to 28 million in 2000. The composition of the foreign-born residents has also changed. The share of foreign-born residents from Europe dropped from 62% to 15%, whereas the share from Asia grew from 9% to 25% and from Latin America from 19% to 51%. Although relatively few of the foreign born are less than 18 years old (10%), the majority (44%) are between the ages of 25 and 44 years (US Department of Commerce, 2000).

The rapidly changing demographics in the United States have important implications, not only for the health of the individuals who comprise these ethnic and racial groups, but also for the overall population. With an increase in the number of ethnic and racial minorities in the United States, the minority will become the majority, and existing barriers are likely to affect an even larger proportion of the population.

## What Causes Health Status Differentials?

The predominant yet largely unsubstantiated explanations for the existence of higher rates of disease or death in ethnic minority populations are that these groups are genetically predisposed to disease, that they make purposeful life choices that are unhealthy (do not eat healthy foods, do not exercise, etc.), that they do not receive adequate health care (for a variety of reasons, including lack of insurance, a lack of willingness to access care, a lack of service availability, and poor quality care). In reality, health inequities are not the result of characteristics or qualities inherent in the population. Genetic characteristics may play a role in the development of specific diseases, but the existence of differential genetic makeup by race is not substantiated by scientific data. Differential expression of adverse genetic characteristics, however, is mediated by adverse environmental and social exposures. These environmental and social exposures may be differentially experienced by different racial/ethnic groupings, as mediated by the prevalent social order in society. Differences exist in the experiences and histories of the minority population in relationship with the majority result in inequities in living environments, levels of resources, and exposure to noxious agents (Krieger, 2000).

Even though personal behaviors may play a role in disparate health status, their role varies by health outcome. When behaviors do play a role, they exist within a social context that can limit the range of behavioral choices among which one has to choose (Tarlov, 1999). For example, women are unlikely to exercise regularly if there is no access to affordable exercise facilities and there are no safe walking areas in the neighborhood. They are less likely to purchase fresh fruits and vegetables if the neighborhood stores do not carry them or if they are overpriced and of low quality (Morland, Wing, Diex-Roux, & Poole, 2002; Morrison, Wallenstein, Natale, Senzal, & Huang, 2000). They are likely to prioritize work, school, or other responsibilities ahead of a health care visit because the former directly affect their economic solvency and the health appointment does not (Mullings et al., 2001). As such, the factors contributing to health disparities cannot be easily explained away by personal choice, health care use, or genetics alone.

The former Director of the National Institutes of Health stated in Congressional testimony that

> The causes of health disparities are multiple. They include poverty, level of education, inadequate access to medical care, lack of health insurance, societal discrimination and lack of complete knowledge of the causes, treatment and prevention of serious diseases affecting different populations. The causes [of health disparities] are not genetic, except in rare diseases like sickle cell. . . . Eliminating health disparities will require a cross-cutting effort, involving not only various components of the Federal government, but the private sector as well. (Kirstein, 2000)

Similarly, the Institute of Medicine (2003), in an extensive review of health care inequities, recognized the predominant role of social and economic factors as a cause of health status differentials overall and although confirming a role of health care factors as a contributor to disparities in health, casts them in a different light:

> Racial and ethnic disparities in health status largely reflect differences in social, socioeconomic, behavioral risk factors and environmental living conditions. Health care is therefore necessary but insufficient in and of itself to redress racial and ethnic disparities in health status. A broad and intensive strategy to address social-economic inequality, concentrated poverty, inequitable and segregated housing and education . . . individual risk behaviors as well as disparate access to medical care is needed to seriously address racial and ethnic disparities in health status.

In a comprehensive review of the literature on health disparity, contributors concluded that it is unlikely race and ethnic disparities will be eliminated in the near future because the current level of disparate health status is "locked in" by poorly understood economic, social, educational, political, and medical inequities existent in the United States today (Kington & Nickens, 2001). Recent research is adding new dimensions to this list of contributing factors by revealing other aspects or effects of long-term social inequities. These factors include *weathering* (cumulative physiologic wear and tear caused by the effects of stress over time), with its adverse physiologic impacts (Culhane et al., 2001; Geronimus, Bound, Waidmann, Hillemeier, & Burns, 1996; McEwen & Seeman, 1999), intergenerational exposures creating inherited disadvantage (Hertzman, 1999), and intrauterine programming of physiologic function adapting to fetal exposures to stress (Foster, Wu, Bracken, Semenya, & Thomas, 2000), leading to increased disease risks across the life course. Overlaying all of these, racism is being studied as a direct and indirect cause of health inequities. The existence of health inequities is seen as a direct indicator of the degree of racism that exists in society because most of the economic and social determinants of health are *inequitably distributed* by race/ethnicity (Clark, Anderson, Clark, & Williams, 1999; Jackson, Phillips, Hogue, & Curry-Owens, 2001; Jones, 2000; Klonoff & Landrine, 2000; LaViest, Keith, & Gutierrez, 1993; Williams, 2001; Williams & Rucker, 2000).

## Inequitable Distribution of Social Determinants of Health

Poverty is disproportionately found among minority populations and could limit the resources available to conduct activities known to maintain health or limit the ability to seek health services. The poverty rate among blacks and Hispanics (22%) is almost three times as high as it is among whites (8%) and over two times the rate for Asians/Pacific Islanders (10.8%) (US Department of Commerce, 2000).

Educational attainment is also disproportionately distributed by population. Eighty-eight percent of whites and 86% of Asians had at least completed high school, whereas 78% of blacks and 57% of Hispanics had completed high school. Although 28% and 44% of Asians and Pacific Islanders received a Bachelor's degree, only 16% of blacks and 11% of Hispanics had completed a 4-year degree (US Department of Commerce, 2000) (Figure 16–1). In addition, African Americans earn less than whites regardless of educational levels attained. Thus, African Americans and their families are more likely to be classified as poor. Data from the US Census 2000 indicate an almost threefold higher level of poverty for black families (22%) compared with white families (8%). Twenty one percent of Hispanic families, 10.8% of Asian, and 11% of Native American families live in poverty (US Department of Commerce, 2000).

Socioeconomic diversity exists across and within the Hispanic population subgroups; among the three main subgroups comprising the Hispanic category, Puerto Ricans have the lowest socioeconomic status (SES) and Cubans the highest as determined by years of formal education, income, and home ownership. Unemployment rates, poverty rates, and the number of households headed by women are the highest among the Puerto Rican individuals.

# HEALTH STATUS OF MINORITY GROUPS

The following section presents selected mortality, morbidity, and trend data for various ethnic and racial groups. When available or appropriate, mortality and morbidity statistics are for the MCH populations within these racial and ethnic groups. Mortality data are used to identify the leading causes of death among the various racial and ethnic groups. By examining sex, age, and cause-specific mortality rates by racial/ethnic groups for important diseases and conditions, public health practitioners can determine how best to achieve the national objectives detailed in *Healthy People 2010* and to improve the health of special populations.

## Infant Mortality

### Infant Mortality Rates

The infant mortality rate, (the number of children who die before their first birthday divided by the total number of live births times 1,000) serves both as a national and an international indicator of the overall status of health of a community or nation. The significance of infant mortality as a key indicator of a nation's health status and well-being is well accepted in social and biomedical sciences (Reidpath & Allotey, 2003; CDC, 1991; Klein & Hawk, 1992; Nersessian, 1988; Singh, Kposawa, & Augustine, 1994; US Department of Health and Human Services, 2000). Although the infant mortality rate for all Americans has been steadily declining since 1980 to a low of 6.8 per 1,000 live births in 2001, these reductions have not led to reductions in disparities in infant mortality rates among race and ethnic groups, especially between whites and blacks (NCHS, 2004). For example, the mortality rate for black infants in 1980 was twice the rate for white infants (NCHS, 1993; NCHS, 2004), but in 2000, the mortality rate for black infants was 2.5 times the rate for white infants (NCHS, 2004). Unfortunately, these statistics represent a long-term trend that has been evident in mortality data collected since 1950 (Singh & Yu, 1996a).

Until recently, the focus on infant mortality was on the differentials between whites and blacks. The failure to show differentials for other racial and ethnic groups was partly due to the small numbers of deaths and the unavailability of reliable population counts for the various sub-groups. In addition, race- and ethnic-specific mortality data contained on death and birth certificates have also been questioned, with claims that the death rates for American Indians and Asians/Pacific Islanders are grossly underestimated (Bennett, 1993; Sorlie, Rogot, & Johnson, 1992). Recent improvements in data collection methods and statistical techniques addressing the issue of small numbers for selected subgroup groups have allowed better and more detailed reports concerning infant mortality rates associated with racial and ethnic subgroups. For example, Singh and Yu (1996b) aggregated 3 years of mortality data to provide stable estimates of infant mortality for various ethnic and racial groups. These researchers found significant differences in rates of infant mortality among subgroups of Asian/Pacific Islanders when rates were reported by nationality, such as Chinese, Japanese, Hawaiian, and Filipinos.

Similarly, periodic reports on infant mortality published by the CDC and other agencies are now more likely to report health data by racial subgroups, although problems related to sparse data still exist. Table 9–2, from the CDC's National Vital Statistics Reports (CDC, 2003), shows infant, neonatal, and postneonatal mortality rates by the standard four race categories—white, black, American Indian, and Asian/Pacific Islanders—and by subgroups of Asian/Pacific Islanders based on nationality. There was wide variation in infant mortality rates by race of mother with the highest rate, 13.3 for infants of black mothers, four times greater than the lowest rate of 3.2 for infants of Chinese mothers. Rates were also high for infants of Hawaiian (7.3) and American Indian (9.7) mothers. Rates were intermediate for infants of non-Hispanic white (5.7) and Filipino mothers (5.5).

Besides the alarming differences among the four standard racial groups regarding these mortality rates, there are also considerable differences in these rates within the Asian/Pacific Islander and Hispanic subgroups, as mentioned previously here. At the same time, there remains a problem with small numbers. The postneonatal mortality rate for Japanese is not reported for this reason.

**Table 9–2** Infant, Neonatal, and Postneonatal Deaths and Mortality Rates by Specified Race or National Origin of Mother: United States, 2001 Linked File

| Race of Mother | Live Births | Number of Deaths** | | | Mortality Rate per 1,000 Births | | |
|---|---|---|---|---|---|---|---|
| | | Infant | Neonatal | Postneonatal | Infant | Neonatal | Postneonatal |
| All Races | 4,026,036 | 27,523 | 18,275 | 9,248 | 6.8 | 4.5 | 2.3 |
| White | 3,177,698 | 18,087 | 12,078 | 6,009 | 5.7 | 3.8 | 1.9 |
| Black | 606,183 | 8,084 | 5,396 | 2,688 | 13.3 | 8.9 | 4.4 |
| American Indian[1] | 41,872 | 404 | 176 | 228 | 9.7 | 4.2 | 5.4 |
| Asian or Pacific Islander | 200,283 | 947 | 624 | 323 | 4.7 | 3.1 | 1.6 |
| Chinese | 31,401 | 100 | 60 | 40 | 3.2 | 1.9 | 1.3 |
| Japanese | 9,048 | 36 | 22 | 14 | 4.0 | 2.5 | * |
| Hawaiian | 6,411 | 47 | 23 | 24 | 7.3 | 3.6 | 3.7 |
| Filipino | 32,470 | 180 | 131 | 48 | 5.5 | 4.0 | 1.5 |
| Other Asian or Pacific Islander | 120,953 | 584 | 388 | 197 | 4.8 | 3.2 | 1.6 |

*Figure does not meet standard of reliability or precision; based on fewer than 20 deaths in the numerator.
[1]Includes Aleuts and Eskimos.
**Infant deaths are weighted so numbers may not exactly add to totals due to rounding. Neonatal is less than 28 days, and postneonatal is 28 days to under 1 year.
Source: CDC (2003).

### Leading Causes of Infant Death

The leading cause of infant death in the United States in 2001 was congenital malformations (deformations and chromosomal abnormalities), accounting for 20% of all infant deaths. Disorders relating to short gestation and low birth weight was second, accounting for 16% of all infant deaths, followed by sudden infant death syndrome (SIDS), accounting for 8% of infant deaths. The fourth and fifth leading causes—newborns affected by maternal complications of pregnancy (maternal complications) and respiratory distress of the newborn—accounted for 5% and 4%, respectively, of all infant deaths in 2001. Together, the five leading causes accounted for 53% of all infant deaths in the United States in 2001 (CDC, 2003).

When differences between infant mortality rates based on congenital malformations were examined by race and ethnicity, infant mortality rates were 21% higher for black than for white mothers. Rates were 12% higher for Mexican mothers and 19% higher for Central and South American mothers than for non-Hispanic white mothers. Differences in infant mortality rates for congenital malformations between American Indian and white mothers were not statistically significant, but were 14% lower for Asians/Pacific Islanders than for white mothers.

Infants of black mothers had the highest infant mortality rates from low birth weight. The rate for black mothers was 3.8 times the rate for white mothers. The rate for Puerto Rican mothers was more than twice that for non-Hispanic white mothers, whereas rates for Mexican mothers were 11% lower than those for non-Hispanic white mothers.

SIDS rates were highest for American Indian mothers—3.2 times those for white mothers. Rates for black mothers were also high—2.5 times those for white mothers. As most SIDS deaths occur during the postneonatal period, the high SIDS rates for infants of black and American Indian mothers account for much of their elevated risk of postneonatal mortality. SIDS rates for Asians/Pacific Islanders mothers were less than half of those for white mothers. For Mexican mothers, the SIDS rate was less than half that for non-Hispanic white mothers, and for Puerto Rican mothers, the SIDS rate was 46% higher than the rate for non-Hispanic white mothers.

An examination of cause-specific differences in infant mortality rates between race and Hispanic-origin groups can help researchers better understand overall differences in infant mortality rates between these groups. For example, 28% of the elevated infant mortality rate for black mothers when compared with white mothers can be accounted for by their higher infant mortality rate caused by low birth weight and prematurity, 9% by differences in SIDS, and 7% by differences in maternal complications. In other words, if black infant mortality rates for these three causes could be reduced to levels for white infants, the difference in the infant mortality rate between black and white mothers would be reduced by 44%.

For American Indian mothers, 25% of their elevated infant mortality rate when compared with white mothers can be accounted for by their higher SIDS rates. Thus, if American Indian SIDS rates could be reduced to levels for white infants, the difference in the infant mortality rate between American Indian and white mothers would be reduced by 25%. Similarly, 33% of the difference between Puerto Rican and non-Hispanic white infant mortality rates can be accounted for by differences in infant mortality rates caused by low birthweight, 9% by differences in respiratory distress, and 8% by SIDS. If Puerto Rican infant mortality rates for these three causes could be reduced to levels of non-Hispanic white infants, the difference in the infant mortality rate between Puerto Rican and non-Hispanic white infants would be cut in half. In addition to helping to explain differences in infant mortality rates between various groups, comparisons such as these can be helpful in targeting prevention efforts (CDC, 2003).

## Childhood and Adolescence

The most recent statistics on the health of the nation's children provides a mixed bag of positive and negative trends with regard to their well-being. For example, there appear to be declining birth rates for adolescents, fewer incidents of violent crime involving young people, and expanded vaccine coverage. However, increases in obesity as well as in infant mortality and low birth weight among minority teen mothers represent major challenges (Federal Interagency Forum on Child and Family Statistics, 2004). Not surprisingly, these and other trends in health and risk behaviors do not affect minority youth in uniform patterns, as disparities in health indicators across race and ethnic groups persist.

### Mortality Rates

As noted by Singh and Yu (1996a) in an examination of data from the National Vital Statistics System, the National Longitudinal Mortality Study and the Area Resource File, Asians and Pacific Islanders 1 to 4 years old have the lowest child mortality rate of all racial and ethnic groups for the periods of 1979 to 1981 and 1989 to 1991. However, mortality varied greatly within the category of Asians and Pacific Islanders. Chinese, Japanese, and Filipino children 1 to 4 years old have lower death rates than Hawaiians and other Asians. This was the case for both boys and girls. Black, American Indian, and Hawaiian male and female children had the highest death rates for the two time periods. Among Hispanics, Cuban children had lower death rates than their white counterparts, and Puerto Rican and Central and South American children had higher rates in both time periods examined.

As in the case of younger children, Asian and Pacific Islander children 5 to 14 years old have the lowest mortality rates. Specifically, Chinese, Japanese, and Filipino children had significantly lower death rates than whites, blacks, Hawaiians, and American Indians (Singh & Yu, 1996b). This was true among female and male children. Black, American Indian, and Hawaiian male and female children had the highest death rate for the periods of 1979 through 1981 and 1989 through 1991, whereas Cuban children had significantly lower rates than other Hispanics (Singh & Yu, 1996b).

**Causes of Death**

An examination of the leading causes of death among children 1 to 4 years and 5 to 14 years indicates that for children 1 to 4 years old, the leading causes of death during 1989 and 1991 were motor vehicle fatalities, other unintentional injuries, congenital anomalies, homicide, cancer, pneumonia and influenza, and HIV. For children 5 to 14 years old, the list contained some of the same causes except that added to this list were suicide, cerebrovascular disease, and pulmonary disease (Singh & Yu, 1996a). Although the classification system for causes of death was modified for 1999 data to date, similar findings are reflected in more current data (Arias et al., 2003; CDC, 1998). The leading health problems affecting preadolescents and adolescents have less to do with the medical etiologies and more with environment, behavior, and lifestyle. For racial and ethnic youth, injuries, intentional and unintentional, are of major concern.

**Birthrates for Adolescents**

Birth rates for adolescents have dropped steadily since 1991, reaching a record low of 23 births per 1,000 females ages 15 to 17 in 2002. The steepest decline has been among black, non-Hispanic adolescents who experienced a decline of more than half between 1991 and 2002 (from 86 to 41 per 1,000, respectively). Declining adolescent birth rates are a direct result of declining adolescent pregnancy rates as evidenced by decreases in not only live births, but in induced abortions and fetal losses as well (Ventura, Abma, Mosher, & Henshaw, 2003).

### Violence

Although the rates of violent incidents involving young people soared in the 1990s, recent reports from the National Crime Victimization Survey and the FBI's Uniform Crime Reports indicate a dramatic decline in the level of violence affecting young people. Substantial declines have been reported for both serious violent crime victimization of youth and offending (perpetration) by youth. After peaking in 1993, serious violent crime victimization rates dropped 74%, from 44 crimes per 1,000 youth ages 12 to 17 in 1993 to 11 in 2002. Likewise, since 1993, serious violent crime offending rates dropped 78%, from 52 crimes per 1,000 youth in 1993 to 11 crimes in 2002 (Federal Interagency Forum on Child and Family Statistics, 2004).

It is in this area of crime victimization that disparities based on race and ethnicity appear to be eroding. In contrast to 1993, when the serious crime victimization rate for black youth was 72 crimes per 1,000 compared with 40 crimes per 1,000 white youth, in 2002, black youth were nearly as likely to be the victims of serious violent crime as white youth. The 2002 serious crime victimization rate for black youth was 17 crimes per 1,000 versus 10 crimes per 1,000 white youth (Federal Interagency Forum on Child and Family Statistics, 2004).

In spite of this highlight, work still needs to be done to address the problem of violence involving young people. According to 2002 victims' reports, 17% of all serious violent crimes involved a juvenile offender, and more than one offender was involved in 57% of all of the serious violent crimes involving youth offenders (Federal Interagency Forum on Child and Family Statistics, 2004).

### Cigarette, Drug, and Alcohol Use

Prevention of cigarette smoking among adolescents is a national public health priority. Data from a National Institute on Drug Abuse survey, Monitoring the Future (Johnston, O'Malley, Bachman, & Schulenberg,

2003), indicate that in 2003, 5% of 8th graders, 9% of 10th graders, and 16% of 12th graders reported that they had smoked cigarettes daily in the past 30 days. These are the lowest rates since the survey began (1975 for 12th graders and 1991 for 8th and 10th graders). However, from 2002 to 2003, the daily use of cigarettes did not decline significantly for students in any grade. As in the past, male and female students continue to have similar rates of daily smoking, and white students continue to smoke at a higher rate than either black or Hispanic students.

Illicit drug use over the past 30 days did not decrease significantly from 2002 to 2003 for students in any grade. Nonetheless, in 2003, illicit drug use was at its lowest point since 1993 among 8th graders (10%), since 1994 among 10th graders (20%), and since 1995 among 12th graders (24%). From 2002 to 2003, heavy drinking remained steady across all age groups; 12% of 8th graders, 22% of 10th graders, and 28% of 12th graders consumed five or more drinks in a row at least once in the past 2 weeks in 2003. The pattern of illicit drug use and heavy drinking by race and ethnicity is similar: both are much more prevalent among white and Hispanic secondary school students than among their black counterparts (Federal Interagency Forum on Child and Family Statistics, 2004).

### Overweight and Obesity

Data from the National Health and Nutrition Examination Survey show that the prevalence of being overweight among US children has increased sharply in recent years. In 1976 to 1980, only 6% of children were over-weight. By 1988 to 1994, this proportion had risen to 11% and contin-ued to rise to 15% in 1999 to 2000 (Figure 9–2). Black, non-Hispanic girls, and Mexican American boys are at particularly high risk of being overweight. In 1999 to 2000, 24% of black, non-Hispanic girls and 29% of Mexican American boys were overweight.

# HIV INFECTION AND AIDS

For minority populations that are already plagued by a variety of indica-tors of poor health status, HIV infection and AIDS are additional handi-caps. Although in the 1990s the majority of AIDS cases in the United States occurred in the white population, recent statistics indicate that may no longer be the case, as individual minority groups are increasingly over-

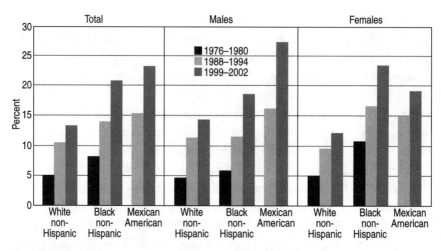

Data for Mexican American children are not available from 1976 to 1980 because of differences in reporting of race and Hispanic origin. Overweight is defined as body mass index (BMI) at or above the 95th percentile of the 2000 CDC BMI-for-age growth charts. BMI is calculated as weight in kilograms divided by the square of height in meters.

Source: Federal Interagency Forum on Child and Family Statistics (2004). *America's children in brief: Key national indicators of well-being, 2004.* Available from: http://childstats.gov [cited] Jan. 5, 2005. Data source: Centers for Disease Control and Prevention, National Center for Health Statistics, National Health and Nutrition Examination Survey, 2003–2004.

**FIGURE 9–2** Percentage of children ages 6 to 18 who are overweight by gender, race, and Hispanic origin, 1976 to 1980, 1988 to 1994, and 1999 to 2002.

represented in AIDS statistics. HIV/AIDS in minority women has made a significant impact on their communities given that infection and disease occur most often in women of childbearing age. Women as well as men of all race and ethnic groups are at increasing risk of HIV contraction as medical and sociocultural approaches to the problem attempt to slow the epidemic.

Table 9–3 shows recent estimates of the number and rates of AIDS diagnoses by race/ethnicity, age, and sex. Non-Hispanic black males and females have by far the largest number of and highest rate of AIDS diagnoses (13,890 diagnoses and a rate of 108.4 per 100,000 people for black males and 7,159 diagnoses and rate of 48.6 per 100,000 people). Among females, Hispanics had the second highest rate, followed by American Indian/Alaska Natives. The rate for black women is more than 23 times the rate for non-Hispanic white women. The numbers and rates for children follow the

**Table 9–3** Estimated Numbers of Diagnoses and Rates (per 100,000 Population) of AIDS, by Persons' Race/Ethnicity, Age Category, and Sex, 2002–United States

| | Adults or Adolescents | | | | | | Children (< 13 Years) | | | |
| | Males | | Females | | Total | | | | Total | |
| Race/ethnicity | Number | Rate | Number | Rate | Number | Rate | Number | Rate | Number | Rate |
|---|---|---|---|---|---|---|---|---|---|---|
| White, not Hispanic | 10,095 | 12.3 | 1,801 | 2.1 | 11,896 | 7.0 | 7 | 0.0 | 11,903 | 5.9 |
| Black, not Hispanic | 13,890 | 108.4 | 7,159 | 48.6 | 21,049 | 76.4 | 57 | 0.7 | 21,106 | 58.7 |
| Hispanic | 5,508 | 39.7 | 1,471 | 11.3 | 6,979 | 26.0 | 19 | 0.2 | 6,998 | 19.2 |
| Asian/Pacific Islander | 397 | 8.6 | 75 | 1.5 | 471 | 4.9 | 1 | 0.1 | 473 | 4.0 |
| American Indian/ Alaska Native | 151 | 16.9 | 54 | 5.8 | 205 | 11.2 | 0 | 0 | 205 | 8.5 |
| Total* | 30,120 | 26.4 | 10,589 | 8.8 | 40,709 | 17.3 | 84 | 0.2 | 40,793 | 14.1 |

These numbers do not represent actual cases in persons with a diagnosis of AIDS. Rather, these numbers are point estimates of cases diagnosed that have been adjusted for reporting delays. The estimates have not been adjusted for incomplete reporting.

Data exclude cases from the US dependencies, possessions, and associated nations, as well as cases in persons whose state or area of residence is unknown because of the lack of census information by race and age categories for these areas.

*Includes 108 persons of unknown or multiple race. Because column totals were calculated independently of the values for the subpopulations, the values in each column may not sum to the column total.

Source: CDC (2002).

same pattern as for the adults, with non-Hispanic black children having the highest rate, more than three times the rate for Hispanics.

With regard to new infections among women in the United States, the CDC estimates that approximately 75% of women were infected through heterosexual sex and 25% through injection drug use. Of newly infected women, approximately 64% are black, 18% are white, 18% are Hispanic, and a small percentage are members of other racial/ethnic groups (CDC, 2001b). The proportion of AIDS cases among women, especially among women of color, continues to rise. During 2001, women represented 26% of new AIDS cases compared with only 11% in 1990 and 6% in 1982 (CDC, 2001b). In areas with confidential HIV reporting, persons 13 to 24 years old accounted for 13% of newly reported HIV cases (not AIDS) from July 1999 to June 2000. Of these persons, females accounted for 47% of the cases in this age group (CDC, 2001b).

The problems women face with regard to HIV infection has been well documented. Women with HIV infection often face problems that HIV-infected men do not. For example, women are less likely to be diagnosed because gynecologic infections and conditions are not always recognized by health professionals as signs of HIV infection (Pizzi, 1992). Also, because in many homes women are the sole providers for their families, women will have to deal with decisions regarding custody of their children in addition to maintaining their physical health (Pizzi, 1992). Because of this, HIV/AIDS has had a devastating impact on minority families and communities. In lower income families, there is a higher risk of HIV infection and a more adverse economic impact because of HIV infection (Mann, Tarantola, & Netter, 1992). Dependent children are the most frequently and most significantly affected by HIV infection in the family. In addition to economic hardships caused by medical bills and lost wages of the sick parent, children are often required to assume the responsibilities of the adult, including that of nurturer (Mann et al., 1992). This has ramifications for children's educational and social futures. It also has psychological ramifications, as children are often forced to experience the early and painful death of one or both parents in a society that has both stigmatized HIV/AIDS and discriminated against its victims.

Although medical advances in HIV diagnosis and treatment are improving the life expectancy and quality of life of those infected, prevention remains the focus of many health educators. However, especially for minority populations, cultural sensitivity is an integral part of delivering effective prevention messages. Cultural sensitivity can mean something as simple as holding educational workshops with same-sex participants to reduce embarrassment or discomfort or providing Native Americans disposable razor blades to use in skin-offering ceremonies (to prevent the reuse of nonsterile razors). The key is identifying the links among culture, healthy behaviors, and effective communication. In recent years, more emphasis has been placed on identifying cultural characteristics and using them to develop more effective intervention and prevention programs.

One such program developed and implemented by and Wechsberg, Zule, Lam, and Bobashev (2004) resulted in a culturally enriched woman-focused intervention for crack-abusing African American women that was grounded in empowerment theory (Wechsberg, 1998) and black feminism (Roberts, Wechsberg, Zule, & Burroughs, 2003). The women's intervention focused on HIV/AIDS risk reduction and emphasized the social and cultural context of these women, including race, gender, and personal power, as they relate to HIV risk. In comparing the effects of this culturally enriched intervention with a standard intervention that put much less emphasis on cultural factors and a control group of women who received no intervention, these researchers found that the woman-focused intervention was effective in reducing crack use and sexual risk among African American women. The enhanced intervention was also effective in increasing self-sufficiency by decreasing homelessness and increasing employment. These findings provide evidence that relatively brief personalized interventions conducted outside of a treatment setting can be effective in empowering women and reducing high-risk sexual behaviors.

## CHRONIC DISEASES

Figure 9–3 shows disparities of age-adjusted mortality rates for categories of major chronic diseases among white and minority group women for 2000. As indicated, the mortality rates for the chronic diseases are not uniformly higher for minority groups than for whites. Asians/Pacific Islanders, American Indians/Alaska Natives, and Hispanics all had mortality rates below those for white Americans, whereas African Americans had rates well above the rates for whites for all conditions except those related to lower respiratory disease. These profiles show that minority groups are quite heterogeneous when it comes to health status, and for the conditions specified in Figure 9–3, not all ethnic and racial groups are at a disadvantage.

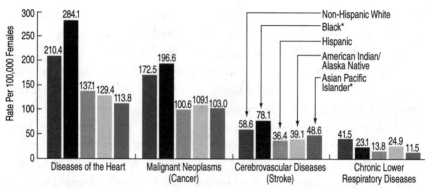

*Does not exclude Hispanic

Source: National Vital Statistics System (CDC, 2003).

**FIGURE 9–3** Age-adjusted death rates from selected conditions for females (all ages) by race/ethnicity, 2000.

Of course, as noted earlier, mortality rates such as those shown here can be artifacts of the classification system used to categorize individuals into racial/ethnic subgroups. For example, it is known that refugees from Southeast Asia have very different health profiles than Japanese Americans, and differences also exist among the major groups making up the Hispanic population. Thus, caution should be exercised when making generalizations about the relative health status of the generally accepted ethnic categories. More issues related to classification are discussed later in this chapter.

# RISK FACTOR CONTRIBUTION TO HEALTH STATUS DIFFERENTIALS

Given the deplorable discrepancies that exist in the health status of some minority groups when compared with whites, one is first compelled to explain these discrepancies in terms of the prevalence of risk factors within these various groups. Two important risk factors among women of child-bearing age, cigarette smoking and alcohol use, are examined in Figures 9–4 and 9–5, respectively. Maternal smoking during pregnancy is associated with ectopic pregnancies, miscarriages, low birth weight, and infant mortality, and drinking alcohol during pregnancy contributes to fetal alcohol syndrome, low birth weight, and developmental delays in children. Figure 9–4 shows that among females who were not pregnant American Indian/Alaska

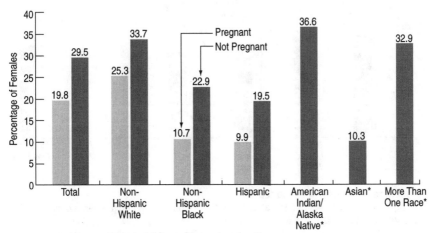

*Low precision, no estimate for pregnant women reported

Source: Women's Health USA (2003a).

**FIGURE 9–4** Females aged 15–44 years reporting past month use of cigarettes, by race ethnicity and pregnancy status, 2000–2001

Native women were most likely to smoke in 2000 to 2001, followed by non-Hispanic white women. Although the prevalence of smoking was lower among pregnant women in all racial and ethnic groups where sufficient data were available, non-Hispanic white women were more than twice as likely to smoke during pregnancy than non-Hispanic black women. There was a slight increase in recent years in the proportion of pregnant women who reported cigarette smoking in the past month, from 18.6% in 1999 to 2000 to 19.8% in 2000 to 2001. Also, this report includes data on women identifying with more than one race. This is a recent trend in statistical reporting that is discussed in a later section of this chapter.

Figure 9–5 shows that among women aged 15–44 who were not pregnant non-Hispanic white and American Indian/Alaska Native women were the most likely to be binge drinkers (22.7% and 21.4%, respectively) compared with other racial/ethnic groups. Non-Hispanic white women were also the most likely to engage in binge alcohol use during pregnancy. In addition to the risk factors mentioned here, minority group members are more likely than whites to report a sedentary lifestyle and being overweight.

Several theories exist as to why the health status of some minority groups is poor relative to whites and other minority groups. All reflect the typical problems of groups that battle poverty, lack of social resources, inadequate

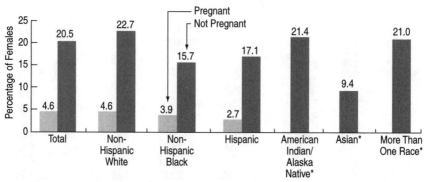

\* Low precision, no estimate reported.

\*\* "Binge" alcohol use was defined as drinking five or more drinks on the same occasion on at least 1 day in the past 30 days.

"Occasion" means at the same time or within a few hours of each other. "Heavy" alcohol use is defined as drinking five or more drinks on the same occasion on each of 5 or more days in the past 30 days; all "heavy" alcohol users are also "binge" alcohol users.

Source: Women's Health USA (2003b).

**FIGURE 9–5** Females aged 15–44 years reporting past month binge alcohol use,\*\* by race/ethnicity and pregnancy status, 2000–2001.

education, and discrimination by mainstream society. Reasons may include differences in medical care-seeking behavior, difference in sexual behavior (Moran, Aral, Jenkins, Petersen, & Alexander, 1989), differences in knowledge about disease transmission (Ford & Norris, 1993), a lack of grass roots organization, and a lack of medical insurance (Perrow & Guillen, 1990). These reasons can be exacerbated by various cultural attitudes that exist in some minority communities. For example, in some black and Hispanic communities, male dominance may lead to couples not using condoms during sexual acts (Perrow & Guillen, 1990; Wechsberg, Zule, Lam, & Bobashev, 2004). An inability of the female partner to insist on the use of condoms may be difficult or next to impossible, as doing so may imply mistrust of the male partner (Wechsberg, Zule, Lam, & Bobashev, 2004; Weeks, Schensill, Williams, Singer, & Grier, 1995). This may be especially true for women whose sexual partners provide financial support (Kline, Kline, & Oken, 1992). It may also reflect the need for improvement of negotiating skills in sexually active women who do not use condoms. Other cultural barriers to safer sex practices and reduced HIV infection are language differences and the fact that, in some minority communities, the mention of sexual practices is taboo outside of the bedroom (Pizzi, 1992).

Removing these barriers and changing attitudes will be crucial steps in preventing future HIV infection in minority women.

A lack of education and living in poverty also has predictably detrimental effects on the health status of minority groups. Illiteracy often prevents mothers from obtaining information about behaviors that can put them or their infants at risk, and poverty too often prevents mothers from seeking treatments for their families until health problems are severe (and more costly to treat). Poverty among children varies greatly by family structure. Children living in female-householder families with no husband present continued to experience a higher poverty rate in 2002 than their counterparts in married-couple families: 39.6% compared with 8.5%. Disparities by race and ethnicity also persist. Children who were black (and no other race) had a poverty rate of 32.1% in 2002; Hispanic children (who could be of any race) had a poverty rate of 28.2%, whereas single-race white, non-Hispanic children had a poverty rate of 8.9% (DeNavas-Walt, Proctor, & Mills, 2004).

To a large extent, the racial gap in mortality is a function of economic inequalities such as poverty, a lack of educational and employment opportunities, substandard housing, and an inability to access health care. However, in addition to the economic inequalities, some, but not all noneconomic factors such as differences in lifestyle, diet, and micro-level or behavioral variables (e.g., substance use) explain the differentials in health status between racial and ethnic subgroups and the white population.

Reasons that have been proposed in an attempt to explain the observed racial and ethnic differences in physician and hospital care access include the lack of health insurance and other economic disadvantages, small number of minority physicians, restrictions in hospital admissions, changes in hospital locations, individual perceptions of symptoms and disease status, long waiting periods, inconvenient hours, racial discrimination, a lack of continuity of care, inadequate privacy, dissatisfaction with physician treatment, and physician bias (Mirvis, Burns, Gaschen, Cloar, & Graney, 1994). A lack of trust may be an issue as a result of the US Public Health Service's 40-year study of untreated syphilis in African Americans at the Tuskegee Veterans Administration hospital (Armstrong, Crum, Rieger, Bennett, & Edwards, 1999; LaViest et al., 1993). Significant differences in physician–patient relationships have been observed between whites and nonwhites. However, it is unclear whether discordance in race or ethnicity between physician and patient ultimately causes differences in care (Weddington & Gabel, 1991).

Compared with white children, African American and Hispanic children are less likely to receive prescribed medication, and they receive fewer medications (Hahn, 1995). That these differences were found to persist after such factors as SES, health status, and number of physicians were controlled suggests that racism may be an independent cause of persons of a different race receiving fewer medical services than whites (Hahn, 1995). Also, African American mothers have been observed to experience inadequate and delayed prenatal care compared with white mothers (LaViest et al., 1993). It was thought that Medicare and Medicaid would narrow racial differences, although race is still observed to be a factor in quality of health care (LaViest et al., 1993).

## HOMELESSNESS

Homelessness represents a daunting national problem affecting hundreds of thousands of individuals and their families every year (National Coalition for the Homeless, 2004), and minority populations appear to be at greater risk of homelessness (Greene, Ringwalt, Kelly, Iachan, & Cohen, 1995; Link et al., 1994; National Coalition for the Homeless, 2004; Urban Institute, 1999). According to the 2000 US Census, minorities represent approximately 27% of the overall US population. However, recent surveys suggest that national minorities represent approximately 60% of the homeless population (Urban Institute, 1999), and in US cities with populations of 100,000 or more, poor blacks are twice as likely to be homeless as poor whites in the same cities (Rosenheck, Leda, Frisman, Lam, & Chung, 1996).

One of the fastest growing segments of the homeless population appears to be homeless families, most of which (84%) are headed by women. Most of these women are in their late 20s with approximately two young children. It is estimated that people in homeless families represent 40% of the total homeless population (US Conference of Mayors, 2003; Urban Institute, 2000) and that 63% of children in homeless families are minorities (Urban Institute, 1999). Of homeless parents, approximately 38% are white non-Hispanic, 43% are black non-Hispanic, 15% are Hispanic, 3% are Native American, and 1% are other races (Urban Institute, 1999).

Too often, both parents and children suffer dire consequences when confronted with problems leading to and associated with homelessness. Parents in homeless families are more likely to suffer from chronic health conditions, mental health problems, and substance abuse problems and to have experienced childhood abuse. Similarly, children in homeless families have been found be more likely to have chronic health problems, mental health issues, food sufficiency issues, and developmental delays (Bassuk et al., 1996). These illnesses have potentially devastating consequences if not treated early. In addition, homeless families are also at high risk for disruption by separation in that some emergency shelters will only accept women and children or adults only, resulting in children being separated from one or both parents.

Although blacks and to a lesser extent Hispanics have received the most attention from researchers regarding homelessness among minorities, the presence of other minorities among the homeless and the documentation of their needs have received minimal attention. More research in this area is sorely needed to understand fully and address this personal tragedy and national crisis.

# THE DEBATE SURROUNDING THE COLLECTION OF RACIAL AND ETHNIC DATA

Our knowledge regarding the reasons for racial and ethnic differences in health outcomes is compromised by some of the challenges associated with collecting data on race and ethnicity. Some of these challenges include debates surrounding the appropriateness of collecting and analyzing data by race and ethnicity, the use of questionable strategies and approaches for collecting data on ethnic and racial subpopulations, and aggregating data for ethnic and racial subpopulations such that one cannot examine the health status of a particular subgroup or the prevalence of a particular health condition. Further confounding our ability to interpret race and ethnic differentials is the failure to supplement standard racial and ethnicity data with the use of culturally sensitive and appropriate instruments.

The collection of data by race and ethnicity is advocated by many because such information can assist in public health efforts to recognize disparities and targeting resources to affected communities and subpopulations. Although few public health practitioners and data users would refute the value in collecting data by ethnic and racial identifiers, some scholars argue that race should not be a variable in health research and that race as a concept should be deleted from all classification schemes. In his classic article, Terris (1973) advocated for an abandonment of the practices of collecting and analyzing data by racial categories. According to Terris (1973), the concept of race is unscientific, accepts unsubstantiated beliefs of biological distinctness, promotes racial discrimination, and obscures the real causes of racial differences in health outcomes.

Terris' position is supported by Osborne and Feit (1992). According to them, when race is used as a variable in research, there is a tendency to assume that the results obtained are manifestations of differences in biology, whereas the confounding effects of other factors are often not made explicit when the data are interpreted. That is, using race as a variable implies that there is a genetic reason for the observed differences in incidence, prevalence, or severity of health conditions. Although widely shared in our society, the belief that races in human populations differ from each other primarily in terms of genetics is without scientific basis (Cavalli-Sforza, Menozzi, & Piazza, 1994; Gould, 1977; Latter, 1981; Lewontin, 1982; Littlefield, Lieberman & Reynolds, 1982). In fact there is more genetic variation within than between races. Lewontin (1982) contends that the fact that we know what race an individual belongs to tells us more about our society than about his or her genetic makeup. Nonetheless, without saying so, researchers and readers of various material discussing racial differences often conclude that certain racial groups have predispositions, risks or susceptibilities to illnesses, conditions, and diseases being studied. According to Terris (1973) and Osborne and Feit (1992), this presupposition is seldom warranted, and comparisons of racial groups, without providing explanations, may represent a subtle form of discrimination and reinforce stereotypes and could lead to political consequences for these groups, such as quarantining and "blaming the victims."

Osborne and Feit (1992) continued by saying that constant attention to racial and ethnic groups being disproportionately affected by certain diseases often leads to the belief that one of the best efforts to reduce or eliminate the observed differentials is to focus primarily on creating and/or revamping health programs for these groups. By doing this, less attention is given to addressing the virulent societal problems such as economic and social inequalities that predispose to those diseases. For example, factors contributing to the high rate of violence among ethnic and racial groups of youth include poverty, joblessness, and interpersonal problems in ethnic and racial families. Race, in and of itself, should not be considered a causal or risk factor for violence. Thus, as noted by Osborne and Feit (1992), to avoid erroneous conclusions, it is essential that researchers and users of racial identifiers in their analyses clarify terms, state clearly the reasons for examining racial disparities, and make clear that race and ethnicity are not risk factors but are instead *risk markers*. Race as a risk marker means that race represents many underlying problems of greater relevance to health, including SES and cultural and behavioral characteristics that are social and not biological in nature.

This debate for and against the collection and use of data on race and ethnicity recently spilled into the public arena in California, as a movement to restrict (with some exceptions) state and local governments from "classifying" (collecting and using) information on an individual's race, ethnicity, color, or national origin was put before voters as Proposition 54. Although the proposition failed, the debate was heated and intense. Many of the arguments echoed the same themes as the debate among researchers described previously here. For example, supporters of the proposition argued the following:

- Labeling people as to their ancestry and racial background without their knowledge and/or consent is an invasion of privacy.
- Government-imposed racial classifications have been used to divide people by emphasizing minor differences rather than common interests and values. We should stop categorizing citizens and create a color-blind society where we are all just Americans.
- The California Constitution forbids state and local governments from discriminating against or granting preferential treatment based on race; therefore, there is no need to classify people by race, ethnicity, color, or national origin.

Opponents of the proposition countered with the following arguments:

- Preventing the collection, analysis, and use of race-related data will hinder the ability to address disparities by race and ethnicity in public health, education, crime prevention, and civil rights enforcement. It also will prevent the identification and tracking of hate crimes.
- The exceptions leave open questions about the scope of the prohibitions, making numerous legal challenges a certainty.

- America is not close to being a color-blind society. We need to understand our differences in order to deal with them in a positive way.

The controversy surrounding Proposition 54 illustrates the extent to which the concept of race has become thoroughly woven into the cultural and political fabric of the United States. It has become an essential element of both individual identity and government policy. Because so much harm has been based on "racial" distinctions over the years, research and policies aimed at correcting such harm must acknowledge the impact of "racial" consciousness among the US populace, regardless of the fact that race has no scientific justification in human biology.

## Strategies and Approaches for Classifying Race

Depending on the data source, collecting racial and ethnic identifiers presents methodological problems. Issues of misclassification come into play in the calculations of rates of any kind because rates require compatible data for the numerator and denominator. Often, however, the numerator and denominator come from different sources. For example, data for demographic estimates at the national level come from vital statistics collected by individual states, which may use different race and ethnicity categories. Often, census data are used as the principal source of numbers for the denominator, which can lead to systematically poor estimation if the collection procedures used for the numerator do not gather data in the same manner as the census. The case of infant mortality is often cited as an example of inaccuracies that result from inconsistent racial and ethnic reporting. Beginning in 1989, births have been categorized by the race of the mother as recorded on the birth certificate. If the mother does not state her race on the certificate, then the baby's race is imputed to be the race of the father. If neither parent's race is reported on the birth certificate, the baby's race is imputed to be that of the mother on the preceding record with known race. However, racial classification of death, unlike births, is designated by an outside party, usually attending physicians or funeral home directors, on the basis of information provided by relatives or their own observation. The reliance on visual identification or the possibility of inadequate information from relatives has resulted in an overassignment of deaths to black and white categories and an underassignment of deaths to American Indian and Asian/Pacific Islander categories. Hahn and Stroup (1994) noted that before the 1989 change in classifying parents of the same race, almost 10% of American Indian infant deaths were incorrectly classified when both parents were American Indians, and the inconsistent assignment of Asian infant deaths varied from almost 20% for Japanese to almost 40% for Chinese. Changes introduced in 1989 whereby infants were assigned the same race as their mothers have failed to reduce the level of incorrect assignment. As a result the infant mortality rates—even when both parents are Asian or American Indian—are substantially lower than the actual levels.

Hahn and Stroup also noted that the level of inconsistent classification of infant death by race is even greater for children of mixed heritage. The result of this inconsistency is only a slight overestimation of black and white infants' mortality rates, as the numbers of births are so large. For the smaller racial and ethnic groups, however, the underreporting of infant mortality rates will produce inaccurate results and have major ramifications for calculations made by Social Security and private insurance industry actuaries. One suggestion for improving or reducing inconsistencies is to collect more data on ancestral background or to institute the same kinds of requirements for data collection across data systems to allow for consistent racial and ethnic identification.

One of the most troublesome issues in the area of minority health is the imprecise nature of many existing classification systems as well as the varying of the categories, such that it is difficult to collect reliable data or to conduct highly targeted and focused analyses of minority populations. In many classification systems, small populations of diverse minority groups are often clustered together under one category, with only whites and blacks being separated. Given the increasing ethnic diversity, data collection using broad and crude racial categories is inadequate. Using broad categories makes it impossible to recognize important differences within racial groups. Because of limitations in detail, within-group heterogeneity cannot be recognized, and differences within racial groups are masked.

The collection of health information by racial and ethnic categories is an important component of public health surveillance. Sources for this surveillance information regarding the health status of the overall population and racial and ethnic subgroups are state agencies and a myriad of federal agencies, including the CDC, the Bureau of the Census, the Indian Health Service, and the NCHS. Census data systems and those from other federal and nonfederal statistical systems are closely related and interdependent. In fact, this interdependence is demonstrated by the use of census data as the denominators for virtually all birth, mortality, and morbidity rates. In turn, these rates are used to develop the Census Bureau's population estimates and projections (Edmonston, Goldstein, & Lott, 1996). Additionally, federal agencies use census data as the baseline for designing sampling frames for their data collection efforts. For example, birth, death, and immigration data are combined to get estimates of postcensal population counts. Census data are also used to assess the completeness of natality registration and survival rates (Hahn & Stroup, 1994).

Currently, official reports disseminated through federal agencies must adhere to Office of Management and Budget [OMB]), Federal Statistical Policy Directive No. 15: "Race and Ethnic Standards for Federal Agencies and Administrative Reporting," *Federal Register* 43:19269–19270, May 4, 1978. New standards were adopted by OMB in October 1997 and will be implemented by all federal agencies no later than January 1, 2003. The OMB sets the standards for federal statistics and administrative reporting on race and ethnicity. The current directive states that in data collection and reporting

- Race will be based on self-identification by the respondent or someone who may be reporting race in his or her absence through a question that asks for an individual race. There are four groups, including white, black, American Indian/Alaska Native, and Asian/Pacific Islander. The directive's categories allow collection of more detailed information as long as it can be aggregated to the specified four categories.
- Hispanic origin will be based on self-identification by the respondent or someone who may be reporting Hispanic origin in his or her absence through a question that asks for an individual's origin or descent. People of Hispanic origin are those who indicated that their origin was Mexican, Puerto Rican, Cuban, Central or South American, or some other Hispanic origin. People of Hispanic origin may be of any race.
- Non-Hispanic refers to all people whose ethnicity is not Hispanic. Race and ethnicity are separate concepts, and thus, the racial categories of white, black, American Indian/Alaska Native, and Asian/ Pacific Islander all contain some people of Hispanic origin. Thus, the term white non-Hispanic is used to indicate the white population minus that part of this group that is of Hispanic origin.

New to the 2000 census method was the option for respondents to report more than one race category. Although this provides the respondent with a better opportunity to express accurately his or her race and ethnic background, it does hold some problems for analysis and interpretation. For example, when selecting multiple race categories, there is no mechanism for the respondent to indicate the extent to which he or she actually identifies with each of the reported racial categories. Thus, if a respondent selects, for example, black and white race, should that person be included in analyses of whites, blacks, both, or a separate category? These issues are likely to result in inconsistent reporting, as different researchers may use different ways of combining data. It will also require that researchers clearly define how all of the racial groups are defined clearly for each analysis in each report.

Research and data collection activities related to ethnic and racial classification currently do a poor job of differentiating race/ethnicity from SES variables in addressing minority populations. The co-mingling of race/ethnicity and SES has important ramifications for understanding and improving the health of minority groups. Race may be a confounding factor that can operate in concert with other factors that are rarely used to measure SES. Because low SES and poverty have been associated with poor health, and minorities are disproportionately represented in low SES groups, then low SES and race have often been used synonymously in the research literature. The inability to sort out the differential impact of these two variables obscures the ability to understand how to intervene and to develop appropriate mechanisms to measure and monitor the effectiveness of interventions, especially in minority populations. Some people have called for a decreased emphasis on race with a corresponding increase in attention to SES. However, such an action is inappropriate for several reasons. First, the widely used SES indicators are not equivalent across races (LaViest, 1992; Williams, 1992). The standard measures of SES are income, education, and occupational status or some combination of the three. These concepts may be misused or misleading when applied to minority populations, and there is a need to identify and use more accurate indicators of SES for racial/ethnic groups. David Williams (1992; Williams & Neighbors, 2001), a sociologist who devotes a great deal of time and attention to this issue of SES and ethnic/racial groups, suggested that African Americans, even though they might have a certain income, might have higher costs in terms of being charged more for food, housing, and other services such as insurance. In addition, middle-class African Americans are often involved in the provision of material support for poorer family members, and a similar pattern exists for other minority groups. Thus, when income status is determined, attention must be given to the extent to which nonhousehold residents are supported by a given household income. Furthermore, the fact that middle-class African Americans are more likely to be the first generation in that status suggests that a disproportionate share of the African American middle class experienced poorer living conditions in childhood.

SES is not stable or constant during the life course, and a measure of current SES does not capture lifetime exposure to deprived living conditions. Krieger, Rowly, Herman, Avery, and Phillips (1993) in their article "Racism, Sexism and Social Class: Implications for Studies of Health and Disease and Well-being" pointed out that we know that black women are twice as likely as white women to experience the loss of their babies before they reach the age of 1 year. To explain this finding, researchers have invoked two well-known facts. First, infant mortality is higher among poor and less well-educated women, and second, black women in the United States have persistently higher levels of poverty than white women. However, on closer inspection of the data, we observe that black women have problematic birth outcomes regardless of their SES. They fare worse than white women at every economic level, and the disadvantage persists even among the most highly educated black women. Thus, a major issue is how socioeconomic status is defined and operationalized. Some people such as Williams (1992) have recommended using a variety of measures, including assets, and measuring SES over time.

Another major challenge to increasing our knowledge and understanding of differentials in health status is the use of culturally insensitive approaches and the development of culturally appropriate instruments for obtaining data from various ethnic and racial groups. A large number of research projects and data collection efforts are being conducted without attention to cultural factors of the minorities and/or racial groups being studied. That is, there is no information collected on ancestral backgrounds, their group-specific attitudes, perceptions, expectations, norms, and values or linguistic preferences. One of the critical issues in national surveys is whether the questions are clearly understood by respondents. Often the survey questions and measurement instruments are not "formed" on minority/racial populations, and there are issues of whether the language of the questions and scales used to measure health events are measuring the same phenomena across all populations. For example, researchers have found marked differences in the way African Americans respond to the words "hypertension" and "high blood pressure" (CDC, 1993a). These two terms have significantly different connotations. It is also clear that there may be significant translation problems in questions intended for the English-speaking/white population. For use with groups having a different culture, it is important that questions that are relevant to health on national surveys be designed specifically to fit the unique lifestyles, histories, and cultures of specific racial and ethnic groups, including mixed heritage or peculiar life experiences. Comparable questions that are theoretically and racially relevant need to be formulated for different racial and ethnic groups to assure that equivalent phenomena are really being measured. Culturally sensitive instruments would also recognize the use of alternative health systems and the extent of identification with one's ethnic and racial heritage, norms, values, and beliefs.

# IMPLICATIONS FOR MCH POLICY, PRACTICE, RESEARCH, AND TRAINING

Current efforts to address and ultimately eliminate health disparities focus on changing individual behaviors, on increasing access to care, and on improving the quality and equality of care received by vulnerable populations. In MCH, we rely almost totally on attendance at prenatal or pediatric health visits to provide women and children with (or link them to) the range of health, education, and medical services in our arsenal. However, given the complex interactions among the multiple factors affecting health disparities, a focus on changing individual and health provider behaviors is a necessary but insufficient strategy to close the health gap. Eliminating health inequities will require a national resolve to redress existent social inequities, requiring intervention at the national, state, community, as well as individual levels. That is, policies, institutions, the environment, and social networks, along with health care and individual behavior, should be simultaneously considered as targets for intervention in strategies to eliminate disparities (Anderson, Fullilove, Fielding, & Task Force on Community Preventive Services, 2003; Hogan, Richardson, Ferre, Durant, & Boisseau, 2001; Hogan, Njoroge, Durant, & Ferre, 2001; Jenkins, 2001; Kington & Nickens, 2001; Office of Behavioral and Social Sciences Research, 2001; Williams, 2001).

## Policy

The initiation of the *Healthy People* health goals and their link to state reporting requirements stimulated efforts in most states to address health disparities. This demonstrates the impact that a statement of national will can have on moving policy progressively forward. Additionally, policy changes can be stimulated by cohesive community advocacy and action. To increase the likelihood of further policy developments in support of elimination of MCH disparities, the following recommendations are presented:

- Ensure that individuals in MCH policy-making positions understand the complexities of health disparity causality and recognize the contribution of social inequities.
- Increase numbers of public health professionals who are trained in health disparity science.
- Actively increase the knowledge base and support the power of communities to articulate and advocate for their needs.

## Practice

Health and medical institutions are the primary contact point linking populations to health resources and, along with government agencies, private research institutes and universities, are the primary institutions for generating new knowledge and implementing solutions to address health disparities. To increase the impact on health disparities, health and medical institutions need to

- Improve quality of care, including providing culturally and socially appropriate care by eliminating unequal treatment.
- Improve access to care, including increased insurance coverage for preventive and palliative care.
- Re-examine process of care delivery. A life course perspective can stimulate new systems and processes for delivering preventive services and education. For example, we can reassess the timing of delivery of care designed to impact perinatal outcomes given that the etiologic development of many adverse perinatal outcomes begins before pregnancy.
- Create institutional change. Although social inequities need to be addressed to achieve progress in disparity elimination, public health and medical institutions cannot create this change alone. Establishing

new institutional relationships, sharing data and research findings, and development of interdisciplinary teams can increase the involvement and effectiveness of others outside of the allied health field in addressing social inequities associated with adverse health. Public health and medical institutions can also play a role in assessing their own structures, history, and processes. For example, racism is such an insidious force, it is sometimes invisible to all but those who are victimized by it. Health care and public health institutions can assess the extent that racism operates within their own systems and make concerted efforts to undo racism where it exists.

## Research

Research frameworks, methods, and analytic tools must continually develop to reflect the complexity and context of the problems being studied. The predominant reductionist public health paradigm, although adequate for understanding many diseases, may be inadequate for understanding diseases that have more complex social correlates and may be inadequate for explaining health inequities. New paradigms may introduce more relevant frameworks, methods, and analytic tools that help to uncover the currently unknown aspects of the context of life that affects the health of vulnerable populations.

Hogue (2002) proposed applying public health's "agent/host/environment" paradigm to guide research and action to eliminate health disparities. This paradigm is useful as a theoretical framework that can model root causes, the affected individual and the social context, within classic epidemiologic analytic models. Kaplan (2004), Krieger (1999), and Savitz and Miller (1999) proposed expanding the tools used both within epidemiology and in addition to epidemiology in order to understand better the complexities of social factors and health and to bridge the gap between biologic and social processes.

Anderson et al. (2000) and the Office of Behavioral and Social Sciences Research (2001) suggested multilevel and interdisciplinary research and the development of analytic tools to conduct this type of research. Multilevel research allows simultaneous assessment of social and biologic factors, at both the individual and community levels of analysis. Raster density modeling is also being developed as a tool to model complex interactions in perinatal health using geocoding and sophisticated statistical techniques (Culhane, Rauh, McCollum, Elo, & Hogan, 2002).

Rowley et al. (1993) proposed using community-partnered approaches and qualitative research as tools within a constructivist paradigm. These tools are more likely to uncover contextual meaning behind observed phenomena and the "causes of causes" that underlie the phenomena we are limited to observe using existing data and existing knowledge. This nuanced understanding can be used to improve the specification of explanatory models in traditional quantitative studies. A constructivist paradigm guides the generation of new knowledge by gathering and synthesizing multiple perspectives rather than limiting observations to the perspective of the dominant group. It is posited that the combined view of multiple perspectives and experiences more closely approximates "truth" than does the perspective of the researcher alone. Finally, community-partnered participatory research is suggested as a framework and a tool to increase the relevance and the quality of conceptualization and interpretation of research. Community-partnered research is used as a means of breaking down traditional power barriers between researcher and subject to allow the fluid entrance and acceptance of multiple perspectives into the research process.

Kington and Nickens (2001) suggested specific topics for research, ranging from research to understand the pathways from acculturation, through the adoption of specific health behaviors, that is, research that bridges biologic and social factors, to population-based intervention studies that assess the effectiveness of changing social relationships on health. Williams (2001) suggested more focused research on measurement of social position and its impact on health. All of these recommendations can be appropriately applied to MCH research.

## Training

In order to change policy and conduct the relevant research to understand health disparities, we must first improve the knowledge base within public health, medicine, and society as a whole with respect to what causes and how we could eliminate health inequities. With their concern for the health and well-being of mothers and children, MCH training programs are well positioned to prepare individuals to play a unique role in research, service, and teaching about health disparities among MCH populations. Given this unique role, the following recommendations are offered for strengthening the information pertaining to improving the health status and health outcomes of these groups and for eliminating the inequitable health divide.

1. Curricula in MCH programs should be expanded to include courses on health disparity and on the expanded array of the tools and methods that support the development of health disparity science.
2. Opportunities should be made available to MCH students, practitioners, and faculty to understand better and have direct exposure to the rapidly changing communities in which they will work, to understand better the culturally determined perceptions of disease and the cultural, social, institutional barriers to adherence to prevention and treatment programs.
3. MCH professionals should be trained to create and validate more culturally sensitive instruments and tools for data collection.
4. MCH programs should expand the pool of minority researchers and the pool of researchers trained in paradigms, methods, and tools relevant to health disparity research. Currently, the number of minority researchers involved in the collection and analyzing data is far too few. Minority students must be encouraged, with the provision of financial support, to pursue their doctorates and become engaged in innovative, important research related to the inequities in health of racial and ethnic minority women and children.

## CONCLUSION

The science of health disparities is still in its relative infancy. Although there is much to be known about health inequities, particularly what contributes to them and how to eliminate them in MCH, there is still much that can be done with what we currently know. Action in the policy, research, and service arenas can do much to advance the state of the science, teaching, and practice.

## REFERENCES

Anderson, L., Fullilove, M., Scrimshaw, S., Fielding, J., Normand, J., Zaza, S., Wright-Deaguero, L., & Higgins, D. (2000). A framework for evidence-based reviews of interventions for supportive social environments. *Annals of the NY Academy of Sciences, 896,* 487–488.

Anderson, L.M., Fullilove, S.S., Fielding, M.T., & Task Force on Community Preventive Services. (2003). The community guide's model for linking the social environment to health. *American Journal of Preventive Medicine, 24*(3 Suppl.), 12–20.

Arias, E., Anderson, R.N., Kung, H.-C., Murphy, S.L., Kenneth D., & Kochanek, K.D. (2003, September 18). Deaths: Final data for 2001. *National Vital Statistics Reports, 52*(3).

Armstrong, T.D., Crum L., Rieger R.H., Bennett T.A., & Edwards, L.J. (1999). Attitudes of African-Americans toward participation in medical research. *Journal of Applied Social Psychology, 29,* 552–574.

Bassuk, E.L., Weinreb, L.F., Buckner, J.C., Browne, A., Salomon, A., & Bassuk, S.S. (1996). The characteristics and needs of sheltered homeless and low-income housed mothers. *Journal of the American Medical Association, 276*(8): 640–646.

Bennett, T. (1993, September). *American Indians in California: Health status and access to health.* San Francisco: Monograph Series, Institute for Health Policy Studies, University of California.

Cavalli-Sforza, L.L., Menozzi, P., & Piazza, A. (1994). *The history and geography of human genes.* Princeton, NJ: Princeton University Press.

Centers for Disease Control and Prevention. (1991). Consensus set of health status indicators for the general assessment of community health status: US. *Morbidity Mortality Weekly Report, 40,* 449–451.

Centers for Disease Control and Prevention. (1993a). AIDS among racial/ethnic minorities: US. *Morbidity Mortality Weekly Report, 43,* 644–647, 653–655.

Centers for Disease Control and Prevention. (1993b). Tuberculosis morbidity: US, 1992. *Morbidity Mortality Weekly Report, 42,* 696–704.

Centers for Disease Control and Prevention. (1998, November 10). "Deaths: Final Data 1996," *National Vital Statistics Report, 47*(9), 25.

Centers for Disease Control and Prevention. (2001b). *HIV/AIDS Surveillance Report, 13*(2).

Centers for Disease Control and Prevention. (2002). *HIV/AIDS Surveillance Report, 14,* 1–40.

Centers for Disease Control and Prevention. (2003, September 15). Infant Mortality Statistics from the 2001 Period Linked Birth/Infant Death Data Set. National Vital Statistics Report, *52*(2).

Clark, R., Anderson, N.B., Clark, V.R., & Williams, D.R. (1999). Racism as a stressor for African Americans: A biopsychosocial model. *American Psychologist, 54,* 805–816.

Culhane, J.F., Rauh, V., McCollum, K.F., Hogan, V., Agnew, K., & Wadhwa, P.D. (2001). Maternal stress is associated with bacterial vaginosis in human pregnancy. *Maternal and Child Health Journal, 5,* 127–134.

Culhane, J.F., Rauh, V., McCollum, K.F., Elo, I.T., & Hogan, V. (2002). Exposure to chronic stress and ethnic differences in rates of bacterial vaginosis among pregnant women. *American Journal of Obstetrics & Gynecology, 187,* 1272–1276.

DeNavas-Walt, C., Proctor, B.D., & Mills, R.J. (2004). US Census Bureau, current population reports, P60-226. *Income, poverty, and health insurance coverage in the United States: 2003.* Washington, DC: US Government Printing Office.

DuBois, W.E.B., Anderson, E., & Eaton, I. (1899). *The Philadelphia Negro: A social study.* New York: Lippencott.

Edmonston, B., Goldstein, J., & Lott, T. (1996). *Spotlight on heterogeneity: The Federal standards for racial and ethnic classification.* Washington, DC: National Academy Press.

England, L., Martin, J., & Hogan, V. (1999). Incidence of preterm birth among singletons: United States 1989–1996. *Morbidity and Mortality Weekly Report, 48*(9), 185–189. Centers for Disease Control and Prevention, Atlanta, GA.

Federal Interagency Forum on Child and Family Statistics. (2004). *America's children in brief: Key national indicators of well-being, 2004.* Available from: http://childstats.gov [cited] Jan. 6, 2005.

Ford, K., & Norris, A.E. (1993). Knowledge of AIDS transmission, risk behavior and perceptions of risk among urban, low-income, African-American and Hispanic youth. *American Journal of Preventive Medicine, 915,* 297–306.

Foster, H.W., Wu, L., Bracken, M.B., Semenya, K., & Thomas, J. (2000). Intergenerational effects of high socioeconomic status on low birthweight and preterm birth in African Americans. *Journal of the National Medical Association, 92,* 213–221.

Geronimus, A.T., Bound, J., Waidmann, T.A., Hillemeier, M.M., & Burns, P.B. (1996). Excess mortality among blacks and whites in the United States. *New England Journal of Medicine, 335,* 1552–1558.

Gould, S.J. (1977). Why we should not name human races: A biological view. In S.J. Gould (Ed.), *Ever since Darwin* (pp. 231–236). New York: Norton.

Greene, J.M., Ringwalt, C.L., Kelly, J.E., Iachan, R., & Cohen, Z. (1995). *Youth with runaway, throwaway, and homeless experiences: Prevalence, drug use, and other at-risk behaviors* (Vols. I and II, final report under Contract No. 105-90-1703 from the Administration on Children, Youth, and Families). Research Triangle Park, NC: Research Triangle Institute.

Hahn, R. (1995). Children's health: Racial and ethnic differences in the use of prescription medication. *Pediatrics, 95,* 727–732.

Hahn, R., & Stroup, D. (1994). Race and ethnicity in public health: Surveillance criteria for the scientific use of social categories. *CDC-Agency for Toxic Substances Disease Registry (ATSDR) Workshop, 109,* 11–15.

Hertzman, C. (1999). The biological embedding of early experience and its effects on health in adulthood. *Annals of the New York Academy of Sciences, 896,* 85–95.

Hogan, V.K., Njoroge, T., Durant, T.M., & Ferre, C.D. (2001). Eliminating disparities in perinatal outcomes: Lessons learned. *Maternal and Child Health Journal, 5*(2), 135–140.

Hogan, V.K., Richardson, J.L., Ferre, C.D., Durant, T., & Boisseau, M. (2001). A public health framework for black addressing and white disparities in preterm delivery. *Journal of the American Medical Women's Association, 56*(4), 177–180.

Hogue, C. (2002). Toward a systematic approach to understanding and ultimately eliminating African American women's health disparities. *Women's Health Issues, 12,* 222–237.

Institute of Medicine. (2003). Unequal treatment: Confronting racial and ethnic disparities in healthcare. Washington, DC: National Academy Press.

Iyasu, S., Becerra, J.E., Rowley, D.L., & Hogue, C.J. (1992). Impact of very low birthweight on the black-white infant gap. *American Journal of Preventive Medicine, 8,* 271–277.

Jackson, F.M., Phillips, M.T., Hogue, C.J.R., & Curry-Owens, T.Y. (2001). Examining the burdens of gendered racism: Implications for pregnancy outcomes among college-educated African American women. *Maternal & Child Health Journal, 5,* 95–107.

Jenkins, R. (2001). The health of minority children in the year 2000: The role of government programs in improving the health status of America's children. In W.W. Smelser, W.J. Wilson, & F. Mitchell (Eds.), *America Becoming: Racial trends and their consequences.* Washington, DC: National Academy Press; pp. 351–370.

Johnston, L.D., O'Malley, P.M., Bachman, J.G., & Schulenberg, J.E. (2003). *Monitoring the Future: National survey results on drug use, 1975-2003: Volume I, Secondary school students* (NIH Publication No. 04-5507). Bethesda, MD: National Institute on Drug Abuse.

Jones, C.P. (2000). Levels of racism: A theoretic framework and a gardener's tale. *American Journal of Public Health, 90,* 1212–1215.

Kaplan, G. (2004). What's wrong with social epidemiology, and how can we make it better? *Epidemiology Review, 26,* 124–135.

Kington, R., & Nickens, H. (2001). Racial and ethnic differences in health. In N.J. Smelser, W.J. Wilson, & F. Mitchell (Eds.), *America Becoming: Racial trends and their consequences* (pp. 235–310). Washington, DC: National Academy Press.

Kirstein, R. (2000). US Department of Health and Human Services Agencies, transcripts on disparities: Testimony before Senate and House Committees. Available January, 2005, from: http://www.hhs.gov/asl/testify.

Klein, J., & Hawk, S. (1992). *Statistical notes, health status indicators, definitions and national data* (Vol. 1, No. 3). Hyattsville, MD: US Public Health Service, National Center for Health Statistics.

Kline, A., Kline, E., & Oken, E. (1992). Minority women and sexual choice in the age of AIDS. *Social Science and Medicine, 34,* 447–457.

Klonoff, E.A., & Landrine, H. (2000). Is skin color a marker for racial discrimination? Explaining the skin color-hypertension relationship. *Journal of Behavioral Medicine, 23,* 329–338.

Krieger, N. (1999). Questioning epidemiology: Objectivity, advocacy, and socially responsible science. *American Journal of Public Health, 89,*1151–1153.

Krieger, N. (2000). Refiguring "race": Epidemiology, racialized biology, and biological expressions of race relations. *International Journal of Health Services, 30,* 211–216.

Krieger, N., Rowley, D.L., Herman, A.A., Avery, B., & Phillips, M.T. (1993). Racism, sexism, and social class: Implications for studies of health, disease, and well-being. *American Journal of Preventive Medicine, 9*(suppl.), 82–122.

Latter, D.H. (1981). Genetic differences within and between populations of the major human subgroups. *American Naturalist, 116,* 220–237.

LaViest, T. (1992). Segregation, poverty, and empowerment: Health consequences for African-Americans: Mapping a new territory. *American Journal of Sociology, 94,* 1080–1095.

LaVeist, T., Keith, V., & Gutierrez, M. (1993). Black/white differences in prenatal care utilization: An assessment of predisposing and enabling factors. *Health Services Research, 30,* 43–58.

Lewontin, R. (1982). Human diversity. In H. Nelson & R. Jarman (Eds.), *Introduction to physical anthropology.* St. Paul, MN: West Publishing.

Link, B.G., Susser, E., Stueve, A., Phelan, J., Moore, R.E., & Struening, E. (1994). Lifetime and five-year prevalence of homelessness in the United States. *American Journal of Public Health, 84,* 1907–1912.

Littlefield, A., Lieberman, L., & Reynolds L. (1982). Redefining race: The potential demise of a concept in physical anthropology. *Current Anthropology, 23,* 641–655.

Mann, J.M., Tarantola, D.J., & Netter, T.W. (Eds.). (1992). *AIDS in the world.* Cambridge, MA: Harvard University Press.

Mayberry, R.M., Mili, F., & Ofili, E. (2000). Racial and ethnic differences in access to medical care. *Medical Care Research and Review, 57*(suppl. 1), 108–145.

McEwen, B.S., & Seeman, T. (1999). Protective and damaging effects of mediators of stress. Elaborating and testing the concepts of allostasis and allostatic load. *Annals of the New York Academy of Sciences, 896,* 30–47.

Meriam, L. (1928). *The problem of Indian administration* (pp. 3–4). Washington, DC: Brookings Institution, Institute for Government Research.

Mirvis, D., Burns, R., Gaschen, L., Cloar, F., & Graney, M. (1994). Variation in utilization of cardiac procedures in the Department of Veterans Affairs health care system: Effect of race. *Journal of the American College of Cardiology, 24,* 1297–1304.

Moran, J.S., Aral, S.O., Jenkins, W.C., Petersen, T.A., & Alexander, E.R. (1989). The impact of sexually transmitted diseases on minority populations. *Public Health Reports, 104,* 560–565.

Moreland, K., Wing, S., Diez-Roux, A., & Poole, G. (2002). Neighborhood characteristics associated with the location of food stores and food service places. *American Journal of Preventive Medicine, 22,* 23–29.

Morrison, R.S., Wallenstein, S., Natale, D.K., Senzel, R.S., & Huang, L.-L. (2000). "We don't carry that": Failure of pharmacies in predominately non-white neighborhoods to stock opioid analgesics. *New England Journal of Medicine, 342,* 1023–1026.

Mullings, L., Wali, A., McLean, D., Mitchell, J., Prince, S., Thomas, D., & Tovar, P. (2001). Qualitative methodologies and community participation in examining reproductive experiences: The Harlem Birth Right Project. *Maternal & Child Health Journal, 5,* 85–93.

National Center for Health Statistics. (1983). *Health, United States, 1983.* Hyattsville, MD: US Dept of Health and Human Services, Public Health Service. (p. 256).

National Center for Health Statistics. (1991). *Healthy People 2000 Review, 1991.* Hyattsville, MD: US Public Health Service.

National Center for Health Statistics. (1993). *Healthy People 2000 Review, 1992.* Hyattsville, MD: US Public Health Service.

National Center for Health Statistics. (2004). *Health, United States, 2004. Chartbook on Trends in the Health of Americans.* Hyattsville, Maryland: US Government Printing Office.

National Coalition for the Homeless. (2004). *Who is Homeless?* Fact Sheet #3. Available from: http://www.nationalhomeless.org/who.html [cited] Jan. 6, 2005.

Nersessian, W. (1988). Infant mortality in socially vulnerable populations. *Annual Review of Public Health, 9,* 361–377.

Office of Behavioral and Social Sciences Research. (2001). *Strategic Plan for Health Disparities Research, FY 2002–2006.* Washington, DC: National Institutes of Health.

Osborne, N.G., & Feit, M.D. (1992). The use of race in medical research. *Journal of the American Medical Association, 672,* 275–279.

Parker, W.D., Hogan, V., Chavez, G., Ferre, C.D., Taylor, D., Martin, J., & England, L. (2000). State specific changes in singleton preterm births among black and white women in the United States 1991 and 1997. *Morbidity Mortality Weekly Report, 49,* 837–840.

Perrow, C., & Guillen, M.F. (1990). *The AIDS disaster.* New Haven, CT: Yale University Press.

Pizzi, M. (1992). HIV infection and AIDS: Tapestries of life, death, and empowerment. *American Journal of Occupational Therapy, 46,* 1021–1027.

Reidpath, D.D., & Allotey, P. (2003). Infant mortality rate as an indicator of population health. *Journal of Epidemiology and Community Health, 57,* 344–346.

Roberts, A.C., Wechsberg, W.M., Zule, W.A., & Burroughs, A.R. (2003). Contextual factors and other correlates of sexual risk of HIV among African-American crack-abusing women. *Addictive Behaviors,* Vol. 28, No. 3, pp. 523–536.

Rosenheck, R.A., Leda, C., Frisman, L.K., Lam, J., & Chung, A. (1996). Homeless veterans. In J. Baumohl (Ed.), *Homelessness in America: A reference book.* Phoenix, AZ: Oryx Press.

Rowley, D.L., Hogue, C.J., Blackmore, C.A., Ferre, C.D., Hatfield-Timajchy, K., Branch, P., & Atrash, H.K. (1993). Preterm delivery among African-American women: A research strategy. *American Journal of Preventive Medicine, 9*(6 Suppl.), 1–6.

Sandefur, G.M., Eggerling-Boeck, J., Mannon, S.E., & Meier, A.M. (2001). An overview of racial and ethnic demographic trends. In W.W. Smelser, W.J. Wilson, & F. Mitchell (Eds.), *America Becoming: Racial trends and their consequences.* Washington, DC: National Academies Press. (pp. 40–102).

Satcher, D. (2000, May 11). *Testimony . . . before the House Commerce Committee, Subcommittee on Health and Environment.* Available from: http://www.os.dhhs.gov/asl/testify/t000511a.html [cited] September 30, 2004.

Savitz, D.P., & Miller, W.C. (1999). Reassessing the role of epidemiology in public health. *American Journal of Public Health, 89,* 1158–1161.

Schulman, K.A., Berlin J.A., Harless, W., Kerner, J.F., Sistrunk, S., Gersh, B.J., Dubé, R., Taleghani, C.K., Burke, J.E., Williams, S., Eisenberg, J.M., Escarce, J.J., & Ayers, W. (1999). The effect of race and sex on physicians' recommendations for cardiac catheterization. *New England Journal of Medicine, 340,* 618–626.

Singh, G., & Yu, S. (1994). *Trends and projections of infant, childhood, adolescent and young adulthood, and maternal mortality by sex, race and ethnicity, education, family income and cause of death, US.* Paper commissioned by the Maternal and Child Health Bureau, Health Resources and Services Administration, USDHHS, for the Fourth National Title V Maternal and Child Health Research Priorities Conference June 24–29.

Singh, G., & Yu, S. (1996a). Childhood mortality 1950 through 1993: Trends and socioeconomic differentials. *American Journal of Public Health, 86,* 505–512.

Singh, G., & Yu, S. (1996b). Adverse pregnancy outcomes: Differences between US- and foreign-born women in major US racial and ethnic groups. *American Journal of Public Health, 86,* 837–843.

Singh, G., Kposawa, B., & Augustine, J. (1994). Comparative analysis of infant mortality in major Ohio cities: Significance of non-biological factors. *Applied Behavioral Science Review, 2,* 63–80.

Sorlie, P., Rogot, E., & Johnson, N. (1992). Validity of demographic characteristics on the death certificate. *Epidemiology, 3,* 181–184.

Tarlov, A. (1999). Public policy frameworks for improving population health. *Annals of the New York Academy of Sciences, 896,* 281–293.

Terris, M. (1973). Desegregating health statistics. *American Journal of Public Health, 63,* 477–480.

Urban Institute, The. (1999, 9 December). *Homelessness: Programs and the people they serve/findings of the national survey of homeless assistance providers and clients.* Available from: http://www.urban.org/UploadedPDF/homelessness.pdf [cited] Jan. 6, 2005.

Urban Institute, The. (2000, February 1). *A new look at homelessness in America.* Available from: http://www.urban.org/url.cfm?ID=900366 [cited] Jan. 6, 2005.

US Conference of Mayors. (2003). *A status report on hunger and homelessness in America's cities.* Washington, DC: Author.

US Department of Commerce, Bureau of the Census. (1990). *Decennial census of population and housing: Public use microdata sample.* Washington, DC: Author.

US Department of Commerce, Bureau of the Census. (1992). Population projections of the US by age, sex, and race, 1992–2050. *Current Population Reports* (Series P25, No. 1092b). Washington, DC: US Government Printing Office.

US Department of Commerce, Bureau of the Census. (2000). *Population profile of the United States: 2000.* Washington, DC: US Census Bureau. (Chapters 1–17).

US Department of Health and Human Services. (1985). *Report of the secretary's task force on black and minority health.* Washington, DC: US Government Printing Office.

US Department of Health and Human Services. (1991). *Healthy people 2000: National health promotion and disease prevention objectives.* Washington, DC: US Public Health Service.

US Department of Health and Human Services. (1992). *Improving minority health statistics: Report of the public health statistics task force on minority health data.* Washington, DC: US Government Printing Office.

US Department of Health and Human Services. (2000, November). *Healthy people 2010* (2nd ed.). With understanding and improving health and objectives for improving health. Washington, DC: US Government Printing Office.

Van Ryn, M., & Burke, J. (2000). The effect of patient race on socio-economic status on physicians' perceptions of patients. *Social Science and Medicine, 50,* 813–828.

Ventura, S.J., Abma, J.C., Mosher, W.D., & Henshaw, S. (2003). Revised pregnancy rates, 1990-97, and new rates for 1998-99: United States. *National Vital Statistics Reports, 52.* Hyattsville, MD: National Center for Health Statistics.

Wechsberg, W.M. (1998). Facilitating empowerment for women substance abusers at risk for HIV. *Pharmacology Biochemistry and Behavior, 61,* 158.

Wechsberg, W.M., Zule, W.A., Lam, W.K., & Bobashev, G. (2004). Facilitating empowerment for African-American women who use crack cocaine: Efficacy of a woman-focused, culturally specific intervention to reduce risk for HIV and increase self-sufficiency. *American Journal of Public Health, 94,* 1165–1173.

Weddington, W.H., & Gabel, L.L. (1991). Racial differences in physicians and patients in relationship to quality of care. *Journal of the National Medical Association, 83,* 569–572.

Weeks, M.R., Schensill, J.J., Williams, S.S., Singer, M., & Grier, M. (1995). AIDS prevention for African-American and Latino women: Building culturally and gender-appropriate intervention. *AIDS Education and Prevention, 7,* 251–263.

Williams, D. (1992). *The concept of race in health services research: 1966–1990.* Presented at the Annual Meeting of the Association for Health Services Research, Chicago, IL.

Williams, D. (2001). Racial variations in adult health: Patterns paradoxes and prospects. In N.J. Smelser, W.J. Wilson, & F. Mitchell (Eds.), *America becoming: Racial trends and their consequences.* Washington, DC: National Academy Press (pp. 371–410).

Williams, D.R., & Rucker, T.D. (2000). Understanding and addressing racial disparities in health care. *Health Care Financing Review, 21,* 75–90.

Williams, D.R., & Neighbors, H.W. (2001). Neighbors, racism, discrimination and hypertension: Evidence and needed research. *Ethnicity and Disease 11,* 800–816.

Women's Health USA (2003a). Maternal and Child Health Bureau. Health Resources and Services Administration. Available February, 2005, from: www.mchb.hrsa.gov/pages/page_25.htm.

Women's Health USA (2003b). Maternal and Child Health Bureau. Health Resources and Services Administration. Available February, 2005, from: www.mchb.hrsa.gov/pages/page_26.htm.

# 10

# Women's Health:
# A Life Cycle

*B. Cecilia Zapata, Anjel Vahratian, and Trude Bennett*

> *We must recognize that, in some large measure, problems with infant ill health are a legacy of women's ill health generally. Cross-disciplinary investigations that can examine the interactions between the general health of women and childbearing are needed urgently.* (Wise, 1993, p. 14)

## INTRODUCTION

Why is there a chapter on women's health in a textbook on maternal and child health (MCH)? This is for a number of reasons. Some MCH practitioners in recent years have been pressing for inclusion in the field of general women's health issues. MCH advocates who approach the field from the maternal perspective seek assurance that broad women's health concerns will be promoted in public health. They note that gender discrimination and inequities may cause women's health to fall through the cracks of other disciplines and research arenas, whether they be specific to populations, diseases, or methods. A logical inclusion to the MCH mission may be health promotion and disease prevention, as well as early diagnosis and treatment, for women throughout the life cycle.

Proponents of a more traditional definition are concerned that the special needs of pregnant women may receive too little emphasis if MCH is defined too broadly. However, recognition of the need for a comprehensive reproductive health framework has been spreading from international to domestic MCH. Maternal outcomes are clearly influenced by a complex web of socioeconomic and environmental influences that precede a woman's pregnancy, perhaps by generations. Chronic illness and underlying health status, including psychologic health, are important elements in the creation or exacerbation of pregnancy-related risks. Exclusion of prepregnancy and nonobstetric factors restricts our understanding of maternal health unnecessarily.

In most women's lives, the period of *childbearing* is much shorter than the duration of *childrearing*. Nevertheless, maternal outcomes are usually measured only by immediate pregnancy consequences. The mental and physical stresses and benefits of the childrearing years are seldom considered as part of maternal health. Furthermore, a growing proportion of US women is delaying childbearing or is choosing not to have children. Over the past 30 years, the mean age at first birth in the United States has increased 3.5 years, from 21.4 years in 1970 to 24.9 years in 2000 (Matthews & Hamilton, 2002). In an analysis of national survey data, Abma, Chandra, Mosher, Peterson, and Piccinino (1997) reported that among the 5.4 million women in the United States who had no children and expected none in the future, 4.1 million women chose not to have children voluntarily. Infertility is a medical problem among US couples as well, as one in six couples experience infertility (Barad & Witt, 2000).

Thus, many more "woman-years" than previously are spent today outside the reproductive domain, and many women never enter the realm of maternity care. Because the United States lacks a universal system of health care, maternity services provide entry for many women into primary care that they might otherwise lack. Women's health concerns in MCH include continuity of care and access to services before, during, after, and independent of childbearing. It seems unreasonable to expect women to invest their trust in a health care system that expresses concern about them only during pregnancy.

An important insight from the international health field has been the critical role of the status of women in determining MCH outcomes. The same situation prevails in the United States. If women are not socially valued, they are likely to face limitations in reproductive decision making and hazards to their general and reproductive health status. Unless women command respect and equity in their roles as daughters, students, wives and partners, and workers, they are not likely to experience the physical and mental health advantages predictive of optimal child health. Some observers view the inclusion of women's health in MCH as yet another attempt to confine women to the maternal definition and role; nevertheless, no one can deny that any improvements in the overall determinants of women's health will benefit their offspring. The opposite, however, is not necessarily the case:

> In discussions of MCH it is commonly assumed that whatever is good for the child is good for the mother. However, not only are the causes of maternal death quite different from those of child death but so are the potential remedies. (Rosenfield & Maine, 1985, p. 83)

Examples exist of developing countries that have experienced impressive improvements in infant mortality while maternal mortality remains tragically high (Table 10–1). This situation has caused commentators to ask, "Where is the M in MCH?" (Rosenfield & Maine, 1985) and to demand a sharper focus on questions of maternal mortality and morbidity. In the United States, the lack of emphasis on the M in MCH is reflected in our poor understanding of the marked differentials in maternal and infant health outcomes according to mothers' socioeconomic status, race, ethnicity, and geographic location. Both women and children would be better served by identifying all of the women's health factors that potentially contribute to pregnancy outcomes.

**Table 10–1** A Woman's Lifetime Chances of Dying Because of Pregnancy/Child Birth-Related Complications Are One in

| | |
|---|---|
| • 11,904 in Spain | • 889 in Russia |
| • 10,417 in Switzerland | • 526 in China |
| • 8,772 in Canada | • 370 in Argentina |
| • 8,333 in Norway | • 303 in Mexico |
| • 6,803 in Sweden | • 159 in Egypt |
| • 6,410 in Italy | • 109 in South Africa |
| • 6,173 in the United Kingdom | • 94 in Philippines |
| • 5,848 in Australia | • 49 in India |
| • 5,102 in Israel | • 37 in Zimbabwe |
| • 3,968 in the United States | • 12 in Mali |
| • 3,922 in France | • 10 in Yemen |
| • 3,704 in Japan | • 9 in Sierra Leone |
| • 3,497 in Germany | |

Source: Neft and Levine (1997).

A more holistic approach to maternal health requires much closer investigation of nonobstetric conditions. In a study of all of the deaths to women ages 15 to 44 years in Boston between 1980 and 1989, Katz, Holmes, Power, and Wise (1995) found that only 7 of the 1,234 total deaths were attributable to causes related to childbearing. These researchers concluded that neglect of the comprehensive health needs of women of reproductive age results in many preventable deaths.

> This study challenges the current view that the health needs of young women should be defined principally in relation to childbearing and instead highlights the concept that these needs transcend reproductive care. (Katz et al., 1995, p. 1138)

A final argument for including women's health in MCH is the importance of considering pregnancy and childbearing as potential risk factors for women's health in later life. This reversal of the usual paradigm creates opportunities for exploring poorly understood aspects of women's health, life expectancy, and quality of life. Beral (1985) and Green, Beral, and Moser (1988) have found that parity appears to present elevated risks for certain chronic and acute diseases in women and protection against other conditions. "These data suggest that there may be residual and cumulative effects of childbearing which influence patterns of disease in the long term" (Green et al., 1988, p. 391).

## THE WOMEN'S HEALTH MOVEMENT

Historically, interest in women's health has revolved around fertility and maternity (i.e., pregnancy, childbirth, and the postpartum period). According to feminist historians, the reproductive life of Western women before the 20th century was embedded in a female culture, which provided women with sympathetic support and guidance throughout their reproductive cycle (Ruzek, 1978). Although social class and culture influenced women's experiences, a common value was shared—women assisted other women through the maternity process (Alexander & LaRosa, 1994). Thus, maternity was part of women's domestic and social responsibilities. Women were bound together in mutual support in order to endure frequent pregnancies and childbirth, breastfeeding, and menopause. Women healers and midwives took care of women's reproductive health from menarche through menopause.

By the mid 18th century, the Western world started to question women's unique role in maternity care. European women began to deliver babies in hospitals with the assistance of midwives under the watchful eyes of physicians who had little experience in childbirth. French physicians took advantage of delivery hospitalizations to study childbirth as a natural process, whereas the English engaged in the development of surgical procedures and technologic tools such as the forceps (Alexander & LaRosa, 1994). By the end of the 18th century, physicians attended deliveries along with midwives. This was the beginning of physician control over birthing.

The female culture lost strength by the 20th century, in part because of the new role of male physicians in women's reproductive lives. In the United States, doctors were able to begin a monopoly in medicine through their new power and prestige. Physicians (men and women) were instrumental in the passing of laws requiring a medical degree for the practice of obstetrics. The new laws replaced midwives with physicians, who were eager to use medications and surgical procedures not fully mastered and understood. More deaths were caused by these procedures at the hands of physicians than by infections in the care of midwives (Alexander & LaRosa, 1994; Ruzek, 1978).

In the United States, medicine became almost exclusively a white male profession by 1920. The Flexner Report (an evaluation of medical schools by the Carnegie Foundation) was responsible for the closure of six of the eight black medical schools and the majority of church-affiliated medical schools, which were more willing to train women. As childbirth moved away from the home to the hospital, women's sense of helplessness and lack of control over their bodies increased. The medical presence brought into maternity care a number of interventions, including drugs, anesthesia, and birthing instruments. This was a major intensification of the medicalization of women's lives. The trend continued uninterrupted until the 1960s, when women began to question and openly express their dissatisfaction with the medical profession's approach to women's reproductive health.

Since the 1960s, a multifaceted women's health movement has framed women's health issues in a variety of ways. The second wave of the women's liberation movement of the 1960s and 1970s, inspired by the civil rights movement, offered a critique of gender inequalities and oppression in all aspects of women's lives. Through the lens of a gendered analysis, grassroots groups all over the country began to question women's treatment by medical professionals. Springing from women's desire to define their own sexuality and to reclaim the birthing experience, many of the earliest challenges focused on reproductive health issues. Groups such as the Boston Women's Health Collective (1984), which authored *Our Bodies, Ourselves*, began to develop their own knowledge base and to encourage women's self-confidence related to health matters.

To combat the unnecessary medicalization of women's lives stemming from the hegemony of the medical profession, the women's health movement spawned numerous self-help activities related to gynecologic health. A national network of Feminist Women's Health Clinics developed new models of self-examination and treatment. A revival of midwifery and home birth was accompanied by pressure on hospitals to allow natural childbirth, partner's presence and participation at births, and other conditions, giving more control to women and their families. Central to the changes enacted by the women's health movement was a salutogenic or health-promoting orientation in contrast with the prevailing disease-oriented medical model. Inherent in the framework of self-education and self-help are notions of prevention including diet, herbal remedies, exercise, and stress reduction techniques to ease the discomforts of conditions ranging from menstrual cramps to menopause.

As in all social movements, the beliefs and methods promoted by the different segments of the women's health movement are widely variable. For example, feminist health advocates disagree about the safety and desirability of many new reproductive technologies. Some groups are working to ban the development and implementation of such technologies, whereas others are working to achieve broader diffusion of expensive infertility treatments. Differences exist in the emphasis on developing alternatives to traditional medicine versus demanding changes in the health care system and the education of health care providers. Some groups have worked to create new models through their own counterinstitutions, whereas others have concentrated their efforts at the legislative level or targeted their demands toward professional associations, hospitals, or drug companies.

The politically charged issue of abortion illustrates the effectiveness of a dual strategy involving both approaches. Before the legalization of abortion in 1973, many women's networks made referrals to providers who were willing to perform abortions and who were known to be competent and trustworthy. At least one group, the Jane Collective in Chicago, became trained as lay abortion providers and helped thousands of women terminate their pregnancies without medical complications or economic exploitation. At the same time, broad coalitions were organizing and demonstrating to change the country's laws in order to achieve legal and safe abortions that would become available to a much broader spectrum of women after 1973.

After abortion was legalized, some women in the abortion rights movement expanded their agenda to encompass more comprehensive reproductive rights. Reproductive rights represented a wide array of needs required for women to decide freely whether or not to have children. True reproductive freedom was understood to imply the guarantee of adequate income, housing, child care, health services, schools, and other necessities for bringing up children. The reproductive rights movement recognized the need to ally with other groups struggling to assure such conditions and attempted to address social disparities in access to health and other services. In recent years, groups such as the National Black Women's Health Project, National Latina Health Organization, Native American Women's Health Education Resource Center, and Asian-Pacific Women for Reproductive Health have provided new leadership to invigorate the reproductive rights movement and expand the agenda of the women's health movement to be more responsive to women in different communities (Fried, 1990; Worcester & Whatley, 1994). Moreover, at the Federal level, the Office of Minority Health (OMH) was established by the US Department of Health and Human Services in 1985 with a mission to improve and protect the health of racial and ethnic minority populations through the development of health policies and programs that will eliminate health disparities. The Office of Minority Health also advises the US Department of Health and Human Services Secretary on public health activities involving racial and ethnic minority populations.

Attention to inequities in health outcomes and access to health care has expanded the purview of the women's health movement beyond reproductive issues and into the areas of health care financing, health care delivery systems, and medical research. The National Women's Health Network and other groups have investigated, developed policy positions, and testified at Congressional hearings on diverse women's health issues. Some of their initial efforts included hormonal replacement therapy and the design of experimental research, testing the effectiveness of the drug tamoxifen in preventing breast cancer, and the inclusion of women in

clinical trials and other medical research. Recent issues of concern have
included access to emergency contraception and affordable prescription
drug coverage. Campaigns to improve maternity care services have
recently branched out into consumer movements to force insurance companies to cover longer postpartum hospitalizations.

The legislative attempt to enact universal health insurance coverage
mobilized activists to advocate for women's needs in health care reform.
Since the failure of health care reform, potential changes in the Medicaid
system have raised alarm about the insurance status and access to care for
low-income women. Medicaid currently finances prenatal care and deliveries for a large proportion of US women, and it also funds family planning and other services for many others. However, the lack of health care
coverage is a threat for many women; the lack of scientific knowledge as
the basis for appropriate health care services also places women in jeopardy. Nearly one in five women ages 18 to 64 years in the United States
are uninsured. Furthermore, many low-income women experience a gap
in health care coverage during the time period after childbearing and
before they are eligible for Medicare. This gap has both short and long-
term implications for the health of this population. In the short term,
these women may not have access to services when they are needed. In the
long term, this lack of coverage may affect the health status of low-income
women over time and increase overall health care expenditures, as limited
access to preventive health services may make this population more vulnerable to illness and disease later in life (Strobino, Grason, & Minkovitz,
2002).

The advantages of a women's health specialty within organized medicine have been hotly debated in professional circles (American Board of
Internal Medicine, 1997). Some think such a new field would legitimize
women's health needs and fill important gaps, whereas others fear it
would "marginalize the care of women and leave the mainstream to men"
(Angell, 1993, p. 272). Presently, the American Board of Internal Medicine
and the American Academy of Family Practice consider the development of
a women's health specialty premature. However, these medical organizations strongly recommend the implementation of competencies in women's
health for their residents (Kwoleck, Witzke, Sloan, & Women's Health
Education Working Group, 1999).

A parallel concern about the marginalization of women asserts the
following:

Clinical research has over the years improperly excluded women. According to this view, women have been discriminated against in three ways: diseases that affect them disproportionately are less likely to be studied; women are less likely to be included as participants in clinical trials; and they are less likely to be senior investigators conducting the trials. (Angell, 1993, p. 271)

Over the past 15 years, several developments have aimed to address these problems. The Society for Women's Health Research, through the General Accounting Office, uncovered the lack of accountability by the National Institutes of Health (NIH) in enforcing its guidelines established in 1986 to include women as subjects in federal funding research (Greenberger & Marts, 2000a). Shortly thereafter, in 1990, the NIH established the Office of Research on Women's Health. The following year, NIH Director Bernadine Healy launched the Women's Health Initiative, "a massive 15-year study of 160,000 women that will cost more than $600 million and include the largest clinical trial ever conducted" (Angell, 1993, p. 271). The Women's Health Initiative represented a national commitment to begin to address the impact on women of all major morbidities, not just reproductive risks.

The NIH Revitalization Act of 1993 led to the publication of "Guidelines on the Inclusion of Women and Minorities as Subjects in Clinical Research" by NIH in 1994 (Federal Register, 1994). These guidelines establish a policy that women as well as minority populations and subpopulations must be included in all human research funded by NIH, unless a compelling reason is given that such inclusion is "inappropriate with respect to the health of the subjects or the purpose of the research." The policy specifically prevents the routine exclusion of "women of childbearing potential" from clinical research. The inclusion of women and the analysis of data based on the sex of the study subjects are essential to understand all aspects of the disease process (Ramasubbu, Gurm, & Litaker, 2001; Vidaver, Lafleur, Tong, Bradshaw, & Marts, 2000). Besides, new approaches, including paradigms for modeling women's reproductive system, are necessary to further our understanding of disease etiology (Harlow et al., 1999). Vidaver et al. (2000, p. 503) reinforced this point in stating that "until potential differences in responses to treatment and interventions between women and men are adequately addressed, we cannot be satisfied that sex-specific adverse events are unlikely to occur."

The development and refinement of these NIH guidelines in the early 1990s have been both a response and a spur to increasing surveillance of women's health needs. In 1994, a national conference was convened under the leadership of the American Psychological Association "aimed at developing a specific agenda to address the psychosocial aspects of women's health care" (Voelker, 1994, p. 7). The Centers for Disease Control and Prevention also announced the opening of an Office of Women's Health. According to Reuben Warren, the Centers for Disease Control and Prevention's Associate Director for Minority Health, "Without an effective women's health movement, the health of the nation cannot improve" (Voelker, 1994, p. 7).

To determine the effectiveness of the NIH Guidelines between the years 1993 and 1998, a survey was conducted on original research published by the *New England Journal of Medicine*, the *Journal of the American Medical Association*, the *Journal of the National Cancer Institute*, and *Circulation* (Vidaver et al., 2000). The survey found that the mandate for the inclusion of women in clinical research was not fully implemented. The statistical analysis of outcomes by sex was lacking, and when conducted, the new information for treatment was reported in a sex-neutral manner, regardless of evidence to the contrary (Vidaver et al., 2000). Additionally, the milestones of the last 15 years do not necessarily guarantee that research on women's health will expand and/or impact critical aspects of the process of health and disease in women. A major challenge is to prioritize scientific opportunities that will close the gap in knowledge and provide tangible benefits for women (Mosca et al., 2001). Mosca et al. (2001) identified several barriers to women's health research; these included a lack of funding, recognition, acceptance, or sensitivity by researchers and a lack of the appropriate infrastructure for interdisciplinary research.

Finally, the US women's health movement has expanded its scope by forging stronger links with international women's health advocacy groups. Consciousness about the interrelationship of women here and abroad has been heightened by issues such as (1) the testing of contraceptives on women in developing countries before Food and Drug Administration (FDA) approval for US distribution and (2) the international targeting of women as potential consumers of exported cigarettes while outreach increases to warn US women about the hazards of smoking. At the same time that US policies endanger the health of women in the developing world, grassroots empowerment efforts by women in many parts of the globe provide inspiration for organizing efforts in the United States.

International gatherings such as the meetings on international population issues in Cairo and on women's rights in Beijing, combined with electronic communication and computer technology, have increasingly united women's efforts to improve their health and social status throughout the world (Table 10–2).

Women's health cannot be adequately understood without discussing the role of gender on the maintenance of health and the prevention and treatment of disease (Pinn, 2003; Strickland, 1988; Verbrugge, 1989; Verbrugge & Wingard, 1987). Since the 1980s, sex and gender have been among the most applied but poorly understood concepts within health research. Sex differentials in morbidity and mortality have been widely researched. Some examples are *health and well-being* (Grimmell & Stern, 1992; Lane & Meleis, 1991; Nakano, 1990; Rathgeber & Vlassoff, 1993; Williams, Weibe, & Smith, 1992), *mental health and stress* (Allgood, Lewinsohn, &

**Table 10-2** Countries with Highest Levels of Achievement in Gender Equality and Women's Empowerment.

| Country | 30% Women's Share of Seats in the National Parliament (Minimum) | Female/Male Ratio Net Secondary School Enrollment (Range 95% to 105%) | Female Enrollment Rate in Secondary School | Female Share of Paid Employment in Nonagricultural Sector (Range 44% to 55%) |
|---|---|---|---|---|
| Sweden | 45.0 | 104 | 98 | 51 |
| Denmark | 38.0 | 103 | 91 | 49 |
| Finland | 36.5 | 102 | 96 | 50 |
| Norway | 36.4 | 101 | 96 | 48 |
| Iceland | 34.9 | 104 | 78 | 52 |
| Netherlands | 31.5 | 100 | 92 | 44 |
| Germany | 31.0 | 101 | 88 | 45 |
| *Very Close to the Highest Levels of Achievement in Gender Equality and Women's Empowerment* | | | | |
| Costa Rica | 35.1 | 113 | 46 | 39 |
| Argentina | 31.3 | 109 | 79 | 43 |
| South Africa | 30.0 | 110 | 95 | n.d. |

Source: United Nations Development Fund for Women (2002).

Hops, 1990; Anson, Levenson, & Bonneh, 1990; Avison & McAlpine, 1992; Barnett & Marshal, 1992; Costello, 1991; Desai & Jann, 2000; Gillespie & Eisler, 1992; Groer, Thomas, & Shoffner, 1992; Janes, 1990; Kane, 1991; Meisler, 1999, 2000; Napholz, 1992; Nuess & Zubenko, 1992; Radke-Yarrow, Nottelmann, Belmont, & Welsh, 1993; Woods, Lentz, & Michell, 1993; Zimmerman-Tansella & Lattanzi, 1991), *cardiovascular disease* (Elliott, 1994; Greenberger, 1999; Helmers et al., 1993; Knox & Follmann, 1993; Ramasubbu et al., 2001; Roger et al., 2000; Suarez, Harlan, Peoples, & Williams, 1993; Theorell, 1991), *musculoskeletal disorders* and *liver diseases* (Greenberger, 1999), and in *use of health care services* beyond pregnancy-related services (Ramasubbu et al., 2001). Most recently, researchers have found sex differences at the basic level of gene expression (Greenberger, 2002; Greenberger & Marts, 2000b), and biomedical research has provided evidence on sex differences in nearly in all organs and systems of the human body (Greenberger & Knab, 2002). Sex and gender have been used as synonymous terms in most of these studies. However, sex and gender have very different meanings and measure very distinct components of the continuum of health and disease.

Sex is biologically determined. It can usually be measured easily by using the biological categories of male and female. The construct of sex is determined by the laws of genetics, through the arrangement of chromosomes that result in phenotypes (groups of people with similar genetically and environmentally produced physical appearances) and genotypes (groups of people with similar genetic structures) (de los Rios, 1994; de los Rios & Gomez, 1992; Gomez, 1990; Kane, 1991). Thus, sex (female or male) has a biologic base and is clearly defined by specific anatomic and physiologic traits.

In contrast, gender is socially determined. It is rooted in the biological differences between the sexes, but it relates to the roles assigned by society to the female and male sexes. As yet, universal measurements of gender are not well defined. Gender is expressed through relationships of power and subordination, which translate into assigned roles, norms, activities, and behaviors expected to be performed by women and men in each society (Alexander & LaRosa, 1994; Amit, Bean, McDonald, Stuart, & Stuart, 1989; Arango, 1992; Canadian Council for International Cooperation, 1991; de los Rios, 1994; de los Rios & Gomez, 1992; Gomez, 1990, 1994, 2000; J.E. Austin Associates and The Collaborative for Development Action, Inc., 1989; Kane, 1991; Moser, 1989; Rathgeber &

Vlassoff, 1993). The conditions of women's and men's daily lives and their positions within society are expressed in beliefs, attitudes, and behaviors (de los Rios & Gomez, 1992; Gomez, 1990; Moser, 1989). To be a man or a woman is to be associated with different behaviors and attitudes in public and private life. The construct of gender has been shaped by historical circumstance and is susceptible to changes in policies associated with social, economic, judicial, and political events. According to de los Rios and Gomez (1992), the core of the gender construct is the sex-based division of labor, which is expressed in the segregation of social functions on the basis of belonging to either the female or male sex. The sexual division of labor is a historical product—not a natural aspect of society (Castellanos, 1987). It is the basis by which societies ensure their social reproduction. It guarantees both the biologic reproduction (childbearing and rearing responsibilities) and the social reproduction of society, which shapes its production mode, social and political institutions, and patterns of social relationships (Castellanos, 1987; de los Rios & Gomez, 1992).

As a means of ensuring the social reproduction of society, women's lives are structured to revolve around multiple social roles, needs, and expectations (J.E. Austin Associates and The Collaborative for Development Action, Inc., 1989; Meleis & Lindgren, 2002). These roles form a dynamic web bringing together sex and gender attributes, including age and physical environments (de los Rios & Gomez, 1992). Age is directly related to the cycles in women's lives that trigger not only biological but also political and social changes at the individual and societal levels (Arango, 1992; Directorate General for International Cooperation, 1989). Throughout the world, the social roles assigned to most women dictate their use of physical space (Arango, 1992; de los Rios & Gomez, 1992; Directorate General for International Cooperation, 1989). The spaces where women spend most of their time are directly influenced by social class, race, ethnicity, and family dynamics. Private and public spaces (e.g., school, home, church, workplace) are the cradles of socialization for girls and women. In addition, physical environments influence women's social support and networks, which can be affective, social, or occupational in nature. However, the separations between the private and public spheres are not as clearly delineated, as 39% of women's fatal injuries in the work place are due to homicide. Many of the homicides are perpetrated by spouses or partners, bringing together the private and public (Meleis & Lindgren, 2002).

The options that shape women's lives, including marital status, religion, and political ideology, are directly linked to gender constructs. Gender relationships and identities are not universal but vary from culture to culture and sometimes from community to community. They are dynamic and change over time (de los Rios & Gomez, 1992; Gomez, 1994). The analysis of gender in research needs to take into account all these aspects as well as women's heterogeneity. The construct of gender assumes specific meaning depending on political milieu, culture, race, ethnicity, and social class (de los Rios, 1994; de los Rios & Gomez, 1992; Gomez, 1994). Despite their heterogeneity, in most societies, women are generally disadvantaged compared with men in relationship to social and sex roles and, subsequently, with regard to services and opportunities. Thus, women are exposed more than men to interpersonal violence, sexual discrimination, social displacement, and poverty (de los Rios & Gomez, 1992; Directorate General for International Cooperation, 1989; Meleis & Lindgren, 2002).

# WOMEN'S HEALTH: A LIFE CYCLE

To do justice in one chapter to women's health throughout the life cycle is an impossible task. Thus, the aim of this section is to highlight aspects of women's health from a life cycle perspective.

The influence of biology, cultural roles and behaviors, and social status on health differs greatly between women and men. Women live longer than men worldwide. In addition, as life expectancy increases for both women and men, the gap tends to widen. However, the biological responsibility for human reproduction has been historically a primary cause of women's morbidity and mortality. This was documented in 1662 by John Graunt, when he stated, "Yes I have heard *Physicians* say, that they have two women patients to one man, which assertion seems very likely; for that women have either the *Greensickness,* or other Distempers, are sick of *Breedings, Abortions, Child-bearing, Sore breasts, Whites, Obstructions, Fits of the Mother and the like*" (quoted by Kane, 1991, p. 1). Graunt concluded that men die because of their vices and women because of the disease of their sex (Kane, 1991). Although reproductive mortality and morbidity are still realities for women in many countries, the differences between women's and men's health exist from the time of conception to death, and human reproduction is only part of the life cycle. The conceptualization of women's health throughout life reflects the interconnection of the different life stages and their relationship to the health of women and future generations.

## In Utero, Infancy, and Childhood

### In Utero

Biologists tell us that the sex ratio estimate at conception (primary sex ratio) is 120 male embryos per every 100 female embryos (Overfield, 1995; Strickland, 1988). Although miscarriages in the first month of pregnancy are thought to be frequent, little is known about their sex distribution. Males are more likely to be stillborn because of difficult labor, birth injuries, and diseases or injuries of the mother, whereas deaths of females in utero are more likely to be caused by congenital malformations (Kane, 1991). In some countries, female fetuses are targets of abortions for the purpose of sex selection. For example, "a report from Bombay in 1984 on abortion after prenatal sex determination stated that 7,999 out of 8,000 of the aborted fetuses were females. Sex determination has become a lucrative business" (World Health Organization, 1992). Most of the clients for this expensive procedure are women from the middle and lower classes. More recently, the discussion of sex selection has moved toward the use of assisted reproductive technologies and the preimplantation selection of embryos. However, its use remains controversial and subject to debate (Gleicher & Karande, 2002; Robertson, 2003). Thus, fetal survival is related to biological and genetic factors and is influenced by maternal health, personal decisions, social values, obstetrical care, and other environmental factors (Bandyopadhyay, 2003).

### Infancy

More males than females are born. The sex ratio of live births (secondary sex ratio) is approximately 101 males to 100 females (World Health Organization, 2004). However, this ratio is not universal. In some Asian countries, including China and India, the ratio is higher than average; in some African countries, it is lower (Kane, 1991; United Nations, 2000; World Health Organization, 2004). The sex ratio difference could be due to ineffective birth registration systems. People may not register births that are followed by the death of the infant (Bandyopadhyay, 2003). Parents may be less likely to register an infant girl in countries where girl

**Table 10-3** Sex Ratio at Birth—Five Countries with Strong Preference for Sons.

| Country | Girls Born per 100 Boys |
| --- | --- |
| China | 88 |
| Egypt | 92 |
| India | 91 |
| Pakistan | 91 |
| Republic of Korea | 88 |

Source: United Nations (2000).

children are less valued than males, as a girl has a lower chance of survival in such countries. Presently, there are 100 million females unaccounted for worldwide, and sex preference may be the reason. The preference for a son is associated with the perception of women's meager economic potential. Both women and men have expressed a strong preference for boys in many countries. However, the son preference is especially prevalent in Hindu, Moslem, and Chinese societies (Bandyopadhyay, 2003; Kane, 1991) (Table 10-3).

Infants of both sexes are at risk of dying during the early weeks after birth. The causes of death are related to complications of pregnancy, childbirth, congenital abnormalities, prematurity, low weight for gestational age, and inadequate postnatal care. Male infants are more likely to die of causes related to low birth weight and congenital abnormalities, indicating that female fetuses with congenital malformations may be more likely to miscarry. Infant mortality in general is also associated with poverty, social inequities, and a lack of access to adequate sources of health care (Kane, 1991).

### Childhood

Death rates begin to fall after the first year of life. The risk of dying is two times higher for children ages 1 to 4 years than children ages 5 to 14 years (Arias, MacDorman, Strobino, & Guyer, 2003; Kane, 1991). However, there are sex differentials in child survival favoring boys. According to the World Health Organization (1992, p. 20), "Gender discrimination is found throughout the world, from birth onwards. Research on disease prevalence, health care utilization and family resource allocation indicates that girls are treated differently from boys, with negative results that last for a lifetime." In societies with son preference, baby girls may be breast-fed for a shorter time and thus may be exposed at an early age to contaminated or poor quality foods. In addition, a daughter may get less food and less medical and preventive health care (Frongillo & Bégin, 1993; Kane, 1991; Shrestha, 1990; Singh, 1990; United Nations, 2000). It has been argued by some that better feeding and caring for boys is not so much discrimination against girls as it is a way to compensate for boys' biological disadvantages. However, it is difficult to accept these practices as an impartial way to deal with boys' vulnerabilities (Table 10–4).

Health information about school-aged children (5 to 14 years old) is limited, as studies and reports rarely address sex differentials among school-age children. Selwyn (1990) found in reviewing community surveys that the incidence rates of acute and upper respiratory infections were only slightly higher for boys than girls, but boys were very often the main users of inpatient or outpatient hospital services for those conditions. In England, boys 0 to 14 years old have higher total rates of hospitalization than girls (Kane, 1991). The main causes of illness and hospitalization

**Table 10–4** Annual Death Rate per 1000 Among 1 to 5 Year Olds by Sex.

| Country | Girls | Boys |
| --- | --- | --- |
| Armenia | 1.2 | 1.3 |
| Bangladesh | 15.7 | 14.2 |
| Egypt | 6.6 | 5.6 |
| India | 42.0 | 29.4 |
| Iran | 3.9 | 5.1 |
| Israel | 0.4 | 0.4 |
| Kazakhstan | 1.7 | 2.2 |
| Kuwait | 0.7 | 1.0 |
| Kyrgyzstan | 3.2 | 3.3 |
| Malaysia | 0.6 | 0.8 |
| Pakistan | 9.6 | 8.6 |
| Philippines | 2.5 | 2.8 |
| Republic of Korea | 0.6 | 0.7 |
| Singapore | 0.5 | 0.4 |
| Tajikistan | 8.5 | 9.0 |

Source: United Nations (2000).

among school-aged children are infectious and parasitic diseases, upper and lower respiratory infections, congenital anomalies, signs, symptoms and ill-defined conditions, and injury and poisoning. Evidence suggests that many countries underreport illness episodes for school-aged girls, suggesting that illness among boys tends to be taken more seriously than sickness among girls (Williams, Baumslag, & Jelliffe, 1994).

Children are frequent targets of violence, abuse, and neglect. In 2001, 3 million children in the United States were the subjects of a child protective services investigation or assessment, of which 30% were found to have experienced or to have been at risk for experiencing abuse or neglect (US Department of Health and Human Services, 2003). With respect to sexual abuse in particular, the situation is much worse for girls (Wong, 1990). According to Alexander and LaRosa (1994, p. 169), "Childhood sexual abuse is estimated to occur in about 40% of girls before the age of 17." Research indicates that as abused children become adolescents, they have elevated risks of substance use, suicide attempts, aggressive behavior, anorexia and bulimia, pregnancy, and running away. Child abuse and neglect cut across gender, race/ethnicity, and socioeconomic lines internationally.

In some countries, girls and young women experience cultural practices that place them at risk of morbidity and mortality (Almroth-Berggren, Almroth, Hassanei, El Hadi, & Lithell, 2001; Toubia, 1994). The practice of female circumcision is one example. Worldwide, approximately 120 million women and girls have undergone genital mutilation (Almroth-Berggren et al., 2001). This practice is widely spread in approximately 40 African countries, Malaysia, Indonesia, Yemen, along the Persian Gulf, parts of Mexico, Brazil, Peru, and among migrants from these regions to Europe, North America, and Australia (Almroth-Berggren et al., 2001; Crossete, 1995). England and France have responded by outlawing genital mutilation.

There is not a set age for this cultural practice, which ranges from infancy to the sixth month of a woman's first pregnancy. The surgical procedures are usually performed by women known to the girl, in her home, and without anesthesia. A few wealthy families have their daughters' operations done by medical personnel under anesthesia. There are three types of female circumcision: clitoridectomy—the removal of the skin over the clitoris or the tip of the clitoris; excision—removal of the entire clitoris and the labia minora without closing the vulva; and infibulation—

encompassing the two previous mutilations plus removing part of the labia majora and stitching it together, leaving just a small opening to allow the release of urine and menstrual fluid (Shell-Ducan & Hernlund, 2000; Smyke, 1993; Toubia, 1994).

Girls and women undergoing these procedures experience short and long term effects. Soon after the surgery, women may experience pain, shock, hemorrhage, retention of urine, infection, fever, or tetanus. Death may be an outcome if the girl or woman does not have appropriate medical care to deal with complications. Throughout the life cycle, women subsequently experience pelvic infections, sometimes so severe that the fallopian tubes get blocked. Urinary tract infections are common, and women develop cysts and scar tissue. Most women experience problems with the flow of menstrual blood. The first intercourse is extremely painful for women who have undergone infibulation. If the vaginal opening is too small, the husband or midwife has to cut the scar to enlarge the opening. These women also tend to have labor complications. The most common is obstructed labor, which may bring additional complications (hemorrhage, tearing of the perineal tissue, urinary or rectal fistulae, and possible prolapsed uterus) (Toubia, 1994). Giving birth does not free infibulated women; they are stitched back into their prebirth status. Though most circumcised women do not feel free to talk about sexual matters, a few understandably have reported unresponsiveness and anxiety connected with intercourse (Toubia, 1994).

Tradition is the main reason for the perpetuation of a practice that inflicts pain, suffering, a sequelae of health problems, and sometimes even death of girls and women. For some women and men, it is a symbol of belonging and shared heritage (Shell-Ducan & Hernlund, 2000). For example, in the western part of Sierra Leone, 90% of women are circumcised (Smyke, 1993). In this region, female circumcision is the ritual of passage into women's secret societies, and the desire to be accepted into the society outweighs any doubt. Another reason often given is religion. However, according to Muslim and Christian scholars, nowhere in the Qur'an or the Bible is there a female circumcision requirement (Smyke, 1993). Parents often state that they have the girl's best interest in mind— a girl who does not undergo the procedure will be socially unacceptable without a chance for marriage. The cultural issue has been challenged by Dr. Nafis Sadikon, who stated at the Fourth World Women's Conference, "The function of culture and tradition is to provide a framework for human well-being. If they are used against us, we will reject them" (Crossete, 1995, p. 18). Many African and Asian women reject the claim that female mutilation must be understood in a cultural context. Furthermore, women health professionals from Africa have been outspoken against the practice of female circumcision. The Inter-African Committee on Traditional Practices Affecting the Health of Women and Children has been established to unite and to empower Africans working to abolish female circumcision and other dangerous cultural practices.

## Teen Years

Adolescence has been recognized as the most turbulent stage in the life cycle because of the extent of physiologic changes and social role development (Cothran & White, 2002; Muuss, 1988). Young women and men go through drastic biological changes during their adolescence. The sex hormones responsible for these major changes—estrogens and androgens—are present in both sexes (Whatley, 1994). Women tend to have higher levels of estrogens than androgens and men the reverse; however, there is not a defined ratio of these hormones, and there is a great deal of individual variation. Unfortunately, much of the emphasis has been placed on the differences and very little on the similarities between adolescent boys and girls. Consequently, sexuality becomes defined in terms of hormones and culturally circumscribed sex roles, instead of common areas such as affection, love, and sexual rights and responsibilities.

Worldwide, there are 1.15 billion adolescents 10 to 19 years of age (United Nations, 2000). Previous reports suggest that adolescents contribute to approximately 14% of all live births (Mahowald, 1993), although the number of births to adolescents varies by geographic region. According to Mahowald (1993), it is important to take into consideration gynecologic and social age as well as chronologic age when evaluating the impact of pregnancy on adolescent women. Gynecologic age determines the biological maturity of the young woman and the number of years between the onset of menarche and pregnancy. Although pregnancy is a natural and healthy process among biologically mature women, inadequate gynecologic age contribute to morbidity and mortality among pregnant adolescent women. Social age relates to the developmental milestones achieved by the teenager. Social age can be detrimental to the well-being of pregnant adolescents because of embarrassment, social ostracism, education interruptions, and economic pressures.

Although the teen years have been associated with the best physical health status within the life cycle continuum, adolescents are notorious for their risk-taking behavior (Banister & Schreiber, 2001). Injury and poisoning are major causes of death in the teen years. Morbidity associated with risk-taking behavior is exemplified by the high rates of sexually transmitted infections (STIs), sexually transmitted diseases, and the spread of HIV/AIDS among young people. In order to be consistent with the new terminology recommended by the World Health Organization, the term sexually transmitted diseases has been replaced with STIs in this chapter.

An estimated 15 million new STI cases occur among the US population each year, of which two thirds occur in people 25 years of age and younger (American Social Health Association, 1998). The most reported STI in the United States is chlamydia, with 3 million annual reported cases (Walsh, Anderson, & Irwin, 2000). Teen females have the highest rate of infection, as young women aged 15 to 19 years account for 46% of chlamydia cases in the United States (Cothran & White, 2002). The cost of the infection is estimated to be $2 million per year. One of the consequences of untreated chlamydia is the subsequent development of pelvic inflammatory disease. Human papillomavirus (HPV) is a common STI in the United States, as it is estimated that 5.5 million new cases are contracted each year (Cothran & White, 2002). Both STIs are preventable, diagnosable, and treatable. Frequent screening has been recommended as to ensure early diagnosis and treatment. Presently, vaccines to prevent low- and high-risk HPV are being developed and tested (Sevin, 1999; Zimet et al., 2000).

STIs present greater risk and complications to women than men. Women experience pain, infertility, increased risk of ectopic pregnancy, pelvic inflammatory disease, and psychologic distress. Because most societies have a sexual double standard for women and men, STIs can be a source of shame and embarrassment for women. When a woman finds out that she has STI, she may experience denial, hurt, feelings of victimization, anger, fear, shame, or loss of control over her sexuality. Infection and the ensuing distress are compounded by the fact that women are more likely than men to live in poverty, and they have less access to comprehensive health care, including diagnostic screening, treatment, and follow-up services for STIs (Williams et al., 1994; World Health Organization, 1992). Worldwide, 1 in 20 adolescents contract an STI each year (World Health Organization, 1998). Moreover, adolescents and young adults account for nearly half of all new HIV infections worldwide (Joint United Nations Programme on HIV/AIDS, 2004).

Teenagers face difficult gender role expectations. Appearance can be a source of unhealthy practices among teenagers. For example, in the US and European cultures, tall and well-muscled physiques are socially desirable for males; women are exhorted to be thin (Alexander & LaRosa, 1994; Hoskins, 2002; Mahowald, 1993). Unfortunately, some adolescents pay a high price for such characteristics and consequently develop serious health problems. Young men may seek growth hormone therapy to increase their height and/or steroidal treatment to increase their muscle mass. Young women may develop anorexia nervosa or bulimia nervosa in attempting to keep their weight down. Both eating disorders are identified with extreme preoccupation with food and body figure and image (Alexander & LaRosa, 1994; Hoskins, 2002). Anorexics may purge after eating even a small portion of food, whereas bulimics tend to starve themselves before a binge. Anorexia is very difficult to cure. It is a physically and psychologically debilitating disease. According to research in the United States, the feeling of being "fat" increases with age among young women from 50% in 14 year olds to 70% in 18 year olds (Mahowald, 1993).

Teenagers today are faced with a range of choices that were not even dreamed of two generations ago. At the same time, adolescents experience high levels of alienation, depression, injuries, and death. Furthermore, teenagers are being targeted as consumers for cigarettes, illicit drugs, alcohol, cars, and daring sports and physical activities. There is an increase in illicit drugs and the use of alcohol, sedatives, and cigarettes among teenagers, including young women (Grunbaum et al., 2004; Worcester & Whatley, 1994). A worrisome fact is the increase in cigarette consumption among teenagers and young women, given that the two well-known risk factors for cervical cancer in otherwise normal women are HPV and cigarette smoking (Sevin, 1999).

## Middle Years

In their middle years, women and men assume a number of new social roles and responsibilities and are the main contributors to the economic well being of their societies. This stage of the life cycle has traditionally been associated with issues of human reproduction, marriage, and career. In the last hundred years, women's time spent in childbearing has been reduced from half to one sixth of their lives. It was not so long ago that women could not expect to live long enough to enjoy their grandchildren. Presently, in many cultures, women survive pregnancy and childbirth and have increased life spans, partly because of the implementation of public health interventions and partly because of access to advances in medicine and medical technology.

One in 10 US women between the ages of 18 and 50 years will develop a health condition that will affect the uterus. Among those conditions are fibroids, endometriosis, heavy bleeding during the menstrual cycle, pelvic pain, and hormonal imbalances (Meisler, 1999). Currently, the medical field has deficient knowledge about these conditions and lacks holistic approaches to effectively deal with them. Furthermore, recent publications suggest that the present health care system has deficient knowledge about treating subpopulations of women, such as lesbian, bisexual, and transgender women and women with disabilities (McDonald, McIntyre, & Anderson, 2003; Roberts, 2001; Solarz, 1999; Thierry, 1998, 2000). However, these recent publications aim to improve knowledge and to stimulate further research in these areas. For example, over the past decade, research on lesbian health emerged as an important field of study. A recent report on lesbian health by the Institute of Medicine identified the gaps in the research and provided recommendations for future directions (Roberts, 2001; Solarz, 1999). Moreover, recent reports from the Office on Disability and Health at the Centers for Disease Control and Prevention provide further insight into the health and well-being of the 26 million women with disabilities in the United States (Thierry, 1998, 2000).

STIs are hidden in the "culture of silence" (Walsh et al., 2000; World Health Organization, 1992). They do not discriminate against women based on their social class, race and/or ethnicity, education, or country of origin. In 1999, there were 177 million cases reported of the four major STIs (trichomoniasis, chlamydia, gonorrhea, and syphilis) among women worldwide (World Health Organization, 2001) (Tables 10–5, 10–6, and

**Table 10–5** Estimated New Cases of Sexually Transmitted Infections Among Adults, 1999.

| Disease | Number of Cases (Million) |
| --- | --- |
| Trichomoniasis | 174 |
| Chlamydia | 92 |
| Gonorrhea | 62 |
| Syphilis | 12 |

Source: World Health Organization (2001).

**Table 10-6** Estimated New Cases of Selected Sexually Transmitted Infections (in Millions) Among Women, 1999.

| Region | Trichomoniasis | Chlamydia | Gonorrhea | Syphilis |
|---|---|---|---|---|
| North America | 3.90 | 2.16 | 0.84 | 0.054 |
| Western Europe | 5.09 | 2.94 | 0.63 | 0.069 |
| North Africa and Middle East | 2.35 | 1.44 | 0.68 | 0.167 |
| Eastern Europe and Central Asia | 6.36 | 3.25 | 1.81 | 0.053 |
| Sub Saharan Africa | 15.93 | 8.24 | 8.84 | 1.683 |
| South and Southeast Asia | 40.06 | 23.96 | 15.09 | 1.851 |
| East Asia and Pacific | 4.91 | 2.74 | 1.68 | 0.112 |
| Australia and New Zealand | 0.29 | 0.17 | 0.06 | 0.004 |
| Latin America and Caribbean | 8.79 | 5.12 | 4.01 | 1.294 |

Source: World Health Organization (2001).

10–7). Untreated STIs are a source of infection and have serious short- and long-term consequences for women's general health. For example, untreated infections and pelvic inflammatory disease are considered to be the major causes of disease-related infertility. Worldwide, there are approximately 50 to 80 million people with infertility problems (United Nations, 2000). Women often bear the burden of infertility and are usually the targets for screening and treatment, even in cases of proven male infertility (World Health Organization, 2002).

Women assume multiple roles in most societies today and comprise at least one third of the world's labor force. In addition, more women are remaining in the labor force during their childbearing years. Women are responsible for 50% of production in industrialized countries and 60% in the developing world. They also contribute $16 trillion dollars to the global economy with their nonremunerated work (Melis & Lindgren, 2002). Furthermore, women work more hours than men, often juggling responsibilities in both paid and unpaid positions. However, women earn less than men, especially in cases in which women are the head of household (United Nations, 2000). International data show a direct relationship between female family headship and poverty (Williams et al., 1994). In the United States, a new trend has developed. The percentage of couples in which the woman earns more than the man has increased from 16% in 1981 to 23% in 1996 (Melis & Lindgren, 2002).

**Table 10–7** HIV/AIDS, by Region, 2002.

| Region | Adults and Children Living with HIV/AIDS | Adults and Children Newly Infected with HIV/AIDS | Adult Prevalence (%) Rate | Percentage of Positive Who Are Women |
|---|---|---|---|---|
| Sub-Sahara Africa | 29.4 Million | 3.5 Million | 8.8 | 58 |
| North Africa and Middle East | 550,000 | 83,000 | 0.3 | 55 |
| South and Southeast Asia | 6.0 Million | 700,000 | 0.6 | 36 |
| East Asia and Pacific | 1.2 Million | 270,000 | 0.1 | 24 |
| Latin America | 1.5 Million | 150,000 | 0.6 | 30 |
| Caribbean | 440,000 | 60,000 | 2.4 | 50 |
| Eastern Europe and Central Asia | 1.2 Million | 250,000 | 0.6 | 27 |
| Western Europe | 570,000 | 30,000 | 0.3 | 25 |
| North America | 980,000 | 45,000 | 0.6 | 20 |
| Australia and New Zealand | 15,000 | 500 | 0.1 | 7 |

Source: United Nations Development Fund for Women (2002).

In general, both having a paid job and being married have health benefits for women and men. Men, however, tend to benefit more from being married (Haber, 1991; Klonoff & Landrine, 1991; Martikainen, 1995; Rosenfeld, 1992). According to Kane (1991), paid work and marriage generally have a synergistic and positive effect on the health status of women and men, but unemployed married men have worse health outcomes than unemployed unmarried men. In contrast, women who are either single and employed or married and unemployed have more acute and chronic disabilities than married and employed women. These findings suggest that multiple roles may be related to women's status in the household. In African and Latin American countries where women are responsible for childbearing, at least 70% of food production, and approximately 50% of animal husbandry, the interaction between overwork, pregnancy, and malnutrition has serious health consequences. Women's work encompasses three roles: social production, social capital, and financial capital (Melis & Lindgren, 2002).

Women everywhere work long hours. The workday of women in most countries is 16 hours. Despite modern appliances, Western housewives spend 56 hours per week working, whereas their counterparts in Pakistan works just 6 hours more (62 hours) per week (Williams et al., 1994). Furthermore, it is important to note that the distribution of health and illness is influenced by social class, race and ethnicity, geographic location, and social indicators such as education, access to health services, occupational hazards, environmental factors, and a range of personal circumstances.

Women are responsible for the biological reproduction of humankind. The United Nations Decade for Women provided an international focus on women's reproductive health issues and the right to reproductive health. The following United Nations conferences have had major impact on women's reproductive lives: Mexico City (1975), Copenhagen (1980), Nairobi (1985), Rio de Janeiro (1992), Vienna (1993), Cairo (1994), Beijing (1995), and New York (2000). For discussions of reproductive health, please refer to the chapters on Mothers and Infants and International Health.

## Transitional Years

Significant changes in women's life patterns have occurred in the last 100 years. As mentioned earlier, women's life expectancy surpasses that of men in most countries, and women currently have approximately 30 years more to live compared with women a century ago. In 1999, there were 50 million women 45 years old and older in the United States. This number is expected to rise to 60 million by 2005 (Hoerger et al., 1999). Approximately 23% of women are between the ages of 54 and 64 years in the United States (McClennan Reece, 2002). An interesting phenomenon impacting women's health is that the increase of women's life expectancy has not changed the average age for the onset of menopause (Baron-Hall & Vidaver, 2000). Women are living one third of their lives without estrogen.

During the transitional years, women experience two biological and social phases: perimenopause—"changes in menstrual flow or frequency during the last 12 months" (Morse et al., 1994, p. 164)—and menopause—"no menses for twelve consecutive months or longer" (Morse et al., 1994, p. 164). It is women at the perimenopausal age that are challenging how society deals with the natural process of aging. It is a major phobia in the United States, whereas in some societies women's status increases with age.

Menopause (natural or surgically induced) has been until recently a social taboo—women talked about it only in whispers (Mingo, Herman, & Jasperse, 2000). Not long ago, physicians viewed menopause as the "death of the woman in the woman" (Braus, 1993). Avis and McKinlay

(1995) conducted the largest and most comprehensive prospective cohort study on menopause. They found that natural menopause did not have a major impact on the health or health behavior of women. The majority of women undergoing menopause did not seek medical help, and their attitudes were overwhelmingly positive or neutral. Some women experienced transitional depression; the rate of depression decreased as women move away from the perimenopausal to the postmenopause stage. These findings were similar to those found by Mingo et al. (2000) in their cross-cultural study.

Endocrine changes of menopause are the main causes of physical and psychological symptoms (e.g., hot flashes, vaginal atrophy, weight gain, insomnia, mood changes, and depression), but not all women experience these symptoms. However, all women do have a drastic decline in estrogen levels. Low hormonal levels have been associated with an increased risk of musculoskeletal system– and cardiovascular system–related diseases. Hormone replacement therapy (HRT) has become the "magic bullet" to combat these risks. It has been argued that HRT maintains the high-density lipoprotein and low-density lipoprotein levels at the premenopausal stage. In 1991, the Women's Health Initiative clinical trials were designed to test the effect of estrogen plus progestin on the risk of coronary heart disease and invasive breast cancer. Between 1993 and 1998, the Women's Health Initiative randomized 16,608 healthy postmenopausal women with an intact uterus to either receive estrogen plus progestin or a placebo (Women's Health Initiative Study Group, 1998). However, this trial was stopped on May 31, 2002, after a mean of 5.2 years of follow-up, when the data and safety monitoring board concluded that

> the evidence for breast cancer harm, along with evidence for some increase in [coronary heart disease] CHD, stroke, and [pulmonary embolism] PE, outweighed the evidence of benefit for fractures and possible benefit for colon cancer over the average 5.2-year follow-up period. (Writing Group for the Women's Health Initiative Investigators, 2002, p. 325)

It is important to note that the trial only tested one drug regimen, conjugated equine estrogen, 0.625 mg/day, plus medroxyprogesterone acetate, 2.5 mg/day, in postmenopausal women with an intact uterus (Writing Group for the Women's Health Initiative Investigators, 2002). The results of this trial has generated an ongoing debate in the scientific literature, the medical community, and in the popular media about whether post-menopausal women should continue to take HRT. Presently, there is insufficient evidence that the results from this trial can be generalized to all forms of hormonal replacement therapy and a lack of consensus in the scientific community about the use of HRT remains (Dixon, 2002; Fletcher & Colditz, 2002; Stevenson & Whitehead, 2002; Warren, 2004).

In general, a paucity of research exists on menopause-related issues. Moreover, it will be several years before the ongoing research will yield results useful to women and health providers. Nevertheless, the results are critical for decision-making regarding issues on the quality of life and health for a growing number of women worldwide.

## Older Women

Older women live longer and are poorer than older men. Worldwide, millions of older women experience poverty, social isolation, and ill health. For example, nearly 60% of women aged 60 years or more are widowed in Northern Africa and Central Asia. In Northern Africa, this trend is due in part to women marrying older men, whereas in Central Asia, it is due in part to higher levels of male mortality (United Nations, 2000). By 2020, women 65 years of age and older are estimated to account for 10% of the world's women (22% in developed regions) (United Nations, 2000).

In 1997, 13% of the US population was 65 years of age and older. By 2030, it is expected that 20% of Americans will be 65 years of age or older (Kramarow, Lentzner, Rooks, Weeks, & Saydah, 1999). Women constitute the majority of the older population and are more likely than men to live alone. Thirteen percent of US women aged 65 years and older live in poverty. However, a higher percent of Latina and African American women age 65 years and over live in poverty (Kramarow et al., 1999). According to Arendell and Estes (1991, p. 62), "Being old, female, and a member of a minority group represents a triple jeopardy." A consequence of long longevity is the onset of diseases such as osteoporosis. Women reach their peak bone mass in their mid to late 20s (Meisler, 2000). This is also the time when women are engaged in dieting and other weight-control activities. Osteoporosis is the major public health risk for 28 million people, and 80% of them are women. Unfortunately, one of every two women over 50 years of age will have an osteoporosis-related fracture in their lifetime. Most of the time it is a hip fracture, which has long-lasting consequences in both quality of life and medical cost (Meisler, 2000).

The lives of older women are affected by cultural attitudes toward women and the older population, economic development, and social organizations. For example, in Fiji, Korea, and the Philippines, only 2% of persons aged 60 years and over live away from their families, whereas in the United States over one third live alone. In the United Kingdom, 80% of all older persons living alone were women (Smyke, 1993).

Societal views on older women are not necessarily shared by the women themselves. Most older women do not consider themselves old if they are in good health (Moen, Dempster-McClain, & Williams, 1992; United Nations, 1985). For this population, health is the key to remaining active and to participating meaningfully in society. Older women are organizing themselves and joining forces with women of all ages to improve their lives and to create a world where women can hold their rightful place in society.

## FINAL THOUGHTS

Because women's health is heavily influenced by socioeconomic, environmental, and political trends as well as gender dynamics and other social relationships, new issues are constantly rising to the forefront. In the last 2 decades, technologic and political changes have had a tremendous impact, making available new means of reproduction such as in vitro fertilization and surrogacy and restricting access to abortion and family planning services as legislative mandates and funding have fluctuated. New legal and ethical dilemmas have arisen with the development and approval of long-acting hormonal contraceptives such as Norplant and Depo-Provera, which offer new forms of coitus-independent protection but also new potential for coercion in reproductive decision making.

Women continue to comprise an increasing proportion of the population affected by HIV infection. The tragedies of women's vulnerability to HIV/AIDS and their role in perinatal transmission have accentuated stark disparities in health—disproportionate numbers of poor women of color and their children are affected by HIV. The plague of substance abuse in these women's communities and soaring rates of other sexually transmitted diseases enhance their risk of HIV infection. Models of appropriate drug treatment services for women now exist, but moral judgments compound class and racial discrimination in restricting resource allocation for such badly needed services.

**Table 10–8** Physical Abuse Against Women by Male Partner.

| Country | Percentage |
|---|---|
| Belgium | 41 |
| Canada | 27–36 |
| Chile | 60 |
| Ecuador | 60 |
| Guatemala | 49 |
| Japan | 59 |
| Kenya | 42 |
| Malaysia | 39 |
| Norway | 25 |
| Netherlands | 21 |
| Sri Lanka | 60 |
| Tanzania | 60 |
| Uganda | 46 |
| United States | 28 |
| Zambia | 40 |

Source: Neft and Levine (1997).

Social prejudices against women have also been identified as barriers to adequate health services for lesbians and to medical responsibility for dealing with violence against women as a public health concern (Table 10–8).

Little is known about the health effects of the combination of work and family responsibilities that most women now assume, and the concentration of women in low-wage, low-status occupations creates additional physical and psychologic stresses. Advocacy by and for women continues to seek redress for health inequities and to pursue the long-term goal of universal health care for all women and their families.

# REFERENCES

Abma, J.C., Chandra, A., Mosher W.D., Peterson, L.S., & Piccinino, L.J. (1997). Fertility, family planning, and women's health: New data from the 1995 National Survey of Family Growth. *Vital Health Statistics, 23,* 1–114.

Alexander, L.L., & LaRosa, J.H. (1994). *New dimensions in women's health.* Boston and London: Jones & Bartlett Publishers.

Allgood, M.B., Lewinsohn, P.M., & Hops, H. (1990). Sex differences and adolescent depression. *Journal of Abnormal Psychology, 99,* 56–63.

Almroth-Berggren, V., Almroth, L., Hassanei, O.M., El Hadi, N., & Lithell, U.-B. (2001). Reinfibulation among women in a rural area of central Sudan. *Health Care for Women International, 22,* 711–721.

American Board of Internal Medicine. (1997). *Core competencies in women's health: What internists need to know.* Philadelphia: Author.

American Social Health Association. (1998). *Sexually transmitted diseases in America: How many cases and at what cost?* Research Triangle Park, NC: Author.

Amit, H.R., Bean, W., MacDonald, A.A., Stuart, C., & Stuart, R. (1989). *A Handbook for social/gender analysis.* Ottawa, Canada: Social and Human Resources Development Division, Canadian International Development Agency.

Angell, M. (1993). Caring for women's health: What is the problem? *The New England Journal of Medicine, 329,* 271–272.

Anson, O., Levenson, A., & Bonneh, D.Y. (1990). Gender and health on the Kibbutz. *Sex-Roles, 22,* 213–235.

Arango, Y. (1992). Autocuidado: Una toma de decisión de la mujer frente a su salud. In Y. Arango (Ed.), *Mujer, salud y autocuidado: Memorial* (pp. 81–101). Washington, DC: Pan American Health Organization.

Arendell, T., & Estes, C.L. (1991). Older women in the post-Reagan era. *International Journal of Health Services, 21,* 59–73.

Arias, E., MacDorman, M.F., Strobino, D.M., & Guyer, B. (2003). Annual summary of vital statistics: 2002. *Pediatrics, 112,* 1215–1230.

Avis, N.E., & McKinlay, S.M. (1995). The Massachusetts women's health study: An epidemiologic investigation of the menopause. *Journal of the American Medical Women's Association, 50,* 45–49.

Avison, W.R., & McAlpine, D.D. (1992). Gender differences in symptoms of depression among adolescents. *Journal of Health and Social Behavior, 33,* 77–96.

Bandyopadhyay, M. (2003). Missing girls and son preference in rural India: Looking beyond popular myth. *Health Care for Women International, 24,* 910–926.

Banister, E., & Schreiber, R. (2001). Young women's health concerns: Revealing paradox. *Health Care for Women International, 22,* 633–647.

Barad, D.H., & Witt, B.R. (2000). Multiple pregnancies and assisted reproductive technologies. *Journal of Women's Health & Gender-Based Medicine, 9,* 101–107.

Barnett, R.C., & Marshal, N.L. (1992). Worker and mother roles, spill over effects, and psychological distress. *Women and Health, 18,* 9–40.

Baron-Hall, D., & Vidaver, R.M. (2000). The first annual conference on sex and gene expression. *Journal of Women's Health & Gender-Based Medicine, 9,* 955–958.

Beral, V. (1985). Long term effects of childbearing on health. *Journal of Epidemiology and Community Health, 39,* 343–346.

Boston Women's Health Collective. (1984). *Our bodies ourselves: A book by and for women.* New York: Simon and Shuster.

Braus, P. (1993, March). Facing M. *American Demographics, 15,* 44–48.

Canadian Council for International Co-operation. (1991). *Two halves make whole: Balancing gender relations in development.* Ottawa, Canada: MATCH International, and Association Québécoise des Organismes de Coopération Internationale.

Castellanos, P. (1987). *Sobre el concepto de salud-enfermedad: Un punto de vista epidemiologico.* Fifth World Congress of Social Medicine. Medellin, Colombia, Mimeo.

Costello, E.J. (1991). Married with children: Predictors of mental and physical health in middle-aged women. *Psychiatry, 54,* 292–305.

Cothran, M.M., & White, J.P. (2002). Adolescent behavior and sexually transmitted disease: The dilemma of human papillomavirus. *Health Care for Women International, 23,* 306–319.

Crossete, B. (1995, December 10). Female genital mutilation by immigrants is becoming cause for concern in the US. *The New York Times,* p. 18.

de los Rios, R. (1994). Gender, health, and development: An approach in the making. In E. Gomez (Ed.), *Gender, women, and health in the Americas* (pp. 3–17). Washington, DC: Pan American Health Organization.

de los Rios, R., & Gomez, E. (1992). Mujer en la salud y el desarrolo. In Y. Arango (Ed.), *Mujer, salud y autocuidado: Memorias* (pp. 107–123). Washington, DC: Pan American Health Organization.

Desai, H.D., & Jann, M.W. (2000). Major depression in women: A review of the literature. *Journal of the American Pharmaceutical Association, 40,* 525–537.

Directorate General for International Cooperation. (1989). Women and health. In *Sector Paper, Women and Development* (No. 3). The Netherlands: Ministry of Foreign Affairs. Available from: http://www.minbuza.nl/default.asp? CMS_ITEM=12E5DC3F5E024ADFB2AA6B315606A627X2X31365X4

Dixon, J.M. (2002). Message about hormone replacement therapy is unclear. *British Medical Journal, 325,* 1036.

Elliott, S.J. (1994). Psychosocial stress, women and heart health: A critical review. *Social Science & Medicine, 40,* 105–115.

Federal Register. (1994). NIH guidelines on the inclusion of women and minorities as subjects in clinical research. *Federal Register, 59,* 4508.

Fletcher, S.W., & Colditz, G.A. (2002). Failure of estrogen plus progestin therapy for prevention. *Journal of the American Medical Association, 288,* 366–368.

Fried, M.G. (Ed.). (1990). *From abortion to reproductive freedom: Transforming a movement.* Boston: South End Press.

Frongillo, E.A., Jr., & Bégin, F. (1993). Gender bias in food intake favors male preschool Guatemalan children. *Journal of Nutrition, 123,* 189–196.

Gillespie, B.L., & Eisler, R.M. (1992). Development of the feminine gender role stress scale: A cognitive-behavioral measure of stress, appraisal, and coping for women. *Behavioral Analysis and Modification, 16,* 426–438.

Gleicher, N., & Karande, V. (2002). Gender selection for nonmedical indications. *Fertility & Sterility, 78,* 460–462.

Gomez, E. (1990). *Perfil epidemiologico de la salud de la mujer en la region de las Americas* (pp. 1–3; 221–237). Washington, DC: Pan American Health Organization.

Gomez, E. (1994). Introduction. In E. Gomez (Ed.), *Gender, women, and health in the Americas* (pp. ix–xviii). Washington, DC: Pan American Health Organization.

Gomez, E.G. (2000). *Equity, gender and health policy reform in Latin America and the Caribbean.* Washington, DC: Pan American Health Organization: Women, Health and Development Program.

Green, A., Beral, V., & Moser, K. (1988). Mortality in women in relation to their childbearing history. *British Medical Journal, 297,* 391–395.

Greenberger, P. (1999). News from the society for women's health research: SAM IX: More information on sex-based differences. *Journal of Women's Health & Gender-Based Medicine, 8,* 1223–1224.

Greenberger, P.E. (2002). Advances in sex-based analysis. *Journal of Women's Health & Gender-Based Medicine, 11,* 199–200.

Greenberger, P.E., & Knab, S. (2002). News from the society for women's health research: Subgroup analysis in clinical trials: Detecting sex differences. *Journal of Women's Health & Gender-Based Medicine, 11,* 7–9.

Greenberger, P., & Marts, S.A. (2000a). Women in NIH-funded research studies: There's good news, and there's bad news. *Journal of Women's Health & Gender-Based Medicine, 9,* 463–464.

Greenberger, P.E., & Marts, S. (2000b). Hormones, chromosomes, and the future of sex-based biology. *Journal of Women's Health & Gender-Based Medicine, 9,* 937–938.

Grimmell, D., & Stern, G.S. (1992). The relationship between gender role ideals and psychological well-being. *Sex Roles, 27,* 487–497.

Groer, M.W., Thomas, S.P., & Shoffner, D. (1992). Adolescent stress and coping: A longitudinal study. *Research in Nursing and Health, 15,* 209–217.

Grunbaum, J.A., Kann, L., Kinchen, S., Ross, J., Hawkins, J., Lowry, R., Harris, W.A., McManus, T., Chyen, D., & Collins, J. (2004). Youth risk behavior surveillance: United States, 2003. *MMWR Surveillance Summaries, 53,* 536.

Haber, L.C. (1991). The effect of employment on the relationship between gender-role preference and self-esteem in married women. *Journal of Advanced Nursing, 16,* 606–613.

Harlow, S.D., Bainbridge, K., Howard, D., Myntti, C., Potter, L., Sussman, N., Van Olphen, J., Williamson, N., & Young, E. (1999). Methods and measures: Emerging strategies in women's health research. *Journal of Women's Health, 8,* 139–147.

Helmers, K.F., Krantz, D.S., Howell, R.H., Klein, J., Bairey, C.N., & Rozanski, A. (1993). Hostility and myocardial ischemia in coronary artery disease patients: Evaluation by gender and ischemic index. *Psychosomatic Medicine, 55,* 29–36.

Hoerger, T.J., Downs, K.E., Lakshmanan, M.C., Lindrooth, R.C., Plouffe, L., Wendling, B., West, S.L., & Ohsfeldt, R.L. (1999). Healthcare use among U.S. women aged 45 and older: Total coast and cost for selected post-menopausal health risks. *Journal of Women's Health & Gender-Based Medicine, 8,* 1077–1089.

Hoskins, M.L. (2002). Girls' identity dilemmas: Spaces defined by definitions of worth. *Health Care for Women International, 23,* 231–247.

Janes, C.R. (1990). Migration, changing gender roles and stress: The Samoan case. *Medical Anthropology, 12,* 217–248.

J.E. Austin Associates and The Collaborative for Development Action, Inc. (1989). *Gender analysis for project design: UNFPA training manual.* Cambridge, MA: Author.

Joint United Nations Programme on HIV/AIDS. (2004). *2004 Report on the global AIDS epidemic: Executive summary.* Available August 30, 2004, from: http://www.unaids.org/bangkok2004/GAR2004_pdf/GAR2004_Execsum_en.pdf

Kane, P. (1991). *Women's health: From womb to tomb.* New York: St. Martin's Press.

Katz, M.E., Holmes, M.D., Power, K.L., & Wise, P.H. (1995). Mortality rates among 15- to 44-year-old women in Boston: Looking beyond reproductive status. *American Journal of Public Health, 85,* 1135–1138.

Klonoff, E.A., & Landrine, H. (1991). Sex roles, occupational roles, and symptom-reporting: A test of competing hypothesis on sex difference. *Journal of Behavioral Medicine, 15,* 355–364.

Knox, S.S., & Follmann, D. (1993). Gender difference in the psychosocial variance of framingham and bortner type A measures. *Journal of Psychosomatic Research, 37,* 709–716.

Kramarow, E., Lentzner, H., Rooks, R., Weeks, J., & Saydah, S. (1999). Health and aging chartbook. *Health, United States, 1999.* Hyattsville, MD: National Center for Health Statistics.

Kwolek, D.S., Witzke, D., Sloan, D.A., & Women's Health Education Working Group. (1999). Assessing the need for faculty development in women's health among internal medicine and family practice teaching faculty. *Journal of Women's Health & Gender-Based Medicine, 8,* 1195–1201.

Lane, S.D., & Meleis, A. (1991). Roles, work, health perceptions and health resources of women: A Study in an Egyptian delta hamlet. *Social Science & Medicine, 33,* 1197–1208.

Mahowald, M.B. (1993). *Women and children in health care: An unequal majority* (pp. 242–254). New York: Oxford University Press.

Martikainen, P. (1995). Women's employment, marriage, motherhood and mortality: A test of multiple role and role accumulation hypotheses. *Social Science & Medicine, 40,* 199–212.

Matthews, T.J., & Hamilton, B.E. (2002). Mean age of mother, 1970–2000. *National Vital Statistics Reports, 51,* 1–13. Available from: http://www.cdc.gov/nchs/data/nvsr/nvsr51/nvsr51_01.pdf

McClennan Reece, S. (2002). Weighing the cons and pros: Women's reasons for discontinuing hormone replacement therapy. *Health Care for Women International, 23,* 19–32.

McDonald, C., McIntyre, M., & Anderson, B. (2003). The view from somewhere: Locating lesbian experience in women's health. *Health Care for Women International, 24,* 697–711.

Meisler, J.G. (1999). Toward optimal health: The experts respond to depression. *Journal of Women's Health & Gender-Based Medicine, 8,* 1141–1146.

Meisler, J.G. (2000). Toward optimal health: The experts discuss chronic fatigue syndrome. *Journal of Women's Health & Gender-Based Medicine, 9,* 477–482.

Meleis, A.I., & Lindgren, T.G. (2002). Man works from sun to sun, but woman's work is never done: Insights on research and policy. *Health Care for Women International, 23,* 742–753.

Mingo, C., Herman, C.J., & Jasperse, M. (2000). Women's stories: Ethnic variations in women's attitudes and experiences of menopause, hysterectomy, and hormonal replacement therapy. *Journal of Women's Health & Gender-Based Medicine, 9,* S-27–S-38.

Moen, P., Dempster-McClain, D., & Williams, R.M. (1992). Successful aging: A life-course perspective on women's multiple roles and health. *American Journal of Sociology, 97,* 1612–1638.

Morse, C.A., Smith, A., Dennerstein, L., Green, A., Hooper, J., & Burger, H. (1994). The treatment-seeking women at menopause. *Maturitas, 18,* 161–173.

Mosca, L., Allen, C., Fernandez-Repollet, E., Kim, C., Lee, M., McAuley, J.W., & McLaughlin, M. (2001). Setting a local research agenda for women's health: The National Centers of Excellence in Women's Health. *Journal of Women's Health & Gender-Based Medicine, 10,* 927–935.

Moser, C.O. (1989). Gender planning in the third world: Meeting practical and strategic gender needs. *World Development, 17,* 1799–1825.

Muuss, R.E. (1988). Carol Gilligan's theory of sex differences in the development of moral reasoning during adolescence. *Adolescence, XXIII,* 229–243.

Nakano, K. (1990). Type A behavior, hardiness, and psychological well-being in Japanese women. *Psychological Reports, 67,* 367–370.

Napholz, L. (1992). Locus of control and depression as a function of sex role orientation [abstract]. *Acta-Psiquiatrica y Psicologica de America Latina, 38,* 205–212.

Neft, N., & Levine A.D. (1997). *Where women stand: An international report on the status of women in 140 countries 1997–1998.* New York: Random House.

Nuess, W.S., & Zubenko, G.S. (1992). Correlates of persistent depression symptoms in widows. *American Journal of Psychiatry, 149,* 346–351.

Overfield, T. (1995). *Biologic variation in health and illness: Race, age, and sex differences* (2nd ed.). Boca Raton, LA: CRS Press.

Pinn, V.W. (2003). Sex and gender factors in medical studies: Implications for health and clinical practice. *New England Journal of Medicine, 289,* 397–400.

Radke-Yarrow, M., Nottelmann, E., Belmont, B., & Welsh, J.D. (1993). Affective interactions of depressed and nondepressed mothers and their children. *Journal of Abnormal Child Psychology, 21,* 683–695.

Ramasubbu, K., Gurm, H., & Litaker, D. (2001). Gender bias in clinical trials: Do double standards still apply? *Journal of Women's Health & Gender-Based Medicine, 10,* 757–764.

Rathgeber, E.M., & Vlassoff, C. (1993). Gender and tropical diseases: A new research focus. *Social Science & Medicine, 37,* 513–520.

Roberts, S.J. (2001). Lesbian health research: A review and recommendations for future research. *Health Care for Women International, 22,* 537–352.

Robertson, J.A. (2003). Extending preimplantation genetic diagnosis: Medical and non-medical uses. *Journal of Medical Ethics, 29,* 213–216.

Roger, V.L., Farkouh, M.E., Weston, S.A., Reeder, G.S., Jacobsen, S.J., Zinsmeister, A.R., Yawn, B.P., Kopecky, S.L., & Gabriel, S.E. (2000). Sex differences in evaluation and outcome of unstable angina. *Journal of the American Medical Association, 283,* 646–652.

Rosenfeld, J.A. (1992). Maternal work outside the home and its effect on women and their families. *Journal of the American Medical Women's Association, 47,* 47–53.

Rosenfield, A., & Maine, D. (1985). Maternal mortality: A neglected tragedy: Where is the M in MCH? *The Lancet, 2,* 83–85.

Ruzek, S.B. (1978). *The women's health movement.* New York: Praeger Publishers.

Selwyn, B.J. (1990). The epidemiology of acute respiratory tract infection in young children: Comparison of findings from several developing countries. *Review of Infectious Diseases, 12*(Suppl. 8), S877.

Sevin, B.-U. (1999). Social Implications of sexually transmitted cancer. *Journal of Women's Health & Gender-Based Medicine, 8,* 759–766.

Shell-Ducan, B., & Hernlund, Y. (2000). *Female "circumcision" in Africa: Culture, controversy, and change.* Boulder, CO: Lynne Rienner Publishers.

Shrestha, N.M. (1990). The girl child. *Asian-Pacific Journal of Public Health, 4,* 205–208.

Singh, I. (1990). Sociocultural factors affecting girl children in Nepal. *Asian-Pacific Journal of Public Health, 4,* 251–254.

Smyke, P. (1993). *Women and health, 2d impression.* Atlantic Highlands, NJ: Zed Books Ltd.

Solarz, A.L., & Committee on Lesbian Health Research Priorities, Neurosciences and Behavioral Health Program, Health Sciences Policy Program, Health Sciences Section, Institute of Medicine (Ed.). (1999). *Lesbian health: Current assessment and directions for the future.* New York: National Academy Press.

Stevenson, J.C., & Whitehead, M.I. (2002). Hormone replacement therapy: Findings of women's health initiative trial need not alarm users. *British Medical Journal, 325,* 113–114.

Strickland, B.R. (1988). Sex-related differences in health and illness. *Psychology of Women Quarterly, 12,* 381–399.

Strobino, D.M., Grason, H., & Minkovitz, C. (2002). Charting a course for the future of women's health in the United States: Concepts, findings, and recommendations. *Social Science & Medicine, 54,* 839–848.

Suarez, E.C., Harlan, E., Peoples, M.C., & Williams, R.B., Jr. (1993). Cardiovascular and emotional responses in women: The role of hostility and harassment. *Health Psychology, 12,* 459–468.

Theorell, T. (1991). Cardiovascular health in women: Results from epidemiological and psychosocial studies in Sweden [abstract]. In M. Frankenhaeuser, U. Lundberg, & M.A. Chesney (Eds.), *Women, work and health: Stress and opportunities.* New York: Plenum Press.

Thierry, J.M. (1998). Promoting the health and wellness of women with disabilities. *Journal of Women's Health, 7,* 505–507.

Thierry, J.M. (2000). Increasing breast and cervical cancer screening among women with disabilities. *Journal of Women's Health & Gender-Based Medicine, 9,* 9–12.

Toubia, N. (1994). Female circumcision as a public health issue. *New England Journal of Medicine, 331,* 712–716.

United Nations. (1985). *UN Decade for Women Bulletin, 11.* New York: United Nations Publishers.

United Nations. (2000). *The world's women 2000: Trends and statistics.* New York: United Nations Publishers.

United Nations Development Fund for Women. (2002). Assessing progress in achieving gender equity. *Progress of the world's women: Gender equality and the millennium development goals.* New York: United Nations Publishers.

US Department of Health and Human Services, Administration on Children, Youth and Families. (2003). Child maltreatment 2001. Washington, DC: U.S. Government Printing Office. Available from: http://www.acf.hhs.gov/programs/cb/publications/cm01/

Verbrugge, L.M. (1989). The twain meet: Empirical explanations of sex differences in health and mortality. *Journal of Health and Social Behavior, 30,* 282–304.

Verbrugge, L.M., & Wingard, D.L. (1987). Sex differentials in health and mortality. *Women & Health, 12,* 103–144.

Vidaver, R.M., Lafleur, B., Tong, C., Bradshaw, R., & Marts, S.A. (2000). Women subjects in NIH-funded clinical research literature: Lack of progress in both representation and analysis by sex. *Journal of Women's Health & Gender-Based Medicine, 9,* 495–504.

Voelker, R. (1994). A new agenda for women's health. *Journal of the American Medical Association, 272,* 7.

Walsh, C., Anderson, L.A., & Irwin, K. (2000). The silent epidemic of *Chlamydia trachomatis*: The urgent need for detection and treatment in women. *Journal of Women's Health & Gender-Based Medicine, 9,* 339–343.

Warren, M.P. (2004). A comparative review of the risks and benefits of hormone replacement therapy regimens. *American Journal of Obstetrics and Gynecology, 190,* 1141–1167.

Whatley, M.H. (1994). Male and female hormones: Misinterpretation of biology in school health and sex education. In N. Worcester & M. Whatley (Eds.), *Women's health: Readings on social, economic, and political issues* (2nd ed., pp. 97–103). Dubuque, IA: Kendall/Hunt Publishing Company.

Williams, P.G., Weibe, D.J., & Smith, T.W. (1992). Coping processes as mediators of the relationship between hardiness and health. *Journal of Behavioral Medicine, 15,* 237–255.

Williams, C.D., Baumslag, N., & Jelliffe, D.B. (1994). *Mother and child health: Delivering the services* (3rd ed.). New York: Oxford University Press.

Wise, P. (1993). Confronting racial disparities in infant mortality: Reconciling science and politics. *American Journal of Preventive Medicine, 9,* 7–16.

Women's Health Initiative Study Group. (1998). Design of the Women's Health Initiative clinical trial and observational study. *Controlled Clinical Trials, 19,* 61–109.

Wong, Y.L. (1990). Girl abuse: The Malaysian situation. *Asian-Pacific Journal of Public Health, 4,* 258–264.

Woods, N.F., Lentz, M., & Michell, E. (1993). The new woman: Health-promotion and health-damaging. *Health Care for Women International, 14,* 389–405.

Worcester, N., & Whatley, M.H. (Eds.). (1994). *Women's health: Readings on social, economic, and political issues* (2nd ed.). Dubuque, IO: Kendall/Hunt Publishing Company.

World Health Organization. (1992). *Women's health: Across age and frontier.* Geneva: Author.

World Health Organization. (1998). *The world health report 1998: Life in the twenty-first century: A Vision for All.* Geneva: Author.

World Health Organization. (2001). *Global prevalence and incidence of selected curable sexually transmitted infections: Overview & estimates.* Geneva: Author.

World Health Organization. (2002). *Current practices and controversies in assisted reproduction.* Report of a meeting on "medical, ethical, and social aspects of assisted reproduction" held at WHO Headquarters in Geneva, Switzerland, 17–21, September, 2001. Geneva: Author. Available August 30, 2004, from: http://www.who.int/reproductive-health/infertility/report_content.htm

World Health Organization. (2004). *Reproductive health indicators for global monitoring of reproductive health.* Available August 26, 2004, from: http://www.who.int/reproductive-health/global_monitoring/RHRxmls/RHRNavigate Screen.htm

Writing Group for the Women's Health Initiative Investigators. (2002). Risks and benefits of estrogen plus progestin in healthy menopausal women: Principal results from the Women's Health Initiative randomized controlled trial. *Journal of the American Medical Association, 288,* 321–333.

Zimet, G.D., Mays, R.M., Winston, Y., Kee, R., Dickes, J., & Su, L. (2000). Acceptability of human papillomavirus immunization. *Journal of Women's Health & Gender-Based Medicine, 9,* 47–50.

Zimmerman-Tansella, C., & Lattanzi, M. (1991). The Ryle Marital Patterns Test as a predictor of symptoms of anxiety and depression in couples in the community. *Social Psychiatry and Psychiatric Epidemiology, 26,* 221–229.

# CHAPTER 11

# Children and Youth with Special Health Care Needs

*Anita M. Farel*

*Despite that moment, the disability movement, unlike other civil rights causes, remains rarely recognized and little celebrated. Yet it is a trailblazing crusade. It quietly offers a renewal of civil rights. And it gives America a model for a more fair society that values the talents of all.* (Shapiro, 1993, p. 339)

## INTRODUCTION

Concern about access to services for children and youth with special health care needs and their families resonates in deliberations about health care policy, long-term care, and program development. Public policies and programs continue to be shaped by increased understanding of the impact of a broad array of childhood chronic conditions and of ways to identify and address the needs of children and their families. This chapter provides an overview of the evolution of public policy guiding the development of programs and laws to meet the needs of this population, the epidemiology of childhood conditions, and persistent and emerging issues.

# EVOLUTION OF PUBLIC POLICY: LEGISLATIVE HISTORY

Maternal and Child Health (MCH) and Crippled Children's Services (CCS) programs were initiated as part of Title V of the Social Security Act in 1935. Since that time, the federal government has played an active role in financing, organizing, and delivering services for children with special health care needs and their families. Although the legislation fostering the development of state CCS programs incorporated a broad vision of how the needs of children with, or at risk for, chronic health conditions could be addressed, funds for the CCS program were originally designated primarily for children who would benefit most from treatment. The program was oriented toward direct services and depended primarily on the private sector to provide specialty care. Decisions about which chronic health conditions could best be treated were left to state discretion. Because the effects of polio were of paramount concern, most of the CCS programs emphasized treatment for orthopedic conditions, such as those that affected child survivors of polio.

Medical advances in the 1940s and 1950s continued to broaden the focus of CCS programs to include newly treatable pediatric conditions, such as rheumatic heart conditions and congenital cardiac anomalies. Through the 1940s, 80% of all children served were treated for orthopedic conditions, but the development of the polio vaccine reduced this to less than 50% by 1959 (Ireys, 1980). Other medical and surgical advances continued to modify the context within which the state CCS programs operated, broadening perceptions about the population that should be served and the range of services that should be offered.

During the first 3 decades of its existence, Title V was the sole source of federal funding for children with special health care needs. The enactment of Medicaid in 1965 (Title XIX of the Social Security Act) provided states with a source of funding for medical care for needy children that absorbed many of the reimbursement and direct service provision functions of CCS programs. State CCS programs were thus relieved of some of the financing concerns that had dominated program planning and consequently were able to focus their efforts on the original Title V mandate to "extend and improve services" through planning programs for children with chronic health conditions. An amendment to Medicaid in 1967, the Early and

Periodic Screening, Diagnosis, and Treatment program, was designed to strengthen Medicaid's preventive care component for children.

Since 1974, the Supplemental Security Income (SSI) childhood disability program (Title XVI of the Social Security Act), administered by the Social Security Administration at the federal level, has provided monthly cash payments to low-income children with disabilities. In almost all states, SSI eligibility qualifies a child for Medicaid benefits. A child (birth to 21 years of age) is considered disabled if the physical, mental, or chronic medical condition has lasted or is expected to last at least 12 months or to result in death. Whereas the Medicaid program directly reimburses providers, the SSI monthly cash benefit can be used to help defray costs incurred in caring for a child with special health needs, such as transportation for specialty care, special equipment, or respite care.

In 1976, funds were provided through the SSI/Disabled Children's Program (SSI/DCP) to assure that low-income children under the age of 7 years receiving SSI cash benefits would be referred to the state's Title V agency for service coordination. Each child's need for services was assessed and an Individualized Service Plan was prepared to guide the coordination of services. Thus, children enrolled in the SSI program were assured both a linkage to Medicaid and to services offered under the state's CCS program. Funding for the SSI/DCP program only included children up to the age of 7 years; however, when the SSI/DCP was folded into the MCH Services Block Grant in 1981, rehabilitative services were extended to all children less than 16 years old.

Although Title V programs continued to develop community-based services for children with chronic conditions, services for children with mental retardation emphasized institutional care. In the 1950s, under the leadership of the Children's Bureau, states instituted child development clinics to provide health and related care by multidisciplinary teams for children with mental retardation. Subsequent appropriations to build University Affiliated Facilities—within which exemplary services, research, and professional training in the treatment and prevention of mental retardation would occur—were based on evidence that a multidisciplinary team approach was the most effective way to serve this population of children and their families. To reduce the incidence of mental retardation, a 5-year program of Maternity and Infant Care special projects grants was implemented in the 1960s by the Children's Bureau to provide prenatal care for low income, pregnant women. In the 1970s, Developmental Disabilities (DD) legislation (Developmental Disabilities Amendments of 1970, PL 91-517; Developmentally Disabled Assistance and Bill of Rights Act of 1975, PL 94-103) generated a multifaceted mandate to organize services for individuals with developmental disabilities and to establish state DD Councils. The population targeted by this program, originally limited to those with disabilities attributable to mental retardation, cerebral palsy, and epilepsy, has since broadened. By 1978, developmental disabilities were defined functionally and included all conditions attributable to mental or physical impairment manifested before the age of 22 years that resulted in substantial functional limitations in three or more areas of major life activity (Rehabilitation, Comprehensive Services, and Developmental Disabilities Amendments of 1978, PL 95-602). Under DD legislation, state DD Councils, composed of individuals with disabilities, parents of children with disabilities, and representatives from diverse state agencies, including Title V, education, and social services, developed a comprehensive state plan identifying services needed by the population with disabilities.

Across the country, deliberate and persistent attempts to integrate children with special needs into schools culminated in a landmark lawsuit in 1972 (*Pennsylvania Association for Retarded Children v. Pennsylvania*, 343 F Supp. 279) (E.D. Pa. 1972). In 1975, a Congressional finding that "more than half of the children with disabilities in the United States do not receive appropriate educational services" (20 U.S.C. § 1400[b][3]) quickened the enactment of the Education for All Handicapped Children Act (1975). Renamed the Individuals with Disabilities Education Act (IDEA) in 1990, the law guarantees a free, appropriate education for all school-age children with disabilities. Multidisciplinary assessments were mandated for all children who may need special services. An Individualized Education Plan, which identifies needed services, must be developed by a multidisciplinary group that includes teachers, counselors, and allied health professionals. Parents or guardians are encouraged to be a part of this process. As a result of this legislation, new collaborative relationships among teachers and health care professionals were forged, and schools began to assume certain responsibilities previously relegated to the health services sector, such as administering medications and treatment regimens.

The *related services* provisions of the Education for All Handicapped Children Act refer to services that are necessary for a child to benefit from special education. Related services (e.g., transportation, counseling services, and assistive technology) must be included in a student's Individualized Education Plan. All decisions about related services must be based on a particular child's needs. Schools are not required to provide health services that are usually conducted during nonschool hours or treatment that must be conducted by a physician or in a hospital setting. Nonetheless, the cost of providing other related services may strain the ability of local school systems (Mesibov, 1994). One of the criteria for whether a child with a chronic health condition would gain from related services is whether the condition is considered, under the law, to be an "other health impairment," such as asthma, sickle cell anemia, epilepsy, diabetes, or lead poisoning that adversely affects a child's educational performance. However, limited guidance to schools and inconsistent criteria for determining the child's functional status undermine consistent implementation of special education services.

Since the passage of special education legislation in 1975, states had been encouraged to plan for extending services from school age to birth based on evidence that potential developmental problems could be prevented or corrected the earlier intervention started. The reauthorization of the special education legislation under (Education of the Handicapped Act Amendments of 1986, PL 99-457) in 1986 required states to serve children between 3 and 5 years of age and encouraged states to apply for funds to plan early intervention (EI) programs. EI services focus on reducing the impact of or eliminating developmental delay and helping identified children and their families make the transition to preschool and kindergarten programs. EI services address the developmental needs of children with disabilities in one or more developmental areas: physical, cognitive, communication, social/emotional, and adaptive development. Multiple funding sources have been tapped to help implement these services. Forty-seven states report using Medicaid to support their state EI programs, and 33 states use this source for preschool special education and related services. Nine states and jurisdictions have incorporated at-risk populations into their eligibility definitions. Several other states include children with multiple risk factors in their definition of developmental delay. Since its reauthorization in 1997, all states and jurisdictions have ensured the provision of a free and appropriate education to all 3 to 5 year olds. All states and eligible jurisdictions provide entitlement to EI services for children from birth through 2 years old. In 28 states, the state health agency takes the lead role in overseeing the implementation of the

EI system (Trohanis, 2002). In recognition of the increasingly broad childhood population with special needs, the program title, CCS, was changed to Children with Special Health Care Needs (CSHCN) programs in 1985. However, continued medical advances, escalating professional specialization, program expansion, and increasingly fragmented services threatened to undermine the ability of state programs to offer comprehensive and continuous services.

The Omnibus Budget Reconciliation Act of 1989 (OBRA'89) redirected the mission of the CSHCN program. This legislation reinforced the leadership role of state Title V programs in developing community-based systems of services for all children with special health care needs, regardless of socioeconomic status, and in implementing the program's mission to promote and provide family-centered, community-based, coordinated, comprehensive, and culturally competent services. Explicitly acknowledging the diverse conditions comprising the population of children with special health care needs, 30% of the MCH Services Block Grant was to be directed toward "children with disabilities; chronic illnesses and conditions; and health-related educational and behavioral problems" (OBRA'89).

OBRA'89 also included the requirement that any medically necessary service required to treat a condition identified through an Early and Periodic Screening, Diagnosis, and Treatment screen must be provided, even if the service were an optional one that the state had not otherwise chosen to cover in its Medicaid program (42 U.S.C. § 1396d [r] [5]).

Although the SSI program experienced periods of heightened attention and languished at other times, it was greatly expanded in the wake of OBRA'89 and the 1990 Supreme Court decision, (*Sullivan v. Zebley*, 1990). As a result of the Zebley decision, the *functional status* of children from low-income families, who had previously not been eligible for SSI because they were evaluated against stricter disability criteria than low-income adults, was included in the disability assessment. Although a child's impairment must be comparable in severity to one that would prevent an adult from working, comparability under the new law was interpreted to mean an impairment that substantially reduces the child's ability to function independently and effectively in an age-appropriate manner (Perrin & Stein, 1991). As a result of the outreach to potentially eligible children and their families mandated by OBRA'89, the increased number of childhood impairment listings (from 4 to 11 general categories), and the rising rate of childhood poverty in the 1990s, there was a threefold increase in the number of children enrolled in

SSI, from 296,000 in 1989 to 893,000 children in 1994 (National Commission on Childhood Disability, 1995). In 1989, approximately 51% of the children enrolled in SSI had physical impairments; by 1994, children with physical impairments comprised approximately 39% of children enrolled, whereas children with mental impairments, including mental retardation, accounted for over 61% of enrollment. Disability determination is based on information solicited from physicians, psychologists, schools, teachers, therapists, social workers, parents, friends, relatives, the child, and others who may be able to provide useful information about the child's impairment(s) and functioning.

Alarmed by the rapidly increasing SSI enrollment, Congress passed the Personal Responsibility and Work Opportunity Reconciliation (Welfare Reform) Act of 1996 (PL 104-193) that dramatically redesigned the SSI program by cutting the cash assistance program for children with disabilities and restricting eligibility. This legislation established a definition of childhood disability based on more restrictive medical listings. In order to qualify for benefits, a child must have a "medically determinable physical or mental impairment which results in marked and severe functional limitations" of substantial duration (Schulzinger, 1998). The Individualized Functional Assessment was eliminated, and maladaptive behavior was deleted from the mental impairment listings.

# EPIDEMIOLOGY OF SPECIAL HEALTH CARE NEEDS AMONG US CHILDREN

Estimates of the number of children with special health care needs have been based on random samples of the population, medical records, demonstration projects, records of social and/or educational services, and reports of clinic enrollment. These disparate sources of data have led, not surprisingly, to widely varying estimates of the prevalence of chronic conditions among children.

## Sources of Data

### National Health Interview Survey—Child Health Supplement

One of the earlier sources of population-based information about chronic health conditions among children and youth was the Child Health

Supplement of the National Health Interview Survey (NHIS-CHS, 1988). The size of the population and the impact of chronic conditions were estimated by analyzing data from household interviews with 17,110 respondents. Using this survey, a study of the prevalence and impact of nine developmental disabilities concluded that 17% of children less than 18 years of age had developmental disabilities (Boyle, Decoufle, & Yeargin-Allsopp, 1994). Children with six conditions—cerebral palsy (prevalence, 0.2%), epilepsy or seizures (0.09%), blindness (0.08%), deafness or trouble hearing (0.18%), stammering or stuttering (0.13%), and other speech defects (0.17%)—considered to be developmental disabilities had substantially more doctor visits, hospital days, school days lost, and repeated grades in school than children without these conditions.

Increasing the number of categories of chronic conditions examined to 19, Newacheck and Taylor (1992) estimated that 31% of children less than 18 years old had one or more chronic conditions based on the NHIS-CHS, 1988. The authors suggest that even these estimates may understate the true size of the population with single and multiple conditions, as the checklist did not include all childhood conditions, particularly those related to mental health. The most prevalent conditions included respiratory allergies (9.7%), asthma (4.2%), eczema and skin allergies (3.3%), frequent or severe headaches (2.5%), and speech defects (2.6%). Diabetes (0.1%), sickle cell disease (0.1%), and cerebral palsy (0.2%) were among the less prevalent conditions. The impact of chronic conditions varied. For example, 20% of the children with chronic illnesses were mildly affected. Nine percent of children experienced more than occasional annoyance or limitation of activity, but not both, and 2% were severely affected.

Not all chronic conditions impose the same burden on the child and family. Some conditions require frequent hospitalizations or are more disruptive for a family, whereas others may be managed more easily. The effect of different conditions on developmental progress would also thus be expected to vary. These considerations have stimulated efforts to classify children with chronic health conditions according to such variables as impact on the family, use of medical services, or the child's functional status. In other words, although they may suffer from distinct illnesses and disabilities, the daily experiences of children with special health care needs and their families may be very similar. For example, diabetes and sickle cell anemia have very different etiologies and treatment protocols, but children affected by these conditions have in common school absences and the need for careful monitoring (Fowler, Johnson, & Atkinson, 1985). Conditions also have different ramifications depending on the age and stage of development of the child. The ramifications of compromised lung development as a result of preterm birth usually require less specialized medical attention as a child gets older, but the developmental delay often associated with this birth outcome may necessitate special education services when the child enters school (Farel, Hooper, Teplin, Henry, & Kraybill, 1998).

### National Health Interview Survey on Disability

In 1994, the Maternal and Child Health Bureau (MCHB) formed a workgroup to develop a definition of children with special health care needs. Definitions based solely on conditions or diagnostic lists were rejected as being too unwieldy. Definitions based on functional status alone were eliminated because they would not include children whose disabilities have been alleviated by treatment or the continued use of special services. The following definition, "Children with special health care needs are those who have or are at increased risk for chronic physical, developmental, behavioral, or emotional conditions and who also require health and related services of a type or amount beyond that required by children generally," achieved consensus (McPherson et al., 1998). Although very broad, this definition is consonant with the population described in diverse federal laws, provides useful guidance for strategic planning, and was the definition applied to data collected in the 1994 National Health Interview Survey on Disability (NHIS-D).

Stein, Bauman, Westbrook, Coupey, and Ireys (1993) developed a conceptual framework that cuts across diagnostic categories and provides a means to estimate the impact of chronic health conditions, including mental health, health, functional status, and family functioning, on children and their families. In lieu of specific diagnoses, the framework uses consequences of "chronic ongoing conditions" to identify children along with such parameters as disability or functional limitation, dependency (e.g., medications, special diets, medical technology, assistive devices, and personal assistance), and needs for services. Items based on this framework were incorporated into the NHIS-D (1994). The NHIS-D includes information for more than 60,000 children, enlarging substantially the 17,000 children surveyed in the NHIS-CHS supplement in 1988.

Deliberately avoiding one definition of disability, the survey identifies children with disabilities or special needs through questions in the following areas: limitation of activity (from the NHIS core), impairments (e.g., vision, hearing, mobility), activities of daily living (children > 5 years old), a condition list, special health care needs, special education services, and early child development (Simpson, 1993). Analyses from this survey suggested that 16% to 18% of children less than 18 years old have chronic physical, developmental, behavioral, or emotional conditions that have some degree of functional impact or require special services.

### National Survey for Children with Special Health Care Needs

The quality of data about the prevalence and impact of special health care needs among children and youth has continued to improve. The National Survey of Children with Special Health Care Needs was conducted from April 2000 to October 2002. Data from this survey provide uniform state and national data on the prevalence and impact on children and youth of chronic conditions, data for generating baseline estimates for federal and state Title V Maternal and Child Health performance measures, *Healthy People 2010* national prevention objectives, and data useful for each state's 5-year Title V needs assessment (van Dyck et al., 2002). Thus, for the first time, each state has data for planning and evaluating programs for children and youth with special needs.

The mechanism used by the State and Local Area Integrated Telephone Survey, which shares the random-digit-dial sampling frame of the National Immunization Survey, was also used to conduct the National Survey for Children with Special Health Care Needs. A CSHCN screener (Bethell et al., 2002) was used to identify and select 750 children from each state and the District of Columbia. Items for the screener were based on the federal MCHB definition of CSHCN (McPherson et al., 1998) and the Questionnaire for Identifying Children with Chronic Conditions (Stein, Westbrook, & Bauman, 1997). Missouri provided funding to double the number of children sampled from that state. Parents, or guardians, completed a battery of questions related to the following 10 domains: demographic information, health and functional status, health insurance coverage, adequacy of health insurance coverage, public program participation, access to care, use of health care services, care coordination, satisfaction with care, and the impact of the special need on the family. The interview was conducted in 12 languages. A total of 372,174 screener interviews and 38,866 interviews of children were completed. Estimates based on the survey indicate that 12.8% of children in the United States have a special need.

Estimates of the number of children and youth with special health care needs derived from the National Survey of Children with Special Health Care Needs will provide baseline estimates for the MCHB Performance Measures and make it possible to strengthen the system of care for this population (US Department of Health and Human Services, 2000) and monitor progress reaching the following four MCHB *Healthy People 2010* Objectives for CSHCN.

1. All CSHCN will receive regular ongoing comprehensive care within a medical home.
2. All families of CSHCN will have adequate private and/or public insurance to pay for services that they need.
3. Services for CSHCN and their families will be organized in ways that families can easily use.
4. Families of CSHCN will participate in decision making at all levels and will be satisfied with the services that they receive.

Data generated by the National Survey will also be useful for tracking and reporting the following MCHB Performance Measures, which are used as benchmarks for state CSHCN program performance (www.mchdata.net).

1. The percentage of state SSI beneficiaries less than 16 years old receiving rehabilitative services from the State CSHCN Program
2. The degree to which the State CSHCN Program provides or pays for specialty and subspecialty services, including care coordination, not otherwise accessible or affordable to its clients
3. The percentage of CSHCN in the state who have a "medical/health home"
4. The percentage of newborns in the state with at least one screening for phenylketonuria, hypothyroidism, galactosemia, hemoglobinopathies (e.g., the sickle cell diseases) combined
5. The percentage of newborns who have been screened for hearing impairment before hospital discharge
6. The percentage of CSHCN in the State CSHCN Program with a source of insurance for primary and specialty care

## Projections of Incidence and Prevalence

The prevalence of childhood chronic conditions leading to special health care needs has been estimated to fall between 9% and 20% (Benedict & Farel, 2003; Newacheck et al., 1998; van Dyck et al., 2002). Increasing numbers of children with chronic conditions include those with HIV infection and children who are dependent on advanced medical technology such as ventilators, gastrostomies, and tracheostomies. Improvements in the ability to diagnose some conditions (e.g., asthma and hearing impairments) and longer survival because of medical advances (e.g., cystic fibrosis) and therapeutic regimens (e.g., HIV) are credited in the increasing prevalence of certain diseases. Changes in prevalence rates for some chronic conditions and disabilities also speak to the success of programs with legislatively mandated outreach and child-find components.

The means for preventing some conditions are known. For example, the large decline in spina bifida has been attributed to daily consumption of folic acid (Centers for Disease Control and Prevention, 2002a). Estimated to affect 1 in 1,000 births, fetal alcohol syndrome, which has been associated with mental retardation, birth defects, central nervous system impairment, and other cognitive and behavioral abnormalities, is preventable if alcohol is not consumed during pregnancy (Centers for Disease Control and Prevention, 2002b). However, the means for primary prevention of most chronic conditions are unknown.

# MINORITY CHILDREN AND YOUTH WITH SPECIAL HEALTH CARE NEEDS

Hispanic and other ethnic minority populations are expected to grow disproportionately. If current trends continue, the Bureau of the Census projects that minority racial and ethnic groups will together account for almost half of the US total population by 2050 (US Census Bureau, 2000).

The commitment to implementing culturally competent service systems requires understanding cultural variations in the use of health care and the impact and prevalence of chronic health and disabling conditions among minority populations. Health care practices and attitudes toward illness and disability vary among different cultures. However, the prevalence of chronic conditions among minority populations is difficult to estimate.

Newacheck et al. (1998) developed an epidemiologic profile of children with special health care needs using the definition of this population disseminated by the MCHB. Data from the 1994 to 1995 disability supplement to the National Health Interview Survey were used to estimate that 18% of all children living in the United States have an existing special health care need. The percentages for white non-Hispanic, non-Hispanic African American children, Hispanic, and other, non-Hispanic children were 18.6%, 19.8%, 15%, and 13%. Thus, African American children were most likely to be categorized as having a special health care need, and Hispanic and other minority children were least likely to be so categorized. These data likely reflect disparities in access to health care services, health care use, and health status among minority populations. Certain health conditions clearly have a disproportionate impact on children in minority populations. For example, asthma is the most common chronic childhood disease and leading cause of disability among children in the United States (Centers for Disease Control and Prevention, 2000). African American children with asthma are less likely to receive adequate asthma therapy compared with white children—a finding that persists for children enrolled in Medicaid (Cooper & Hickson, 2001). In 1997, 67.5% of black children diagnosed with asthma reported having an asthma attack in the past year compared with 52.2% of white, non-Hispanic children and 51.3% of Hispanic children. Disparities in activity limitation caused by asthma are even more significant for black children living in poverty (Centers for Disease Control and Prevention, 2000).

Newacheck, Hung, and Wright (2002) used the 1994 to 1995 NHIS-D to examine whether disparities in access and use were discernible among black, white, and Hispanic children identified as having special health care needs. Of the 57,553 parent interviews, 17.7% of the children had a special health care need. Hispanic and black children were significantly more likely than white children to lack health insurance (13.2% vs. 10.3%), to be without usual source of care (6.7% vs. 4.3%), and to report inability to get needed medical care (3.9% vs. 2.8%). White children with special health care needs were more likely to have used physician services (88.6% vs. 85.0%), although black and Hispanic children were more likely to have been hospitalized in the previous year (97.6% vs. 6.3%). Taking into account family income, insurance coverage, health status, differences were reduced but remained significant for the following measures: no usual source of care, receipt of care outside a doctor's office or health maintenance organization

(HMO), no regular clinician no doctor contacts in past year, and "volume" of doctor contacts. This report concluded that disparities between white and minority children persist, especially among Hispanic children.

Multivariate analysis of 1999 to 2000 NHIS data revealed that differences in disability prevalence rates among black and white non-Hispanic children could be entirely explained by socioeconomic status (Newacheck, Stein, Bauman, & Hung, 2003). The prevalence of disability increased for both black and white children over the 40-year period studied—possibly the result of an increase in disease prevalence and severity, changes in awareness of health problems, better detection and ascertainment of health conditions by health professionals and educators, shifts in attitudes and beliefs about health limitations, and other factors. However, largely because of their exposure to poverty, black children had higher rates of disability. Although race was not independently associated with the prevalence of disability, racial differences persisted in the prevalence of disability.

A recent study by Akinbami, LaFleur, and Schoendorf (2002) reported that differences in asthma prevalence rates among black and white children diminished after adjusting for socioeconomic factors. However, black children with asthma experienced more hospitalization, emergency room services, and death caused by asthma than white children with asthma. Poor black children had the lowest level of ambulatory care; white nonpoor children had the highest level. Some of this disparity may be related to differential use of health care services. These authors assert that morbidity is a more profound factor behind the disproportionate impact of asthma on black and poor children than prevalence.

Nonfinancial factors also contribute to reduced access and use of health services by minority CSHCN. Such factors include language barriers, attitudes and cultural beliefs, level of cultural competence among providers, and perceived racial discrimination (Williams, 2000). Language barriers limit parents' access to health services and may affect their understanding of their child's condition. These factors may play a significant role in the health of minority CSHCN in the United States, particularly those Latino CSHCN whose parents may not read or speak English proficiently (Zambrana & Logie, 2000).

In addition to differences in language, minority groups may vary in their attitudes and beliefs about disability, standard medical practice, and use of professional services. In an effort to conduct a cultural validation of a measure of disability among children living in Puerto Rico, Gannotti and

Handwerker (2002) assessed Puerto Rican parents' understanding of their child's disability. Although Puerto Rico must provide educational and rehabilitation services to infants, toddlers, and children with disabilities under IDEA, shortages of qualified professionals, accessible buildings, equipment, and transportation undermine the implementation of services (Mulero & Font, 1997). The authors found that parental expectations and child care customs delayed mastery of diverse skills compared with children with disabilities in the United States. Puerto Rican children may have appeared to their parents as more disabled than might be expected given their actual level of impairment. For example, parents assumed that children with a disability would be more dependent on their parents for many activities of daily living and therefore put relatively little emphasis on facilitating their child's independence through EI. Although a goal of EI is to make children with disabilities more capable and independent, constraints on achieving this goal may be imposed by the assumptions and orientation of parents. Because these assumptions are associated with the parents' cultural context, interventions, to be effective, must take account of this context.

Latinos constitute the fastest growing minority group in the United States. Latinos currently comprise approximately 11% of the population and will reach 14% by 2020. It is estimated that by the year 2020, one in five children in the United States will be Latino (Zambrana & Logie, 2000). Access to health care for children in the United States is influenced by insurance status, family income, and health status. Thus, in addition to being at risk for reduced access to health and other community services and support, Latinos living in the United States also have reduced access to services for children with disabilities, such as specialized medical services and adaptive devices (Moore & Hepworth, 1994).

Despite high poverty rates among Latinos living in the United States, disability rates among Hispanic children are reported to be lower than among white and black children (Newacheck et al., 1998). Hernandez and Charney (1998) acknowledged that "an accurate assessment of the prevalence of chronic health conditions and disability among children in immigrant families does not exist for the most part" (p. 68). Given the complexity of services typically required by CSHCN and the level of skill and knowledge required to navigate the health care system, barriers for Latino immigrant families with CSHCN are likely to be formidable.

Newacheck, Hung, and Wright (2002) noted that the lack of information about services and culturally competent providers who are trained to deal with differences in language may also affect the health of minority CSHCN and their use of services. The National Early Intervention Longitudinal Study followed 3,338 infants and toddlers with disabilities and their families from the time they entered EI services until the child completed kindergarten. A report based on this study (Frank Porter Graham Child Development Institute, SRI International, 2003) indicated that minority families had more difficulty identifying and enrolling in EI services. They were also less likely than white families to be satisfied with their involvement in the decision-making process regarding their child when working with professionals. Spanish-speaking families were less satisfied than English-speaking families with their level of communication with professional staff. African American and Hispanic families in this study were also less likely than white families to report that EI professionals respected their values and cultural backgrounds, considered their opinions, or made them feel hopeful about their child's future. The results of this study indicate differences in the experiences of minority families with EI services when compared with white families. The authors note that many cultural factors may have contributed to the differences observed in this study, including differences in minority parents' perceptions of their child's needs and expectations for care, lack of familiarity about EI services among minority communities, and lack of interpreter services and culturally competent EI providers.

Disentangling the relative contribution of income and racial or ethnic background to disparities in health outcomes for CSHCN has significant implications for program and policy development. For minority families, obstacles such as lack of transportation and language barriers may result in missed appointments, reliance on episodic health care, emergency room visits, and nonadherence to treatment regimens. Analysis of recent data sets (e.g., National Survey of Children with Special Health Care Needs), which take into account changes in access after the implementation of more recent public programs such as State Children's Health Insurance Program (S-CHIP), may provide a more accurate picture of how minority CSHCN obtain access and use health services.

# MENTAL HEALTH

Mental health conditions generate substantial disability in childhood and account for almost a third of all disabling childhood conditions. Mental health conditions are among the fastest growing of childhood conditions and contribute to the growing trend in childhood disabilities for a substantial portion of children who are affected by a chronic disabling condition (Newacheck & Halfon, 1998). In 1999, the US Surgeon General reported that as many as 11% of all children in the United States have a mental disorder that significantly undermines their day-to-day functioning (US Department of Health and Human Services, 1999).

## National Health Interview Survey

Defining disability as "the long-term reduction in a child's ability to perform social role activities, such as school or play as a result of his/her mental health condition," Halfon and Newacheck (1999) used data from the National Health Interview Survey to describe the prevalence and impact of parent-reported disabling mental health conditions. On the basis of a combined sample from 3 years of the NHIS (1992 to 1994), they estimate that approximately 2.1% of all children in the United States live with a mental health condition that interferes with their ability to conduct their usual activities. In the NHIS, respondents (usually parents) are asked the extent to which the child is limited in activity, ranging from complete inability to carry out their usual activity to no limitation at all. An NCHS coding manual based on the International Classification of Diseases coding system (NCHS, 1988) and the International Classification of Diseases, 9th Revision (Centers for Disease Control and Prevention, 1988), was used to generate broad groupings of conditions. Condition categories included autism, neurotic, anxiety and affective disorders, adjustment reaction, conduct disorder, attention deficit hyperactivity disorder (ADHD), developmental delay, learning disability, mental retardation, and other (e.g., childhood schizophrenia and other psychotic disorders). The most common reported causes of disability included mental retardation (10.1/1,000), ADHD (5.0/1,000), and learning disabilities (2.8/1,000).

The prevalence of disabling mental health conditions increases with age and affects approximately 3% of school-age children and youth. Disabling mental health conditions were reported at significantly higher rates for boys, children from low-income families, and children living in families with one parent and were inversely related to educational level of the head of household. Schools play a significant role in the early detection of psychiatric disorders and are a catalyst for mobilizing resources to evaluate and treat children with serious emotional and behavioral problems. Eighty percent of all school children with disabling mental health conditions were in special education classes.

The 1% rate of mental retardation reported in this study is similar to the rate of 1.2% reported for children aged 0 to 21 years who are enrolled in federally supported programs for children with disabilities in schools. Data from this study are also consistent with studies indicating that mental retardation is more prevalent in low-income families and in families in which the level of education is low (Richardson & Koller, 1994). Rates of ADHD and learning disabilities were slightly more prevalent among white, non-Hispanic children.

The impact of disability among children living in residential treatment facilities, almost all of whom live with a range of severe mental disorders, was not measured. Aron, Loprest, and Steurle (1995) estimated that 92,000 of the children and adolescents who live in health-related residential institutions were diagnosed with severe mental retardation or other mental illness. Maguire and Pastore (1999) reported a 3.7% rate for youth (age of 10 years through upper age of jurisdiction) incarcerated in the correctional system.

The rate of mental illness increases dramatically when data from adolescents are included. Kataoka, Zhang, and Wells (2002) analyzed three national household surveys and estimated that one of every five children and adolescents in the United States has a mental disorder. Using the National Survey of American Families, the National Health Interview Survey, and the Community Tracking Survey, rates of mental health service use by children and adolescents 3 to 17 years of age and differences by ethnicity and insurance status were analyzed. From 1996 to 1998, 2% to 3% of children 3 to 5 years old and 6% to 9% of youth 6 to 17 years old used mental health services. The rate of unmet need was reported to be greater among Latino than white children and among uninsured than publicly insured children. This research study, which largely affirmed the findings from of earlier studies (Flisher et al., 1997) and reports, found that 7.5 million children likely have an unmet need for mental health services in the United States.

# GREAT SMOKY MOUNTAIN STUDY OF YOUTH

Other efforts to establish the prevalence and impact of mental health conditions among children and adolescents in the United States have relied on population-based surveys conducted in more defined geographic regions. Although diagnostic instruments vary, conclusions from these studies suggest that between 17% and 22% of children (0 to 17 years) live with some form of diagnosable mental illness (e.g., Burns et al., 1995). Initiated in 1993, the Great Smoky Mountains Study (GSMS) used a representative sample of 4,500 children who were 9, 11, and 13 years old, identified through the Student Information Management System of the public school systems of 11 counties in western North Carolina, to conduct an ongoing, longitudinal study of psychiatric disorders and need for mental health services among children. A screening questionnaire, consisting mainly of questions about behavior problems, was administered by telephone or in person to a parent. All children scoring above a predetermined cutoff were recruited for detailed interviews. Native American children who attend reservation schools were not included in the original sample. Consequently, all 9-, 11-, and 13-year-old Native American children ($n = 431$) living in the area who attended reservation schools were recruited for the interview phase.

The Child and Adolescent Psychiatric Assessment was administered to parents and children. Approximately 89% of the sample was white; 30% lived below the federal poverty rate. Almost 40% of the sample met criteria for a diagnosis or impairment, and an additional 15% met the criteria for serious emotional disturbance (SED) (Costello et al., 1996).

Approximately 16% of children surveyed in the GSMS received some kind of mental health service. Among children with both diagnosis and impairment, approximately 37% had received some type of service (Burns et al., 1995). The most common diagnoses among youth in the GSMS were anxiety disorders (5.7%), enuresis (5.1%), tic disorders (4.2%), conduct disorder (3.3%), oppositional defiant disorder (2.7%), and hyperactivity (1.9%). The prevalence of psychiatric disorders in this rural sample was similar to rates reported in other studies. Poverty was the strongest demographic correlate of diagnosis in both urban and rural children (Costello et al., 1996).

The high rate of co-morbidity in the sample is noteworthy. One third of the children with a diagnosis had more than one condition. Co-morbidity of emotional and behavioral disorders was almost three times as common in boys as in girls. There were no significant differences in age or race, although boys were at higher risk for all psychiatric disorders, attributable primarily to their higher rates of behavioral disorders. The children from the poorest families were at increased risk for every type of diagnosis except for tic disorders. Poor children had both emotional and behavioral conditions at three times the rate of other children (Costello et al., 1996). Rates and correlates of childhood psychiatric disorder were similar to those found in studies in urban areas.

Rates and correlates of childhood psychiatric disorder were similar to those found in studies in urban areas. The Dunedin, NZ, longitudinal study (Anderson, Williams, McGee, & Silva, 1989) documented a high rate of learning difficulties and other problems in adolescents who had some types of psychiatric co-morbidity in childhood. Studies of adults have shown that those with multiple disorders in the course of a lifetime are at higher risk of having "severe" disorders (psychoses or disorders requiring hospitalization or causing severe role impairment) and of substance abuse (Costello et al., 1996). This study replicated other reports in finding that depression, in particular, is highly likely to be accompanied by other disorders.

Burns et al. (1995) examined the roles of mental health, education, health, child welfare, and juvenile justice in providing mental health services for children enrolled in this study. Between 70% and 80% of children ages 9 to 13 years who received services for a mental health problem were seen in the school setting, the sole source of care for many of these children. The authors argue that schools may function as the de facto mental health system for children and adolescents.

Although poverty and minority status have both been associated with risk for child psychiatric disorder, poverty was not strongly associated with child psychiatric disorders in the rural area sampled by the GSMS. Risk factors for both white and African American youth included family mental illness, multiple household and probably school moves, a lack of parental warmth, neglect, and harsh punishment (Costello, Keller, & Angold, 2001). Although white children were three times as likely as African American children to be living in poverty, white students were more likely to have depressive disorders (4.6% vs. 1.4%) and were more likely to use school services (6.1% vs. 3.2%). The results of the GSMS were comparable to those of studies of urban areas, suggesting strongly that urban life per se is not a risk factor in severe emotional disturbance in children. These data suggest that white children are more vulnerable than black children, but the data are possibly confounded by the greater barriers between minority populations and health care resources.

The prevalence of psychiatric disorders, social and family risk factors for disorders, and met and unmet needs for mental health care among Native American children (9 to 13) was examined in the GSMS (Costello, Farmer, Angold, Burns, & Erkanli, 1997). The prevalence of psychiatric disorders was similar to those of white and Native American children. Substance use was more common in Native American children (9.0% vs. 3.8%) than in white children, as was co-morbidity of substance use and psychiatric disorder (2.5% vs. 0.9%). Poverty, family adversity (e.g., parental unemployment, welfare dependency), and family deviance (parental violence, substance abuse, and crime) rates were all higher, but the rate of family mental illness, excluding substance abuse, was lower. Cherokee children were protected from the direct impact of poverty because, under the Indian Health Service, they did not have financial barriers to mental health care. Similarly, the association of poverty, family adversity, and deviance with child psychiatric disorders was significant for the white community but not for the Native American community, likely reflecting the impact of services targeting Native Americans. A possible explanation offered for these findings is that, although Native American families have low personal incomes, social services provided by the federal government and the tribe provide a safety net mitigating many of the effects of poverty.

## SYSTEMS OF CARE

In 1969, growing concern about the unmet needs of children with SED generated a national *system-of-care* approach for delivering community-based, comprehensive, integrated services for this population of children and their families. Depending on the type of condition, rates of severe emotional disturbance range from 1% to 8% (Friedman, Kutash, & Duchnowski, 1999). The Comprehensive Community Mental Health Services for Children and Their Families Program, the largest federal investment in mental health services for children, provides grants to states, territories, and communities to improve and expand their systems of care for children and youth with SED and their families. Children, who during the past year, had a mental, behavioral, or emotional disorder of sufficient duration to meet DSM-IV diagnostic criteria and result in functional impairment that substantially interfered with or limited one or more major life activities were considered to have SED. This definition reinforces the importance of services for children with functional impairment in addition to a diagnosis. However, there is not consensus about how children with a diagnosable disorder demonstrate significant impairment in day-to-day functioning. Reports of the high rate of stability and persistence of SED have implications for developing appropriate services and support as children make transitions to adult services (Burns, 1999). A cross-site evaluation initiated in 1994 is expected to illuminate whether improvements in children's behavior and functioning can be attributed to systems of care compared with traditional service delivery systems (Center for Mental Health Services, 1999).

# TRANSITION FOR YOUTH WITH SPECIAL NEEDS

Achievements in medical technology and public attitudes that have improved survival and community responsiveness to many children with chronic conditions have not been translated into comprehensive services for adolescents with special needs. Chronic health conditions or disabilities that continue through adolescence compound the complex tasks of achieving independence.

A paramount concern for adolescents who live with chronic conditions is making a successful transition from school to work, achieving a maximum level of independence, securing financial support, completing job training, and having adult health care services. As a result, it is essential to ensure continued access to health care and benefits and to strengthen coordination among the public programs with legal responsibilities for serving this population. The Healthy and Ready to Work Initiative, initiated by the MCHB of the Health Resources and Services Administration in 1996, funded active demonstration projects to develop systems of health care, education, vocational rehabilitation, and other community-based programs to promote successful transitions from school to work, home to independent living, and from pediatric-based care to adult-based care for youth with special needs. Each of the Healthy and Ready to Work projects emphasizes different features of transition such as the impact of culturally diverse backgrounds and employers. One project developed a model for transition planning between the state's Title V program for children with special needs and managed-care organizations. A goal consistent with *Healthy People 2010* is for all youth with special health care needs to receive the services that are necessary to make a productive transition to all aspects of adult life, including adult health care, work, and independence.

# CIVIL RIGHTS FOR CHILDREN AND YOUTH WITH SPECIAL HEALTH CARE NEEDS

Several legislative initiatives address specifically the civil rights of individuals with disabilities and have implications for protecting the interests of children and youth with special needs. Section 504 of the Rehabilitation Act of 1973 (PL 98-112) is neither an education law nor a federal grant program. Paralleling the language in the Civil Rights Act of 1964, Section 504 established rights and entitlements for persons with disabilities. For example, under this law, acts of discrimination and failure to provide an appropriate public education to eligible students are perceived as violations of basic civil rights and can be addressed through this legislation. Section 504 has the potential to cover a broader spectrum of students and scope of activities than IDEA. The definition of who qualifies as an "individual with a disability" is more inclusive than IDEA, and many children who are not considered eligible for special education or related services under IDEA are covered under Section 504. Students who fit the Section 504 definition are those with a disability (physical or mental) that substantially limits one or more major life activities. Students who "have a history of" or are "regarded as" having a disability are included. For example, students with ADHD, or students with physical disabilities or sensory impairments who may only need accommodations for physical access or alternative methods of communication, qualify for services through Section 504 even if they do not meet the criteria specified under special education legislation.

In amendments to DD legislation in 1975, Congress established Protection and Advocacy systems in every state to pursue legal, administrative, and other appropriate remedies to protect the rights of persons with disabilities. Over the course of the implementation of special education legislation, some families have used state Protection and Advocacy programs to assist with developing an Individualized Education Plan for their children.

The Americans with Disabilities Act of 1990 was designed to protect people with mental or physical disabilities from discrimination based on disability. The Americans with Disabilities Act requires public facilities, including child care centers, to make reasonable modifications in policies, practices, and procedures to accommodate individuals with special needs. Necessary changes for child care centers may include curriculum adaptations, removal of physical barriers, additional staff training, alteration of staffing patterns, and adaptive equipment.

# FINANCING CARE

The burden of illness falls disproportionately on those who lack resources to marshal and pay for health care services. Insurance coverage is essential for ensuring appropriate and timely access to care for children and youth with special health care needs. An array of public programs, including SSI, Medicaid, and the S-CHIP, provide an important source of support for children with special health care needs. Although almost one third of children with special health care needs are likely covered by these programs, many more are eligible but not enrolled (Kaiser Commission on Medicaid and the Uninsured, 2002). Currently, Medicaid offers the most comprehensive package of benefits. A few children are covered by both public and private insurance, and many children who are privately insured receive some services, such as special education, through the public sector.

## Health Insurance

Newacheck, McManus, Fox, Hung, and Halfon (2000) analyzed data from the 1994 to 1995 NHIS-D to assess the influence of health insurance on access to care and use of services by children with special health care needs. Children below the poverty level or whose family incomes were less than twice the poverty level were more than four times as likely to be uninsured as children whose family incomes were higher. Uninsured children were four times more likely to have unmet medical or mental health needs, and only 25% of uninsured children had seen a physician in the previous year. These authors assert, however, that inadequate access to services occurs even among children with private insurance, although to a lesser extent. The authors argue that expanding eligibility and enrollment in both private and public insurance are urgent to ensure that children with special health care needs obtain needed services. Children with special health care needs who were uninsured were disproportionately represented among low-income families (below 200% of the federal poverty level)— the target population for S-CHIP.

Using data from the recent National Survey of Children with Special Health Care Needs, Mayer, Cockrell, and Slifkin (2004) assessed the prevalence of unmet needs for routine and specialty care among CSHCN. Among respondents who reported a need for specialty care, 7.2% said they could not obtain all that they needed; 3.2% who needed routine care could not obtain it. African American children, multiracial children, and children whose mothers had not finished high school had twice the odds of having an unmet need for routine care. Similarly, children living below the federal poverty level and uninsured children were more likely to report an unmet need for routine care than children who were continuously insured. Consistent with the findings of Newacheck et al. (2000), the analysis presented by Mayer et al. (2004) emphasized the urgent need for insurance coverage that can lower financial barriers to needed care.

## S-CHIP

The S-CHIP has great potential for improving access to care for children with special health care needs by expanding access to insurance. In 1997, the S-CHIP extended health insurance to children in families with incomes below 200% of the federal poverty level that are not eligible for Medicaid, 17% of whom are estimated to have special health care needs. In passing this legislation, Congress gave states substantial flexibility in designing their programs. For example, states can choose to use Medicaid or a separate state health plan, or a combination of both, to expand insurance coverage. Within certain guidelines, states can choose eligibility levels, benefit coverage, and other program characteristics. As a result, there is wide variation in the approaches taken across states.

Schwalberg, Hill, and Mathis (2000) analyzed alternative models for insuring CSHCN under S-CHIP among five states and compared their ability to meet the needs of this population. For each site, eligibility, enrollment, identification, and referral of CSHCN; benefits; service delivery systems; payment mechanisms; and quality assurance and monitoring strategies were examined. The four models included (1) a mainstream approach that includes all enrolled children in a single system with common benefits, (2) a wrap-around model that offers a set of health care benefits that are provided in addition to a package of basic benefits, (3) a service carve-out that excludes specific services from a benefit package, and (4) a specialized system of care that was designed specifically for CSHCN and other individuals with disabilities. The authors concluded that although aimed at providing comprehensive care for all children the mainstream approach could not identify CSHCN or monitor their care. Wrap-around models offered rich benefits to CSHCN but depended on providers to identify eligible children. To date, these providers have reported few referrals. Service carve-outs present challenges for care coordination but preserve long-standing specialty systems of care for CSHCN. The authors found that specialized systems of care offer the most promise for comprehensive, coordinated care to CSHCN, despite presenting challenges for capitation. The authors conclude that comprehensive benefits, including medical and support services and care coordination, are critical features of insurance coverage and access to care. They also urge that the responsibilities of providers and service delivery systems be clearly delineated, and they note that family involvement can produce significant improvements in systems of care. The most important recommendation emerging from this study, however, is that states need clear definitions of CSHCN and methods for identifying and enrolling this population. All states found that the proportion of children enrolled in S-CHIP programs having a special need fell far below the 17% projections derived from national studies. The authors suggest that the definition of CSHCN promulgated by the MCHB is very broad and describes a range of conditions that may require services beyond strictly medical care. Thus, the 17% estimate may not be as useful for a medical insurance program, and many CSHCN may be underinsured rather than uninsured. The usefulness of S-CHIP for underinsured families with CSHCN is an area that must be explored. Although the results of this five-state study may not pertain to other S-CHIP programs, the authors argue that there are valuable lessons to be learned from this documentation about the early implementation of S-CHIP for CSHCN.

## CONCLUSION

A growing number of children and youth have special health care needs. Improved understanding of this diverse population of children and their families has generated clearer understanding of the characteristics of appropriate services and has inspired legislative, policy, and programmatic commitments to the health and welfare of these children. This understanding has reinforced the urgency of improving linkages among health, mental health, education and social services, partnerships between the private and public sectors, and support for the development of community-based services. Affirmation of the importance of comprehensive and continuous care at each developmental stage in the lifespan requires that current deliberations and decisions about the financing of care for this population are monitored and that leadership roles at state and community levels are reinforced.

# REFERENCES

Akinbami, L.J., LaFleur, B.J., & Schoendorf, K.C. (2002). Racial and income disparities in childhood asthma in the United States. *Ambulatory Pediatrics, 2,* 382–387.

Anderson, J.C., Williams, S., McGee, R., & Silva, P.A. (1989). Cognitive and social correlates of DMS-III disorders in preadolescent children. *Journal of American Academy of Child and Adolescent Psychiatry, 28,* 842–846.

Aron, L.Y., Loprest, P.J., & Steurle, C.E. (Ed.). (1995). *Serving children with disabilities: A systematic look at the programs* (p. 182). Washington, DC: Urban Institute Press.

Benedict, R.E., & Farel, A.M. (2003). Identifying children in need of ancillary and enabling services: A population approach. *Social Science & Medicine, 57,* 2035–2047.

Bethell, C.D., Read, D., Neff, J., Blumberg, S.J., Stein, R.E.K., Sharp, V., & Newacheck, P.W. (2002). Comparison of the children with special health care needs screener to the questionnaire for identifying children with chronic conditions. *Ambulatory Pediatrics, 2,* 49–57.

Boyle, C.A., Decoufle, P., & Yeargin-Allsopp, M. (1994). Prevalence and health impact of developmental disabilities in US children. *Pediatrics, 93,* 399–403.

Burns, B.J. (1999). A call for a mental health services research agenda for youth with serious emotional disturbance. *Mental Health Sciences Research, 1,* 5–20.

Burns, B.J., Costello, E.J., Angold, A., Tweed, D., Stangl, D., Farmer, E.M., & Erkanli, A. (1995). Children's mental health service use across service sectors. *Health Affairs, 14,* 147–159.

Center for Mental Health Services. (1999). *Annual report to Congress on the evaluation of the comprehensive community mental health services for children and their families program, 1999.* Atlanta, GA: ORC Macro.

Centers for Disease Control and Prevention. (1988). *International Classification of Diseases, 9th Revision, Clinical Modification ICD-9CM.* National Center for Health Statistics. Available from: http://www.cdc.gov/nchswww/about/otheract/icd9/abticd9.htm

Centers for Disease Control and Prevention. (2000). Measuring childhood asthma prevalence before and after the 1997 redesign of the national health interview survey: United States. *Morbidity Mortality Weekly Report, 49,* 908–911. Available March 23, 2004, from: http://www.cdc.gov/mmwr/preview/mmwrhtml/mm4940a2.htm

Centers for Disease Control and Prevention. (2002a). Folic acid and prevention of spina bifida and anencephaly, 10 years after the U.S. public health service recommendation. *Morbidity and Mortality Weekly Report, 51*(RR-13), 1–3.

Centers for Disease Control and Prevention. (2002b). Alcohol use among women of childbearing age: United States, 1991–1999. *Morbidity Mortality Weekly Report, 51*(13), 273–276.

Cooper, W., & Hickson, G.B. (2001). Corticosteroid prescription filling for children covered by Medicaid following an emergency department visit or a hospitalization for asthma. *Archives of Pediatrics and Adolescent Medicine, 155,* 1111–1115.

Costello, E.J., Angold, A., Burns, B.J., Stangl, D.K., Tweed, D.L., Erkanli, A., & Worthman, C.M. (1996). The Great Smoky Mountains Study of youth goals, design, methods, and the prevalence of SMI-III-R disorders. *Archives of General Psychiatry, 53,* 1129–1136.

Costello, E.J., Farmer, E.M.Z., Angold, A., Burns, B.J., & Erkanli, A. (1997). Psychiatric disorders among American Indian and white youth in Appalachia: The Great Smoky Mountains Study. *American Journal of Public Health, 87,* 827–832.

Costello, E.J., Keller, G.P., & Angold, A. (2001). Poverty, race/ethnicity, and psychiatric disorder. *American Journal of Public Health, 91,* 1494–1498.

Developmental Disabilities Services and Facilities Construction Amendments of 1970, Pub. L. No. 91-517, 84 Stat. 1316.

Developmentally Disabled Assistance and Bill of Rights Act, Pub. L. No. 94-103, 89 Stat. 486 (1975).

Education for all Handicapped Children Act, PL 94-142 (1975).

Education of the Handicapped Act Amendments of 1986, Public. L. No. PL 99-457, 100 Stat. 1145.

Farel, A.M., Hooper, S., Teplin, S., Henry, M., & Kraybill, E.N. (1998). Very-low birthweight infants at seven years: An assessment of the health and neurodevelopmental risk conveyed by chronic lung disease. *Journal of Learning Disabilities, 31*(2), 118–126.

Flisher, A.J., Kramer, R.A., Grosser, R.C., Alegria, M., Bird, R., Bourdon, K.H., Goodman, S.H., Greenwald, S., Horwitz, M., Moore, R.E., Narrow, W.E., & Hoven, C.W. (1997). Correlates of unmet need for mental health services by children and adolescents. *Psychological Medicine, 27,* 1145–1154.

Fowler, M.G., Johnson, M.P., & Atkinson, S.S. (1985). School achievement and absence in children with chronic health conditions. *Journal of Pediatrics, 106,* 683–687.

Frank Porter Graham Child Development Institute, SRI International. (2003). *National early intervention longitudinal study: Families' first experience with early intervention.* Available from: http://www.sri.com/neils/FE_Report.pdf

Friedman, R.M., Kutash, K., & Duchnowski, A.J. (1999). Prevalence of serious emotional disturbance: An update. In R.W. Manderscheid & M.J. Henderson (Eds.), *Mental Health, United States, 1998* (pp. 110–112). Rockville, MD: Department of Health and Human Services.

Gannotti, M.E., & Handwerker, W.P. (2002). Puerto Rican understandings of child disability: Methods for the cultural validation of standardized measures of child health. *Social Science & Medicine, 55,* 2093–2105.

Halfon, N., & Newacheck, P.W. (1999). Prevalence and impact of parent-reported disabling mental health conditions among U.S. children. *Journal of American Academy of Child and Adolescent Psychiatry, 38,* 600–609.

Hernandez, D.J., & Charney, E. (Eds.). (1998). From *Generation to generation: The health and well-being of children in immigrant families.* Washington, DC: National Academy Press.

Ireys, H.T. (1980). *The crippled children's service: A comparative analysis of four state programs.* Mental Health Policy Monograph Series No. 7. Nashville, TN: Vanderbilt Institute for Public Policy Studies, Vanderbilt University.

Kaiser Commission on Medicaid and the Uninsured. (2002, February). *Health insurance coverage in America: 2000 data update.* The Henry J. Kaiser Family Foundation. Available from: http://www.kff.org/uninsured/4007-index.cfm

Kataoka, S.H., Zhang, L., & Wells, K.B. (2002). Unmet need for mental health care among US children: Variation by ethnicity and insurance status. *American Journal of Psychiatry, 159,* 1548–1555.

Maguire, K., & Pastore, A.L. (Eds.). (1999). *Sourcebook of criminal justice statistics, 1999.* US Department of Justice, Bureau of Justice Statistics, Washington, DC: US Government Printing Office.

Mayer, M.L., Cockrell, A.S., & Slifkin, R.T. (2004). Unmet need for routine and specialty care: Data from the national survey of children with special health care needs. *Pediatrics, 113,* e109–e115.

McPherson, M., Arango, P., Fox, H., Lauver, C., McManus, M., Perrin, J.M., Shonkoff, J.P., Strickland, B. (1998). A new definition of children with special health care needs. *Pediatrics, 102,* 137–141.

Mesibov, L. (1994, Summer). What's so special about special education? *School Law Bulletin.*

Moore, P., & Hepworth, J.T. (1994). Use of perinatal and infant health services by Mexican-American Medicaid enrollees. *Journal of American Medical Association, 272,* 297–304.

Mulero, A., & Font, A. (1997). Pediatric physical therapy services in Puerto Rico. *Pediatric Physical Therapy, 7,* 172–174.

National Commission on Childhood Disability. (1995, October). *Supplemental Security Income for children with disabilities report to Congress.* Washington, DC: US Government Printing Office.

National Health Interview Survey-Child Health Supplement. (1988). Rockville, MD: National Center for Health Statistics.

National Health Interview Survey-Disability Supplement. (1994). Rockville, MD: National Center for Health Statistics.

Newacheck, P.W., & Halfon, N. (1998). Prevalence and impact of disabling chronic conditions in childhood. *American Journal of Public Health, 88,* 610–617.

Newacheck, P.W., & Taylor, W.R. (1992). Childhood chronic illness: Prevalence, severity, and impact. *American Journal of Public Health, 82,* 364–370.

Newacheck, P.W., Strickland, B., Shonkoff, J.P., Perrin, J.M., McPherson, M., McManus, M., Lauver, C., Fox, H., & Arango, P. (1998). An epidemiologic profile of children with special health care needs. *Pediatrics, 102,* 117–123.

Newacheck, P.W., McManus, M., Fox, H.B., Hung, Y., & Halfon, N. (2000). Access to health care for children with special health care needs. *Pediatrics, 105,* 760–766.

Newacheck, P.W., Hung, Y.Y., & Wright, K.K. (2002). Racial and ethnic disparities in access to care for children with special health care needs. *Ambulatory Pediatrics, 2,* 247–254.

Newacheck, P.W., Stein, R.E.K., Bauman, L., & Hung, Y.Y. (2003). Disparities in the prevalence of disability between black and white children. *Archives of Pediatrics and Adolescent Medicine, 157,* 244–248.

Omnibus Budget Reconciliation Act of 1989, Sec. 501. [42 U.S.C. 701].

*Pennsylvania Association for Retarded Children v. Pennsylvania,* 343 R Supp. 279 E.D. Pa. (1972).

Perrin, J., & Stein, R.E.K. (1991). Reinterpreting disability: Changes in Supplemental Security Income for children. *Pediatrics, 87,* 1047–1051.

Personal Responsibility and Work Opportunity Reconciliation Act of 1996, Pub. L. No. 104-193, 110 Stat. 2105.

Rehabilitation, Comprehensive Services, and Developmental Disabilities Amendments of 1978, PL 95-602, 92 Stat. 2955.

Richardson, S.A., & Koller, H. (1994). Mental retardation. In I.B. Pless (Ed.), *The epidemiology of childhood disorders.* Oxford: Oxford University Press.

Schulzinger, R. (1998). *Advocates guide to SSI for children* (3rd ed.). Washington, DC: Judge David L. Bazelon Center for Mental Health Law.

Schwalberg, R., Hill, I., & Mathis, S.A. (2000). New opportunities, new approaches: Serving children with special health care needs under S-CHIP. *Health Services Research, 35*(5) Part III, 102–111. Available from: http://www.hospitalconnect.com/hsr/Volume35.html

Section 504 of the Rehabilitation Act of 1973, PL 98-112, 29 U.S.C. 794.

Shapiro, J.P. (1993). *No pity: People with disabilities forging a new civil rights movement.* New York: Times Books, Random House.

Simpson, G. (1993, January). *Determining childhood disability and special needs children in the 1994–95 NHIS survey on disability.* Paper presented at the winter meeting of the American Statistical Association, Fort Lauderdale, FL.

Stein, R.E.K., Bauman, L.J., Westbrook, L.E., Coupey, S.M., & Ireys, H.T. (1993). Framework for identifying children who have chronic conditions: the case for a new definition. *Journal of Pediatrics, 122,* 342–347.

Stein, R.E.K., Westbrook, L., & Bauman, L. (1997). The questionnaire for identifying children with chronic conditions: A measure based on a noncategorical approach. *Pediatrics, 99,* 513–521.

*Sullivan v. Zebley,* 88-1377 (US Supreme Court, 20 February) (1990).

Trohanis, P. (2002). *Progress in providing services to young children with special needs and their families* (NECTAC Notes No. 12). Chapel Hill: University of North Carolina, FPG Child Development Institute, National Early Childhood Technical Assistance Center.

US Census Bureau, Population Division, Population Projections Branch. (2000). *Projections of the resident population by race, Hispanic origin, and nativity: Middle series, 1999 and 2000.* Available March 23, 2004, from: http://www.census.gov/population/www/projections/natsum-T5.html

US Department of Health and Human Services. (1999). *Mental health: A report of the Surgeon General.* Rockville, MD: Substance Abuse and Mental Health Services Administration, Center for Mental Health Services, NIH, National Institute of Mental Health.

US Department of Health and Human Services. (2000, November). *Healthy People 2010: Understanding and improving health* (2nd Ed.). Washington, DC: US Government Printing Office. Available March 23, 2004, from: http://www.health.gov/healthypeople/

van Dyck, P.C., McPherson, M., Strickland, B.B., Nesseler, K., Blumberg, S.J., Cynamon, M.L., & Newacheck, P.W. (2002). The national survey of children with special health care needs. *Ambulatory Pediatrics, 2,* 29–37.

Williams, D.R. (2000). Understanding and addressing racial disparities in health care. *Health Care Financing Review, 21,* 75–90.

Zambrana, R.E., & Logie, L.A. (2000). Latino child health: Need for inclusion in the US national discourse. *American Journal of Public Health, 90,* 1827–1833.

# 12

# Issues in Maternal and Child Health Nutrition

*Janice Dodds and Barbara Laraia*

*Our lives are not in the lap of the gods, but in the lap of our cooks.*
(Lin Yutang, 1937)

## INTRODUCTION

Nutrition is a critical component in any discussion of the health status of the maternal and child health (MCH) population. Physical growth is anticipated and desired in all subgroups of children and among pregnant women. Women who are between pregnancies or who do not become pregnant during their child-bearing years focus on achieving or maintaining their optimal nutrition status. Good nutrition is biologically central to growth in that it provides the elements for building and repairing tissue and is required for the metabolic processes that mediate tissue development. If there is not adequate repair or growth, the body becomes dysfunctional. An inadequately nourished child becomes a sick child, one who listens poorly in or is absent from school. If prolonged, inadequate nutrition during pregnancy and early childhood can affect the brain's development and functioning. In older children and adults, malnutrition can give rise to cardiovascular disease, and an excess of certain nutrients can accelerate the disease process in cancer-prone sites.

Underlying the following discussion, but beyond the scope of this textbook, is basic nutrition assessment methods, including dietary intake, growth status, and tissue levels of nutrients. Measures of dietary intake include 3-day food records, food frequency, 24-hour recall, and dietary history techniques. Measures of growth, such as height and weight, can be combined into a body mass index (BMI) or compared with a growth chart. There are also tissue measures such as bioelectrical impedance to measure fat and muscle, bone densitometry, and biochemical measures of serum levels such as hemoglobin, hematocrit, cholesterol, triglycerides, vitamin A, protein, and glucose.

The knowledge base of nutrition is expanding at an accelerated rate with the application of technology to all phases of research into metabolism, food composition, dietary intake, and food behavior. Each of these areas is relevant to MCH issues. The reader is referred to the maternal and child nutrition texts noted in the bibliography, which are regularly updated for a discussion of the full range of nutrition topics in these populations.

The chapter begins with three salient MCH nutrition issues. Historically, getting enough calories in amount and type that support health has been a problem in the United States. One continues to see hunger among families with children confronting a variety of social and environmental problems, including poverty, absent nutrition education, the disintegration of families and communities, and inadequate accessibility to service programs. An even greater problem in terms of frequency is childhood obesity. Although the federal government has established in *Healthy People 2010* (US Department of Health and Human Services [US DHHS], 2000a) that the United States should decrease obesity among children and adults by the year 2010, in 2000, it continues to rise. Many combinations of factors support this trend and are discussed in this chapter, including sedentary lifestyles, widespread food availability, and a bewildering variety of food products. Finally, this section closes with the issue of breastfeeding. The evidence of the positive impact of breastfeeding for any length of time continues to mount; nevertheless, the prevalence of breastfeeding in the United States is inadequate. The issue of breastfeeding provides an excellent example of the problems and potential of population-level strategies to support the individual nutrition decisions that families make. Without community support for breastfeeding, mothers and families would find it difficult to sustain.

Food and nutrition policies and programs are built from two dietary strategies, the Estimated Average Requirements and food guides. The Estimated Average Requirements provide the scientific foundation for all judgments about the adequacy of dietary intake. A food guide is the consumer information that advises people about their food selection over the course of a day. The Basic Four Food Groups were the prevailing instructions for a number of years but were replaced in 1993 by the Food Guide Pyramid, which is being revised in 2005. Government food and nutrition programs also articulate national policy. Three such programs, heavily used by women and children—the Special Supplemental Nutrition Program for Women, Infants, and Children (WIC), School Meal Programs, and the Food Stamp Program (FSP)—are described later here.

Food and nutrition problems are often difficult to solve because of the number of factors that play a role in their etiology and maintenance. The Social Process Model described at the end of this chapter is an ecologic model that when applied to food and nutrition systems can describe the diverse factors that may be thwarting or impeding solutions. The model describes three processes in sociological systems—the economic, the political, and the cultural. When the Social Process Model is used to describe the food and nutrition systems, the absence or overactivity of a process can illuminate the source of a problem.

# THREE MCH NUTRITION ISSUES

## Hunger in America

### Hunger from the 1930s to 1960s

Hunger has existed throughout US history. The nation has grappled with being hungry as the pioneers built this country, through war and famine, and as a result of poverty. It is in more recent history—1930s to present— that the country has struggled to make sense of why a nation with so much still cannot meet the needs of the least of its citizens.

It was during the Depression of the 1930s that federal domestic food assistance was first developed as a way to meet the needs of the unemployed and to answer the emotional outrage that the problem of hunger created. Communities battled the problem by starting soup kitchens, canneries, gleaning projects, and food baskets. However, this was not enough.

The agricultural sector had been concerned about large food surpluses throughout the 1920s. In the 1930s, food rotted, whereas many Americans went hungry. The government tried to control the agricultural problem by price depressing farm surpluses. Finally came the disposal of farm surpluses, backed by the Agriculture Department, to maintain the income of large-scale commercial farmers. The Agriculture Committees in Congress appropriated money, coined "farmers' money," to support this disposal. This became "the paradox of want amid plenty."

The first attempt at federal food assistance was through the Red Cross during the Hoover Administration (1929–1933). This measure was resisted by both Hoover and the Congress until they were confronted by the cost of surplus storage; the waste caused by rodents, insects, and decay; and the outrage of the American people. Finally, wheat from the Farm Board was distributed to the unemployed.

During the Roosevelt Administration (1933–1945), a continuous food assistance program was created. Congress had made many unsuccessful attempts at trying to deal with the problems of both hunger and surplus food. In the end, Roosevelt announced that the government would purchase a "wide variety" of surplus and have it distributed to the unemployed. The surplus commodity procurement and distribution project was formed and lasted for 30 years. Even today the fundamental problem exists of focusing on surplus crops and not on the nutritional needs of the citizenry (Poppendieck, 1992).

During the 1930s, 1940s, and 1950s, the government continued to address hunger and nutrition through the distribution of surplus agricultural commodities (Table 12–1). After World War II, hunger was ignored until President Kennedy, in response to a campaign promise, outlined a program to expand food distribution by piloting the FSP in eight counties. In 1964, under President Johnson, the FSP became permanent, and in 1966, the School Breakfast Program was established.

The 1960s brought about much change, but the single most powerful event that caused the public to refocus its concern over hunger was the release by the Field Foundation of *Hunger, USA* in 1968 (Citizens Board of Inquiry into Hunger and Malnutrition in the US, 1968). This report, and its accompanying television documentary, showed widespread malnutrition and hunger in the rural South, and once again, this raised national recognition of hunger.

**Table 12-1** Selected Events in the History of Federal Policies to Address Hunger in the United States

| | |
|---|---|
| 1930 | US Department of Agriculture (USDA) and Federal Emergency Relief Administration distribute surplus agricultural commodities as food relief through Federal Surplus Relief Corporation. |
| 1933 | Congress creates the Agricultural Adjustment Administration to control farm prices and production and the Federal Surplus Relief Corporation to distribute surplus farm products to needy families. |
| 1935–1942 | Congress provides for continued operation of Federal Surplus Commodities Corporation, which under USDA, purchases commodities for distribution to state welfare agencies. |
| 1936–1942 | The Amendments to Agricultural Act permit food donations to school lunches. |
| 1939–1943 | The Federal Surplus Commodities Corporation initiates an experimental FSP. |
| 1946 | The National School Lunch Program is established. |
| 1954 | Special Milk Program is established. |
| 1955 | The USDA determines that the average low-income family spends one third of after-tax income on food. |
| 1961 | President Kennedy expands use of surplus food for needy people at home and abroad and announces eight pilot FSPs. |
| 1964 | Congress establishes the national FSP. The Social Security Administration establishes poverty line at three times the cost of USDA's lowest cost Economy Food Plan. Since 1969, values are adjusted according to the Consumer Price Index. |
| 1966 | The Child Nutrition Act passes. President Johnson outlines Food for Freedom program. |
| 1968–1977 | The Senate establishes Select Committee on Nutrition and Human Needs to lead nation's antihunger efforts. |
| 1968–1970 | Ten-State and Preschool Nutrition Surveys and *Hunger, USA* report evidence of malnutrition among children in poverty. |
| 1969 | President Nixon announces the "war on hunger" and holds a White House Conference on Food, Nutrition, and Health. The USDA establishes the Food and Nutrition Service to administer federal food assistance programs. |
| 1971 | Results of the Ten-State Survey released to Congress indicate a high risk of malnutrition among low-income groups. |
| 1972 | Congress authorizes the Special Supplemental Food Program for WIC. |
| 1975 | School Breakfast Program is initiated and becomes permanent. |
| 1977 | Food and Agricultural Act and Child Nutrition and National School Lunch Amendments are passed. |
| 1981 | The USDA establishes a small demonstration project for commodity distribution, the Special Supplemental Dairy Distribution Program. |

*continues*

**Table 12-1** Selected Events in the History of Federal Policies to Address Hunger in the United States (continued)

| | |
|---|---|
| 1981–1982 | Congress passes the Omnibus Budget Reconciliation Acts, Omnibus Farm Bill, and Tax Equity and Fiscal Responsibility Act, which eliminate, restrict, and reduce food and income benefits. |
| 1983 | The Special Supplemental Dairy Distribution Program becomes institutionalized as the Temporary Emergency Food Assistance Program. |
| 1984 | President's Task Force on Food Assistance finds little evidence of widespread or increasing undernutrition but concludes that hunger exists and is intolerable in the United States. |
| 1986 | The General Accounting Office finds that method flaws discredit findings of the Physician Task Force on Hunger that hunger is prevalent in counties with low food stamp participation rates. |
| 1988 | The US DHHS publishes *Surgeon General's Report on Nutrition and Health*, which states that lack of access to an appropriate diet should not be a health problem for any American. Congress passes the Hunger Prevention Act, increasing eligibility and benefits for Food Stamps, Child Care, and Temporary Emergency Food Assistance Program programs. |
| 1989 | The House Select Committee on Hunger holds hearings on food security in the United States. |
| 1991 | Mickey Leland Childhood Hunger Relief Act (HR-1202, S-757) is introduced. |

Source: Nestle & Guttmacher (1992a).

### Hunger Held in Abeyance—1970s

The Select Committee on Nutrition and Human Needs, chaired by Senator George McGovern, was appointed by the Senate the same year that *Hunger, USA* was released. Its charter was to eliminate hunger. Food assistance for families, children, and the older population was expanded. The Special Supplemental Food Program for WIC and congregate and home-delivered meal programs were initiated, and the school lunch program was expanded. In 1978, the Field Foundation sent its hunger investigation teams back to the same sites they had visited in 1968–1969. They found that hunger had greatly diminished and that nutrition programs were reaching the at-risk communities they had studied. As a result, hunger was considered to be virtually abolished in America during the 1970s (Brown & Allen, 1988; Nestle & Guttmacher, 1992b).

### Re-emergence of Hunger—1980s

During the early 1980s, many studies and reports documented a resurgence of hunger in America, especially among families with children.

Among the organizations reporting on hunger were the US Conference of Mayors, the USDA, the US General Accounting Office, the United Church of Christ, the Salvation Army, the Working Group on Hunger and Poverty of the National Council of Churches, Bread for the World, the Citizens Commission on Hunger in New England, Save the Children Foundation, Second Harvest, the Food Research and Action Center (FRAC), and the Physicians' Task Force on Hunger in America. A faltering US economy, accompanied by cuts in federal assistance programs, had increased the demand on emergency food during this time.

President Ronald Reagan appointed a Task Force on Food Assistance in 1983 as a result of the attention that many of these studies and reports drew to this issue. The task force confirmed that serious hunger exists in America but stated that it could not determine to what extent (Brown & Allen, 1988).

One of the largest obstacles in studying hunger was the lack of a clear definition and an acceptable measure of hunger. In 1984, the Connecticut Association for Human Services—with the help of a distinguished panel of child health and research experts—developed a scientifically valid design for a study of hunger among low-income families with children under the age of 12 years. A national replication of this study, known as the Community Childhood Hunger Identification Project (CCHIP), was initiated in 18 sites across the United States under the coordination of FRAC (Food Research and Action Center, 1995).

## Current Research

Beginning in the late 1980s, advocates, academics, and government officials worked to define, operationalize, and measure the extent of hunger in the United States. The first CCHIP study was conducted between February 1989 and August 1990. What made it unique was the use of a uniform definition of hunger applied to a nationwide study. Hunger was defined as "the mental and physical condition that comes from not eating enough food due to insufficient economic, family or community resources" (Food Research and Action Center, 1995, p. 2). An eight-item indicator was used to estimate the prevalence of hunger among US children. Twelve percent of families with children younger than 12 years old in the United States experienced hunger, with an additional 28% of families estimated to be at-risk of hunger. The series of CCHIP studies found child hunger to be associated with poor school attendance, poor concentration, fatigue, irritability, dizziness, frequent headaches, ear infections, frequent colds, and unwanted weight loss (Food Research and Action Center, 1995).

In 1990, the Office of Life Science published the definitions for food security, food insecurity, and hunger. Working with these definitions, questionnaires were developed to assist in the measurement of child and household hunger (Table 12–2).

The Cornell/Radimer scale was also created during this time and was developed from qualitative studies with low-income women from upstate New York. Three dimensions of food insecurity were identified: physiologic, social, and psychologic. Indicators of food insecurity included worrying about having enough meals, skipping meals, and being able to acquire foods in socially acceptable ways and defined hunger as "the inability to acquire or consume an adequate quality or sufficient quantity of food in socially acceptable ways, or the uncertainty that one will be able to do so" (Radimer, Olson, Greene, Campbell, & Habicht, 1992, p. 395). The CCHIP and Cornell/Radimer questions were piloted with other questions in the 1995 Current Population Survey. An 18-item scale was created that could categorize households as food secure, food insecure, food insecure with moderate hunger, and food insecure with severe hunger (Carlson, Andrews, & Bickel, 1999; Hamilton et al., 1997) (Table 12–3).

Since the piloting of the 18-item food security scale, the USDA has monitored the prevalence of food security in the United States. In 1995, there was a 12% prevalence rate of food insecurity. Of that, 4% were food insecure with hunger. In 2002, the prevalence rates were not much better;

---

**Table 12–2** Definitions of Food Security, Food Insecurity, and Hunger

*Food security* is the access by all people at all times to enough food for an active, healthy life. Food security includes at a minimum: (1) the ready availability of nutritionally adequate and safe foods and (2) an assured ability to acquire acceptable food in socially acceptable ways (e.g., without resorting to emergency food supplies, scavenging, stealing, and other coping strategies).

*Food insecurity* exists whenever the availability of nutritionally adequate and safe foods or the ability to acquire acceptable foods in socially acceptable ways is limited or uncertain.

*Hunger* is the uneasy or painful sensation caused by a lack of food. Hunger and malnutrition are potential, although not necessary, consequences of food insecurity.

Source: Anderson (1990, p. 1560).

---

### Table 12–3  USDA Core Food Security Module

1. "I worried whether our food would run out before I got money to buy more." Was that *often* true, *sometimes* true, or *never* true for your household in the last 12 months?
2. "The food that I bought just didn't last, and I didn't have money to get more."
3. "I couldn't afford to eat balanced meals."
4. "I relied on only a few kinds of low-cost food to feed our children because we were running out of money to buy food."
5. "I couldn't feed our children a balanced meal because I couldn't afford that."
6. "Our children were not eating enough because we just couldn't afford enough food."
7. In the last 12 months, did you ever cut the size of your meals or skip meals because there wasn't enough money for food?
8. How often did this happen—almost every month, some months, or only 1 or 2 months?
9. In the last 12 months, did you ever eat less than you felt you should because there wasn't enough money to buy food?
10. In the last 12 months, were you ever hungry but didn't eat because you couldn't afford enough food?
11. In the last 12 months, did you lose weight because you didn't have enough money for food?
12. In the last 12 months, did you ever not eat for a whole day because there wasn't enough money for food?
13. How often did this happen—almost every month, some months, or only 1 or 2 months?
14. In the last 12 months, did you ever cut the size of any of the children's meals because there wasn't enough money for food?
15. In the last 12 months, did any of the children ever skip meals because there wasn't enough money for food?
16. How often did this happen—almost every month, some months, or only 1 or 2 months?
17. In the last 12 months, were the children ever hungry but you just couldn't afford more food?
18. In the last 12 months, did any of the children ever not eat for a whole day because there wasn't enough money for food?

---

Source: Hamilton et al. (1997).

11.1% of US households are food insecure, and of that portion, 3.5% experience food insecurity with hunger (Nord, Andrews, & Carlson, 2003). Twenty percent of US children live in these food insecure households (Bickel, Carlson, & Nord, 1999).

Food insecurity has several consequences in childhood. Food insufficiency has been associated with poor dietary intake, frequent headaches, and stomachaches among children (Alaimo, Briefel, Frongillo, & Olson, 1998). In addition, it is associated with repeating a grade, poor cognitive ability, poor academic performance, and poor mental health among children and adolescents (Alaimo, Olson, & Frongillo, 2001a; Alaimo, Olson, Frongillo, & Briefel, 2001b). Food insecurity has inconsistently been associated with overweight among children (Aliamo, Olson, & Frongillo, 2001c; Casey, Szeto, Lensing, Bogle, & Weber, 2001; Jones, Jahns, Laraia, & Haughton 2003).

Food insecurity has also been associated with *increased* body mass (Olson, 1999) and an increase in overweight and a risk of obesity among women (Adams, Grummer-Strawn, & Chavez, 2003; Townsend, Peerson, Love, Achterberg, & Murphy, 2001). Depending on the measure used, this relationship does not always hold up. Using a one-item "concern about having enough food" from the Behavior Risk Factor Surveillance System, concern about enough food and overweight has been inconsistently associated (Laraia, Siega-Riz, & Evensen, 2004; Centers for Disease Control and Prevention, 2003). An association between food insecurity and being overweight has not been found for men; however, food insecurity has been associated with being underweight in men (Vozoris & Tarasuk, 2003). Food security has been associated with poor diabetes management, especially with the loss of food stamps (Nelson, Brown, & Lurie, 1998). It has also been associated with mental health among women (Casey et al., 2004). The phenomenon of food insecurity in US households seems to be one that influences health in a variety of ways, although the pathways are not clearly understood.

### Suggestions/Interventions

Hunger affects children physically, mentally, emotionally, and psychologically. If hunger persists, potential health care needs and the decrease in productivity that accompany prolonged hunger. Combating hunger starts at the local level. People can do several things to help fight against hunger: find out where soup kitchens and Food Banks are located; investigate other food programs, such as gleaning projects and food rescue programs; and most importantly, know that although people do not want to be poor and hungry, they often need professionals' support to break barriers. A qualitative study of hunger conducted in North Carolina found that barriers to getting help and relieving hunger included pride, the stigma of poverty, transportation, staff attitudes at social services, and discrimination. During the focus groups that the North Carolina Hunger Project held, participants frequently cited the desire for all of the public assistance programs to be more supportive of men and women who are making an effort. They also stated that as soon as they "get ahead" their benefits are cut immediately, often leaving them further behind.

## The Other Extreme—Obesity in America

Once a sign of wealth, obesity is a growing concern in most industrialized countries because it is a risk factor for many chronic diseases. Obesity is associated with coronary heart disease, hypertension, non–insulin-dependent diabetes mellitus, certain cancers, and gallbladder disease. Obesity is also associated with psychosocial problems.

### Prevalence and Incidence

Being overweight and obesity have rapidly increased over the past 3 decades to reach epidemic proportions (Flegal, Carroll, Kuczmarski, & Johnson, 1998; Mokdad, Serdula, Dietz, Bowman, Marks, & Koplan, 1999). Obesity is rising in all age and ethnic groups and in both sexes; it disproportionately affects low-income and ethnic minorities (Drewnowski & Specter, 2004; Flegal et al., 1998). Overweight is usually defined by a BMI of at least 25 to 30 kg/m$^2$. By this definition, more than 55% of adults in the United States are considered overweight. Severe overweight is indicated by a BMI of greater than 30 kg/m$^2$. Between 1976 and 1994, the number of cases of obesity alone increased more than 50%—from 14.5% of the adult population to 22.5%. Current data show that nearly 31% of adults 20 years of age and over—nearly 59 million people—have a BMI of 30 or greater compared with approximately 23% in 1994. Approximately 33% of US adult females and 28% of US adult males are obese (US Department of Health and Human Services, National Center for Health Statistics, 2002; US DHHS, 2000b).

The prevalence of overweight in the US adult population is alarming because of its impact on health, and it leads us to assess the risk of obesity among children. The prevalence of overweight among children and adolescents has more than doubled between 1980 and 1999–2002. It has increased from an estimated 7% to 16% among children ages 6 to 11 years old, whereas it has risen from 5% to 16% among adolescents ages 12 to 19 years old (National Center for Health Statistics, 2004). Obese children may be at increased risk of becoming obese adults. In a 1993 study, approximately a third (26% to 41%) of obese preschool children were obese as adults, and approximately half (42% to 63%) of obese school-age children were obese as adults. For all studies and across all ages, the risk of adult obesity was at least twice as high for obese children as for nonobese children. The risk of adult obesity was greater for children who were at higher levels of obesity and for children who were obese at older ages (Serdula et al., 1993).

Because obesity has a potentially lasting effect from childhood, the difference between overweight and overfat is important for purposes of counseling and treatment (Dietz & Robinson, 1993). Overweight is defined by a 20% increase in weight for height above ideal weight. However, weight for height does not directly measure body fat. Therefore, excess weight may be due to a large body frame and may not represent a long-term problem. Body fat is measured by triceps skinfold thickness; obesity is defined as a triceps skinfold measurement greater than the 85th percentile for age. A child who is overweight but has triceps skinfold thickness measurements within normal limits should be counseled differently than one who is overfat.

Epidemiologically, obesity occurs more in the Northeastern part of the United States, followed by the Midwest, then the South, and finally the West. The environmental effects that are strongest are found within the family. Family patterns of inactivity, parental obesity, increased socioeconomic class, higher parental education, and smaller family size are all associated with childhood obesity. Sixty to seventy percent of obese adolescents have one or both parents who are obese. Furthermore, 40% of obese adolescents have obese siblings. Many people think that obese children may have "metabolic" or "glandular" disorders, but in reality, less than 1% has these severe types of problems (Dietz & Robinson, 1993).

## Theories of Etiology

There is no clear understanding of why obesity occurs, and unfortunately, there is no one successful treatment for obesity. Many theories purport to account for the increase in obesity in recent history, and most are sketchy at best. The majority of these cite both a genetic and an environmental component to obesity. One theory is that obesity has increased with an increase of available calories per capita while there has been a decrease in energy expenditure. Available calories increased from 3,100 calories per capita from 1950 to 1959 to 3,800 calories in 2000. During this time, the percentage of calories available from fat remained consistently 40% to 43% of the diet. The per capita consumption of meats, fats, flour, and caloric sweeteners has increased between 1970 and 2000. Per capita egg consumption decreased until the mid 1990s, at which point it leveled off and dairy consumption has declined by 38% since the 1950s, mostly because of a decrease in milk consumption. Although fruits and vegetables have all increased during this same period, the greatest increase in per capita consumption has been in caloric sweeteners. Americans have become conspicuous consumers of sugar and sweet-tasting foods and beverages. Per capita consumption of caloric sweeteners—mainly sucrose (table sugar made from cane and beets) and corn sweeteners (notably high-fructose corn syrup)— increased 39%, between 1950–1959 and 2000 (USDA, 2004). The increase in the amount of food available and the increase in the amount of food consumed have a direct impact on weight management in America.

Studies have shown diet to be directly linked to obesity, to chronic diseases such as cardiovascular disease, and to some cancers. Although for most of its history the United States has been concerned that its citizens get enough food, the concern now focuses on "optimal" intake, which may be less food. Current dietary recommendations suggest no greater than 30% of calories in the diet be from fat. Moreover, studies show that a diet containing less than 20% of calories from fat can reverse disease processes. Needless to say, this greatly differs from the 40% to 43% fat diet that Americans currently are eating. It has been suggested that a clear definition of "optimal" intake reflecting a lower percentage of dietary fat might help to direct public policy in combating the ill effects of obesity and some chronic diseases (Wynder, Weisburger, & Ng, 1992).

An example of how focusing on lower "optimal" intake could help modify policy can be found in the school lunch program. As of 1993, the dietary assessment of school meals showed an average lunch contains 38% fat and 15% saturated fat. In 1995, the USDA revised the nutritional requirements of National School Lunch Program meals. Averaged over a week, school lunches must contain no more than 30% of calories from fat and less than 10% of calories from saturated fat. Schools must conform by 1996 to 1997 unless they received a waiver (USDA, 2004). The fat content of school lunches exceeds current dietary recommendations of 30% or less total fat and 10% or less saturated fat. They contain an estimated 39% of energy from total fat and 21% of energy from saturated fat. A menu that often contains ground beef is a major contributor to the total fat. A study by Snyder et al. (1994) showed a reduction in total and saturated fat by cooking, draining, and rinsing the meat with water. Draining and washing allowed an additional 25% to 30% reduction in fat after cooking while maintaining nutritive values of iron and niacin in school lunch ground beef. Innovations such as these can contribute to the reduction of the fat content of school meal programs (Snyder et al., 1994).

The greatest environmental influences on children are their parents. In a study by Klesges et al. (1991), the impact of parental influences on food selection in young children was evaluated. A wide range of foods was offered to children for lunch independent of their mothers, then again with the understanding that their mothers would monitor their selection, and finally, mothers were allowed to modify the choices of their children. This study showed that when children chose foods freely, their diets were less nutritious than when there was a threat of their mothers' watching or when their mothers modified the diet. Twenty-five percent of calories came from added sugar when children selected their own lunches. The meals were more nutritious when modified by the mothers. These were lower in total calories, lower in calories from saturated fats, and had lower sodium content. Nevertheless, even though these meals were lower in total calories and saturated fat, foods highest in nutrient content still were not selected. The overall results reveal first that children do not chose nutritious foods on their own and second that mothers focus on lowering calories but not on increasing high nutrient-dense foods (Klesges et al., 1991). Beyond food selection, parents influence children's eating behavior in other ways. Verbal prompting at mealtime, adult eating behavior, and the use of food for rewards and punishments all directly influence behavior.

Inactivity and a sedentary lifestyle also contribute to obesity. Studies by Gortmaker, Dietz, and Cheung (1990) and Kotz and Story (1994) show that increased television viewing increases the prevalence and severity of obesity. This may be explained by an increase in the number of inactive hours, as well as the effect on children of televised high-calorie food commercials. Viewing time has increased from 18 hours per week in 1968 to 25 hours per week in 1983. Viewing time may currently be as high as 40 hours per week, not including video movies, video games, or computer games (Gortmaker, Dietz, & Cheung, 1990). A study by Kotz and Story (1994) reviewed a total of 997 commercials selling a product during 52.5 hours of Saturday morning children's television. Of the commercials, 56.6% were for food, 33% were for toys, and 10.2% were for other items. Of the food advertisements,

43.6% were for foods that contained fats and sweets; 35.7% were for breads, cereals, rice, and pasta. Of the latter group, 23% were for high-sugar cereals. Fast-food restaurants comprised 10.8% of the commercials, and milk, cheese, yogurt, meats, eggs, nuts, and frozen meals totaled less than 10% of all commercials. Needless to say, the overall picture of food commercials does not comply with the USDA Food Guide Pyramid's recommendations. Food commercials encourage consumption of the foods that are least necessary in one's diet, namely, fats and sweets. Television viewing has been associated with not only an increased consumption of advertised foods, but an increase in children's requests for and parents' purchase of these foods.

### Consequences

As mentioned, obesity is associated with coronary heart disease, hypertension, non–insulin-dependent diabetes mellitus, certain cancers, and gallbladder disease. Both adults and children can experience hypercholesterolemia, hypertriglyceridemia, Blount disease and other bone diseases, and respiratory complications directly related to obesity. Obesity is also associated with psychosocial problems.

Problems with body image and discrimination have been well documented. A study conducted by Stunkard and Burt (1967) showed that the development of a negative body image takes place most often during adolescence. Although other studies have shown that overweight individuals have no greater psychologic disturbances than do nonobese persons, all studies have shown evidence of a strong prejudice against obese persons as young as 6 years old. Children have reported words such as "lazy," "dirty," "stupid," "ugly," and "lies" when describing silhouettes of obese children (Wadden & Stunkard, 1985). Discrimination against the obese was revealed in a 1966 study by results that showed less obesity in colleges than in high schools even though obese and nonobese high school students showed no differences in academic criteria or application rates (Canning, Mayer, & Mayer, 1966). Gortmaker, Must, Perrin, Sobol, and Dietz (1993) found social and economic consequences of obesity in adolescence. Obese women were less often married, had lower incomes and a higher rate of poverty than nonobese women when controlling for socioeconomic status and aptitude.

### Interventions

Studies have shown that there is no easy treatment for obesity. One of the most effective approaches thus far is a family-based behavioral intervention, which employs nutrition, exercise, and parent/child involvement (Epstein, Valoski, Wing, & McCurley, 1990). Another approach in the SHAPEDOWN program, which incorporates cognitive, behavioral, and affective techniques to help make small modifications in the diet (Mellin, Slinkard, & Irwin, 1987).

The absence of a successful treatment for obesity makes preventive measures even more important. Reducing excessive caloric intake by reducing fat in school lunches, decreasing television viewing time, and implementing nutrition education for families is a good beginning. Furthermore, the amount of exercise must also increase. Daily physical education during primary and secondary school is very important. Decreasing the amount of television viewing time will aid in a decrease in sedentary activity and lower exposure to inappropriate food commercials. Interactive nutrition education during school can help to reinforce and shape a child's eating habits. Having children involved in the solution is necessary in order to create the most effective change possible. Optimal diet and exercise are still the best preventive tools!

## The Issue of Breastfeeding

The issue of breastfeeding has become very complex in America's recent history. Although no longer an established practice in the United States, breastfeeding is widely agreed to be the best form of nourishment for a baby. Not only does breast milk have all of the necessary nutrients in the correct proportion, it also has antibacterial factors and immunoglobulins to protect the infant. These biologically active constituents of breast milk are absent from formula. Since the advent of formula at the turn of the century, the use of breastfeeding has fluctuated greatly. The industrial revolution, urbanization, glass bottles, rubber nipples, pasteurization, and refrigeration are only some of the forces that have influenced the increased use of "artificial" feeding. Whereas 58% of Americans were still breastfeeding in 1911, this figure had declined to only 38% by 1946 and was 52% in 1989 (Worthington-Roberts & Williams, 1989). The focus of this section is to review the multiple barriers to successful breastfeeding that have prevented this country from reaching the national goal of 75% breastfeeding among new mothers (US DHHS, 2000b) and to offer some suggestions for changing and combating these barriers. Contraindications to breastfeeding are also reviewed.

## Background

Despite all that is known about the benefits of breastfeeding, the practice has declined among women in the United States (Worthington-Roberts & Williams, 1989). At one point, there had been an increase in breastfeeding prevalence from the all-time low of 18% in 1966 to approximately 59% in 1984. In 1988, there were reported declines to 55% (Rassin et al., 1993; Worthington-Roberts & Williams, 1989) and to 52% in 1989 (Rassin et al., 1993). The Ross Laboratories Mother Surveys in 1984 found that determinants of breastfeeding were race, maternal education, maternal age, and geographic region. Namely, college-educated and white women and those in western states breastfed more; black women, those younger than age 20 years, and those with less education breastfed less often. The breastfeeding incidence is also declining among Hispanic women in spite of their strong cultural belief in this practice (John & Martorell, 1989; Worthington-Roberts & Williams, 1989). Rassin et al. (1993) found a decrease in breastfeeding among Hispanics with increased acculturation in the United States.

Currently, the American Academy of Pediatrics (AAP), the American Dietetic Association (ADA), and the Surgeon General all endorse breastfeeding as the optimal feeding method for healthy infants. The breastfeeding objective in *Healthy People 2010: Understanding and Improving Health* is to increase the proportion of mothers who breastfeed their babies to 75% from 64% in 1998 and to increase the proportion of mothers who breastfeed at 6 months to 50% from 29% in 1998. The baseline for black mothers was 45% at discharge from birth site and 19% at 6 months old in 1998, and for Hispanic mothers the baseline was 66% and 28%, respectively (US DHHS, 2000a). Since the new objectives were published, breastfeeding has remained constant and possibly decreasing among black mothers (Li & Grummer-Strawn, 2002; Li, Zhao, Mokdad, Barker, & Grummer-Strawn, 2003).

The AAP supports exclusive breastfeeding for the first 6 months of life. The definition of exclusive breastfeeding is that no other form of milk or food be used for the first 4 months and that breast milk be used until 1 year (or until the infant is weaned). In other words, no formula, cow's milk, or other milk substitute is recommended during the first year of life. Many studies have looked at breastfeeding using loosely constructed definitions; any breastfeeding, breastfeeding and bottle feeding, or breastfeeding for 3 to 6 months are all considered "breastfeeding." To see the effect of breastfeeding more clearly, however, many studies have used the more narrow definition of exclusive breastfeeding.

There are many reasons that the AAP so strongly encourages exclusive breastfeeding. Among them are the aforementioned properties of breast milk that protect infants against disease in general and infectious disease in particular. The protective action of breast milk is well documented during the first year of life. The potential long-term protective effects are not known. One topic of current research is to investigate the relationship between breastfeeding or bottle feeding and childhood obesity. Work done by Prentice, Lucas, Vasquez-Velasquez, Davies, and Whitehead (1988) suggested that the British DHSS and the Food and Agriculture Organization/World Health Organization/United Nations University (FAO/WHO/UNU) both recommend dietary allowances for children that overestimate energy need. The DHSS and FAO/WHO/UNU used estimates based on modified Atwater factors derived from adult diets and by the assumption that breast milk was 20% more energy dense than currently is known to be the case. Then the FAO used a 5% inflation factor above these estimates. This led to an 8% to 17% increase in energy allowance, between 1 month and 3 years, compared with what Prentice et al. (1988) found by directly measuring energy expenditure through the use of doubly labeled water ($^2H_2$ $^{18}O$).

### Barriers to Breastfeeding

Many of the initial barriers to breastfeeding occur before a woman becomes pregnant and while she is pregnant. Studies show that the sooner a woman makes a decision to breastfeed the more likely she is to breastfeed (Freed, Jones, & Schanler, 1992). Studies also show that this decision is oftentimes not encouraged or supported properly by the woman's health care provider and is influenced greatly by her "significant other." Many health care practitioners agree that "breast is best" but send a double message when they do not counsel on breastfeeding during prenatal visits.

Information is often given in the form of educational materials that may reinforce fears and frustrations associated with breastfeeding. These materials may use well-dressed, attractive models that in turn reinforce the idea that only confident, affluent women are successful at breastfeeding (Bryant, Coreil, D'Angelo, Bailey, & Lazarov, 1992). Often, information regarding breastfeeding is not consistent. Advice may vary from "don't feed any supplement" to "top off each breastfeed with a bottle" or from "feed for 10 minutes on each breast" to "let the baby feed as long as he or she wants" (Ellis, 1992a, p. 5553). A new mother can be left feeling vulnerable when she receives varied information from several sources.

Furthermore, hospital policies can greatly deter any decision to breast-feed once the baby is born. The most negative policies are "separation of mothers and infants, regular feeding intervals, timed feeds, routine or sporadic supplementation with artificial feeds, exclusion of lay support people, and the provision of equivocal information, either oral or written, regarding infant feeding" (Ellis, 1992b, p. 5554). Policies such as giving a free formula gift at discharge are not consistent from one hospital to another. Snell, Krantz, Keeton, Delgado, and Peckham (1992) found a significant decline in breastfeeding among Hispanic women who were given a free formula sample. Additional studies have been cited that show a significant decrease in breastfeeding in the first month when formula samples were given and significant declines in women who are from lower socioeconomic backgrounds, who are less educated, and who experience postpartum illness. However, at least three studies have shown no difference in breastfeeding between women who received a gift pack at hospital discharge and those who did not (Snell et al., 1992).

Other hospital policies, such as separating baby and mother after birth, lead to a more difficult time breastfeeding. The early introduction of bottles has been shown to interfere with the prolactin reflex and also to reduce the duration of breastfeeding. Prolactin is the hormone that stimulates the breast's milk-producing alveoli and is released in response to its stimulation. This "let-down" reflex may be interrupted because of interference with "proper" sucking. The sucking movement has been said to be different for a bottle and for a breast, leading to difficulty or "nipple confusion" for the baby. Poor suckling may also occur when a baby is more easily rewarded by the rapid emptying of a bottle (Newman, 1990).

The WHO/UNICEF's (World Health Organization/United Nations International Children's Emergency Fund) "Ten Steps to Successful Breastfeeding" can be used by hospitals and birthing centers as a standard of practice for more successful breastfeeding outcomes. Based on these guidelines and other criteria (such as no free formula samples), a hospital can work toward a "Baby Friendly" UNICEF designation. First, a self-appraisal tool is used to establish how baby friendly an institution is to start. This assessment tool can then be used to work toward a more baby-friendly state. After the majority of the questions of the assessment tool are answered "yes," the institution can proceed with an external assessment conducted by a multiprofessional team with expertise in breastfeeding and lactation. After the team observes and questions the administrators, staff, and patients, the institution can be designated a baby-friendly place by UNICEF. If the institution does not meet the baby-friendly external assessment criteria, which are an 80% adherence to the UNICEF criteria (Table 12–4) and at least a 75% exclusive breastfeeding rate, the administrators can sign a certificate of commitment to put in place the necessary changes by a specified date (Jones & Green, 1993).

In a meta-analysis by Pérez-Escamilla, Pollitt, Lonnerdal, and Dewey (1994), hospital-based breastfeeding interventions, such as the ones that follow the WHO/UNICEF recommendations, are found to have a beneficial effect on lactation success. This was found strongly among first-time mothers. Their results showed that commercial discharge packs had a negative effect on successful breastfeeding. Rooming-in and breastfeeding support had a positive effect on breastfeeding among first time mothers. Finally, breastfeeding on demand had a positive effect on successful lactation (Pérez-Excamilla et al., 1994).

Apart from hospital policies and protocols, societal and political influences also have a bearing on breastfeeding success. The value placed on

---

**Table 12–4** Ten Steps to Successful Breastfeeding

1. Have a written breastfeeding policy that is routinely communicated to all health care staff.
2. Train all health care staff in skills necessary to implement this policy.
3. Inform all pregnant women about the benefits and management of breastfeeding.
4. Help mothers initiate breastfeeding within one hour of birth.
5. Show mothers how to breastfeed and how to maintain lactation, even if they should be separated from their infant.
6. Give newborn infants no food or drink other than breastmilk, unless medically indicated.
7. Practice rooming-in—that is, allowing mothers and infants to remain together, 24 hours a day.
8. Encourage breastfeeding on demand.
9. Give no artificial teats or pacifiers (also called dummies or soothers) to breastfeeding infants.
10. Foster the establishment of breastfeeding support groups and refer mothers to them on discharge from the hospital or clinic.

Source: UNICEF (n.d.).

breastfeeding is reflected in workplace policies and state legislation. The presence of women in the work force has increased since the Industrial Revolution, and it continues to climb at a fast pace. In 1977, 32% of women with a child who is younger than 1 year of age worked outside the home. In 1989, the percentage had increased to 52%, and by 1998, the number rose to 59%. Employment of mothers of infants and young children could be detrimental to successful breastfeeding. However, a paucity of conclusive evidence shows that this is true. What has been shown is that some types of work interfere with breastfeeding more than others. A study by Kurinij, Shiono, Ezrine, and Rhoads (1989) of women from Washington, DC, showed that both black and white women returning to a professional job had a longer duration of breastfeeding after leaving the hospital compared with women returning to sales or technical jobs. The author suggests that professional women have more control over their situation and can achieve a balance between the demands of the job and the demands of breastfeeding, whereas the women who hold clerical, sales, or technical positions have little control over their environment and have more difficulty acclimating to the demands of the job and of breastfeeding (Kurinij et al., 1989).

A study by Moore and Jansa (1987) surveyed 29 Fortune 500 companies and phone interviewed 12 of the companies known to support breastfeeding to examine the types and prevalence of policies that help to support women who breastfeed. The study was small and not generalizable. It did, however, find that of the 25 who responded to the mailed surveys, 48% had refrigeration, 14% allowed infants to breastfeed at work, 14% had health care professionals on site, and 5% had electric breast pumps. None had either day care or breaks for breastfeeding. Of the 12 companies interviewed by phone, 63% had refrigeration, 43% provided space to breastfeed, 75% had health care professionals, and 50% had electric pumps. Again, none had either daycare or breaks for breastfeeding. The authors note that there is not generalized support for breastfeeding, nor is there a national parental leave policy for this purpose. Because the country is without a standard of procedure for maternity leave and breastfeeding practice, obtaining the goal of increasing breastfeeding incidence to 75% by the year 2000 will be very difficult. Additionally, more research, with the involvement of institutions, needs to be conducted in this area to measure effectiveness of breastfeeding programs (Moore & Jansa, 1987).

Beyond the hospital and the workplace, social influences on breastfeeding can include the use of the law. Currently, four states protect the right of women to breastfeed in public: Florida, New York, North Carolina, and California. Until 1994, when Florida passed a law to enhance breastfeeding services in hospitals, encouraging baby-friendly designations and permitting breastfeeding in public, breastfeeding was officially viewed as indecent exposure by this state, as it is in many others. New York, North Carolina, and California have followed Florida's example.

Within the Hispanic population in the United States, there has been a marked decline in breastfeeding. The strongest association with this decline is with increased acculturation. The Mexican American component of the Hispanic Health and Nutrition Examination Survey was used to study the incidence and duration of breastfeeding. It was shown that English-speaking Hispanic households, which reflect a high degree of acculturation, had a lower rate of breastfeeding than did Spanish-speaking households. Furthermore, when the head of the household identified himself or herself as a Mexican American, another indicator of acculturation, there was a negative association with breastfeeding compared with those designating themselves as Mexican, Hispanic, Chicano, Puerto Rican, Cuban, or of another country (John & Martorell, 1989). A study by Rassin et al. (1993) also found that individuals with a lower level of acculturation—as measured by language, time in the United States, and association with other Hispanic people—breastfed more. Clearly, modern American society works in a myriad of ways to discourage breastfeeding, even among those culturally predisposed to breastfeed. Effecting change and promoting breastfeeding challenge the public health establishment and the nation.

## Contraindications

Physiologically, almost all women can breastfeed. Ninety-nine percent of women who try breastfeeding are successful. There are very rare instances when a woman cannot breastfeed because of pathophysiologic reasons. There are other reasons, however, that a woman may not be able to breastfeed or should be advised against breastfeeding. Four such contraindications are most notable. The first three are that breastfeeding is not appropriate when a mother is addicted to drugs, such as cocaine or PCP, when a mother takes more than a minimal amount of alcohol, or when a mother is receiving certain therapeutic or diagnostic agents, such as radioactive elements and cancer chemotherapy.

In addition, women infected with human immunodeficiency virus (HIV) should not breastfeed to avoid transmission of HIV to a child who may not be infected (Anonymous, 1993). However, this is not the case in situations in which there is an otherwise high infant morbidity and mortality due to infectious diseases and malnutrition (Anonymous, 1993; Kennedy et al., 1990). A meta-analysis of four studies of women who seroconverted to HIV positivity postnatally, either through blood transfusion at birth or by heterosexual transfer, showed that the estimated risk of transmitting HIV through breast milk is 29% (95% CI, 16% to 42%). This study also revealed that breastfeeding, when there was a positive HIV status prenatally, increased the risk of transmission in utero or during delivery by 14% (95% CI, 7% to 22%) (Dunn, Newell, Ades, & Pechkham, 1992). The exact mechanism of transmission is not known. Transmission may take place after contact with the HIV before the mother makes antibodies or when the mother is manifesting disease symptoms. In any case, where high infant death rates are attributable to infectious diseases, namely diarrhea, the mortality rate from bottle feeding can be as high as 15/100,000, with a relative risk of 4, producing twice as many deaths (Kennedy et al., 1990). Therefore, because the risk of not breastfeeding outweighs the risk of infection with HIV, breastfeeding should be promoted, even where the HIV epidemic is severe (Dunn et al., 1992; Goldfarb, 1993; Kennedy et al., 1990). Additional investigation is needed to define clearly the risks attributable to breastfeeding and the timing of transmission through breastfeeding (ADA, 2001).

## POLICIES AND PROGRAMS

Nutrition policy and programs are influenced by agriculture policy, food policy, and politics. The issue of food access and availability has become emotionally, morally, and economically based. This section reviews the history and application of two nutrition policies—the Food Guide Pyramid and the Estimated Average Requirement. Furthermore, two examples of program delivery to achieve these policies are illustrated in the context of MCH.

There are two primary nutrition program strategies in the United States: education or dietary guidance and the delivery of food, in bulk or prepared. Nutrition programs usually consider both. Generally, if food is delivered, it is not without dietary and nutrition information. In the recent past, nutritionists emphasized nutrition in education strategies; however, there is a growing trend to emphasize making food nutritious, tasty, convenient, and easy to prepare. Such messages are more likely to be received with enthusiasm and to succeed in terms of participation and dietary change.

## Dietary Guidance

Within the discipline of nutrition, two central tools are the basis of food and nutrition education: the food guide and the Estimated Average Requirement. The food guide describes the type of food and amounts for daily consumption. Currently, the Food Guide Pyramid (Figure 12–1),

# A Guide to Daily Food Choices

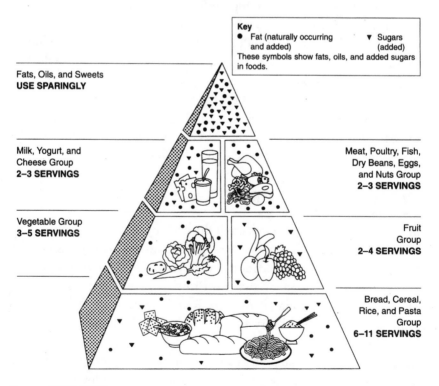

Source: DHHS (1992).

FIGURE 12–1 The food guide pyramid.

which divides food into five categories with a sixth being foods to avoid or eat in small amounts, is the basis of the US government's nutrition education policy.

## Food Guides

### History and Purpose

Food guides were first developed in the United States in the 1923 and consisted of five groups. They were developed to help lay people ascertain whether they were eating enough of the right foods to prevent nutrition deficiencies. During the war years, food was scarcer, and careful planning was necessary in order to maintain nutrition adequacy in the population. In fact, it was the discovery after the war that more men than expected failed their physical examinations because of undernutrition that led to the establishment of the national school lunch and milk programs to prevent this problem in the future.

In the 1950s, when the food guide grouping was reorganized and simplified from seven groups to four, it became known as the Basic Four and was central for nutrition education in schools. Nearly every adult was taught the Basic Four, and it was used by food companies in advertising and packaging. It was not until the early 1970s that nutritionists recognized that excess food intake rather than deficiencies was the primary dietary problem in the United States. Because the Basic Four did not include fat or sugar, people assumed that they could eat as much of these as they wanted. The shift to address excess dietary intake began with the publication of Dietary Goals by the Senate Select Committee on Hunger in 1977 (US Senate Select Committee, 1977). It was not until the 1980s, when the administrative arms of the government, the USDA and the US DHHS, officially released the Dietary Guidelines, establishing them as policy, that programs began to teach moderation energetically. However, the Dietary Guidelines are not helpful in planning a meal, a day's intake of food, or a weekly food list. For that reason, the USDA released the Food Pyramid in 1992, which provides dietary guidance to those who wish to eat for their own health and to assist others in doing so (Figure 12–1).

### Policy and the Pyramid

As mentioned earlier, nutrition policy is influenced by agriculture policy, food policy, and politics. The changes in the Food Guide Pyramid were scrutinized and debated at every turn. Agricultural interests had a substantial influence on the changes (Nestle, 1993). Two commodity groups—dairy and meat—resisted the efforts to limit consumption of their foods even though scientific evidence showed a strong association between animal fat, notably saturated fat, and cardiovascular disease. Initially, dietary cholesterol alone was the focus for dietary change, and people were advised to eat no more than three or four eggs a week. As studies demonstrating the relationship between saturated fat and cardiovascular disease proliferated, nutritionists began advising individuals to reduce cholesterol and saturated fat by selecting reduced fat milk, preferably skim milk, and low-fat yogurt and limiting meat intake to two to three servings of two to three ounces per day, red meat only three times a week. By 1990, meat consumption was down from 158.7 pounds per capita in 1970 to 130.2 pounds per capita (Raper et al., 1992). Egg consumption has also decreased from 39.2 pounds per capita in 1970 to 29.6 per capita in 1990. In the mid 1980s, meat consumption leveled off as a result of a high-visibility media campaign but resumed its decline after 1985. The beverage milk trend is toward lower fat milk. Whole milk represented 92% of all beverage milk (plain, flavored, and buttermilk) in the 1950s, but its share dropped to 36% in 2000. The dairy industry now offers several reduced fat products containing 1% milk fat or less. During 1970 to 1979, the average whole-milk consumption in the United States was 21.7 gallons per capita. In 1998, it was 8.3. Low-fat milk went from 8.1 gallons per capita to 15.4 during the same time period.

### Implications for MCH

Nutrition has become one of four factors that consumers use in selecting food products, the others being taste, convenience, and price (Food Marketing Institute, 1995). For this reason, after the release of the pyramid, it quickly appeared on food packages. Consumer materials produced by the food industry and trade associations appeared even before USDA materials. The adoption of this new dietary guidance material was immediate and pervasive. The categories of the pyramid are based enough on visible characteristics that children can learn them as well as adults. It can be used both to categorize items in a snack or meal and as a basis for art activities and trips to stores, expanding children's familiarity with foods. The pyramid is the basis of team games in school and the content of games modeled after television quiz shows. The *Journal of Nutrition*

*Education and Behavior* publishes reports of these applications regularly. These can be accessed through PubMed.

## Nutrient Intake Standards

### History and Purpose

The second tool integral to food and nutrition education in the United States are the Dietary Reference Intakes (DRIs). The DRIs differ from the Food Guides with a focus on specific nutrient intakes instead of food portion sizes. The Recommended Dietary Allowances (RDAs), the precursor to DRIs, were adopted in 1941 after the National Nutrition Conference and were published by the Food and Nutrition Board of the National Academy of Sciences. They are reviewed every 10 years. They are the standard against which to measure dietary adequacy and include the vitamins, minerals, and calories for which there are enough data to establish a recommended daily dietary intake for various age and gender groups. One or two nutrients are added with each revision as the scientific literature provides adequate evidence of the critical role of those nutrients and the amount the human body requires.

### Characteristics

In the most recent publication of the DRIs, there were 30 nutrients that were discussed in eight volumes. The reference values published included five new values—the Estimated Average Requirement, Estimated Energy Requirement, Adequate Intake, Acceptable Macronutrient Distribution Range, and Tolerable Upper Intake Level—and one familiar value, the Recommended Dietary Allowance.

### Issues

Although the field of nutrition describes the nutritional status of the population more precisely each year, the food supply is changing at a rapid pace. Computer technology is providing the system to distribute quickly new information about the nutrient content of foods. The Food Labeling Act of 1992 mandated a rapid change in the nutrition information required on food labels, and food composition analysis technology and rapid information exchange made implementation possible within the proposed time frame of 2 years. With the advent of methods to substitute noncaloric sweeteners for sugar and to introduce fat substitutes with acceptable texture and flavor compounds, food product innovations multiplied in food markets.

Research studies have shown associations between dietary intake and certain disease conditions. Scientists often assume that the nutrient they know something about is the factor that is making the difference. However, this is not always the case. For example, studies show an inverse association between cruciferous vegetables and the development of cancer. Scientists assumed that beta-carotene, which was high in those vegetables, was the factor that made the difference. A clinical trial was mounted among a large population in New England where one group received a large dose of beta-carotene, and another group did not. In preliminary results, the experimental group did not do any better or worse than the control. Very likely, there are other constituents in the vegetables and combinations of constituents that make the difference. Because of issues such as these, the best dietary recommendation to the public is to eat whole foods, close to where they were grown.

### Implications for MCH

The DRIs are used as the criteria for nutrient adequacy in the meals served in the School Meals Program and for menu systems used in the FSP. There are several caveats for the use of these standards. They are for healthy individuals. They are for groups of people, and they should be compared with dietary data that include several days of intake or a large sample (see Chapter 3 for further discussion of nutrition problems among women and Chapters 4, 5, and 6 for nutrition problems among children and adolescents).

## Three Food and Nutrition Programs

### Special Supplemental Food Program for WIC

#### History

Assurance of food availability to low-income or disenfranchised populations is a growing concern in the United States (see the Hunger Section). Nutrition problems—either deficiencies or excesses—have been identified but are difficult to combat because of the many barriers to food access. There may not be enough money to purchase the food or the population may live in a neighborhood where the food is not sold or is too high priced. These factors are described in more detail previously here. At the 1969 White House Conference on Food, Nutrition, and Health, this problem was made very clear and led to the expansion of the FSP and to the Special Supplemental Food Program for WIC, renamed in 1994 to the Supplemental Nutrition Program for WIC. Studies have demonstrated the effect of inadequate nutrition during pregnancy on birth outcomes, including lower birth weight and prematurity. Inadequate nutritional intake by newborns and older infants also puts normal development at risk because of the rapid brain growth that occurs from birth until the age of 2 years. Along with the possibility of nutritionally compromised brain growth, the most common nutrient deficiency of children below 5 years of age, iron deficiency, may further jeopardize cognitive development. Therefore, children less than 5 years of age are included in WIC population because of the potential harm that undernutrition has on growth and learning.

### Characteristics

The WIC program was designed to give a woman and/or a child's caretaker a voucher or "check" with a list of approved foods and amounts to be purchased at participating food stores. A certain amount of food is approved for the certified person for 6 months, at which time she needs to return for recertification. For pregnant women and children, those foods are milk, eggs, cheese, cereal, and fruit juice. The food store has a list of brands that are acceptable for purchase. The determination is based on their concentration of the target nutrients—protein, iron, calcium, and vitamin C. Breastfeeding mothers may continue to get food supplements for up to 6 months postpartum. Infants may be given the infant formula that meets their needs, and foods are added progressively up to age 1 year old. Each participant or caretaker in the program must have two nutrition education program contacts every 6 months, when she must return to the agency for recertifications. If the food supply is not limited among these participants, after 6 or 12 months on the program, the nutritional risk is often rectified. However, if the participant leaves the program, she is likely to be back in several months because her low income puts her at nutritional risk again.

Eligibility for WIC is met in most states if the pregnant woman, infant, or child has an income below 185% of poverty and has a nutritional risk factor that includes specific medical conditions or an inadequate diet;

47% of all babies born in the United States participate in WIC. Of all eligible, it is currently estimated that WIC has achieved full coverage of all eligible infants. In 1993, approximately 54% of eligible pregnant women were being served, 93% of eligible infants, and 49% of eligible children (Food Research and Action Center, 1995). The WIC program requires referral for medical services, and thus, many programs are associated with primary health care for children and women.

### Policy Implications/Evaluation

WIC was controversial from its inception (Brown, Gershoff, & Cook, 1992). Although the purchase of foods included in the program supported domestic agriculture, critics of the program protested the "free lunch" appearance. In order to answer questions about the benefits of the WIC program, a large, national evaluation was funded by USDA and was designed and conducted by Dr. David Rush and the Research Triangle Institute. The study demonstrated that infants whose mothers were on the WIC program weighed an additional 28 grams at birth, a statistically significant difference. In addition, other studies showed that a $1 investment in WIC was worth $3 of Medicaid money saved in hospital costs that the lower weight infants would have incurred without WIC (Buescher, Larson, Nelson, & Lenihan, 1993).

Whether a food was included in the WIC Program became big business because of the volume of food being purchased by program participants each month. Breakfast cereals were fortified with the nutrients to the level that made them eligible to be included on the WIC-approved food lists. Iron was the most important nutrient. Infant formula vouchers were sought by mothers, and as infant formula steadily rose in price, the vouchers became very valuable. In addition, the WIC market share of infant formula was one third of the total sales. Infant formula rebates, which began in 1988, forced the formula companies to bid for a state's business for 1 to 5 years. With three and later four formula companies putting in competing bids, the WIC Program in the state could save substantial funds that could then be used to add more clients to the program.

### Implications for MCH

Participants in WIC like the program, and thus, it becomes a good drawing card for the population that MCH programs want to serve. For this reason, immunization, injury prevention, and early intervention programs are pairing up with WIC to increase its health promotion potential. Sometimes abuse of the program or lack of participation by eligible people may come to the attention of an MCH staff person. Referral of eligible people and notification of possible abuses to the WIC staff can lead to important improvements in the program. If a health facility for children or pregnant women does not have a WIC program or does not know where to refer clients to find one, advocacy by MCH personnel on behalf of the program is needed.

## School Nutrition Programs

### History

Congress established the National School Lunch Program in 1946, recognizing that a large proportion of children were not receiving an adequate lunch and possibly less than desirable breakfasts and dinners. It passed laws and allocated funds to establish a program to make low-priced milk available in all schools and a hot lunch in as many schools as possible. This program has grown so that 25,073,570 children in public and private schools participate in the National School Lunch Program. School districts are subsidized for all lunches. Some children receive a free lunch and some a reduced price lunch based on the ability to pay. Forty-four percent of the children pay the "full charge," but even those lunches are subsidized a small amount.

### Characteristics

Until 1995, participating school districts planned menus that followed the USDA criteria, and they were evaluated for approval by the State Education Agency. The guidelines required that a menu consist of five items—a protein food, bread, vegetable or fruit, dessert, and milk. In the 1970s, plate waste (food being thrown away) in the school meal program was reaching unacceptable levels. There were efforts to design menus that children liked; however, this did not totally rectify the problem. Now the school meal regulations allow children to select three of the five items on the menu rather than requiring them to take all five, knowing that they are going to throw away at least two. Since 1995, school meal managers have been able to plan their menus using the food groups or to meet a nutrient standard—for example, one third of the RDA requirement for each required nutrient. This will require a nutrient calculation of each menu that is now feasible with computerized nutrient analysis software. However, implementation of the nutrient method will require training of school food service managers because a significant proportion of them across the country will be unfamiliar with the analytical procedure.

The impetus for this change is again a problem of excess rather than deficiency. The fat, salt, and sugar content of school meals has grown to unacceptable levels. In an effort to serve food that children will eat, school food managers have found that this is most likely to be pizza, french fries, hamburgers, hot dogs, and a la carte items such as ice cream, cookies, and candy. However, these foods are all high in one or more of the items to avoid. Although this is a dilemma for the school meal program, the problem extends well beyond the schools. This means that there are a substantial number of young people now and there will be more in the future who have poor food habits. They will not try new foods. They have developed a one or two taste palate, and they have no idea how to start or where to go if they want to try new foods. The reason fat, salt, and sugar are problems is because their high satiety value (feeling full) moves other nutrients out of the diet. Indeed, the population with these food habits is deficient in vitamins and minerals that are critical for their health and the health of children they will raise. It also makes them more susceptible to cardiovascular disease and cancer at an early age. This is a problem that every MCH professional needs to deal with whether through parents, teachers, physicians, or the children themselves.

Even if the school meal program were one that nutritionists could endorse, one that offered foods that school children liked, those children who receive free or reduced price meals have to deal with the stigma attached to their participation by virtue of the payment arrangement. The only way to do away with the stigma is to give everyone a free meal, or have everyone pay the same low price by first getting the money into the hands of the poor children.

## The FSP

### Purpose

The FSP is the primary government program designed to improve the nutrition of low-income individuals and families. In general, households with incomes below 135% of poverty are eligible for food stamps. The amount is revised each year after July when the annual poverty income guidelines are released by the Department of Labor. At the food stamp office, the household's net income is calculated, and the program assumes that 30% of the income is spent on food. The difference between the amount of money available and the cost of the Thrifty Food Plan prepared by USDA is the value of the food stamps issued to the household (Cleveland & Kerr, 1988). "Certification" of the household can be for 1 to 24 months. Before the expiration of the certification, the household is notified, and a household member may make an appointment with the program to apply for recertification.

### Characteristics

Food stamps can be used to purchase most foods at participating stores. They may not be used to purchase items such as diapers, cigarettes, household cleaning supplies, pet food, prepared foods, or alcoholic beverages. Participating stores are interviewed and monitored by the USDA. If a store is found to be violating the rules, it will be discontinued from the FSP. If the store also redeems WIC vouchers, the WIC program becomes discontinued automatically.

### Issues

Two ongoing issues exist with the FSP. One is the stigma associated with using the coupons, and the second is fraud. The more common acts of fraud are selling food stamps for cash and the use of food coupons for disallowed items. Theft is a personal hazard for recipients. Currently, a number of states are using the results of pilot studies to implement a debit card issuance system. The debit card minimizes the sale for cash and theft because an identification verification will be necessary for its use. A recipient will receive a debit card to use at the food store in place of food stamp coupons. This will also decrease stigma because debit cards are becoming available for use in food stores generally. Many stores are already using credit cards. The threat of being discontinued from the program is the incentive for food stores to not overcharge the FSP. Nutrition education, keeping cost and health in mind, is necessary for food stamp recipients so that they will receive the largest nutritional benefit from the food purchased.

The amount of money issued to the recipient is also a problem. The program assumes that the difference between the Thrifty Food Plan amount and the food stamp value issued is spent on food. In fact, the money available in a household is frequently used for emergencies that arise such as transportation to employment or to a health appointment, school fees for trips or special services, and household bills such as telephone, heat, and/or power. In addition, the Thrifty Food Plan requires economical food purchasing, planning, and time for preparation as many of the menus use recipes requiring preparation "from scratch." The estimated value per meal per person is approximately 84 cents (Cleveland & Kerr, 1988). When middle- or upper-class individuals follow the menus and recipes prescribed for food stamp participants, their comments include that they are possible to do, but that the menus are boring, there is no allowance for eating out, every household member must carry lunch made at home, and that preparing the meals required too much time.

Periodically, it is recommended that the program be "cashed out," that is, included in the welfare benefit a household receives. However, recipients, particularly mothers, insist that the program retain the food coupons or debit cards so the benefit must be spent on food; therefore, the recipient could not be forced to yield to pressures that it be spent on other expenses. As it is now, the value of the food stamp benefit issued is less than the cost of the Thrifty Food Plan, and thus, it is not surprising that households, particularly those who are eating at emergency food locations, report that the food stamps do not last the month.

# THE SOCIAL PROCESS MODEL: AN APPLICATION

The ultimate objective of public health nutrition programs is to maintain and improve the nutritional well-being of the population. As a professional, one will often focus on a subgroup of the population, such as pregnant women and infants, school children, or all of the people in a geographic area whether a neighborhood or a state. Food, the basic component of nutrition, is consumed differently by different people for a number of reasons. As a professional whose purpose it is to see that every person knows what he or she should eat and how one can purchase or grow and/or prepare it, one will need to review a number of factors in the population in order to determine whether the population's nutritional well-being is adequate. A model was developed that addresses and organizes three factors, or "basic dynamics," of a society—the Social Process Model (Figure 12–2) (Jenkins & Jenkins, 1997).

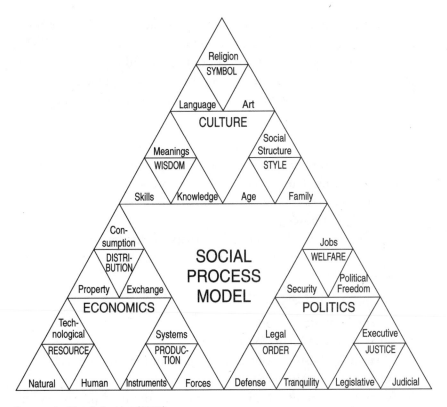

Source: Jenkins & Jenkins (1997).

FIGURE 12–2 The social process model.

The basic dynamics from which the Social Process Model is constructed include economic, political, and cultural processes. Each of the processes in turn includes three underlying activities: the economic process (resources, production, and distribution), the political (order, justice, and welfare), and the cultural process (wisdom, style, and symbols).

The Social Process Model is a basic organizational tool used to extend the description of a community from one dimension to a nine dimensional design. It is brief enough to be remembered but inclusive enough to expand a discussion or plan to be multidimensional. It triggers the user to see the "big picture," to identify network possibilities, and to form well-rounded coalitions for stronger program impact. Thinking from a multidimensional context leads to more effectively integrated programs, and the synergy from this connected activity energizes participants and programs. Breadth is critical in nutrition planning, as discussed later here, because even when people know what they should eat, this knowledge alone cannot improve nutritional well-being (Foster, 1992). Foods needed may not be available in the stores where people shop or sell for a price they can afford. People may not have money to buy the food or may not know how to prepare it. Perhaps their family is unfamiliar with the food and will not eat unknown foods.

## Economic Process

A community's economic, political, and cultural processes are present in community systems. The *Economic Process* in a community is the system that delivers resources (material and human), processes them into usable products, and distributes them throughout the community. One can use the process to describe the economic activity of the population or community that affects the food and nutrition systems. The questions include the following:

1. What is the rate of employment?
2. Where do residents work?
3. What are the residents' occupations?
4. What major businesses or employers are in the community?
5. What is the number of employees at each?
6. What are the transportation systems that the food producers, distributors, and consumers depend on?

## Political Process

The *Political Process* in the community is the system that maintains order and justice in the community and responds to the community's concerns and needs, including systems that provide for the general welfare of the citizens (both resources and services) such as those that assure the availability of health services and housing for the community. The elected representatives as well as government agencies are obligated to allocate public revenues in a way that meets the community's needs and is responsive to the will of the majority. The model describes a community's political process by supplying specific data that answer the following questions:

1. Who are the elected representatives of the area?
2. Who are the food, welfare, or health legislative aides?
3. Which public agencies provide income maintenance services, and where are they located?

4. What are the health facilities in the community—acute care, preventive care, extended care facilities?
5. Are there public residential facilities—correctional, rehabilitation, or psychiatric?
6. What citizen committees are there advising local or state health services? Who are the people on the committees? Do they have a nutrition committee? Who are the staff people for these committees?
7. What is the housing stock like in the area?
8. Is there a local newspaper? What is its reach, number of subscribers? Is there a food and nutrition column?
9. Which newspaper and which column are most popular in the community?

## Cultural Process

The *Cultural Process* in the community that affects nutrition includes the educational systems for all ages; social groups, based on (but not limited by) ethnicity, age, occupation, and gender; and symbolic activities, which include art, language, and religious institutions. As with economic and political processes, data about the cultural process will answer the following questions:

1. What are the agencies (with a contact person) that provide child daycare both in homes and in centers?
2. Who is on the community school board?
3. Who are the superintendent, the school lunch supervisor, and the principal of the schools?
4. What is the reading level of each grade? What is done and when with children who are not reading at grade level?
5. How are children who do not speak English handled?
6. Are there computers in the schools?
7. How much television do children watch? Do they have homework?
8. What recreation is there?
9. What is the educational level of the adults in the community?
10. How many children are in an average family? How many single parent families are there?
11. Are there different neighborhoods that hold to ethnic traditions? What are they? Where are they, and what are some of their centers of community activities?

12. What happens to old people? What happens to teenagers? Are there gangs? Are children left unsupervised?
13. What happens to the women? Do they work?
14. What professional groups are there for people to be a part of? What voluntary/civic groups are there, and who can join?
15. How many religious buildings are there? What faiths are represented and what are their numbers?
16. Are there libraries? Art galleries? Are there murals in the community? What does the space look like? Is it cluttered, lush, clean, or filthy? Are there litter barrels or only litter? Do the drains in the street work? Are there parks? What condition are they in? Who uses them?

## Application of the Social Process Model to Food and Nutrition Systems

Within each of the economic, political, and cultural processes described previously here, there are food and nutrition systems. The food supply system of the community is part of the *Economic Process* and is described by answering these questions:

1. Are there food-producing areas in the vicinity—farms, gardens?
2. From how far away does the food come? From where and how much?
3. Are there farmers' markets? Is the food warehoused, and if so, where and for how long?
4. How does the food get into the area?
5. Where are the major distribution points? Are they in the vicinity or outside the area?
6. What is the profile of retail food stores, including specialty shops such as bakeries, fruit and vegetable stores, meat shops? Are there thrift stores?
7. Are there large national chain supermarkets? Are there local chain food markets? Are there small groceries?
8. How do prices on several common food items, such as milk, bread, dry cereal, and apples, compare? Are some small groceries more costly than others?
9. What is the quality of the food?
10. Describe the restaurants of the area, and categorize them as inexpensive, midrange, or expensive in price.

- Do people outside of the area come to the area to eat?
- Are there diners, coffee shops, or low-cost ethnic restaurants?
- What restaurant chains are in the community?
- What are the prices of several common items such as hamburgers, milk, soda, fries, and salad?

Several of the food and nutrition programs whose data are collected in the *Political Process* have been discussed, specifically WIC and school nutrition programs. They are categorized as political because they are directly controlled by the electoral process, not the free enterprise system that controls the market place. However, because these programs provide a source of food, they are indirectly included in the food supply system. In the political process, the focus is on the location and number of nutrition personnel. Beyond food and nutrition education programs requiring nutritionists, the primary location of nutritionists is in health care services and residential units. Nutritionists may be found in extension, private nutrition practices, physician practices, ambulatory care facilities, health centers, health departments, health maintenance organizations, acute care hospitals, residential institutions such as correctional and child care, and special rehabilitative residences, such as for alcohol abuse, psychiatric illness, and other chronic health problems. Additionally, nutritionists are employed by social service agencies and agencies for the older population. The following questions can be asked:

1. Do all stores take food stamps and WIC vouchers?
2. Who are the nutritionists in the area? Where do they work?

Within the *Cultural Process*, there are multiple mechanisms, organizations, and institutions whereby nutrition information can be delivered, including regular meetings or informal gatherings. The schools are a natural setting for disseminating information, both in classrooms and lunch rooms. The following questions are asked to assess where nutrition information is or can be disseminated:

1. Is there a district curriculum coordinator of nutrition, science, or health who can facilitate the use of nutrition curriculum materials by teachers?
2. Is there a nutrition committee that makes recommendations about lunch items and a system to better meet the needs of students and teachers? Have the schools had some special food and nutrition events?

3. Have the older population meal programs, the day care programs for preschoolers, and after-school programs had nutrition education events?
4. Are there a local dietetic association, food and nutrition members of the local home economics association, a Society for Nutrition Education affiliate or members, or local food and nutrition councils that serve as a source of nutrition information and resource people?
5. Are there nutrition professional training programs that would be a source of student trainees who could carry out programs in the community?
6. What ethnic events occur in the community, and what are the most popular foods served at them?
7. Are there religious organizations and service organizations that offer free public gathering space in the community? Are they available for nutrition education events?
8. Is there an artists' group that has shown an interest in food and food-related themes in its work or other activities?
9. Is there dramatic activity in which food might be a theme? Could food be related to the dramatic activities?

With this description of the community, a professional can develop a plan, set priorities, select areas of work, and recruit community members and leaders to develop interventions in some detail. The Social Process Model can assist in the analysis of a community as well as provide a framework for organizational purposes. The *Economic Process* in nutrition includes agriculture and the issues of environmental tradeoffs to produce foodstuffs required by a population. For example, in the 1960s, there was a shift to vegetarian practices when consumers realized that it took 16 bushels of grain to produce one pound of meat (Lappe, 1982). Food-processing issues include the energy used to process a food and ship it from parts quite distant to the consumption point. Finally, there are issues surrounding the retailing of food, from advertising, location of grocery stores, quality of product provided, and point of purchase education to transportation and storage.

Nutrition and the *Political Process* centers on accessibility and availability of the food supply. There are examples of inequity of access that occur due to class, race or ethnicity, gender, and age. Based in the political process, food assistance programs also relate to distribution of food (economic) and the knowledge and acceptability of the program (cultural).

There are issues of access to information that appear in the numerous barriers confronted when accessing the welfare system (political). Electronic and mail systems to provide information are integral to the proper operation of the political process.

The *Cultural Process* has historically been the primary focus of nutrition professionals. This includes nutrition education regarding knowledge and skills about nutrients and cooking. Where the food is eaten—home, school, or restaurants—is critical for the design of interventions. The reasons why people eat and the meaning the food has for a person are critical. Food can be symbolic, representing something such as celebration, love, repentance, or guilt. To the extent that it does represent something cultural, food becomes a critical component in communication or art.

# REFERENCES

Adams, E.J., Grummer-Strawn, L., & Chavez, G. (2003). Food insecurity is associated with increased risk of obesity in California women. *Journal of Nutrition, 133,* 1070–1074.

Alaimo, K., Briefel, R.R., Frongillo, E.A., & Olson, C.M. (1998). Food insufficiency exists in the United States: Results from the Third National Health and Nutrition Examination Survey (NHANES III). *American Journal of Public Health, 88,* 419–425.

Alaimo, K., Olson, C.M., & Frongillo, E.A. (2001a). Food insufficiency and American school-aged children's cognitive, academic, and psychosocial development. *Pediatrics, 108,* 44–53.

Alaimo, K., Olson, C.M., Frongillo, E.A., Jr., & Briefel, R.R. (2001b). Food insufficiency, family income, and health in US preschool and school-aged children. *American Journal of Public Health, 1,* 781–786.

Alaimo, K., Olson, C.M., & Frongillo, E.A. (2001c). Low family income and food insufficiency in relation to overweight in US children. *Archives of Pediatrics and Adolescent Medicine, 155,* 1161–1167.

Anderson, S.A. (1990). Core indicators of nutritional state for difficult-to-sample populations. *Journal of Nutrition, 120,* 1559S–1600S.

Anonymous. (1993). Position of the American Dietetic Association: Promotion and support of breast-feeding. *Journal of the American Dietetic Association 93,* 467–469.

American Dietetic Association (ADA). (2001). Breaking the barriers to breast-feeding: Position of ADA. *Journal of the American Dietetic Association, 101,* 1213.

Bickel, G., Carlson, S., & Nord, M. (1999). *Measuring food security in the United States: Household food security in the United States 1995–1998 (advanced report).* Washington, DC: Food and Nutrition Service, USDA.

Brown, J.L., & Allen, D. (1988). Hunger in America. *Annual Review of Public Health, 9,* 503–526.

Brown, J.L., Gershoff, S.N., & Cook, J.T. (1992). The politics of hunger: When science and ideology clash. *International Journal of Health Services, 22,* 221–237.

Bryant, C.A., Coreil, J., D'Angelo, S.L., Bailey, D.F.C., & Lazarov, M. (1992). A strategy for promoting breastfeeding among economically disadvantaged women and adolescents. *NAACOG's Clinical Issues, 3,* 723–730.

Buescher, P.A., Larson L.C., Nelson, M.D., Jr., & Lenihan A.J. (1993). Prenatal WIC participants can reduce low birth weight and newborn medicine costs: A cost-benefits analysis of WIC participants in North Carolina. *Journal of the American Dietetic Association, 93,* 163–166.

Canning, H., Mayer, A.B., & Mayer J. (1966). Obesity: Its possible effect on college acceptance. *New England Journal of Medicine, 275,* 1172–1174.

Carlson, S.J., Andrews, M.S., & Bickel, G.W. (1999). Measuring food insecurity and hunger in the United States: Development of a national benchmark measure and prevalence estimates. *Journal of Nutrition, 129*(2S Suppl), 510S–516S.

Casey, P.H., Szeto, K., Lensing, S., Bogle, M., & Weber, J. (2001). Children in food-insufficient, low-income families: Prevalence, health, and nutrition status. *Archives of Pediatrics & Adolescent Medicine, 155,* 508–514.

Casey, P., Goolsby, S., Berkowitz, C., Frank, D., Cook, J., Cutts, D., Black, M.M., Zaldivar, N., Levenson, S., Heeren, T., & Meyers, A. (2004). Children's Sentinel Nutritional Assessment Program Study Group. Maternal depression, changing public assistance, food security, and child health status. *Pediatrics, 113,* 298–304.

Centers for Disease Control and Prevention. (2003). Self-reported concern about food security associated with obesity: Washington, 1995–1999. *Morbidity and Mortality Weekly Report MMWR, 52,* 840–842.

Citizens Board of Inquiry into Hunger and Malnutrition in the US. (1968). *Hunger, USA.* Boston: Beacon Press.

Cleveland, L., & Kerr, R.L. (1988). Development and uses of the USDA food plans. *Journal of Nutrition Education, 20,* 232–238.

Dietz, W.H., & Robinson, T.N. (1993). Assessment and treatment of childhood obesity. *Pediatrics in Review, 14,* 337–343.

Drewnowski, A., & Specter, S.E. (2004). Poverty and obesity: The role of energy density and energy cost. *American Journal of Clinical Nutrition, 79,* 6–16.

Dunn, D.T., Newell, M.L., Ades, A.E., & Pechkham, C.S. (1992). Risk of human immunodeficiency virus type 1 transmission through breastfeeding. *Lancet, 340,* 585–588.

Ellis, D.J. (1992a). The impact of agency policies and protocols on breastfeeding. *NAACOG's Clinical Issues, 3,* 5552–5559.

Ellis, D.J. (1992b). Supporting breastfeeding: How to implement agency change. *NAACOG's Clinical Issues, 3,* 560–564.

Epstein, L.H., Valoski, A., Wing, R.R., & McCurley, J. (1990). Ten-year follow-up of behavioral, family-based treatment for obese children. *Journal of the American Medical Association, 264*, 2519–2523.

Flegal, M.C., Carroll, R.J., Kuczmarski, R.J., & Johnson, C.L. (1998). Overweight and obesity in the United States: Prevalence and trends, 1960–1994. *International Journal of Obesity Related Metabolic Disorders, 22*, 39–47.

Food Marketing Institute. (1995). *Trends in the U.S.* Washington, DC: Research Division, The Institute.

Food Research and Action Center. (1995). *Community Childhood Hunger Identification Project: A Survey of Childhood Hunger in the US.* Washington, DC: Food Research and Action Center.

Foster, P. (1992). *The world food problem: Tackling the causes of undernutrition in the Third World.* Lynne Rienner Publishers, Boulder, CO.

Freed, G.L., Jones, T.M., & Schanler, R.J. (1992). Prenatal determination of demographic and attitudinal factors regarding feeding practice in an indigent population. *American Journal of Perinatology, 9*, 420–429.

Goldfarb, J. (1993). Breastfeeding: AIDS and other infectious diseases. *Clinical Perinatology, 20*, 225–243.

Gortmaker, S.L., Dietz, W.H., & Cheung, L.W.Y. (1990). Inactivity, diet, and the fattening of America. *Journal of the American Dietetic Association, 90*, 1247–1252.

Gortmaker, S.L., Must, A., Perrin, J.M., Sobol, A.M., & Dietz, W.H. (1993). Social and economic consequences of overweight in adolescence and young adulthood. *New England Journal of Medicine, 329*, 1008–1012.

Hamilton, W.L., Cook, J.T., Thompson, W.W., Buron, L.F., Frongillo, E.A., Olson, C.M., & Wehler, C. (1997). *Household food security in the United States in 1995: Summary report of the Food Security Measurement Project.* Alexandria, VA: US Department of Agriculture, Food and Consumer Service.

Jenkins, J., & Jenkins, M. (1997). *The Social Process Triangles.* Grohingen, The Netherlands: Imaginal Training.

John, M., & Martorell, R. (1989). Incidence and duration of breast-feeding in Mexican-American infants, 1970–1982. *American Journal of Clinical Nutrition, 50*, 868–874.

Jones, F., & Green, M. (1993). Baby friendly care. *The Canadian Nurse, 89*, 36–39.

Jones, S.J., Jahns, L., Laraia, B.A., & Haughton, B. (2003). School-aged food insecure children who participate in food assistance are less likely to be at risk of overweight: Results from the PSID-CDS. *Archives of Pediatric and Adolescent Medicine. 157*(8):780–4.

Kennedy, K.I., Fortney, J.A., Bonhomme, M.G., Potts, M., Lamptey, P., & Carswell, W. (1990). Do the benefits of breastfeeding outweigh the risk of postnatal transmission of HIV via breast milk? *Tropical Doctor, 20*, 25–29.

Klesges, R.C., Stein, R.J., Eck, L.H., Isbell, T.R., & Klesges, L.M. (1991). Parental influence on food selection in young children and its relationships to childhood obesity. *American Journal of Clinical Nutrition, 53,* 859–864.

Kotz, K., & Story, M. (1994). Food advertisements during children's Saturday morning television programming: Are they consistent with dietary recommendations? *Journal of the American Dietetic Association, 94,* 1296–1300.

Kurinij, N., Shiono, P.H., Ezrine, S.F., & Rhoads, G.G. (1989). Does maternal employment affect breast-feeding? *American Journal of Public Health, 79(9),* 1247–1250.

Lappe, F.M. (1982). *Diet for a Small Planet.* New York: Ballantine.

Laraia, B.A., Siega-Riz, A.M., & Evensen, K.R. (2004). Self-reported overweight and obesity are not associated with concern about food among adults in New York and Louisiana. *Preventive Medicine, 38,* 175–181.

Lin Yutang. (1937). *The Importance of Living.* New York: William Morrow and Company.

Li, R., & Grummer-Strawn, L. (2002). Racial and ethnic disparities in breast-feeding among United States infants: Third National Health and Nutrition Examination Survey, 1988–1994. *Birth, 29,* 251–257.

Li, R., Zhao, Z., Mokdad, A., Barker, L., & Grummer-Strawn, L. (2003). Prevalence of breastfeeding in the United States: The 2001 National Immunization Survey. *Pediatrics, 111*(5 Pt 2), 1198–1201.

Mellin, L.M., Slinkard, L.A., & Irwin, C.E. (1987). Adolescent obesity intervention: Validation of the SHAPEDOWN program. *Journal of the American Dietetic Association, 87,* 333–338.

Mokdad, A.H., Serdula, M.K., Dietz, W.H., Bowman, B.A., Marks, J.S., & Koplan, J.P. (1999). The spread of the obesity epidemic in the United States, 1991–1998. *Journal of the American Medical Association, 282,* 1519–1522.

Moore, J.F., & Jansa, N. (1987). A survey of policies and practices in support of breastfeeding mothers in the workplace. *Birth, 14,* 191–195.

National Center for Health Statistics. (2004, Dec. 16). *Prevalence of Overweight Among Children and Adolescents: United States, 1999–2002.* Available January 17, 2005, from: http://www.cdc.gov/nchs/products/pubs/pubd/hestats/overwght99.htm#Table%201.

Nelson, K., Brown, M.E., & Lurie, N. (1998). Hunger in an adult patient population. *Journal of the American Medical Association, 279,* 1211–1214.

Nestle, M. (1993). Food lobbies, the food pyramid, and US nutrition policy. *International Journal of Health Services, 23,* 483–496.

Nestle, M., & Guttmacher, S. (1992a). Hunger in the US: Policy implications. *Nutrition Reviews, 50,* 242–245.

Nestle, M., & Guttmacher, S. (1992b). Hunger in the US: Rationale, methods, and policy implications of state hunger surveys. *Journal of Nutrition Education, 24,* 18S–22S.

Newman, J. (1990). Breastfeeding problems associated with the early introduction of bottles and pacifiers. *Journal of Human Lactation, 6,* 59–63.

Nord, M., Andrews, M., & Carlson, S. (2003). *Household food security in the United States, 2002*. Washington, DC: Economic Research Service, USDA.

Olson, C.M. (1999). Nutrition and health outcomes associated with food insecurity and hunger. *Journal of Nutrition, 129*, 512S–524S.

Pelto, G.H. (1991). Ethnic minorities, migration and risk of undernutrition in children. *Acta Paediatrica Scandinavica Supplement, 371*, 51–57.

Pérez-Escamilla, R., Pollitt, E., Lonnerdal, B., & Dewey, K.G. (1994). Infant feeding policies in maternity wards and their effect on breast-feeding success: An analytical overview. *American Journal of Public Health, 84*, 89–97.

Poppendieck, J.E. (1992). Hunger and public policy: Lessons from the Great Depression. *Journal of Nutrition Education, 24*, 6S–11S.

Prentice, A.M., Lucas, A., Vasquez-Velasquez, L., Davies, P.S.W., & Whitehead, R.G. (1988). Are current dietary guidelines for young children a prescription for overfeeding? *Lancet, 2*, 1066–1068.

Radimer, K.L., Olson, C.M., Greene, J.C., Campbell, C.C., & Habicht, J.P. (1992). Understanding hunger and developing indicators to assess it in women and children. *Journal of Nutrition Education, 24*, 36S–44S.

Raper, N., et al. (1992) Nutrient content of the U.S. food supply, 1909–1990. Washington, DC: USDA, Home Economics Research Report No. 50.

Rassin, D.K., Markides, K.S., Baranowski, T., Bee, D.E., Richardson, C.J., Mikrut, W.D., & Winkler, B. (1993). Acculturation and breastfeeding on the United-States–Mexico border. The *American Journal of the Medical Sciences, 306*, 28–34.

Serdula, M.K., Ivery, D., Coates, R.J., Freedman, D.S., Williamson, D.F., & Byers, T. (1993). Do obese children become obese adults? *Preventive Medicine, 22*, 167–177.

Snell, B.J., Krantz, M., Keeton, R., Delgado, K., & Peckham, C. (1992). The association of formula samples given at hospital discharge with the early duration of breastfeeding. *Journal of Human Lactation, 8*, 67–72.

Snyder, M.P., Obarzanek, E., Montgomery, D.H., Feldman, H., Nicklas, T., Raizman, D., Rupp, J., Bigelow, C., & Lakatos, E. (1994). Reducing the fat content of ground beef in a school food service setting. *Journal of the American Dietetic Association, 94*, 1135–1139.

Stunkard, A., & Burt, V. (1967). Obesity and the body image: II: Age at onset of disturbances in the body image. *American Journal of Psychiatry, 123*, 1443–1447.

Townsend, M.S., Peerson, J., Love, B., Achterberg, C., & Murphy, S.P. (2001). Food insecurity is positively related to overweight in women. *Journal of Nutrition, 131*, 1738–1745.

UNICEF (n.d.). *The baby-friendly hospital initiative*. Available January 17, 2005, from: http://www.unicef.org/nutrition/index_24806.html.

US Department of Agriculture, Food and Nutrition Services. *National School Lunch Program Fact Sheet*. Available May 1, 2004, from: http://www.fns. usda.gov/cnd/lunch/AboutLunch/NSLPFactSheet.htm

US Department of Health and Human Services. (1992). *FDA Consumer*, Vol. 26, No. 6 July–August.

US Department of Health and Human Services. (2000a, November). *Healthy People 2010: Understanding and improving health: Chapter 16: Maternal, infant and child health* (2nd ed.). Washington, DC: US Government Printing Office. Available June 6, 2004, from: http://www.healthypeople.gov/document/html/volume2/16mich.htm#_Toc494699661.

US Department of Health and Human Services, Public Health Service. (2000b). *Healthy People 2010: National health promotion and disease preventions objectives.* Boston: Jones and Bartlett Publishers.

US Department of Health and Human Services, National Center for Health Statistics. (2002, October 8). *Obesity Still on the Rise, New Data Show.* Available, January 17, 2005, from: http://www.cdc.gov/nchs/pressroom/02news/obesityonrise.htm.

US Senate Select Committee on Nutrition and Human Needs. (1977). *Dietary goals for the US.* Washington, DC: Government Printing Office.

Vozoris, N.T., & Tarasuk, V.S. (2003). Household food insufficiency is associated with poorer health. *Journal of Nutrition, 133,* 120–126.

Wadden, T.A., & Stunkard, A.J. (1985). Social and psychological consequences of obesity. *Annals of Internal Medicine, 103,* 1062–1067.

Worthington-Roberts, B., & Williams, S.R. (1989). *Nutrition in pregnancy and lactation* (4th ed.). St. Louis: Times Mirror/Mosby College Publishing.

Wynder, E.L., Weisburger, J.H., & Ng, S.K. (1992). Nutrition: The need to define "optimal" intake as a basis for public policy decisions. *American Journal of Public Health, 82,* 346–350.

# CHAPTER 13

# International Maternal and Child Health

*Sian Curtis, Shelah Bloom, and Elizabeth Sutherland*

> *We have an opportunity to focus global attention on what should be obvious: every mother, and every child, counts. They count because we value every human life. The evidence is clear that healthy mothers and children are the bedrock of healthy and prosperous communities and nations.* (Lee, 2005)

## INTRODUCTION

Over six billion people now live on earth, the majority of whom live in less developed countries. In 2002, just under 30% of the world's population were less than 15 years old, and approximately 25% were women of reproductive age (15 to 49 years old) (US Census Bureau, 2004). Women and children are often the most vulnerable members of society, and the health of this population serves as a marker for wider development. Infant, child, and maternal mortality remains high in many parts of the world, fueled by poverty, political instability, environmental degradation, gender discrimination, economic crises, poor public infrastructure, inadequate health systems, and new threats such as HIV/AIDS. At the same time, considerable progress has been made in many countries.

Given the breadth and complexity of international maternal and child health (MCH), this chapter provides only a very general overview. We aim to provide the reader with a basic knowledge of levels and trends in international MCH indicators and of international MCH program strategies. The chapter begins with a historical perspective on international health. The global MCH program strategies and health outcomes are reviewed. The next sections review specific program areas: maternal health, child health, family planning and reproductive health, and HIV/AIDS. We then conclude with a brief discussion of equity concerns.


# BACKGROUND AND HISTORICAL CONTEXT[1]

The history of international health is closely linked to global political history, war, colonialism, and trade. During the colonial period, a number of schools of tropical medicine were established in Western Europe. Their focus was on the nature, origin, and transmission of diseases that were new and dangerous to Europeans. They were not concerned about the introduction of European diseases (e.g., measles and smallpox) to the colonies, and it was some time before tropical medicine and public health interventions were extended to the native population.

At the same time, growth in world trade led to concerns about transmission of diseases between countries through trading vessels and reciprocally to concerns about the impact of disease outbreaks on international trade. Ships were quarantined to prevent the spread of infections such as cholera and plague, but it was not until the First Sanitary Conference in Paris in 1851 that European nations adopted a common sanitary code to improve the sanitation in ports and establish fair and consistent quarantine measures to protect their respective populations. In the Americas, the Pan America Sanitary Bureau was established in 1902, leading to the development of a Pan-American Sanitary code.

Tropical medicine was never really adopted in the Americas, probably because of its close association with colonialism in Western Europe. The term international health appeared after the establishment of the Inter-

---

[1]This section summarized from Zapata, B.C., & Godue, C.J.M. (1997). International maternal and child health. In J.B. Kotch (Ed.), *Maternal and child health: Programs, problems, and policy in public health* (1st ed.). Gaithersburg, MD: Aspen Publishers, Inc.

national Health Commission (the Commission) of the Rockefeller Foundation in 1913. The Commission operated on the assumption that disease was the main impediment to social and economic development. It focused on controlling or eliminating specific diseases such as yellow fever and bubonic plague that had a high impact on trade because of the associated paralysis of affected ports. Similarly, malaria and ankylostomiasis were targeted because of their affects on the productivity of workers, and the Commission played a major role in the eradication of hookworm disease. The Commission focused on Latin America and China and developed a network of schools of public health in the region.

The United Nations was created in the aftermath of World War II as a vehicle for peace and conflict resolution between nations. The political institutions of the United Nations dealt with security, whereas the specialized agencies attached to it fostered cooperation necessary to address common problems in the specialized area. The World Health Organization (WHO) was founded in 1948 to promote and protect the health of all people. The United Nations International Children's Emergency Fund (UNICEF) was created the same year to assist the thousands of orphans and abandoned children resulting from the war in Europe. The WHO is intended to function as an intergovernmental institution. The World Health Assembly is the supreme decision-making body for WHO. It generally meets in Geneva in May each year and is attended by delegations from all 192 member states. Its main function is to determine the policies of the organization. The Secretariat of WHO has the responsibility to implement the resolutions and to deliver appropriate technical assistance to achieve common goals.

Many of the bilateral aid agencies were also established in the post-World War II era, including those in the United States and Canada. For example, the history of the United States Agency for International Development goes back to the Marshall Plan's reconstruction of Europe after World War II and the Truman Administration's Point Four Program. In 1961, President John F. Kennedy signed the Foreign Assistance Act into law and created the United States Agency for International Development.

Recent developments such as increasing globalization have profound health implications that can be broadly summarized as increased mobility and health transfer risks between countries, increased exchanges of goods and information between countries in response to health problems, and changing roles of national governments and international organizations in the health sector. Recent illustrations of the truly global nature of health threats in today's world include the emergence and global spread of Severe Acute Respiratory Syndrome in 2003, the re-emergence of tuberculosis (TB) as a growing public health threat in the industrialized world, and the emergence of the global HIV/AIDS pandemic. In addition, societies and subpopulations within societies are becoming increasingly polarized between those who can make it in today's highly competitive global environment and those who cannot, raising growing concerns about health equity.

# THE MILLENNIUM DEVELOPMENT GOALS

The member nations of the United Nations unanimously adopted the Millennium Declaration at the conclusion of the Millennium Summit held in New York in September 2000. The Millennium Declaration contains a statement of values, principles, and objectives for the international agenda for the 21st century and includes deadlines for collective action. Accompanying the Millennium Declaration is a set of clearly defined goals and associated targets to be achieved by 2015. The eight Millennium Development Goals cover a broad definition of development. Although all of the Millennium Development Goals are relevant to international MCH, three of the goals explicitly refer to health. These three goals and associated targets are listed in Table 13–1.

**Table 13–1**  Millennium Development Health Goals

Goal 4: Reduce child mortality
Target for 2015: Reduce by two thirds the mortality rate among children.

Goal 5: Improve maternal health
Target for 2015: Reduce by three quarters the ratio of women dying in childbirth.

Goal 6: Combat HIV/AIDS, malaria and other diseases
Targets for 2015:
  · Halt and begin to reverse the spread of HIV/AIDS.
  · Halt and begin to reverse the incidence of malaria and other major diseases.

Source: United Nations (2004).

# GLOBAL MCH PROGRAM STRATEGIES

Global MCH program strategies can be broadly split into two categories: disease-specific interventions and broad community-based strategies typified by primary health care (PHC) initiatives (Claeson & Waldman, 2000). Examples of disease-specific programs include attempts to eradicate malaria in the 1950s, 1960s, and 1970s, the campaign to eradicate smallpox, and the current campaign to eradicate polio. These initiatives are highly focused and aim to have a dramatic impact on a single disease. The campaign to eradicate smallpox was a success. The last case of human-to-human transmission of smallpox was reported in 1977, but the campaign to eradicate malaria failed and was abandoned in the mid 1970s. Global attempts to eliminate polio are close to achieving success, although the original aim to eradicate polio by the year 2000 has not been achieved.

Dissatisfaction with highly vertical disease-focused interventions fueled by the failure of the malaria eradication program led to a shift toward a broader, community-based PHC strategy in the late 1970s. The seminal concept of "health for all by the year 2000" achieved through PHC was proclaimed at a conference convened by WHO and UNICEF in Alma Atta in 1978. PHC emphasizes the provision of universal MCH services, family planning, improved sanitation and clean water supplies, achieved through equitable distribution of resources, community participation, emphasis on preventive rather than curative services, and a multisectoral approach.

Subsequent debates about the feasibility of achieving PHC objectives with limited resources led to the emergence of "selective primary health care" (SPHC) (Warren, 1988). SPHC aims to prioritize health problems that have a high impact in terms or mortality or morbidity and for which cost-effective interventions that can be applied in resource-poor environments are available. They were advocated as an interim strategy to improve the health of the largest number of people in the short to medium term. One of the early examples of a SPHC program was UNICEF's GOBI program (growth monitoring, oral rehydration, breastfeeding, and immunization). SPHC programs use available technology but also recognize that in order to be successful, such programs require functioning health structures at all levels and community acceptance and participation. Advocates of the original concept of PHC have, however, been highly critical of SPHC

(Newell, 1988; Rifkin & Walt, 1986). They argue that a fundamental element of PHC is lacking in SPHC: the involvement of the community in identifying health priorities and choosing solutions.

# THE STATE OF GLOBAL MCH

The availability of good quality information on international MCH is an ongoing challenge. Therefore, the quality of data is an important concern, especially when making comparisons between countries or over time within a country because variations in data collection procedures, definitions, and data quality can significantly distort conclusions. In developed countries, vital registration systems provide the data required to monitor mortality levels, causes of death, and fertility rates. Such systems are typically not functional in most developing countries. Coverage is generally very incomplete and tends to be biased toward the more affluent and educated segments of the population who also tend to experience better health outcomes. Even when data are available, they are often not reported in a timely manner and may be of poor quality. Sample vital registration systems provide improved data in some countries such as India and China, but such systems are not available everywhere. Therefore, population-based surveys such as the Demographic and Health Surveys (DHS) and UNICEF Multiple Indicator Cluster Surveys remain an important source of information on MCH globally. The widespread implementation of good quality household surveys since the 1970s has allowed global trends in MCH outcomes and behaviors to be documented and greatly added to the international MCH knowledge base. Nevertheless, household surveys suffer from several limitations, and many significant knowledge gaps remain.

Table 13–2 shows four key indicators of MCH for different regions of the world. These regional estimates mask large variations between countries within regions but serve to illustrate the magnitude of global inequity in MCH. Maternal mortality ratio (MMR) estimates vary from 12 deaths per 100,000 live births in industrialized countries to 1,100 deaths per 100,000 live births in sub-Saharan Africa. Similarly, the under-5 years mortality rates vary from seven deaths per 1,000 live births in industrialized countries to 173 deaths per 1,000 live births in sub-Saharan Africa. Sub-Saharan Africa typically has the poorest MCH outcomes, followed by South Asia, whereas industrialized nations have the best outcomes. MCH

**Table 13-2** Selected Indicators of MCH by Region

| Region | MMR | Under-5 Mortality Rate | Stunting Prevalence (%) | Total Fertility Rate |
|---|---|---|---|---|
| Sub-Saharan Africa | 1,100 | 173 | 41 | 5.7 |
| Middle East and North Africa | 360 | 61 | 23 | 3.7 |
| South Asia | 430 | 98 | 45 | 3.5 |
| East Asia and Pacific | 140 | 43 | 21 | 2.0 |
| Latin America and Caribbean | 190 | 34 | 16 | 2.6 |
| CEE/CIS and Baltic States | 55 | 37 | 16 | 1.6 |
| Industrialized countries | 12 | 7 | NA | 1.6 |
| World | 400 | 82 | NA | 2.7 |

Source: UNICEF (2004).
MMR: Number of maternal deaths per 100,000 live births. Figures are for 1995.
Under-5 Mortality Rate: Number of deaths of children under 5 years of age per 1,000 live births. Figures are for 2001.
Stunting Prevalence: Percentage of children under 5 years old whose height is below two standard deviations from the median height for age of the WHO recognized international reference population. Estimates are for 2000.
Total Fertility Rate: Expected number of life-time births at current fertility rates. Estimates are for 2000.
NA: not available.

outcomes are highly correlated with economic development both between and within countries.

# MATERNAL HEALTH

International maternal health has been evolving in earnest since the Safe Motherhood Conference in Nairobi in 1987 (Cohen, 1987). In 2000, it was estimated that 529,000 women died from maternal causes (AbouZahr & Wardlaw, 2000); adequate maternal health care could have prevented 90% to 95% of these deaths (Ransom & Yinger, 2002). Although mortality remains a formidable problem, it constitutes only a small portion of the maternal health arena. For every maternal death, it is estimated that there are at least 100 acute morbidity episodes that occur during pregnancy, childbirth, and the postpartum period (Koblinsky, Campbell, & Harlow, 1993). Many factors have an impact on maternal health, but the provision of adequate health services is key to decreasing pregnancy-related morbidity and mortality (Koblinsky, 1995).

Monitoring maternal health status has been problematic because of the difficulty in measuring its key indicators. The International Classification of Diseases defines a maternal death as the death of a woman during pregnancy or within 42 days of its termination, regardless of the duration and site of the pregnancy, from any cause related to or aggravated by the pregnancy or its management, but not from accidental or incidental causes. Direct obstetric deaths, accounting for approximately 80% of maternal deaths, are those resulting from complications of pregnancy and birth. Indirect obstetric deaths are caused by an underlying illness or one that developed during pregnancy that was aggravated by the physiologic effects of pregnancy (WHO, 1993). The most common measure of maternal death is the MMR, defined as the number of maternal deaths during a given time period per 100,000 live births during the same time period. The MMR indicates the risk of death to a woman once pregnant. The maternal mortality rate is the number of maternal deaths in a given time period per 100,000 women during the same time period. It reflects the frequency that women are exposed to the risk of death through fertility. The lifetime risk of maternal death is based on the probability of becoming pregnant along with the probability of dying as a result of pregnancy across a woman's reproductive years (AbouZahr & Wardlaw, 2000).

Identifying maternal deaths in developing countries is problematic because in many countries the majority of women give birth and are treated for complications outside of medical facilities. Then because a maternal death is a relatively rare event, even in areas where the risk is high, obtaining a sound estimate requires a study population so large that it is impractical. A number of field and statistical methods have been devised in recent years to improve the accuracy of measures of the risk and level of maternal death. (Hill, AbouZahr, & Wardlaw, 2001). Generally, the MMR should not be used to monitor and evaluate maternal health programs because of the potential inaccuracies in its estimation (Buekens, 2001).

Despite these problems, estimates of the magnitude of maternal mortality are still considered vital to the field of maternal health because they call our attention to one of the largest ongoing health tragedies of the present era. The risk of maternal death represents the greatest health disparity between developed and less developed countries. For example, the MMR in France is 10/100,000 live births, compared with 98/100,000 in

Panama, 238/100,000 in the Philippines, 826/100,000 in Nepal, and 1497/100,000 in Chad (Hill, AbouZahr, & Wardlaw, 2001).

Some variation exists by region and setting in the proportion of deaths due to each cause, but generally, direct obstetric deaths result from hemorrhage (34%), obstructed labor (11%), hypertensive disorders of pregnancy (16%), and unsafe abortions (18%). Most indirect maternal deaths result from aggravated conditions such as malaria, anemia, and diabetes (Ransom & Yinger, 2002). Although the occurrence of conditions leading to a maternal death cannot be predicted, the vast majority of deaths can be prevented with adequate obstetric care at the time of an emergency. Thaddeus and Maine (1994) posited this in a conceptual model defining three phases of delay in obtaining appropriate maternal health care: the delay in the decision to seek care, the delay in getting to a facility, and the delay encountered once reaching the facility. Each of these phases is influenced by a set of factors that ultimately pose barriers to care. The proportion of maternal deaths resulting from unsafe abortion ranges from 12% to 33% around the world. Most of these deaths occur in places where there are varying levels of legal restrictions on abortion. In these countries, women resort to illegal procedures that are often performed by unskilled practitioners. Women in need of help after such a procedure are hampered by the same obstacles faced by women in need of emergency obstetric care, with the addition that both they and their practitioners may face legal consequences (Ransom & Yinger, 2002).

Maternal morbidity conditions—illnesses or injury arising from pregnancy, birth, or its management—result from the same set of causes linked to mortality and can be acute or chronic in nature (Ashford, 2002). It is estimated that 30% to 40% of pregnant women develop long-term disabilities such as obstetric fistula, genital prolapse, severe anemia, and reproductive tract infections. Measuring maternal morbidity is also very difficult, as many women do not enter the formal health care system. During the 1990s, many studies were undertaken to estimate the magnitude of maternal morbidity based on women's self-reports and to determine the validity and reliability of these estimates. Although some conditions such as eclampsia and severe bleeding could be reliably measured by asking a specific algorithm of questions on a survey, findings generally indicated that the sensitivity and specificity for the majority of morbidity conditions were low, making it inadvisable to use self-reports (Tsui, Wasserheit, & Haaga, 1997).

The same set of interventions will prevent both maternal death and disability, as the causes of both conditions are the same. Although some women are at higher risk for developing complications of pregnancy and childbirth, most maternal emergencies and morbidities are unpredictable. It is recommended that for every 500,000 persons there should be at least four facilities offering basic emergency obstetric care (BEOC) and one that has comprehensive emergency obstetric care (CEOC). BEOC includes the ability to administer certain drugs, such as ergometrine to stop uterine bleeding, and perform life-saving procedures, such as manual removal of the placenta. CEOC includes the ability to perform surgery, anesthesia, and blood transfusions, as well as the management of conditions such as anemia and hypertension (Ransom & Yinger, 2002).

Because many women in rural areas do not live close to a facility with either BEOC or CEOC, good referral and transport networks need to be in place to assure access to care. This may include training traditional birth attendants to recognize the danger signs of developing complications and helping to integrate them into the referral and transport systems to the formal medical infrastructure. Access to family planning services will reduce unintended pregnancies and lower women's lifetime risk for pregnancy-related death and disability by lowering fertility and reducing the need for abortion. Safe abortion services can be provided with relatively simple technology and will reduce complications of abortion. Postpartum and postabortion care will ensure that the complications developing after birth and abortion—whether safe procedures are available or not—will be managed properly (Ashford, 2002). Finally, although the benefits of antenatal care have been difficult to measure in maternal outcomes because of the unpredictable nature of the development of the most severe complications, the provision of antenatal care is considered as an essential component of a comprehensive maternal health system because visits during this time allow an opportunity for the treatment and management of sexually transmitted infections, malaria, hypertension, and other conditions that may arise, as well as for educating women about family planning, nutrition, child care, and sexually transmitted infection prevention (WHO, 2004).

The Safe Motherhood Initiative (SMI) was launched at the 1987 Nairobi conference by a host of international organizations. The SMI mission was to draw attention to the magnitude of maternal mortality. Over the years, the SMI has become a global partnership of governmental and nongovernmental agencies, donors, and women's health advocates.

Recommendations have been evidence based and now include the prevention and management of unwanted pregnancy and unsafe abortion, the need for every woman to have skilled care during pregnancy and childbirth, and the importance of access to referral care when complications arise. The Making Pregnancy Safer Initiative is a recent offshoot of the SMI, becoming an integral component of its missions and implementation. It aims to prevent the half-million maternal deaths that occur each year by reducing unwanted pregnancies and unsafe abortion, implementing best practices in the care of pregnant women, increasing the proportion of women assisted by a skilled birth attendant as part of an efficient referral system, reducing neonatal mortality and stillbirth rates, and establishing and providing access to CEOC facilities (WHO, 2004).

Given the difficulties and resulting inaccuracies in the outcome measures of maternal mortality, process measures are recommended to monitor progress of these programs toward the goal of reducing maternal death and disability. Two measures have been proposed to act as a proxy for the level of maternal death and disability. These are the proportion of births attended by a skilled health care worker, meaning a doctor, nurse, or midwife (not including traditional birth attendants), and the rates of caesarian delivery (proportion of births delivered by caesarian section). The higher the proportion of attended deliveries the better, and caesarian section rates should not fall below 5% (AbouZahr & Wardlaw, 2000).

In sub-Saharan Africa in the late 1990s, caesarian section rates were less than 5% in all countries except Kenya and less than 2% in Burkina Faso, Madagascar, Niger, and Zambia. Furthermore, between the early and late 1990s, there was little change overall, indicating that access to caesarian section in sub-Saharan Africa is not improving. In many countries, the proportion of singleton births delivered by a trained attendant also decreased over the 1990s (Buekens, Curtis, & Alayon, 2003). In other areas of the world, caesarian section rates stayed more or less stable over the 1990s, but substantial improvements were observed in the proportion of deliveries attended by health professionals in North Africa, the Middle East, and Asia (AbouZahr & Wardlaw, 2000). In some regions, particularly in some countries of Latin America, caesarian section rates are higher than 15%, indicating that the procedure is being overused. Although the caesarian section can be a life-saving procedure when medically indicated, in cases in which it is not, the procedure unnecessarily increases the health risks for both the mother and baby, as well as increasing the costs associated with childbirth. In the late 1990s, 12 Latin American countries, accounting for 81% of deliveries in the region, had national caesarian section rates above 15%. In Brazil and Chile, rates of 27% and 40% were observed, respectively (Belizan, Althabe, Barros, & Alexander, 1999). In resource-strained settings such as sub-Saharan Africa, increased access to caesarian section will improve maternal health outcomes, whereas in regions such as Latin America, an overuse of caesarian section drives up the rate of maternal morbidity.

# CHILD HEALTH

Mortality is the ultimate indicator of poor child health outcomes. Childhood mortality rates are commonly reported for different age ranges: early neonatal (0 to 6 days), neonatal (0 to 27 days), postneonatal (28 days to 11 months), infant (0 to 11 months), toddler (12 to 23 months), child (2 to 4 years), and under 5 years (0 to 4 years). The mortality rates are typically calculated as the number of deaths occurring in the age interval in a given period divided by the number of children entering the age interval. For infant and under-5 mortality rates, this is the number of deaths under the age of 1 year or under the age of 5 years, respectively, divided by the number of live births. These two rates represent the probability that a newborn child dies before their first and fifth birthdays, respectively. As child mortality declines, deaths at older ages (1 to 4 years) typically fall first. Therefore, in high mortality settings, there will tend to be a large difference between the infant and under-5 mortality rates, whereas in low mortality settings, the two measures will be quite similar because deaths among 1 to 4 year olds are so few. The under-5 mortality rate is the most widely used summary measure of child health outcomes for international purposes because it captures the entire high-risk period in high-mortality settings. UNICEF described it as "a critical indicator of the well-being of children" and ranked countries by their estimated under-5 mortality rate in its annual State of the World's Children publications (UNICEF, 2003). The exact method used to calculate childhood mortality rates varies depending on the data source and should be considered when comparing published estimates from different sources.

Considerable progress has been made in reducing child mortality over the last several decades. The estimated global under-5 mortality rate has declined from almost 200 deaths per 1,000 live births in 1960 to 82 deaths per 1,000 live births in 2000 (Table 13–3). However, declines have not been uniform. Sub-Saharan Africa has seen less improvement than other areas of the world. Furthermore, there is evidence that the rate of decline of child mortality has slowed in recent years and that child mortality rates are increasing in some countries, most notably in Southern Africa (Ahmad, Lopez, & Inoue, 2000). The reasons for the slow down in the decline vary across countries. In some areas (e.g., industrialized countries), mortality rates are very low, and thus, further reductions are difficult to achieve. In other areas (e.g., some countries in North Africa, the Near East, Latin America, and the Caribbean), mortality rates have declined rapidly from high to relatively low levels, limiting the potential for further rapid reductions. Of concern are countries in which the pace of mortality decline is slowing at high levels of mortality, most notably in sub-Saharan Africa. The emergence of the HIV/AIDS epidemic has contributed to the slowdown in childhood mortality decline in sub-Saharan Africa and increasing child mortality in countries hardest hit by the epidemic. The role of HIV/AIDS in global MCH is discussed in more detail later here.

The 2000 global under-5 mortality rate of 82 deaths per 1,000 live births translates into approximately 10 million deaths of children under 5 years old each year. These deaths are concentrated in less developed countries, with approximately 90% of them occurring in 42 countries. The largest numbers of child deaths occur in India, Nigeria, China, and Pakistan, but the highest mortality rates occur in Sierra Leone, Niger, Angola,

**Table 13–3** Trends in Under-5 Mortality by Region, 1960–2000

| Region | 1960 | 1970 | 1980 | 1990 | 2000 |
| --- | --- | --- | --- | --- | --- |
| Sub-Saharan Africa | 253 | 223 | 194 | 180 | 174 |
| Middle East and North Africa | 250 | 196 | 132 | 81 | 62 |
| South Asia | 244 | 206 | 176 | 128 | 100 |
| East Asia and Pacific | 212 | 125 | 77 | 58 | 44 |
| Latin America and Caribbean | 153 | 123 | 84 | 54 | 36 |
| CEE/CIS and Baltic States | 103 | 76 | 58 | 44 | 38 |
| Industrialized countries | 37 | 26 | 14 | 9 | 7 |
| World | 197 | 147 | 117 | 93 | 82 |

Source: UNICEF (2004).

and Afghanistan, where more than 25% of children die before their fifth birthday (Ahmad et al., 2000; Black, Morris, & Bryce, 2003). In the United States, less than 1% of children die before their fifth birthday.

Reliable data on cause of death are very difficult to obtain in developing countries. The WHO estimates that globally under-5 deaths are due to the following causes: diarrhea (13%), pneumonia (19%), malaria (9%), measles (5%), AIDS (3%), neonatal causes (42%), other causes, including noncommunicable diseases, and injuries (9%) (Black et al., 2003). Causes of death vary by region and by the level of mortality. Malaria is a significant cause of death in some countries, mostly in sub-Saharan Africa. AIDS deaths among children are concentrated in East and Southern Africa. However, in countries with relatively high levels of child mortality diarrhea, pneumonia, and neonatal causes account for the majority of deaths. As mortality declines, deaths from infectious diseases such as diarrhea, pneumonia, and vaccine-preventable diseases such as measles tend to fall first. This pattern results in an increasing concentration of deaths in the neonatal period and a shift in the cause of death profile toward neonatal causes such as birth asphyxia and low birth weight. In low child mortality settings, under-5 deaths are mostly due to neonatal conditions (e.g., congenital anomalies, conditions arising in the perinatal period) and injuries.

Many proven prevention and treatment interventions to improve child survival can be implemented in resource-poor environments. These include exclusive breastfeeding; immunization; micronutrient supplementation (particularly vitamin A and zinc); complimentary feeding; antibiotics for pneumonia, dysentery, and sepsis; oral rehydration therapy for diarrhea; antimalarial drugs; and insecticide-treated bednets to name a few. Jones, Steketee, Black, Bhutta, and Morris (2003) estimated that achieving global coverage of existing interventions could prevent approximately 63% of the 10 million child deaths that occur each year. The challenge is to achieve global coverage with these interventions in resource-poor environments with weak public health infrastructure. Coverage of key child survival interventions was only approximately 50% globally in 2003 (Jones et al., 2003). The barriers to scaling up child survival interventions to achieve high coverage are the same as those for other health interventions in these settings: high staff turnover, poor management and supervision, and inadequate funding to name a few. Furthermore, in populations in which contact with health services is infrequent, delivery strategies that focus only on the delivery of services without addressing demand for services at the community level will be ineffective in achieving high coverage.

Many global initiatives have been aimed at reducing child mortality and morbidity. The WHO Expanded Programme on Immunization and Diarrheal Disease Control Programme are among those considered to have been effective in achieving high coverage and measurable impacts on mortality (Bryce et al., 2003; Claeson, Gillespie, Mshinda, Troedsson, & Victora, 2003). The Expanded Programme on Immunization, launched in 1974, focused on immunizing children against six major infectious diseases (diphtheria, pertussis [whooping cough], tetanus, tuberculosis, polio, and measles) before their first birthday. Coverage of these vaccines was estimated to be less than 5% when the initiative was launched but had reached 73% for DPT3 (third dose of diphtheria-pertussis-tetanus) vaccine by 1999 and 72% for measles (UNICEF, 2004). However, these global figures mask wide differences between countries. For example, 14 countries, mostly in sub-Saharan Africa, still had measles coverage levels below 50% in 1999. In addition, there is growing evidence that progress stalled in the late 1990s, as evidenced by stagnation in DPT3 coverage rates globally and declines in some regions most notably sub-Saharan Africa and South Asia (Bryce et al., 2003).

More recently, there has been a move toward broader approaches to child survival programs. Integrated Management of Childhood Illnesses (IMCI) was launched by WHO in the mid 1990s and was being implemented in more than 100 countries in 2003. The strategy is based on the fact that most sick children presenting at health facilities have signs and symptoms related to more than one of the major conditions that account for most child deaths. The IMCI strategy has three main components: improvements in the case management skills of health staff through the provision of locally adapted guidelines and activities to promote their use, improvements in the health system to support effective management of childhood illnesses, and improvements in family and community practices (Tulloch, 1999). The IMCI approach is currently being evaluated; however, initial reports show mixed results, and hopes that the introduction of IMCI would lead to general improvements in the health system have not been supported by the initial findings (Bryce et al., 2003). However, many countries are still in the early stages of implementing IMCI.

There has been a growing recognition that further large reductions in child mortality will require large reductions in neonatal mortality. As noted previously, 42% of child deaths globally are associated with neonatal causes, and deaths become increasingly concentrated in the neonatal period as child mortality declines. In poor populations, many neonatal deaths are associated with poor maternal nutritional status and maternal infections during pregnancy (such as malaria and syphilis), which contribute to low birth weight and increased risk of preterm delivery. Unsafe delivery care and inappropriate care of the newborn after delivery also contribute significantly to preventable newborn deaths. A number of low-cost interventions are effective in reducing neonatal mortality and can be applied in low resource settings. These include antenatal care, birth preparedness, safe delivery care, including attendance by skilled health professionals, and postnatal care for the newborn and the mother. Antenatal care should include tetanus immunization for mothers to prevent neonatal tetanus, iron and folic acid supplementation for women of reproductive age, antimalarial drugs and use of insecticide-treated bednets to prevent malaria during pregnancy, and screening and treatment for syphilis. Postnatal care of the newborn should include prevention and management of hypothermia by drying and wrapping the entire baby right after delivery, encouraging immediate breastfeeding, clean cord care, and timely management and antibiotic treatment of infections. Family planning is also an important newborn health intervention, as it increases the intervals between births and reduces births to very young and very old mothers whose newborns are at particular risk. Integrating essential newborn care into existing safe motherhood and child health initiatives is key to improving newborn health and survival and ultimately achieving sustained reductions in child mortality.

# INTERNATIONAL REPRODUCTIVE HEALTH

The changing landscape of human reproduction in the latter half of the 20th century and at the turn of the millennium has been characterized as a global "reproductive revolution." This revolution has been marked by dramatic declines in fertility rates around the world and equally remarkable increases in the use of contraception. The world's total fertility rate (TFR) has declined from an estimated 5.4 children per woman in 1974 to 2.8 children per woman today. Contraceptive prevalence in developing countries in 1960 was just 9% of married women of reproductive age, whereas today it is estimated that 55% of reproductive age married women in these countries are using contraception (Caldwell, 2001; Zildar et al., 2003).

These global patterns are striking, but there has been considerable variation between and within regions in fertility decline and the adoption of contraception (Caldwell, 2001; Zildar et al., 2003). In the interval between 1974 and today, fertility in Sub-Saharan Africa has fallen from 6.5 children per woman in 1950 to 1955 to an estimated 5.9 children per woman today. In contrast, the TFR in Latin America and the Caribbean has declined from 5.9 children per woman in 1950 to 1955 to an estimated 2.7 children per woman today. Southern Europe, a region with an already low TFR of 2.7 in 1950 to 1955, has also shown a decline in fertility, with a TFR of only 1.4 children per woman today. Replacement level fertility is considered to be a TFR of 2.1 children per woman, a level of fertility below which no region fell before 1960. Today, East Asia and all regions in Europe are experiencing below replacement fertility.

Trends in contraceptive use show similar variation across world regions. In developing countries, contraceptive prevalence varies from a low of 15% in sub-Saharan Africa to a high of 68% in Latin America and the Caribbean, a rate comparable to the industrialized country average. The popularity of different contraceptive methods also varies across regions. The four most popular methods of contraception in developing countries are female sterilization (the most popular method in Latin America and the Caribbean), oral contraceptives (the most popular method in sub-Saharan Africa), injectables, and the intrauterine device (the predominant method in North Africa and the Near East). Together, these four methods comprise 75% of all methods used in less developed regions (Zildar et al., 2003). Female sterilization and to a lesser extent the intrauterine device are especially good methods for limiting family size, whereas injectables or oral contraceptives can be used to limit or space births. Method selection is a function of regional variations in method availability, social norms, method costs, and awareness of different methods. Cultural and political contexts can also affect method use. Until recently, many former Soviet countries relied predominantly on legal and institutionalized abortion as a means of fertility regulation, at least partly as a result of a lack of widespread and efficient distribution of contraceptives under the Soviet regime.

International policy regarding fertility and contraceptive use has also changed over time, although it is difficult to be sure how much these policies incited change as opposed to merely reflecting trends that were already established.

In the late 1960s and 1970s, policy makers became concerned about the specter of global overpopulation. This time period saw the establishment of the first national population policies designed to curtail population growth. The controversy in policy circles at the time was a question of whether there was a "population problem" and if so how best to bring about a decline in fertility (Sinding, 2000). One suggested method was a focus on economic growth and development that would lower fertility preferences and postpone marriage. A second strategy was the widespread introduction of contraception. Over time, as contraceptive use has skyrocketed and fertility plummeted, the focus has increasingly been on access to family planning on a voluntary basis, moving away from demographic targets, and offering family planning as part of a comprehensive reproductive health program. The focus on economic development and growth has shifted to an emphasis on gender equality and the empowerment of women and girls (McIntosh & Finkle, 1995).

This shift can be plainly seen in the changing policy language coming out of the United Nations' World population conferences. At the 1974 World Population Conference in Bucharest, developing countries joined with the Soviet bloc to protest the global demographic goals proposed by Western nations. At Bucharest also, arguments began about appropriate means for encouraging fertility decline: development or family planning. In 1984 in Mexico City, at the International Conference on Population, the debate became less polarized, with Western countries and the developing world agreeing, or at least neutral, to the idea that rapid population growth could impede development and that family planning was an appropriate response to unwanted fertility. This watershed conference set the stage for what is often referred to as the Cairo "consensus," or the Program of Action, set forth in the 1994 International Conference on Population and Development in Cairo, Egypt. Cairo was a defining moment in international population policy. For the first time, development and population linkages were specifically addressed in the title of the conference. Furthermore, a heavy feminist involvement at Cairo shifted the focus from overall economic growth to gender inequalities (McIntosh & Finkle, 1995). Traditional development schemes, it was argued, ignore and can be harmful for women. Furthermore, there was concern that family planning programs in concert with demographic targets are unfair to women and that family planning should be offered on a voluntary basis together with comprehensive reproductive health services.

As the international reproductive health community moves past Cairo and into the new millennium, many questions regarding population trends remain. In countries with limited resources, hard decisions must be made regarding how many and what kinds of reproductive health services should be offered in addition to family planning. Although much of Africa is just beginning the transition to low levels of fertility and increasing levels of contraceptive use, European policy makers are struggling with concerns over fertility levels that many consider too low. A final question that the international reproductive health community is facing is to what extent "consensus" will lead to shifting attention and complacency that may slow the trends in fertility and contraceptive use that we have witnessed over the past 30 years of heated debate and controversy.

# HIV/AIDS

The Joint United Nations Programme on HIV/AIDS (UNAIDS) estimates that worldwide there were 40 million people living with HIV/AIDS, 5 million new infections, and 3 million AIDS deaths in 2003. Sub-Saharan Africa is by far the worst affected region of the world, with approximately 26.6 million people estimated to be living with HIV/AIDS and approximately 2.3 million AIDS deaths in 2003. HIV prevalence in sub-Saharan Africa was estimated to be approximately 8% in 2003 compared with approximately 1% globally. Within sub-Saharan Africa, adult HIV prevalence is estimated to range from less than 1% in Mauritania to almost 40% in Botswana, with Southern Africa most badly affected (UNAIDS and WHO, 2003).

Considerable uncertainty surrounds estimates of HIV prevalence and AIDS mortality due to data deficiencies in most countries. Traditionally, estimates of HIV prevalence in populations with generalized epidemics are obtained from antenatal surveillance systems in which pregnant women in selected sites are anonymously tested for HIV. The quality and coverage of these systems varies across countries and over time within countries, complicating comparisons. Countries are, increasingly, including HIV testing in population-based surveys such as the DHS. Such surveys have the advantage of wider representation of the population, including men, and typically better representation in rural areas than antenatal surveillance systems. However, they can be subject to high non-response rates for HIV testing, which has serious implications for the quality of the estimates obtained, especially if nonresponse is associated with HIV status. Estimates of HIV prevalence therefore should be interpreted cautiously. However, they still provide an essential basis for tracking the epidemic and identifying general patterns and trends.

The HIV/AIDS epidemic has numerous implications for global MCH. First, HIV directly affects many of the populations of most interest in MCH: women of reproductive age, adolescents, and children. Approximately half of the estimated 40 million people living with HIV/AIDS are women. New infections occur disproportionately among young adults aged 15 to 24 years, and in sub-Saharan Africa, new infections occur disproportionately among girls and young women. Women are particularly vulnerable to HIV infection because traditional gender roles make it difficult for them to refuse sex or to negotiate safer sex. They are often infected by husbands or other stable partners in situations in which it is acceptable for men to have multiple partners, and HIV infection is strongly linked to experience of gender-based violence (Dunkle et al., 2004). Women are also biologically more vulnerable to HIV infection; the rate of male to female transmission is estimated as approximately twice that of female to male transmission.

HIV is associated with an increased risk of child mortality and morbidity through both direct and indirect mechanisms. Mother-to-child transmission of HIV can occur during pregnancy, childbirth, or breastfeeding. Available evidence indicates that in the absence of antiretroviral therapy approximately 30% of children born to HIV-positive mothers will be infected and that 60% of infected children will die before their fifth birthday (Spira et al., 1999). Indirect effects are many and varied, but most prominently involve illness and death of parents, which in turn are associated with reduced parental care and support, reduced food production at the household level, reduced access to health services for children, and dissolution of households when death occurs. In low-resource settings, already weak health services are further strained by the burden imposed to treat HIV-infected patients, reducing staff and financial resources for other services, including MCH services. At the same time, HIV/AIDS affects working-age adults, resulting in increased staff shortages in health facilities as qualified staff becomes sick and unable to perform their duties. A recent cross-national review of DHS and HIV prevalence data found that most countries in sub-Saharan Africa with high HIV prevalence (5% or more of adults seropositive) also experienced increased under-5 mortality rates (Adetunji, 2000).

The political and financial commitment to fighting HIV/AIDS has increased in the early part of the 21st century through initiatives such as the Global Fund to Fight AIDS, TB, and Malaria, the United Nations General Assembly Special Session on HIV/AIDS declaration, the US Government President's Emergency Plan for AIDS Relief, and the WHO "3 by 5" Initiative. Several of these initiatives include an emphasis on providing ARV treatment and care and support to individuals living with HIV/AIDS. For example, the WHO "3 by 5" Initiative aims to put 3 million HIV-infected people on ARV therapy by 2005, whereas the US Government President's Emergency Plan for AIDS Relief aims to provide treatment to 2 million HIV-infected people and provide care to 10 million people infected by HIV/AIDS, including orphans and vulnerable children. At the same time, prevention efforts focus on the "ABC" messages (Abstinence, Be faithful, Correct and Consistent Condom use), along with voluntary counseling and testing and prevention of maternal to child transmission (PMTCT). The WHO PMTCT framework takes a holistic view of PMTCT and includes four main strategies: (1) primary prevention of HIV in young women, (2) avoidance of unintended pregnancies among HIV-infected women, (3) provision of ARVs targeted at preventing HIV transmission from HIV-infected women to their infants, safe delivery, counseling, and support for safer infant feeding practices, and (4) providing care and support for mothers and their families.

The increased emphasis on HIV/AIDS globally has both positive and negative implications for broader MCH programs. Certainly, the attention to HIV/AIDS is urgently needed given the very high levels of HIV infection throughout the world and the potential for emerging epidemics in areas such as the Caribbean, China, India, Central Asia, and Eastern Europe to explode. PMTCT programs are clearly linked to wider maternal and newborn health services such as antenatal care, safe delivery care, and family planning, with the potential to improve these services for all women, not just those infected with HIV. However, in severely resource-constrained settings, the heavy emphasis on a single disease could draw human and financial resources away from other health areas. For example, in 2003 and 2004, the US Government reduced budgets for international

MCH while increasing funds for AIDS, TB, and malaria. Although fighting HIV/AIDS is clearly a burning global health priority, meeting global targets in MCH will require more than fighting a single disease (Claeson et al., 2003; Walker, Schwartlander, & Bryce, 2002).

# INEQUALITIES IN INTERNATIONAL MCH

A recurrent theme throughout this chapter has been the striking regional variation in global MCH outcomes. However, stark differentials in health outcomes exist between and within the countries in each of these regions. For example, sub-Saharan Africa has the highest number of child deaths in the world, accounting for 41% of all deaths to children less than 5 years old worldwide. However, within sub-Saharan Africa, under-5 mortality rates vary from 120 deaths per 1,000 live births in Kenya to 316 deaths per 1,000 live births in Sierra Leone (Black et al., 2003). Within Kenya, the under-5 mortality rate among the poorest fifth of the nation's population is more than three times the rate in the richest fifth (Victora et al., 2003). In this section, we briefly discuss some sources of inequality in health outcomes within and among countries worldwide, with a particular focus on three major factors: socioeconomic status, gender, and education.

## Socioeconomic Status

In virtually every country in the world, the poor have a lower use of antenatal and delivery care, lower rates of contraceptive use, and higher fertility. Poor women are also more likely than wealthy women to have complications from an unsafe abortion. Poor women and children are at greater risk for disease as a result of poor sanitation, crowding, and undernutrition. Furthermore, poor women and children are less likely than their wealthy peers to receive either preventive health or appropriate and timely treatment for illness and maternal complications (Shiffman, 2000; Victora et al., 2003). Socioeconomic differentials in MCH outcomes are not limited to the poorest, least industrialized countries and regions in the world. Data from 19 of the wealthiest countries in the world show that wage inequalities within a country are positively and significantly correlated with the infant mortality rate (Macinko, Shi, & Starfield, 2004).

## Gender

In many areas of the world, such as Asia and Northern Africa, cultural norms dictate a low status for women and a strong preference for sons. This is translated in some areas into differences in survival between boy and girl children. The selection for boy children can take two major forms. The first is through sex-selective abortion made possible through ultrasound technologies. Abnormally high sex ratios at birth have been observed in Northern India, China, and parts of East Asia, indicating the use of sex-selective abortion in these populations. The second is through infanticide and neglect of female children, which leads to a higher mortality rate. Evidence for these practices has been found, for example, in India, where a girl is 40% more likely to die before her fifth birthday than a boy (Victora et al., 2003). In the absence of strong gender preferences, girls are typically less likely than boys to die in childhood. Even within India there are important regional variations, with female child mortality being higher in North India, where women have lower status and a dowry tradition makes girl children more expensive.

Low status for women creates health risks for females from childhood through their reproductive years (Blanc, 2001; Shiffman, 2000). Women with low status tend to have less education and are at higher risk for gender-based violence than their counterparts (Blanc, 2001). Low status also confers a greater risk for maternal mortality, in part due to a lower likelihood for receiving appropriate health care, lower contraceptive use, higher fertility, and an earlier age at marriage (Shiffman, 2000). Women who have less power in sexual relationships are less likely to have the power to negotiate safe sexual practices and are at greater risk for sexually transmitted infections such as HIV (Dunkle et al., 2004).

## Education

Education, particularly female education, is strongly and consistently associated with MCH outcomes. Educated women and their children are less likely to die than their less educated counterparts, with higher levels of education conferring additional advantage. The pathways by which female education influences MCH outcomes have not been conclusively identified, but several hypotheses are generally accepted. Education is thought to provide women with information and the ability to obtain and act on information on their and their children's health, resulting in improved domestic health care and hygiene and increased use of health services. It is also thought that education may enable women to communicate and negotiate more effectively with health providers. Education increases the status of the women, strengthening her position within the household and her ability to obtain resources for herself and her children. It also increases the socioeconomic status of the woman both by allowing her to make a more favorable marriage and to work in higher paid occupations (Cleland & van Ginneken, 1988).

### Reducing Inequities

Obviously, socioeconomic standing, women's status, and female education are neither mutually exclusive nor exhaustive explanations for global disparities in MCH outcomes. Research about the role of these factors in health outcomes is complicated by the fact that socioeconomic status and gender roles are difficult constructs to measure and model, as they are often relative and culturally determined. Furthermore, institutional factors also play a role in reducing inequality in MCH outcomes. The majority of child and maternal deaths are preventable if women and children receive appropriate and timely health care interventions (Bryce et al., 2003; Jones et al., 2003; Shiffman, 2000). The most important of these are immunization, antenatal care, and delivery care with a skilled attendant. How do poor countries, and for that matter rich countries, ensure that essential health care is available and used by all people—rich and poor, male and female, educated and uneducated? What is the best way to allocate scarce resources to maximize the efficiency of the existing health care infrastructure? Many questions still remain to be answered. Nevertheless, continued attention to these dilemmas and to the sources of inequality in MCH will help us to understand better why these inequalities exist and how they are best to be reduced or even eliminated.

## CONCLUSIONS

This chapter has provided a broad overview of international MCH. Considerable progress has been achieved in the latter part of the 20th century, but much remains to be done. At the current rate of progress, the millennium development goals listed in Table 13–1 will not be achieved. Many countries lag behind, particularly those in sub-Saharan Africa, and large differentials exist within countries. Addressing these challenges will not be easy. It will require leadership, sustained political and financial commitment, and an emphasis on building strong health systems, as well as fighting specific diseases. The early part of the 21st century has seen large increases in international political commitment and resources for AIDS, TB, and malaria and a call to action for child survival (Claeson et al., 2003). At the same time, the commitment to reproductive health appears to be dwindling (Gillespie, 2004). It remains to be seen what impact these international MCH developments will have on the health of women and children worldwide.

# REFERENCES

AbouZahr, C., & Wardlaw, T. (2000). *Maternal mortality in 2000: Estimates developed by WHO, UNICEF, and UNFPA.* Geneva: World Health Organization.

Adetunji, J. (2000). Trends in under-5 mortality rates and the HIV/AIDS epidemic. *Bulletin of the World Health Organization, 78,* 1200–1206.

Ahmad, O.B., Lopez, A.D., & Inoue, M. (2000). The decline in child mortality: A reappraisal. *Bulletin of the World Health Organization, 78,* 1175–1191.

Ashford, L. (2002). *Hidden suffering: Disabilities from pregnancy and childbirth in less developed countries.* Washington DC: Population Reference Bureau.

Belizan, J.M., Althabe, F., Barros, F., & Alexander, S. (1999). Rates and implications of caesarean sections in Latin America: Ecological study. *British Medical Journal, 319,* 1397–1400.

Black, R.E., Morris, S.S., & Bryce, J. (2003). Where and why are 10 million children dying every year? *Lancet, 361,* 2226–2234.

Blanc, A.K. (2001). The effect of power in sexual relationships on sexual and reproductive health: An examination of the evidence. *Studies in Family Planning, 32,* 189–213.

Bryce, J., el Arifeen, S., Pariyo, G., Lanata, C., Gwatkin, D., & Habicht, J. (2003). Reducing child mortality: Can public health deliver? *Lancet, 362,* 159–164.

Buekens, P. (2001). Is estimating maternal mortality useful? *Bulletin of the World Health Organization, 79,* 179.

Buekens, P., Curtis, S., & Alayon, S. (2003). Demographic and health surveys: Caesarean section rates in sub-Saharan Africa. *British Medical Journal, 326,* 136.

Caldwell, J. (2001). The globalization of fertility behavior. *Population and Development Review, 27*(Suppl), 93–115.

Claeson, M., & Waldman, R. J. (2000). The evolution of child health programmes in developing countries: From targeting diseases to targeting people. *Bulletin of the World Health Organization, 78,* 1234–1245.

Claeson, M., Gillespie, D., Mshinda, H., Troedsson H., & Victora C. (2003). Knowledge into action for child survival. *Lancet, 362,* 323–327.

Cleland, J.G., & van Ginneken, J. K. (1988). Maternal education and child survival in developing countries: The search for pathways of influence. *Social Science & Medicine, 27,* 1357–1368.

Cohen, S. (1987). The Safe Motherhood Conference. *International Family Planning Perspectives, 13,* 68–70.

Dunkle, K.L., Jewkes, R.K., Brown, H.C., Gray, G.E., McIntyre, J.A., & Harlow, S.D. (2004). Gender-based violence, relationship power, and risk of HIV infection in women attending antenatal clinics in South Africa. *Lancet, 363,* 1415–1421.

Gillespie, D.G. (2004). Whatever happened to family planning and, for that matter, reproductive health? *International Family Planning Perspectives, 30,* 34–38.

Hill, K., AbouZahr, C., & Wardlaw, T. (2001). Estimates of maternal mortality for 1995. *Bulletin of the World Health Organization, 79,* 182–193.

Jones, G., Steketee, R.W., Black, R.E., Bhutta, Z.A., & Morris, S.S. (2003). How many child deaths can we prevent this year? *Lancet, 362,* 65–71.

Koblinsky, M.A. (1995). Beyond maternal mortality: Magnitude, interrelationship, and consequences of women's health, pregnancy-related complications and nutritional-status on pregnancy outcomes. *International Journal of Gynecology & Obstetrics, 48,* S21–S32.

Koblinsky, M.A., Campbell, O., & Harlow, S.D. (1993). Mother and more: A broader perspective on women's health. In M. Koblinsky, J. Timyan, and J. Gays (Eds.), *The health of women.* Boulder, CO: Westview Press.

Lee, J.W. (2005). A personal invitation to celebrate World Health Day, World Health Day 2005. Geneva, Switzerland: World Health Organization. Available February 9, 2005, from: http://www.who.int/world-health-day/2005/dg_invite/en/.

Macinko, J.A., Shi, L.Y., & Starfield, B. (2004). Wage inequality, the health system, and infant mortality in wealthy industrialized countries, 1970–1996. *Social Science & Medicine, 58,* 279–292.

McIntosh, C.A., & Finkle, J.L. (1995). The Cairo conference on population and development: A new paradigm. *Population and Development Review, 21,* 223–260.

Newell, K.W. (1988). Selective primary health-care: The counter revolution. *Social Science & Medicine, 26,* 903–906.

Ransom, E., & Yinger, N. (2002). *Making motherhood safer: Overcoming obstacles on the pathway to care.* Washington DC: Population Reference Bureau.

Rifkin, S.B., & Walt, G. (1986). Why health improves: Defining the issues concerning comprehensive primary health-care and selective primary health-care. *Social Science & Medicine, 23,* 559–566.

Shiffman, J. (2000). Can poor countries surmount high maternal mortality? *Studies in Family Planning, 31,* 274–289.

Sinding, S.W. (2000). The great population debates: How relevant are they for the 21st century? *American Journal of Public Health, 90,* 1841–1845.

Spira, R., Lepage, P., Msellati, P., Van De Perre, P., Leroy, V., Simonon, A., Karita, E., & Dabis, F. (1999). Natural history of human immunodeficiency virus type 1 infection in children: A five-year prospective study in Rwanda. *Pediatrics, 104, e56.*

Thaddeus, S., & Maine, D. (1994). Too far to walk: Maternal mortality in context. *Social Science & Medicine, 38,* 1091–1110.

Tsui, A.O., Wasserheit, J.N., & Haaga, J.G. (1997). *Reproductive health in developing countries: Expanding dimensions, building solutions.* Washington, DC: National Academy Press.

Tulloch, J. (1999). Integrated approach to child health in developing countries. *Lancet, 354,* S16–S20.

UNAIDS and WHO. (2003). AIDS epidemic update, December 2003. *UNAID/03.39E.* Geneva: UNAIDS.

UNICEF. (2003). State of the world's children. Geneva: United Nations.

UNICEF. (2004). *End of the decade databases.* Available March 6, 2004, from: http://www.childinfo.org/index2.htm

United Nations. (2004). *Millennium development goals.* Available May 16, 2004, from: http://www.un.org/millenniumdevelopmentgoals

US Census Bureau. (2004). *Global population profile 2002.* Available June 6, 2004, from: http://www.census.gov/prod/2004pubs/wp-02.pdf

Victora, C.G., Wagstaff, A., Schellenberg, J.A., Gwatkin D., Claeson, M., & Habicht J.P. (2003). Applying an equity lens to child health and mortality: More of the same is not enough. *Lancet, 362,* 233–241.

Walker, N., Schwartlander, B., & Bryce J. (2002). Meeting international goals in child survival and HIV/AIDS. *Lancet, 360,* 284–289.

Warren, K.S. (1988). The evolution of selective primary health-care. *Social Science & Medicine, 26,* 891–898.

World Health Organization. (1993). *International statistical classification of diseases and related health problems* (Vol. 2, 10th ed.). Geneva: World Health Organization.

World Health Organization. (2004). Safe motherhood and making pregnancy safer. Available May 30, 2004, from: http://www.who.org

Zildar, V., Gardner, R., Rutstein, S., Morris, L., Goldberg H., & Johnston, K. (2003). The reproductive revolution continues (Series M, no. 17). *Population reports.* Baltimore, MD: Johns Hopkins University Bloomberg School of Public Health INFO Project.

# Maternal and Child Health Skills

# 14

# Research Issues in Maternal and Child Health

*Greg R. Alexander, Donna J. Petersen, Martha Slay Wingate, and Russell S. Kirby*

> *It is often said that science has destroyed our values and put nothing in their place. What has really happened of course is that science has shown in harsh relief the division between our values and our world.* (Bronowski, 1967)
>
> *She blinded me with science.* (Dolby & Kerr, 1982)

## RESEARCH IN MATERNAL AND CHILD HEALTH

### The Need for Research in Maternal and Child Health

Maternal and child health (MCH) is the field that focuses on the determinants, mechanisms, and systems that promote the health, safety, well-being, and appropriate development of children and their families (Alexander, 2003a; Alexander et al., 2002). Research is an essential cornerstone of the MCH field. MCH is a collaborative, multidisciplinary specialty area of public health and uses the research tools of other public health, social science, and public administration disciplines (including epidemiology, biostatistics, policy analysis, health services research, medical sociology, and geography) to (1) explore the etiology, determinants and distribution of disease, injury, disability, and death; (2) assess needs, along with expanding crucial surveillance and data systems; (3) develop cost-effective prevention and intervention approaches; (4) plan for and monitor the implementation, administration, and functioning of systems of care; (5) evaluate the process and outcomes of programs and policies; and (6) guide effective, responsible advocacy and the dissemination of information and new knowledge.

Although public health and MCH research are traditionally valued for increasing our understanding of the determinants of the health status and health care use of the MCH population, it further offers well-established methods to identify need priorities, to select an appropriate course of action among alternative interventions, and to assess the cost-effectiveness and impact, both intended and otherwise, of our chosen response. As rooted as the MCH field is in public health practice, MCH professionals must continually assess the evolving needs of the MCH population in light of ongoing developments in our health care and social service systems and a changing physical and social environment. In order to make needed policy and programmatic decisions regarding the allocation and targeting of limited resources, MCH professionals must rely on scientifically rigorous and defensible data to guide their choices, thereby assuring accountability and maintaining credibility. Research provides the means to distinguish efficacious, evidence-based practices from those that may only be fads with insufficient evidence to support their being touted as best practice. Indeed, the hallmark of responsible advocacy to inform the choices of the public and policy makers is its strict reliance on research-based evidence.

The funding of new research and practice initiatives in the MCH field is largely based on the submission of demonstration, research, or training grants. Applications for funding typically contain detailed descriptions of study objectives, aims, and hypotheses, along with plans for the execution of the project, the monitoring of its implementation and conduct, and the evaluation of its impact based on stated and measurable objectives. From carefully constructed research trials to demonstration projects that describe the feasibility of a practice approach, the application of research methods assures a more valid and systematic assessment of the conduct and end products of these efforts.

As market-driven health care in the United States continues to alter the face of public health and re-emphasize its basic core functions of assessment, assurance, and policy/advocacy, the importance of fostering and maintaining a viable and growing research capacity in MCH is critical to supporting state and local efforts to carry out those core functions. Without a continuing investment into research and the training of future MCH researchers, the MCH field will not be able to achieve its historic mission for children and their families nor will it be able to enhance the future health and welfare of society and subsequent generations.

## Pressing Research Needs

The MCH field faces a number of pressing research needs, some ongoing and others emerging. In recent times, the more persistent MCH research needs to involve the further development of key MCH health and health care use indicators and the refinement of methods for need assessment and systems evaluation. Nonetheless, there are many areas where there is an acute need to understand the basic etiology and determinants of disease and development. Although any list of the most critical MCH research needs is open to debate and may quickly become outdated, candidates for a list of pressing MCH research need areas follows.

### Measuring Key MCH Concepts

MCH is rich in the use of highly abstract concepts, for example, primary care, to describe desired approaches to caring for the needs of children and families (Grason & Wigton, 1995; Johansen, Starfield, & Harlow, 1994; Starfield, 1992; Alexander 1996). In addition, abstract terms that are frequently employed in MCH but are still less than adequately defined include "systems," "cultural competency," "family centered," "community based," "medical home," etc. Research measurement approaches are invaluable to MCH in order for the field to document progress and assess the performance of its programs, policies, and practitioners. Our ability to advocate for and assure coordinated, comprehensive, and continuous systems of care depends in part on our ability to measure current levels of health status and use and track changes that we propose will result from specified policies and leadership efforts. The old adage "that which can't be measured can't be changed" underscores the importance to MCH of improving our research measurement capacity and thereby improving its ability to assess health status and health care use needs more completely.

### Assessing Needs, Evaluating Solutions, and Monitoring Performance

Within the statutory requirements of Title V of the Social Security Act is the 5-year needs assessment that every state and territory must complete and report (PL 74-271, 1935; PL 101-239, 1989). Beyond the 5-year needs assessment, state MCH programs are expected to engage in ongoing needs assessments as part of a rational planning cycle linked to policy development, program design, budgets, resource allocation, and evaluation (MCHB, 2004). Despite the importance of needs assessment to MCH, the scientific knowledge base necessary to inform program leaders about the most rigorous, productive, and cost-effective approaches to address persistent need areas remains underdeveloped (Alexander & Petersen, 2004). There is a critical need to evaluate rigorously the current intervention and prevention programs and to expand the evaluation literature relevant to MCH in order to increase the effective use of our available resources to impact health status and health care use favorably. Similarly, in response to the Government Performance and Results Act of 1993 and various states' performance-based budgeting initiatives, state MCH programs must be prepared to articulate a set of performance measures that capture the depth and breadth of their efforts in ways that are reasonable and realistic but not potentially detrimental to the viability of the programs (PL 102-63, 1993). This becomes a delicate balancing act, fraught with challenges, including how to handle mandated programs, how to address politically sensitive activities, how to consider politically popular programs, and how to maintain focus on less popular but fundamentally important areas of MCH. Although needs assessment methods have continued to develop, the science of performance monitoring is not far behind. Nevertheless, performance measurement and monitoring deserves increased attention from researchers interested in supporting the capacity of programs not only to survive but also to lead responsibly and effectively.

### Assessing Child Health and Development at the Population Level

The vital records system in the United States provides an extraordinary resource for researchers interested in events surrounding perinatal health. Unfortunately, as a field, we have been unable to capitalize on this opportunity to track and monitor the health of children, on a population basis, as they grow. In fact, from a research population database perspective, we know very little about early childhood with the exception of mortality and immunization status. In some states, we may be able to monitor blood lead levels, hospitalizations, and injuries, but this is not uniform across the country. After school entry, some states require physical examinations, yet these data are not captured for further study. With recent concern about nutritional status and obesity, some states are exploring ways to record and monitor body mass index measurements on children. As researchers, we must make the argument that data on our children are critically important to monitor effectively trends and explore issues that affect their health, in order to advocate for needed policy and programmatic initiatives in the promotion of child health. In spite of some recent efforts toward population-wide surveys and surveillance of child health parameters, much more must be accomplished.

## Evaluating Health Services Systems

The failure to achieve a national health plan in the 1990s left the US health system in relative disarray and without an overarching roadmap or a strategic plan. Individuals attempt to access needed health care services for themselves and their children through a tattered and confusing patchwork of health insurance plans, provider networks, and managed-care plan rules and restrictions. The state-level health reform plans of the 1980s and 1990s failed to achieve their goals of increased quality and access at reduced costs. Health care costs continue to rise, straining not only corporate budgets but also the budgets of states struggling to maintain an effective workforce within state fiscal constraints. Changes contemplated by the White House and the Congress to Medicaid, the State Child Health Insurance Program, and related regulations such as the Employee Retirement Income Security Act (ERISA) demand vigorous scrutiny by MCH professionals and advocates and require a rich repository of research evidence to support or refute proposed initiatives. Data systems to support such research are also in need of development.

## Investigating Determinants of Racial Disparities

Despite advances in health care in recent decades and improvements in health status for many Americans, certain racial/ethnic minorities experience disparities in health outcomes and health care compared with non-minorites. Although these disparities are quite evident among adult populations for stroke, heart disease, and other conditions, they also exist among children. Despite the reduction of overall infant mortality, African Americans are still more than twice as likely as whites to die in the first year of life (Alexander & Slay, 2002). Moreover, disparities related to access to care continue, although not always in anticipated ways (Institute of Medicine, 2002). Health care disparities, often related to geography, immigrant status, cultural and linguistic barriers, etc., disproportionately impact minority populations and are associated with more negative outcomes. The need for continued research regarding these disparities in outcomes and in health services access is evident. Efforts at federal, state, and local levels are in place, working to close the gap, but more information is needed about their effectiveness. The Initiative to Eliminate Racial and Ethnic Disparities in Health by the US Department of Health and Human Services Office of Minority Health provides funding to numerous state and local programs aimed at improving the health of minority populations (*HHS Disparities Initiative*, 2001). The Maternal and Child Health Bureau's strategic research agenda also includes a focus on health disparities (*Maternal and Child Health Bureau Strategic Plan*, 2003). The *Healthy People 2010* objectives include two overarching goals of increasing the quality and years of life as well as eliminating racial and ethnic disparities (*Healthy People 2010*, 2000; US Department of Health and Human Services, 2000). Although improvement has been noted in some health outcomes, certain ones continue to be immutable. The increasing racial disparity in infant mortality is a noteworthy example in which much research attention has been given to the disparities in preterm birth, a key risk factor for infant death among African American infants, but no "silver bullet" has been identified (Alexander, 2003b; Alexander & Kogan, 1998). Continued research is critical in identifying, understanding, and eliminating these disparities.

# FUNDAMENTAL CONCEPTS OF SCIENCE AND RESEARCH

## *Measurement, Order, and Classification*

From a philosophical point of view, we use research and the scientific method to understand better the workings of world around us (e.g., understanding the mechanisms underlying the distribution and spread of disease) and to better predict the probability of events to come. Testing and falsification are the hallmarks of this approach in that we propose research questions such that, through experimentation, we can find evidence, within the limitations of our study design and data, that argues against (rejects) or does not refute (fails to reject) our preconceived notions (hypotheses and theories) about reality. Fundamental to this research process is the classification or ordering of events and observations into identifiable categories of likes and dislikes (Bronowski, 1967). Practically speaking, research measurement entails our ability to identify cases from controls correctly, those with disease from those without, those who use health care services from those who do not, and those with specific risk characteristics from those who may be free of those attributes. The precise definition and measurement of ideas, concepts, or variables are critical steps in all scientific research. As such, the importance and value of studies that seek to develop new or refine existing measurement approaches should not be overlooked, particularly in a research field as relatively new as MCH. Furthermore, studies conducted on MCH-related topics require the same rigor and necessity of solid measurement as any other scholarly discipline.

## Validity and Reliability of Measurement

To bring order to our concepts about health problems, risk factors, and at-risk populations, our observations are typically categorized using various measurement approaches. The basic ways of ordering include *categorical* and *continuous* measures. Categorical measures consist of *dichotomous* (two mutually exclusive categories), *nominal* (more than two mutually exclusive categories), *ordinal* (ordered qualitative categories), and *interval* (categories with a "natural," equal interval between values). Continuous variables are those with an interval scale with a true zero point so that ratios between values are meaningful (Isaac & Michael, 1995).

Errors in the classification of individuals or observations into one group or another are inherent to the process of grouping data and call into question the validity of the measurement approach employed. *Validity of measurement* asks this question: "Is this measuring what it claims?" In the strictest sense, to be valid, the measures should reflect true differences among groups on the characteristics or concepts that are measured and not be result of systematic or nonrandom errors in classifying. Validity of measurement is concerned with several types of validity, including *criterion validity* (also known as predictive validity), which asks whether the measure is a good predictor or "validator" of an outcome or criterion of interest; *content validity*, involving questions about breadth and adequate coverage of what it claims to measure; and *construct validity*, which asks whether the concept that is being measured truly exists and whether the measure is really measuring it (Carmines & Zeller, 1979; Isaac & Michael, 1995; Nunnally, 1978).

The *reliability of measurement* is an equally important consideration in research and is directed at identifying measurement errors, mainly random or chance errors, related to the consistency and stability of scoring observations in a series of measurements. In other words, it entails assessing the accurate repeatability of a measurement approach or the agreement between multiple measurement approaches, that is, the yielding of the same results. Various different methods are available for assessing the degree of reliability, all involving comparisons between multiple measures, for example, retest, alternate forms, and split-halves method (Carmines & Zeller, 1979; Isaac & Michael, 1995; Nunnally, 1978). In relationship to validity, a measure may be reliable but not valid, that is, an invalid result (one that does not appropriately measure the given concept, etc.) yet can be repeated (Isaac & Michael, 1995).

The assessment of measurement validity and reliability is a primary starting point for developing and assessing any research study. For example, studies about preterm birth should clearly describe the measurement of gestational age, including identifying and addressing out-of-range or implausible data, the treatment or imputation of missing data, and the combination of various approaches for measuring gestational age (e.g., ultrasound, duration of pregnancy, obstetric vs. pediatric methods). Appropriately, there is a considerable body of literature directed at reliability and validity of measurement, and the indicated references provide a starting point for further reading about these essential measurement issues (Carmines & Zeller, 1979; Isaac & Michael, 1995; Nunnally, 1978).

## Causality, Association, and Chance

Beyond bringing order to our observations, scientific research seeks to reveal the mechanisms that underlie the way the world works, for example, what is the cause of disease, low birth weight, or preterm delivery. By better understanding the relationships between occurrences and characteristics, we are better able to describe the flow of events that we see around us and predict with greater accuracy the expected consequences of actions. Moreover, we are better able to develop effective interventions and understand how modifying the environment, behaviors, and conditions might change the course of future events and thereby improve the future for children and their families. Nevertheless, the utility of science to reveal the causal nature of the surrounding environment and universe at large has been subject to ongoing debate. Beyond the scope of this chapter, grounding in the philosophy of science is instructive to understand better the language of research and the distinct attention that is paid to the cautious use of the term "causality" (Bronowski, 1967; Popper, 1965; Rothman, 1986). Causality is generally used to indicate that a relationship exists between two concepts or events and that one is believed to determine the specific occurrence of the other. At issue with this notion is the recognition of chance and probability, the belief that although future events may for the most part be predictable within an interval of confidence, there is always some uncertainty. In research, there is always some component of chance for which we use statistics to assess the probability of relationships and outcomes.

Recognizing the role of chance in science, researchers have taken a more circumscribed approach to the use of the term "causality" to describe research on hypothesized relationships. Various benchmarks have been advanced to differentiate whether an association should be considered causal versus noncausal, including (1) biologic plausibility, (2) a time-sequenced relationship (the predictor always precedes the outcome), (3) the strength and type of the association (strong, dose-response), and (4) a necessary (nonsubstitutable), sufficient, and consistent relationship between predictor and outcome (Hill, 1965; Rothman, 1986). Although the development of absolute criteria for causality continues to be as elusive as the scientific search for "truth," these benchmarks do emphasize the need for prudence in the interpretation of research findings. It cannot be stressed enough that science does not prove what is and will always be true. It instead offers a pathway for life-long learning, relearning, and intellectual adaptation in an uncertain and changing world.

In MCH, much of the research conducted is epidemiologic in nature and seeks to find potential risk factors and associations of particular characteristics with a given disease or outcome. Rarely is the intent of MCH research to reveal causal associations. For example, research on teen pregnancy typically reveals that infants born to mothers who are less than 18 years of age are at increased risk of being low birth weight. This association is well established, although it may not exist in every population and could possibly change in terms of the strength of the association. For very young teens, less than 15 years old, there may be biologically plausible reasons why young, still-developing mothers are more likely to have smaller babies. Nevertheless, it is important to note that a teen mother is not the *cause* of a low birth weight infant, and most infants born to teen mothers are not low birth weight.

# BUILDING BLOCKS OF RESEARCH

## *Theories, Hypotheses, and Operational Definitions*

*Theories* are used to drive the direction of research and scientific inquiry. Theories are sets of interrelated propositions that are collectively used to explain some aspect of reality. They may have stated boundaries, for example, populations and time frames, that circumscribe the limits of the theory. They are neither true nor false and are useful only if they are accurately descriptive or predictive. Theoretical development typically begins with logical descriptions of phenomena and progresses to testable hypotheses, using empirical measures. Findings from these empirical studies can only support theories, not prove them.

*Hypotheses* and *operational definitions* are the empirical basis for examining theories and exploring whether there are relationships between two or more concepts. Hypotheses are used to test theories at the empirical level, and as they are used for testing, they must provide propositional statements that are falsifiable. To be further useful, hypotheses should have available operations to measure variables and collect data in concrete situations (Miller, 1991). Hypotheses are generally stated in the "null" form and suggest that there will be no difference or change in one concept variable, given a variation on another. Similar to theories, boundary statements may be used to define the populations, time period, or geographic area to which the hypothesis is limited.

Operational definitions are used to measure concepts found in hypotheses. In order to make sense of a concept, one must operationalize it so that it will be evident to others. For example, for a study on child abuse (a concept), a measurement tool must be developed to assess if it occurred and to which study participants. The measurement tool, possibly a survey, interview form, or case report, documents to other researchers the definition and procedures used to determine child abuse cases. Therefore, operational definitions employ empirical indicators, for example, questions, a scale, and test scores, to define and measure the existence and extent of observable events or characteristics that measure the concepts used in the hypothesis. Operational definitions need to be abstract enough to be able to be used in different time and space settings while still providing a sufficient description of measurement procedures to be replicable and therefore to help standardize research. Within the MCH field, there are many commonly used operational definitions employed for research on such concepts as use of prenatal care, premature birth, and unintentional pregnancy. Conventions have been developed for measuring these concepts; for example, the R-GINDEX has been employed to measure adequacy of prenatal care use (Alexander & Kotelchuck, 1996), and the use of these measurement conventions facilitates comparing research results and synthesizing of the current evidence on a particular topic.

## Modeling Hypothesized Relationships

Modeling is a useful technique for organizing thoughts while developing research ideas and for visually describing the proposed relationships between concepts used in hypotheses. It allows for a visual depiction of the relationships of predictor variables to the outcome variables of interest. Variables are the primary components of hypotheses, and before constructing a theoretical model, the dependent and independent variables need to be identified. *Dependent variables* measure the outcome(s) of interest. Implicit in their label, change in the values of the dependent variable will depend on the values of the independent variables. *Independent variables* are the proposed predictors of the outcome, the variables that are potentially associated with changes in the dependent variable's values. For the purposes of modeling and developing stated hypotheses, two types of independent variables can be differentiated: the main independent variable(s), whose relationship with the dependent variables are of primary interest, and the other independent variables, which will be taken into account or controlled for in the analysis because of their perceived relationship with the main independent variables and the dependent variables.

The following is a schematic example for a theoretical model (Figure 14–1). The three types of variables are identified, and the directions of the

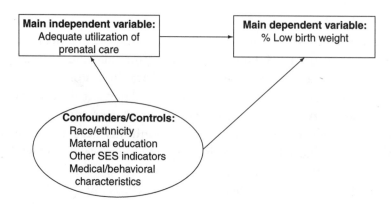

**FIGURE 14–1** Boundary statement among US resident women <133% poverty.

relationships among the variables are specified by the directions of the arrows. Pluses or minuses could be noted by each arrow to signify a possible positive or negation association. The example model provides a boundary statement and indicates that there will be a relationship between the independent variable and the dependent variable after controlling for the potential confounders. This model depicts the following formally stated null hypothesis. Among US resident women less than 133% of poverty (boundary statement): "There will be no change in the proportion of women delivering a low birth weight infant (dependent variable) by adequacy of prenatal care utilization (main independent variable), after taking into account maternal race/ethnicity, education, socioeconomic status and medical and behavioral risk factors (control independent variables)." In order for this hypothesis to be tested, the variables listed in the model still require specific concrete operations definitions, for example, the percentage of low birth weight (less than 2,500 grams), adequate use of prenatal care (R-GINDEX), maternal education (less than 12 years, 12 years, or more than 12 years), etc. (Piper, Ray, & Griffin, 1990).

## TYPES OF RESEARCH

Choosing an appropriate design for a research study is critical. This early-stage decision can influence the overall conclusions that can be made regarding the research findings. For much of the research in the MCH field, study designs fall into three general categories: nonexperimental, experimental, and health services research. These are described in greater detail later here.

## Nonexperimental Designs

*Nonexperimental designs* characterize those types of research in which there is only observation and no manipulation of the variables (Bordens & Abbott, 2002). These types of studies can also be referred to as *epidemiologic studies*, consisting of both descriptive and analytical studies. *Descriptive studies* are those concerned with general distributions of disease and health status. *Case studies* are in-depth studies of single cases. *Case series* use a number (series) of cases in which the disease/outcome of interest is observed in order to evaluate whether any common features are shared. These observations, often obtained through questionnaires, data from records, etc., can be retrospective or prospective. Both case studies and case series are useful in generating hypotheses and developing new measurement strategies (Ellis, 1994).

Cross-sectional studies and *screening surveys*, both based on a representative sample questioned at one point in time, are also descriptive studies. Cross-sectional studies aim to assess the prevalence of a disease or condition and associated factors. Screening surveys are useful in potentially identifying individuals or populations at high risk for some disease or condition so that some health care intervention or promotion can be implemented. The final descriptive epidemiologic study described in Table 14–1 is *ecological*. These studies aim to assess the relationship between an exposure and disease/mortality. The unit of study is a group of people (Bowling, 2002).

*Analytic studies* include *case-control* and *cohort studies* that, although nonexperimental, are concerned with the cause and prevention of disease. These types of studies typically compare population groups based on exposure to a given risk factor or disease/condition. The case-control study starts by identifying a group with a condition/disease of interest and comparing it with a reference group (controls) to determine whether there is a difference in exposure to a hypothesized risk factor or factors. The aim of this type of study is to assess which factors occur more or less often among cases compared to controls in order to identify potential means of reducing risk factors for disease or increasing protective factors. This analysis allows for calculation of an odds ratio, an approximation of

**Table 14–1**   Research Designs: Nonexperimental

| | | Nonexperimental: No Manipulation of Variables; Observational Only | |
|---|---|---|---|
| **Types of Research** | | **Research Design** | **Description** |
| Epidemiologic | Descriptive | Case study | It involves in-depth study of single cases and is useful for generating hypotheses. |
| | | Case series | It observes a series of cases with certain characteristics/conditions to determine any shared features; it is useful for generating hypotheses. |
| | | Screening surveys and case finding | It is conducted in order to detect individuals or populations at high risk for disease/condition. |
| | | Cross-sectional survey | It is based on a sample or subsample of a population that is questioned at one point in time. |
| | | Ecological | The aim is to assess the exposure and disease/mortality. |
| | Analytical | Case-control | Involves a comparison of a group with a condition/disease of interest or who have been exposed to a risk factor with a comparison or reference group; the aim is to identify factors that occur more or less often in the cases than in the controls; retrospective. |
| | | Cohort | Intended to assess the incidence of disease and the potential causative agents of a disease; division into "exposed" and "unexposed" groups occurs naturally, with no manipulation from the investigator; prospective. |

relative risk, that can measure the association of a risk factor and a disease. These studies are typically retrospective, although the case-control design can be applied to subjects accrued prospectively (Bowling, 2002).

Cohort studies are longitudinal or "follow-up" studies of the occurrence of disease in a group of subjects chosen on the basis of exposure in comparison to that of individuals in a group not exposed to a risk factor of interest. They are intended to assess the incidence of disease and the potential causative agents. The division into the "exposed" and "unexposed" groups often occurs naturally, with no manipulation (Bowling, 2002; Ellis, 1994; Handler, Rosenberg, Kennelly, & Monahan, 1998; Miller, 1991).

Each of the nonexperimental designs can be applied to descriptive or cross-sectional data sets. For example, a study of risk factors for placenta previa by race of mother using national public use birth certificate files is a case-control design of a cross-sectional study population.

## Experimental Designs

*Experimental designs* involve the manipulation of the main independent variable and the control of other independent, confounding, or covariate variables. Table 14–2 describes experimental research designs. Included as true experimental design are *randomized control trials*, which involve two or more randomly assigned groups, each treated differently. In its most basic form, the experimental group receives the treatment, and the control group, although treated exactly like the experimental group in every other way, is not exposed to the treatment (Hulley et al., 2001). *Quasi-experimental designs* include natural, field, and community-intervention experiments. *Natural experiments* are those in which an independent

**Table 14–2 Research Designs: Experimental**

| | Experimental: Manipulation of Main Independent Variable and Control of Other Independent, Confounding or Covariate Variables | |
|---|---|---|
| **Type of Research** | **Research Design** | **Description** |
| True experimental | Randomized controlled trial | Involves two or more groups that are randomly assigned to groups and each group is treated differently; the investigator must have control over treatment and group assignment. |
| Quasi-experimental | Natural experiment | Aims to assess a situation in which the independent variable is manipulated by the investigator or by natural occurrences. |
| | Field experiment | Entails research studies in a natural situation in which one or more variables are manipulated by the investigators. |
| | Community intervention experiment | Involves a community-wide intervention on a collective basis, rather than an individual basis. |

variable is manipulated by natural or man-made occurrences not under the control of the investigator (Isaac & Michaels, 1995). A classic public health example is the Dutch Famine Winter of 1944 to 1945 for studies of nutrition and pregnancy outcome. *Field experiments*, or clinical trials, are research studies occurring in a natural situation in which one or more variables are manipulated by the researcher(s). Studies using these designs typically examine individuals in relationship to some preventive health measure targeted at individual health behaviors (Friis & Sellers, 1999). This differs from *community intervention experiments* with a collective or community focus rather than an individual basis. The overall goal of the experiment or research is to assess the impact on the community as a whole. (Table 14–2)

## Health Services Research

Table 14–3 describes some types of research applicable to MCH but outside of the epidemiologic or experimental realm. These study types include those relevant to leadership, administration, and management. *Needs assessment* aims to gather information related to the health of a population or community and serves as the foundation for the development of programmatic and policy directives, as well as the allocation of resources to achieve strategic objectives. This is the initial step in developing or establishing objectives (Kettner, Moroney, & Martin, 1990; Petersen & Alexander, 2001a). *Evaluation* is equally critical to the success of any public health or MCH program. This component serves as the assessment of a program to evaluate whether the measurable, clearly stated goals and objectives were achieved and activities were completed. *Process evaluation* investigates whether the specific program objectives of the program or intervention were achieved. It considers both the scope and nature of the activities conducted. *Outcome evaluation* aims to evaluate whether the program or intervention achieves the decided outcomes or meets the overall goal of the program (Rossi & Freeman, 1993; Shadish, Cook, & Leviton, 1991; Weiss, 1972) (see Chapter 18). *Performance monitoring* is rooted in the basic concept of evaluation, in that it aims to assess progress and/or performance against stated objectives. Many MCH programs, particularly Title V, use performance measures, which are measurable outcomes linked to funding sources (Petersen & Alexander, 2001a) (see Chapter 17).

*Systems evaluation* involves documentation of the elements of systems that involve interrelated components working toward a common goal or

**Table 14-3** Research Designs: Health Services Research

| Type of Research | Health Services Research Research Design | Description |
|---|---|---|
| Needs assessment | Needs assessment | Aims to gather information related to the health of a population or community as the foundation for the development of programmatic and policy directives and the allocation of resources to achieve strategic objectives; initial step in developing or establishing objectives. |
| Evaluation | Process evaluation | Investigates to ensure the specific objectives of the program or intervention are met; considers both the nature and scope of activities conducted. |
| | Outcome evaluation | Investigates whether the program or intervention achieves the decided outcome or meets the overall goal of the program; assess results of activities of program. |
| | Performance monitoring | Rooted in the basic concepts of evaluation; assessing progress/performance against stated objectives; performance measures are measurable outcomes sometimes linked to funding sources. |
| | Systems evaluation | Involves documentation of the elements of systems that involve interrelated components working toward a common goal or outcome objective; emerging area in public health; numerous barriers (time intensive, measurement issues). |
| | Policy analysis | Aims to assess the impact of policy development and works to enhance the public process. |
| Economic | Financial and service delivery use analysis | Includes a number of specific research study designs that focus on use and service delivery (resource allocation; cost-forecasting, and cost reduction impact assessment; cost-effectiveness and benefit assessment; quality assurance; risk adjustment; patient flow and satisfaction). |
| Action | Community-based participatory | Requires community demand for research to address locally identified needs; communities as active participants in the research process. |

outcome objective. This is an emerging area in public health and MCH (Petersen & Alexander, 2001b; Platt & Hill, 1995). *Policy analysis*, which can greatly enhance the policy process, aims to assess the impact of policy development. The next research category is that of *financial and service delivery use analysis*. Included in this category are numerous types of study designs that focus on use. These include resource allocation (also linked to needs assessment), cost forecasting and cost-reduction impact assessment, cost-effectiveness and benefit assessment, quality assurance, risk adjustment, and patient flow/satisfaction.

The final health service research type described in Table 14–3 is *action research*, specifically, *community-based participatory* research, which is a "collaborative process of research involving researchers and community representatives; it engages community members, employs local knowledge in the understanding of health problems and the design of interventions, and invests community members in the processes and products of research. In addition, community members are invested in the dissemination and use of research findings and ultimately in the reduction of health disparities" (Agency for Healthcare Research and Quality, 2001). This partnership approach to research equally involves community members, organizational members, and researchers in all aspects of the research process. Partners guide the process with their expertise and share responsibility in order to improve the health of the community (Eisinger & Senturia, 2001; Felix-Aaron & Stryer, 2003; Freudenberg, 2001; O'Toole, Feliz-Aaron, Chin, Horowitz, & Tyson, 2003).

## *Validity of Inference*

When compared with nonexperimental and quasi-experimental designs, experimental research designs remain less frequently employed by MCH researchers. Nevertheless, experimental designs sit at the top of the hierarchy of evidence supporting evidence-based practice. There is a growing call for public health practitioners to improve the decision-making capacity of the field through application of more rigorous analytical research methods and study designs (Brownson, Baker, Leet, & Gillespie, 2003). Meta-analyses and comprehensive, systematic reviews of experimental research designs provide the highest level of evidence, followed by experimental, well-controlled research studies (Petitti, 2000). Cohort studies and carefully conducted case-control studies sit lower in the hierarchy, with descriptive studies (case series, cross-sectional and ecological analyses, case-control study designs applied to administrative or single center databases) still lower in the hierarchy of evidence. Irrespective of the research design of a study, researchers must take pains to ensure study validity, both in terms of external generalizability (relevance of study conclusions to other populations and settings) and internal validity (scientific integrity of research protocol implementation). Validity of inference is not directly related to the hierarchy of evidence, although generally research designs at higher levels of evidence tend to provide more valid results. A cautionary note should be made in regards to external generalizability. Typically, experimental research designs make some sacrifice of external generalizability in the zeal to make the strongest possible case for the internal validity of their findings. Cross-sectional study designs often provide limited internal validity, but their results, within the context of the study questions posed, can be more broadly generalizable.

At state and local public health levels, MCH practitioners, in order to address myriad emerging need priorities, are routinely faced with selecting an intervention strategy from a host of highly touted "best practices" and must rely on the professional literature to provide a rational basis for their decision making. When there are conflicting reports in the literature as to the effectiveness of an intervention, a method is needed to determine whether greater weight should be given to some studies as compared with others. Assessing each report's study design in terms of potential threats to validity of inference is a well accepted approach (Cooper, 1989). The application of experimental research designs to MCH studies and the completion of well-structured meta-analyses and systematic reviews to address pressing issues of health policy and risk factor epidemiology will assure that public health actions are based on scientific evidence and thereby increase accountability.

# DATA: TYPES AND SOURCES

A crucial step in the development of a research or evaluation design is the selection of the data source(s). Researchers must decide whether to collect their own data or to use an existing database. Good quality secondary databases, covering in detail a wide array of MCH populations and topics, are increasingly available to researchers at a time when research funding for primary data collection is being constrained (Gable, 1990). Not only must researchers choose between using primary and secondary data, they must also be prepared to justify their choice in terms of data acquisition costs, study duration costs, the quality, completeness and availability of needed data elements, and the potential validity and broad generalizability of results.

Secondary data for research is attractive for several reasons. The extended time required for the collection of primary data is saved, and the costs associated with data collection are accordingly diminished (Stewart, 1984). To the extent that a secondary database can answer the same research question more quickly and at lower cost, the funder of the research receives better value for the research investment. Moreover, secondary databases can often provide extensive information on a large number of cases. Population-based secondary data, such as vital records, provide multiyear data on entire populations. Nationally representative surveys, for example, the Maternal and Infant Health Survey, offer extensive collections of variables (Sanderson, Placek, & Keppel, 1991). The results of studies using these databases have broad generalizability compared with the more limited representativeness of studies using primary data collected from a single local population. Therefore, secondary data analysis may confer several advantages during times of fiscal constraints on research dollars. A list of secondary databases and potential sources of secondary data is provided in Table 14–4.

Notwithstanding these attributes, several problems are associated with the use of secondary data. The analysis of secondary databases requires access to and mastery in the use of computer hardware and statistical analysis software. Although mainframe computers are often required to analyze large secondary databases, this is rapidly changing with the development of more advanced personal computers and the availability of data sets on CD-ROM. These advancements have reduced the costs of secondary data analysis but have not lessened the level of statistical computing and research methods skills needed to manage, analyze, and interpret these data sets.

Being restricted to the variables contained on the data set is a basic limitation of secondary data. The primary collection of data affords researchers the opportunity to select their own variables of interest and to decide how these variables will be measured, collected, and coded. This allows researchers to proceed from a theoretical or conceptual model to

## Table 14–4  MCH-Related Secondary Data Sources

A. National Vital Records (National Center for Health Statistics [NCHS])
   1. Live Births
   2. Fetal Deaths
   3. Induced Abortions
   4. Infant Deaths
   5. Marriages
   6. Divorces
   7. Linked Live Birth-Infant Death Files
   8. Matched Linked Multiple Pregnancy Files
B. National Health and Medical Records Surveys (NCHS)
   1. National Hospital Discharge Survey
   2. Family Planning Reporting Survey
C. National Population-based Surveys (NCHS)
   1. National Health Interview Survey
   2. National Health and Nutrition Examination Survey
   3. Hispanic Health and Nutrition Examination Survey
   4. National Survey of Family Growth
   5. Ambulatory Medical Care Survey
   6. Nursing Home Survey
   7. Medical Care Utilization and Expenditure Survey
   8. Survey of Personal Health Practices and Consequences
   9. National Maternal and Infant Health Survey, 1988
   10. Longitudinal Follow-up to the National Maternal and Infant Health Survey
D. Other Sources of National Data
   1. Census Bureau
   2. Centers for Disease Control and Prevention
      a. Pregnancy Risk Assessment and Monitoring System
      b. Pregnancy and Infancy Nutrition Survey
      c. Behavior Risk Factor Surveys
      d. Developmental Disability Surveillance
      e. Teenage Pregnancy Surveillance
      f. Birth Defects Surveillance
      g. Assisted Reproductive Technology
      h. State and Local Area Integrated Telephone Survey
   3. Consumer Product Safety Commission
   4. FBI: Uniform Crime Reports
   5. National Institute for Occupational Health and Safety
      a. Traumatic Occupational Fatality

*continues*

---

**Table 14–4** MCH-Related Secondary Data Sources (continued)

---

      b.  Fatal Accident Circumstances

    6.  United States Department of Agriculture: Special Supplemental Food Program for Women, Infants, and Children; Pregnancy Nutrition Surveillance System; Pediatric Nutrition Surveillance System

    7.  Indian Health Service

E.  State and Local Data Sources

    1.  State and local health and social service programs

        a.  Prenatal Care Programs

        b.  Special Supplemental Food Program for Women, Infants, and Children

        c.  Immunization

        d.  Child Abuse Reporting

        e.  Foster Care

        f.  Juvenile Corrections

        g.  Social Services

        h.  Adoptions

        i.  Child Health

        j.  Newborn Screening and Hearing Screening

        k.  Children with Special Health Care Needs

        l.  Child Lead Exposure

    2.  State Medical Societies

    3.  State Hospital Associations

    4.  School Systems

    5.  Community Health Centers

    6.  Poison Control Centers

    7.  State Registries: Tumor, cancer, birth defects, head trauma, spinal cord injury, pregnancy-associated mortality

    8.  State Medicaid

    9.  State Vital Records

    10.  Medical Registry Boards

    11.  Police and Fire departments

    12.  Wildlife, Hunting, and Boating departments

F.  Other Data Sources

    1.  Insurance Companies

    2.  Private medical records

    3.  Hospital and Health Maintenance Organization medical records

---

the determination of the operational definitions that will be employed to collect specific data elements or values from each individual case. In contrast, researchers using a secondary database must work with the data elements that are available. This presents a scientific and creative challenge.

In order to move beyond simply documenting and describing the contents of an existing database, researchers using secondary data must also start from a theoretical base with specific research hypotheses in mind. Being unable to specify the operational definitions of their research constructs, they must move backward from the available data elements to determine whether the existing variables can be used, manipulated, or combined in such a manner as to provide conceptually valid indicators that will be useful for their own research purposes. This task involves both science and ingenuity. For example, the reported biological age initially collected on a database can be reformulated in a secondary analysis as a measure of legal status or age of majority. Income and occupation variables can be combined into a measure of status inconsistency. The art of secondary data analysis entails the creative reconceptualization and manipulation of existing variables into cogent new measures. When elegantly done, it would almost appear that the original data elements were collected for the specific purpose of the secondary analysis.

## BIAS AND THREATS TO VALID INTERPRETATION OF DATA AND RESULTS

Secondary databases can be very important for research, planning, evaluation, and needs assessment in MCH. These databases can provide powerful evidence for new policy initiatives or justification for ongoing program activities. However, it should also be stressed that the use of these databases entails complex measurement issues. Knowledge of the database and the coding of the variables contained therein are essential to the prevention of simplistic and erroneous interpretations of the data. In drawing attention to inherent problems in secondary databases like vital records, we run the risk of damping enthusiasm for their use. However, these data are extremely useful. In particular, vital record data sets may offer benefits not available in hospital or medical record databases because of their coverage of entire populations over time and the increasing application of error checking programs by states.

Of major concern in the use of secondary data is the difficulty inherent in using and interpreting data elements that have been collected, coded, and recoded by others. In order to analyze appropriately secondary data or to interpret the results of such analyses, a good working knowledge of the database is essential. This includes an understanding of variable definitions, reporting completeness and accuracy, and variable recoding strategies. As decisions about data measurement may produce unexpected biases, the credible use of secondary data for research and policy requires an in-depth assessment of the data, a careful and detailed documentation of the data coding procedures, and a cautious interpretation of the results (Kirby, 2001).

There are many potential threats to the accurate interpretation of secondary data. Although these threats are not different from those found in primary data, the "finished" appearance of a secondary database or analysis might make them less apparent. The remainder of this chapter is devoted to identifying a number of the fundamental threats to the accurate interpretation of these data. These fundamental threats to accurate data interpretation include these issues:

- Missing data
- Out of range data
- Bivariate inconsistency
- Interpreting small and large numbers
- Concept validity
- Equating risk or association with cause

Several state vital record databases will be used to illustrate examples of these threats. State vital record data, specifically, Certificates of Live Birth and Infant Death, are probably the most commonly used data for MCH research, evaluation, and needs assessment efforts. Although many questions have been raised regarding their accuracy, these vital record data continue to be widely used for MCH program planning and evaluation.

## Missing Data

The first threat to accurate data interpretation involves the completeness of data reporting and the treatment of missing data. Missing or incomplete data can create major interpretation problems as it is uncertain whether cases with missing data are similar to or markedly different from those with completely recorded information. Often at issue is whether it is appropriate to calculate rates and percentages from only those records or cases where data exist. There are good reasons to assume that cases with missing data are different from those with complete data. For example, several studies have noted that women whose birth certificates are missing gestational age data are more likely to have lower educational attainment and other indicators of lower socioeconomic status (Buekens, Delvoye, Wollast, & Robyn, 1984; David, 1980; Taffel, Johnson, & Heuser, 1982;

Wenner & Young, 1974). As these women may have a higher risk of preterm delivery, we may suspect that cases with missing gestational age information may actually have a different gestational age distribution than those with this information reported.

Sometimes the issue of missing data is obscured by the way in which data are combined or presented. A notable example is the Institute of Medicine's "Index of Adequacy of Prenatal Care" (Kessner, Singer, Kalk, & Schlesinger, 1973). In this index, cases with missing prenatal care data were traditionally classified as receiving inadequate prenatal care, whereas cases with missing gestational age data were excluded from the index. Using Minnesota data from 1990 to 1991 (Table 14–5), we observed that, depending on the treatment of missing cases, the proportion of infants with mothers adequately using prenatal care is either 62.9% or 74.5%. If the 15.7% with missing data have the same pattern of prenatal care use as those with completed data, then the 74.5% figure may be a good estimate of adequate prenatal care use. However, if cases with missing data are slightly less likely to adequately use prenatal care, then the 75% would be an overestimate.

Having missing data on the date of last normal menses (DLNM), needed for the calculation of the gestational age interval, which in turn is used to compute adequacy of prenatal care indices, is a well-recognized problem. Nationwide, an appreciable percentage of birth certificates have missing or incomplete DLNM data. A previous report on Region III states indicated variations in missing DLNM data ranging from approximately 5% to 30% (Alexander, Petersen, Tompkins, Zinzeleta, & Jones, 1990a). Reporting also varies by year. In South Carolina, the percentage missing DLNM data was 31% in 1974 and less than 3% in 1990 (Alexander, Tompkins, & Cornely, 1990b). As the percentage of missing adequacy of prenatal care data will exceed the percentage of missing gestational age data, an abrupt change in the proportion missing DLNM data, or major

---

**Table 14–5** Adequacy of Prenatal Care, 1990–1991 Minnesota Live Births

| All Cases | Only Complete Cases |
|---|---|
| 62.9% Adequate | 74.5% Adequate |
| 21.4% Less than adequate | 25.5% Less than adequate |
| 15.7% Missing | |

differences in the percentage missing between population groups, can lead to the misinterpretation of prenatal care statistics (Alexander, Tompkins, Petersen, & Weiss, 1991). In secondary analyses, careful attention must be given to the proportion missing and the treatment of cases with missing values in the computation of new variables, and indices should be clearly reported.

One accepted method for dealing with missing DLNM data is to impute a gestational age. There are two commonly used methods for this: the Day 15 method and the Preceding Case method (Alexander et al., 1990b). The choice of which, if any, imputation method to use is not without consequence. An investigation of 12-year trends in preterm delivery contrasted preterm percentages based on no imputation and by each of these imputation schemes (Alexander et al., 1990b). Different trends emerged. The preterm percentages based on no imputation increased over the period. The Preceding Case method preterm percentages exhibited little if any change, whereas the Day 15 method preterm percentages decreased over time.

## Out-of-Range Data

Out-of-range data present another fundamental problem for secondary data analysis. The proportion of out-of-range data is often not reported, as a convention for defining such data may not exist. Out-of-range data are those considered biologically implausible or those outside the normally expected range. This is mainly a problem with continuous variables. The problem with defining out-of-range data is determining the specific values that define the limits of the valid range. For example, although 10 to 50 years may seem like a reasonable range to use to define valid ages of mother, recent reports of live births to an 8-year-old and to older women have increased the difficulty in selecting these cut points. As some health status measures are typically described in terms such as "< 2500 grams" for low birth weight or "< 37 weeks" for preterm delivery, improbable and clearly erroneous values may be inadvertently included in the calculation of these percentages unless precise limits are set that define the data values considered plausible. If cases with out-of-range values are included in the calculation of percentages and rates, for example, preterm and very low birth weight, the resulting rates may be inflated.

Out-of-range data are a particular concern for investigations of cases at the extreme tails of distributions, for example, very low birth weight, macrosomia, very preterm and postterm delivery, preteen pregnancy, and intrauterine growth. When secondary data are used for investigations of these topics, decisions made regarding the treatment of out-of-range data should be well documented.

## Bivariate Inconsistency

A data value may appear accurate until compared with another; then it may become apparent that one is incorrect. This threat to accurate data interpretation is known as bivariate inconsistency. A fairly typical example of this is a case with a birth weight of 3,700 grams and a gestational age of 22 weeks. Such combinations are a little more than unusual. Tables have been developed to identify cases with implausible or inconsistent birth weight and gestational age values (Alexander, Himes, Kaufman, Mor, & Kogan, 1996). Other combinations of variables that can be checked for inconsistency include maternal age and parity and age and education. Checking for bivariate inconsistency is a good strategy when employing a secondary database and can reveal important information about the potential accuracy of the data that would not be evident from merely assessing the proportion missing or out of range.

## Interpreting Small and Large Numbers

The next threat to accurate data interpretation involves large and small numbers. One attractive attribute of vital record databases is that they represent entire populations and, as such, contain a large number of cases from which to draw inferences. Nevertheless, in spite of the large numbers involved, many of the health status indicators monitored, for example, infant deaths, are relatively rare events. Infant death rates, either based on a small number of births or a small number of deaths, are subject to considerable fluctuation. Highs and lows may not be reflective or typical of prevailing trends.

Large numbers are also a problem. Reliance on statistical tests can interfere with the appropriate interpretation of the data. It must be remembered that statistical testing is most useful for samples. For large populations, the majority of statistical comparisons will be significant based on large numbers alone. Although "significant," they may not signify a meaningful public health concern. For example, using data from Hawaii (Table 14–6), we note that the infant mortality rates vary sig-

**Table 14-6** Infant Mortality Rates by Military Status and Ethnicity, 1979–1989 Single Live Births to Adult, Married Hawaii Resident Women

|  | White | Black |
|---|---|---|
| Military | 6.8 | 9.7 |
| Nonmilitary | 5.1 | 16.8 |
| Significance | $p < 0.01$ | NS |
| N | 52,720 | 5,333 |

nificantly by military status among whites, although the actual difference is relatively moderate. Among African Americans, the difference in infant mortality rates by military status is quite marked, but not significant. The differences in the number of live births among military status and ethnic groups underlie the results of the significance tests.

## Construct Validity

The selection of a health status indicator for research, evaluation, or needs assessment involves a good conceptualization about what the indicator measures. At issue here is construct validity, a fundamental predicament in interpreting data. For example, gestational age refers to a unit of time between conception and birth, but this term is commonly used to refer to a host of other measures of fetal and newborn physical and neurologic maturity that are highly correlated with but conceptually distinct from gestational age (Alexander, Tompkins, Hulsey, Petersen, & Mor, 1995; Alexander & Allen, 1996). Furthermore, the use of neonatal and post-neonatal time periods to differentiate endogenous–exogenous causes of death has been a hallmark in perinatal research but has been soundly criticized as no longer a conceptually valid approach (Kirby, 1993).

Sometimes the stated title of the indicator may seem out of line with the strategy employed to measure it. The term teen pregnancy is a good example of a health status indicator without a well-established measurement convention. Thirteen to 19 years of age is technically the teenage years, but less than 18, the age of majority, is often used in research. As seen in the US national data presented in Table 14–7, the risk of low birth weight to the infant of a 19-year-old mother is quite distinct from that of a 13 year old. The inclusion of 18- and 19-year-old mothers in the teenage group

**Table 14-7** Low Birth Weight by Age of Mother, 2001–2002, Single Live Births to US Residents

| Age of Mother | Number | Percentage of Low Birth Weight |
|---|---|---|
| 11 | 44 | 29.6 |
| 12 | 399 | 16.3 |
| 13 | 2,483 | 13.8 |
| 14 | 11,977 | 11.9 |
| 15 | 38,379 | 10.5 |
| 16 | 87,279 | 9.8 |
| 17 | 154,313 | 8.9 |
| 18 | 240,948 | 8.6 |
| 19 | 336,104 | 7.8 |
| < 18 | 294,874 | 9.6 |
| < 20 | 871,926 | 8.6 |

greatly inflates the numbers and percentages of teenage mothers while reducing the level of the associated risks observed to the group.

One focus of investigations into the impact of prenatal care use is a discussion of the conceptual premise for the various indices that are used to describe prenatal care use (Alexander & Kotelchuck, 1996, 2001). In Table 14–8, low and very low birth weight percentages are displayed by two different indices: (1) a modification of the original Institute of Medicine (IOM) index developed in the 1960s and (2) an updated version of this index using the latest standards for prenatal care visits recommended by the American College of Obstetrics and Gynecology. The strength of the relationship between adequacy of prenatal care and birth weight is dependent on the index used. The American College of Obstetricians and Gynecologists ACOG index results in a lower proportion of cases in the adequate category and the adequate category no longer has the lowest percentage of moderately low birth weight infants. There is little relationship to very low birth weight by either index.

Construct validity should not be confused with content validity. Some indices or measures do not provide full coverage of the concept they measure. For example, prenatal care use indices only address the quantity of visits and do not consider the quality or content of care received. These indices may also exclude other forms of prenatal care.

**Table 14–8** Very Low (VLBW) and Moderately Low Birth Weight (MLBW) Percentages by Two Measures of Adequacy of Prenatal Care Use, 2001–2002, Single Live Births to US Residents

| | MODIFIED IOM* | | | ACOG** | | |
|---|---|---|---|---|---|---|
| | Percent | % VLBW | % MLBW | Percent | % VLBW | % MLBW |
| Adequate | 71.88 | 0.93 | 4.36 | 46.64 | 1.42 | 5.81 |
| Intermediate | 17.61 | 1.16 | 6.12 | 38.95 | 0.53 | 3.53 |
| Inadequate | 4.08 | 0.87 | 7.30 | 7.98 | 0.50 | 5.31 |
| No care | 1.00 | 6.26 | 13.31 | 1.00 | 6.26 | 13.31 |
| Missing | 5.43 | 2.43 | 6.24 | 5.43 | 2.43 | 6.24 |
| | 100.00 | | | 100.00 | | |

*IOM (Institute of Medicine)
**ACOG (American College of Obstetricians and Gynecologists)

## Equating Risk or Association with Cause

Another threat to data interpretation involves delineating between causal factors and risk factors. Rarely are we investigating causal relationships, for example, a relationship where a variable is a direct biological precursor. Most investigations focus on risk factors, for example, factors that are associated with an increased chance of a poor outcome. Although a characteristic may be a risk factor, not all individuals with that factor will experience negative outcomes.

In these national data (Table 14–9), low birth weight percentages by age of mother and prenatal care use are examined. Teen mothers (less than 18 years of age) have a higher percentage of low birth weight (9.56%) than adult mothers (5.95%). Nevertheless, nearly 95% of total low birth weight births occur to adult mothers. If all teen pregnancies could have been eliminated, the number of total low birth weight infants during this period would only have been reduced by 6%.

Similarly, note the higher low birth weight percentages to mothers with no or inadequate prenatal care. Over 80% of the low birth weight infants are to mothers with adequate or intermediate use of prenatal care. Certainly, the young age of mother and no prenatal care use, as measured here, are associated with a low birth weight. Still, it cannot be concluded that even the elimination of both of these risk factors will reduce as much as 10% of the low birth weight problem.

**Table 14–9** Low Birth Weight (LBW) by Age of Mother and Prenatal Care, 2001–2002, Single Live Births to US Residents

| Age of Mother | % Distribution | % LBW* | % LBW Distribution |
|---|---|---|---|
| < 18 | 3.79 | 9.56 | 5.96 |
| 18+ | 96.21 | 5.95 | 94.04 |
| **Prenatal Care** | | | |
| Adequate | 71.88 | 5.29 | 62.49 |
| Intermediate | 17.61 | 7.28 | 21.07 |
| Inadequate | 4.08 | 8.18 | 5.48 |
| No care | 1.00 | 19.57 | 3.22 |
| Missing | 5.43 | 8.67 | 7.74 |

*LBW (low birth weight: < 2500 grams)

# ETHICS

Although research should follow the highest ethical standards, the history of public health research in the United States has not lived up to that goal. Research, concerned as it is with the pursuit of knowledge and truth, must be equally concerned with the integrity and purity of the research process. Ethical considerations must be paramount in all phases of the research process from conceptualization through study design, data gathering, analysis, and reporting of results. Although it is essential that all researchers maintain vigilance in assuring the highest ethical quality of their own work in order to retain credibility in individual studies, it is important for the entire field of science that research be conducted in the most scrupulous manner in order to contribute accurate information to the larger knowledge base in a way that it will be believed and ultimately used in the promotion of health and quality of life.

Because of the importance of research in MCH, research must be undertaken within accepted standards of ethical conduct. Unethical conduct in research includes falsifying data, deliberately misclassifying study subjects and controls, deliberately mishandling data, and failing to disclose fully how data were manipulated (e.g., how missing or outlier variables were handled). Mistakes can happen in research, and even these can call into question the credibility of the result. Deliberate misconduct can cast doubt on the entire scientific profession and result in public reluctance to accept research findings.

In MCH, issues germane to the field of study warrant particular attention even beyond these concerns over general misconduct. Research involving children and pregnant women is always subject to a higher degree of scrutiny because of the vulnerability of the population under study. Researchers must be very careful in considering how to assure informed consent with these populations, how to treat subjects justly, how to maintain the confidentiality of the data collected, and how to minimize harm to the research subjects. Institutional review boards pay particular attention to these issue when the research subjects include children or pregnant women because of the potential for harm from the research study itself, harm from the intentional or inadvertent disclosure of information, or harm from insufficient attempts to fully explain the nature of the study when seeking consent to participate. The fact that infants and children cannot consent for themselves makes them uniquely vulnerable to ethical lapses.

The issues surrounding research with human subjects are so important to the integrity of the research process that the National Institutes of Health (NIH), the largest government research entity in the country, has a website devoted to resources on bioethics in research and on the use of human subjects (www.nih.gov/sigs/bioethics/). For example, read the NIH policy announcement provided below that was placed on NIH website for Bioethics Resources. Every federally funded research institution in the United States requires this education, and every institution maintains an active institutional review board designed to review thoroughly every research proposal generated within the institution for its adherence to research ethics and standards relating to human subjects in research.

> Policy: *Beginning on October 1, 2000, the NIH will require education on the protection of human research participants for all investigators submitting NIH applications for grants or proposals for contracts or receiving new or non-competing awards for research involving human subjects.* (This announcement is placed on the NIH website for Bioethics Resources: www.nih.gov/sigs/bioethics/)

# REVIEWING THE LITERATURE

MCH practitioners, as well as students and faculty, are often faced with making decisions based not on their own knowledge or research but solely on information available in the professional literature. Their ability to review and synthesize the literature is therefore a critical part of their decision-making process. Equally important is the quality of the literature itself. Here again, the MCH professional plays an invaluable role by serving as a reviewer for peer-reviewed, professional journals and by contributing manuscripts describing scientifically rigorous research.

A fundamental part of gaining research experience is reviewing the research of others. The use of a systematic approach to reviewing a scientific research article allows the reviewer to critically assess variable measurement issues, study design, statistical analysis, and ethics. It also provides a structure for the development of manuscripts that report research. The following outline provides a structure for reviewing articles and organizing materials into a manuscript for submission for publication (Alexander, in press). For each section of the traditional format of a research article, key questions are identified for the reviewer and also serve as a reminder to authors of aspects to consider.

## Title, Abstract, and Keywords

The importance of a good title and an interesting abstract cannot be overstated during the period of transition toward electronic journals. As search engines increasingly help direct us to the individual research studies based on keywords, either specifically indicated as such or contained in titles, an author's choice of these may appreciably determine whether interested readers find their study among the multitude of articles contained in the ever growing number of journals available to us electronically. Therefore, selection of keywords for a study is a serious business. Moreover, it is also critical that the title and abstract be interesting and provide a faithful, clear, and concise summary of the article.

## The Introduction

The introduction of a manuscript should provide a statement of the general problem to be addressed by the article, followed by a description of the specific focus of the research, for example, infant mortality rates in the United States and the growing racial disparity in those rates. Highlights from the literature should be referenced and existing theories, controversies, and unresolved issues discussed. The introductory discussion should make evident why this topic and study is important (based on rates, numbers involved, costs, potential for spread, long-term consequences, etc.) and what populations are involved. Finally, the study purpose, that is, what the study hopes to accomplish, should be stated. At a minimum, a reviewer/reader should find the following in the introduction:

- A clear and succinct statement of the problem and its relevance
- Germane references and essential background information to place study in context and to establish its importance
- A clear statement of study purpose and hypotheses

## The Methods/Data

The methods section of an article should be comprehensive enough that the reviewer/reader has a clear picture of the study in terms of data collection, variable measurement, study design, and data analysis. The methods section should provide a sufficient description of the study to assure the readers understand what the researcher did and, within reason, could potentially replicate the study elsewhere. In addition to assessing if there is a complete description of the study methods, reviewers should also consider whether the data, measurement, study design, and statistical analysis methods are appropriate, given the study purpose. Finally, there should be a description of the actions taken to assure that human subjects concerns have been reviewed and addressed. Depending on their applicability to the study, items in the following list should be detailed in the methods section:

- Source of data
- Study/research design
- Case selection criteria
- Sampling techniques
- Number of cases
- Definition and measurement of important variables
- Statistical analysis methods
- Human subjects review

## The Results

The results section presents the findings of the study. Tables and figures are typically used to depict exact findings, and the text of the results section needs not duplicate those other than describing and providing an example of how to read these displays. The following are key considerations for reviewing a results section:

- Logical presentation of results
- Clear, complete, and accurately labeled tables and figures
- Neutral description of results with interpretations left for the discussion/conclusions section

## Discussion/Conclusions

The final section of the text of the article, the discussion or conclusions, provides a concise summary of the findings of the research and should tie the findings back to the study purpose (e.g., was the study hypothesis rejected, or did the findings provide support for the study's underlying theoretical premise?). It is appropriate to discuss whether the research findings concurred with the findings of similar studies. In this section, authors may offer their interpretations and speculations on the impact of the study findings on current research controversies, but these should be scholarly and within reason. Future research directions can be provided, and these are often helpful for advancing research and guiding students and new researchers looking for research topics to pursue. In the MCH field, it is often important that relevant policy/program implications be discussed. Finally, the section may typically end with a restatement of the main take-home points and final concluding statement. Aspects for a critical assessment of this section include the following:

- Conclusions clearly provided and related to the stated study purpose and hypotheses
- Conclusions supported by results
- Restrictions to generalization of findings indicated
- Study limitations described

## References

The reference section of the article provides the citations for studies to which this study refers. This section provides the reader a roadmap to related studies on the topic matter. As such, the following characteristic of the reference section are important:

- Accurate citation of references (e.g., correct journal, volume, page numbers, year)

- Valid citation of references (e.g., the referenced quote is actually what the original reference stated)
- Current references (although the key old ones should not be left out)
- Unbiased selection of references (i.e., articles from both sides of a controversy should be unbiasedly selected and cited)

### General Issues for Reviewers

In addition to the points previously raised, there are some general issues of concern for reviewers of articles for professional scientific journals. The following aspects are important for researchers to consider when preparing their manuscript for submission and when deciding which journal would be best to publish their manuscript:

- Originality of the topic
- Original use of data and methods
- Current importance to field
- Length of article
- Grammar and style
- An impartial and unbiased presentation
- Interest to readership
- Interest to multiple disciplines

## CONCLUSION

Although MCH's traditional orientation to public health practice, policy, and advocacy lends an applied focus to MCH research, it is supported and given credibility by an underpinning of scientific evidence. In a culture that demands evidence-based accountability, the MCH practitioner and MCH researcher are now interdependent and need a basic background in each other's domains in order for our research to be relevant and our practice to be cost-effective. The importance of communication between MCH researchers and practitioners for the dissemination and application of scientific information is highlighted by the popular slogan "from data to action." This phrase describes part of a needed cycle of collaboration that can be drawn full circle for the benefit of the MCH population by adding "from action to research" to our vision to assure that we evaluate what we do and continually refine and, as needed, retarget our practice and policy endeavors.

The fundamental elements of science and research (i.e., hypothesis testing, empirical data measurement, study design, statistical analysis) are the same for MCH as for any other field within public health. Advanced graduate level training in the principles and tools of research is often initially compartmentalized by discipline with study design falling within epidemiology courses, statistical analysis techniques coming from biostatistics, and measurement theory sometimes being taught by health behavioral sciences. Nevertheless, these different elements of research are interconnected in the actual practice of research. Like legs of a tripod, a failure in one may seriously compromise the ultimate utility of a study. Strength in one area, for example, an experimental study designed to limit possible threats to validity of inference, cannot fully compensate for clear weakness in another, for example, poor reliability and validity of measurement of the key variables. Inevitably, no research study is without flaw. Thus, the strength of our scientific method comes from its emphasis on persistent testing and retesting. Occasionally, one study makes a breakthrough, but overall, lasting advances are based on the contributions of many researchers whose work at exploring, replicating, and refining new approaches may stretch across several careers from mentor to students to the next generation, all pursuing a similar research agenda.

The complexity of many of the health status and health care use concerns facing MCH is such that it is unlikely that these seemingly intractable problems will be resolved in one generation of research. For example, the topic of racial disparities in perinatal health is hardly new and has attracted research attention for over 50 years. Such intractable problems highlight the need for the MCH field to maintain a strong emphasis on research and research training to assure that there will be an ongoing cadre of MCH investigators committed to the important research issues and health problems of the MCH population.

# REFERENCES

Agency for Healthcare Research and Quality. (2001). Background. In *Community-based participatory research: Conference summary.* Available Jan. 17, 2005, from: http://www.ahrq.gov/about/cpcr/cbpr/cbpr1.htm.

Alexander, G.R. (1996). *A Population-based maternal and child health status surveillance system for the state of Arizona.* Technical report prepared for Health

Systems Research, Inc. and the Community and Family Health Section of the Arizona Department of Health Services. Available from: http://www.hsrnet.com/pdf/az-rpt.pdf.

Alexander, G.R. (2003a). Maternal and child health. In Stahl, M.J. (ed). *Encyclopedia of Health Care Management.* Knoxville, TN: Sage Publications.

Alexander, G.R. (2003b). Our legacy for leadership in MCH. *Maternal and Child Health Journal, 7,* 145–150.

Alexander, G.R. (2005, in press). A guide for reviewing the literature. *Maternal and Child Health Journal, 9(1).*

Alexander, G.R., & Allen, M.C. (1996). Conceptualization, measurement and use of gestational age: I: Clinical and public health practice. *Journal of Perinatology, 16,* 53–59.

Alexander, G.R., & Kogan, M.D. (1998). Ethnic differences in birth outcomes: The search for answers continues. *Birth, 23,* 210–213.

Alexander, G.R., & Kotelchuck, M. (1996). A comparison of prenatal care indices: Classification of adequacy of prenatal care use. *Public Health Reports, 111,* 408–418.

Alexander, G.R., & Kotelchuck, M. (2001). Assessing the role and effectiveness of prenatal care: History, challenges, and directions for future research. *Public Health Reports, 116,* 306–316.

Alexander, G.R., & Petersen, D.J. (2004). MCH needs assessment capacity shows improvement; but, meager MCH evaluation capacity may impede performance (editorial). *Maternal and Child Health Journal, 8,* 103–105.

Alexander, G.R., & Slay, M. (2002). Prematurity at birth: Trends, racial disparities, and epidemiology. *Mental Retardation and Developmental Disabilities Research Reviews, 8,* 215–220.

Alexander, G.R., Petersen, D.J., Pass, M.A., Slay, M., Chadwick, C., & Shumpert. (2002). *Maternal and child health/public health milestones, history and philosophy* (Vol. I–XII). The MCH Leadership Skills Training Institute, Department of Maternal and Child Health, University of Alabama at Birmingham. Available May 2002 from: http://www.soph.uab.edu/mchcontent.asp?ID=587

Alexander, G.R., Petersen, D.J., Tompkins, M.E., Zinzeleta, E., & Jones, M.D. (1990a). *The region III perinatal data and chart book.* Baltimore, MD: Region III Perinatal Information Consortium Special Report.

Alexander, G.R., Tompkins, M.E., & Cornely, D.A. (1990b). Gestational age reporting and preterm delivery. *Public Health Reports, 105,* 267–275.

Alexander, G.R., Tompkins, M.E., Petersen, D.J., & Weiss, J. (1991). Sources of bias in prenatal care utilization indices: Implications for evaluating the Medicaid expansion. *American Journal of Public Health, 81,* 1013–1016.

Alexander, G.R., Tompkins, M.E., Hulsey, T.C., Petersen, D.J., & Mor, J.M. (1995). Discordance between LMP-based and clinically estimated gestational age: Implications for research, programs and policy. *Public Health Reports, 110,* 395–402.

Alexander, G.R., Himes, J.H., Kaufman, R., Mor, J., & Kogan, M. (1996). A U.S. national reference for fetal growth. *Obstetrics & Gynecology, 87,* 163–168.

Bordens, K.S., & Abbott, B.B. (2002). *Research design and methods: A process approach* (5th ed.). Boston: McGraw-Hill.

Bowling, A. (2002). *Research methods in health: Investigating health and health services* (2nd ed.). Philadelphia: Open Press.

Bronowski, J. (1967). *The common sense of science.* Cambridge: Harvard Press.

Brownson, R.C., Baker, E.A., Leet, T.L., & Gillespie, K.N. (2003). *Evidence-based public health.* Oxford: Oxford University Press.

Buekens, P., Delvoye, P., Wollast, E., & Robyn, C. (1984). Epidemiology of pregnancies with unknown last menstrual period. *Journal of Epidemiology and Community Health, 38,* 79–80.

Carmines, E.G., & Zeller, R.A. (1979). *Reliability and validity assessment: Quantitative Applications in the Social Sciences Series, Number 07-017.* Beverly Hills, CA: Sage Publications.

Cooper, H.M. (1989). Integrating research: A guide for literature reviews (2nd ed.). *Applied social research methods series* (Vol. 2). Newbury Park, CA: Sage.

David, R.J. (1980). The quality and completeness of birth weight and gestational age data in computerized birth files. *American Journal of Public Health, 79,* 964–973.

Dolby, T. & Kerr, J. She blinded me with science. The golden age of wireless. Capitol Records, March 1982.

Eisinger, A., & Senturia, K. (2001). Doing community-driven research: A description of Seattle partners for healthy communities. *Journal of Urban Health, 78,* 519–534.

Ellis, L. (1994). *Research methods in the social sciences.* Madison, WI: Brown & Benchmark.

Felix-Aaron, K., & Stryer, D. (2003). Moving from rhetoric to evidence-based action in health care. *Journal of General Internal Medicine, 7,* 589–591.

Freudenberg, N. (2001). Case history of the center for urban epidemiologic studies in New York City. *Journal of Urban Health, 78,* 508–518.

Friis, R.H., & Sellers, T.A. (1999). *Epidemiology for public health practice* (2nd ed.). Gaithersburg, MD: Aspen Publications.

Gable, C. (1990). A compendium of public health data sources. *American Journal of Epidemiology, 131,* 381–394.

Grason, H., & Wigton, A. (1995). *Review of the literature and measurement strategies related to key principles in the development of systems of care for children and youth.* Baltimore, MD: Child and Adolescent Health Policy Center, The Johns Hopkins University.

Handler, A., Rosenberg, D., Kennelly, J., & Monahan, C. (1998). Analytic methods in maternal and child health. Health Resources and Services Administration (HRSA), Maternal and Child Health Bureau (MCHB).

*Healthy People 2010 Goals and Initiatives.* (2000). Available May 5, 2004, from: http://www.healthypeople.gov/About/.

*HHS Disparities Initiative.* (2001). Office of Minority Health Resource Center. Available from: http://www.omhrc.gov/rah/indexNew.htm.

Hill, A.B. (1965). The environment and disease: Association or causation? *Proceedings of the Royal Society of Medicine, 58,* 295–300.

Hulley, S.B., Cummings, S.R., Browner, W.S., Grady, D., Hearst, N., & Newman, T.B. (2001). *Designing clinical research* (2nd ed.). Philadelphia: Lippincott.

Institute of Medicine. (2002, March). *Unequal treatment: Confronting racial and ethnic disparities in health care.* Washington, DC. Available from: www.iom.edu.

Isaac, S., & Michael, B.W. (1995). *Handbook in research and evaluation for education and the behavioral sciences* (3rd ed.). San Diego: EdITS.

Johansen, A.S., Starfield, B., & Harlow, J. (1994). *Analysis of the concept of primary care for children and adolescents: A policy research brief.* Baltimore, MD: Child and Adolescent Health Policy Center, The Johns Hopkins University.

Kessner, D.M., Singer, J., Kalk, C.W., & Schlesinger, E.R. (1973). *Infant death: An analysis by maternal risk and health care.* In *Contrasts in Health Status* (Vol. I). Washington, DC: Institute of Medicine, National Academy of Sciences.

Kettner, P.M., Moroney, R.M., & Martin, L.L. (1990). *Designing and managing programs: An effectiveness-based approach.* Newbury Park, CA: Sage.

Kirby, R.S. (1993). Neonatal and postneonatal mortality: Useful constructs or outdated concepts? *Journal of Perinatology, 13,* 433–441.

Kirby, R.S. (2001). Invited commentary: Using vital statistics databases for perinatal epidemiology: Does the quality go in before the name goes on? *American Journal of Epidemiology, 154,* 889–890.

*Maternal and Child Health Bureau Strategic Plan: FY 2003–2007.* (2003). Available from: http://www.mchb.hrsa.gov/about/stratplan03-07.htm#2.

MCHB (Maternal and Child Health Bureau), HRSA (Health Resources and Services Administration). Maternal and Child Health Needs Assessment and State Performance Measures DHSC Technical Assistance Workshop. (2004). Available from: http://128.248.232.90/archives/mchb/needs2004/index.htm and http://128.248.232.90/archives/mchb/needs2004/workshop.htm.

Miller, C.D. (1991). *Handbook of research design and social measurement* (5th ed.). Newbury Park, CA: Sage.

Nunnally, J.C. (1978). *Psychometric theory* (2nd ed.). New York: McGraw-Hill Book Company.

O'Toole, T., Felix-Aaron, K., Chin, M.H., Horowitz, C., & Tyson, F. (2003). Community-based participatory research: Opportunities, challenges and the need for a common language. *Journal of General Internal Medicine, 8,* 592–594.

Petersen, D.J., & Alexander, G.R. (2001a). *Needs assessment in public health: A practical guide for students and professionals.* New York: Kluwer Academic/Plenum Publishers.

Petersen, D.J., & Alexander, G.R. (2001b). Integrating the roles of health surveillance, performance monitoring and systems evaluation. In H.M. Wallace, G. Green, K. Jaros, L. Paine, & M. Wallace. (Eds.), *Family health and health and welfare reform in the 21st century: An interdisciplinary perspective* (2nd ed.). Sudbury, MA: Jones and Bartlett Publishers.

Petitti, D.B. (2000). *Meta-analysis, decision analysis, and cost-effectiveness analysis: Methods for quantitative synthesis in medicine* (2nd ed.). Oxford: Oxford University Press.

Piper, J.M., Ray, W.A., & Griffin, M.R. (1990). Effects of Medicaid expansion on prenatal care and pregnancy outcome in Tennessee. *Journal of the American Medical Association, 264,* 2219–2223.

PL 74-271. (1935). Social Security Act of 1935, Title V: Grants to States for Maternal and Child Welfare. Available from: http://images.main.uab.edu/isoph/MCH/Tech_Reports.

PL 101-239. (1989). Omnibus Reconciliation Act of 1989, Title V, Subtitle C, MCH Block Grant Program. Available from: http://images.main.uab.edu/isoph/MCH/Tech_Reports.

PL 102-63. (1993). The Government Performance and Results Act of 1993. Available from: http://www.whitehouse.gov/omb/mgmt-gpra/index.html.

Platt, L.J., & Hill, I. (1995, June). *Measuring systems development in Wyoming: Instruments to assess communities' progress.* Washington, DC: Health Systems Research.

Popper, K.R. (1965). *The logic of scientific discovery.* New York: Harper & Row.

Rossi, P.H., & Freeman, H.E. (1993). *Evaluation: A systematic approach.* Newbury Park, CA: Sage.

Rothman, K.J. (1986). *Modern epidemiology.* Boston/Toronto: Little, Brown and Company.

Sanderson, M., Placek, P.J., & Keppel, K.G. (1991). The 1988 national maternal and infant health survey: Design, content and data availability. *Birth, 18,* 26–32.

Shadish, W.R., Cook, T.D., & Leviton, L.C. (1991). *Foundations of program evaluation.* Newbury Park, CA: Sage Publications.

Starfield, B. (1992). *Primary care: Concept, evaluation and policy.* New York: Oxford University Press.

Stewart, D.W. (1984). *Secondary research: Information sources and methods: Applied social research methods series* (Vol. 4). Beverly Hills, CA: Sage Publications.

Taffel, S., Johnson, D., & Heuser, R. (1982). *A method of imputing length of gestation on birth certificates.* US Department of Health and Human Services. Vital & Health Statistics. Data Evaluation and Methods Research Series 2, No. 93.

US Department of Health and Human Services. (2000, November). *Healthy People 2001: Understanding and improving health* (2nd ed.). Washington, DC: US Government Printing Office.

Weiss, C.H. (1972). *Evaluation research.* Englewood Cliffs, NJ: Prentice Hall.

Wenner, W.H., & Young, E.B. (1974). Nonspecific date of last menstrual period: An indication of poor reproductive outcome. *American Journal of Obstetrics and Gynecology, 120,* 1071–1079.

# CHAPTER 15

# Planning Maternal and Child Health Programs

*Mary D. Peoples-Sheps*

> *Planning remains at the nexus of health care policy and regulatory choices as we enter a new century. At its core, health planning promotes the active participation of stakeholders and the public in efforts to improve the system. . . Ultimately planning promotes efficiency, equity, and security by providing a voice for the uninsured and the under-served in our communities. The enduring challenge of making the health care system more accountable to ordinary citizens remains.* (American Health Planning Association, 2005)

## INTRODUCTION

Program planning skills are essential to the practice of maternal and child health (MCH). Regardless of political climate, economic context, or cultural milieu, MCH professionals are called on repeatedly to plan and implement intervention programs. As the practice of public health has undergone serious scrutiny during the past decade, program planning has been recognized consistently as an essential public health service (Institute of Medicine [IOM], 1988, 2003; Turnock, 1997). Virtually all public health practitioners engage in planning processes at one time or another; some focus primarily on planning, whereas others incorporate planning tasks into such primary professional activities as health administration, health care delivery, and epidemiology. MCH professionals are no exception. Six of the 10 *Essential Public Health Services to Promote Maternal and Child Health in America* relate directly to program planning (Grason & Guyer, 1995).

Program planning is a process through which interventions to improve health outcomes are developed. The model of program planning most often used in public health is derived from rational decision-making processes that use analytic techniques to link the determinants of a problem to an intervention, which in turn, is expected to improve the problem (Gilbert & Specht, 1977; Kettner, Moroney, & Martin, 1999). The process is considered rational because the means (interventions) correspond with the ends (outcomes in terms of problem improvement) as well as existing knowledge and circumstances permit. Program planning is carried out through a series of integrated steps shown in the center of Figure 15–1. The steps are presented in a circular format to show that the process is continuous; that is, the last step, evaluation, produces information required to inform problem assessment, the first step in the next planning cycle. The circular model is also intended to demonstrate that there are at least six points of entry to the planning process. The most appropriate place to start depends on the stage of development of the program. For example, planning to address an emerging problem begins with assessment of the problem, whereas planning in the context of well-understood problems and ongoing programs might begin with setting new objectives or adjusting the program to stay on track.

In addition to having multiple points of entry and continuity from one round to the next, the planning process is also iterative. There is movement back and forth among the steps as new information provides opportunity for revision and refinement of earlier steps. Iteration assures that each step uniquely influences and is influenced by the steps that both precede and follow it. The greater the amount of iteration in the planning process, the closer the plan comes to being truly rational.

Figure 15–1 also identifies a number of factors that interact with the program planning process. The political, social, and organizational environments in which planning is conducted influence whether and how a problem is perceived, the types of interventions that are acceptable, and the community assets available to synergize the entire planning endeavor (McKnight, 2000). Financial resources are essential to support planning activities and the interventions that are ultimately generated by them.

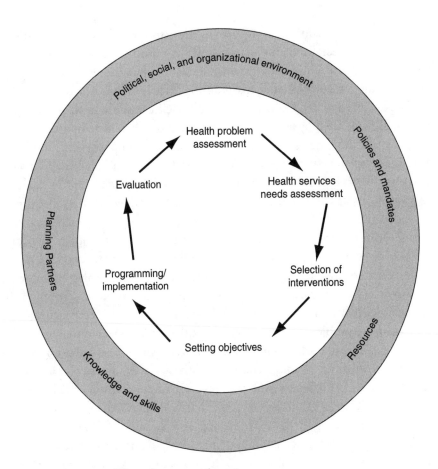

**FIGURE 15–1** The program planning process.

Policies and mandates of the organizations involved in the process set parameters on acceptable program functions.

Effective programs depend on a planning process in which the public health measurement sciences, theories of human and organizational behavior, decision-making strategies, and state-of-the-art knowledge about health conditions and management practices are seamlessly woven together to affect changes in population health. Extensive knowledge and well-honed skills are necessary requirements for this job. Analytic expertise, including capabilities in epidemiology, biostatistics, decision analysis, cost analysis, and evaluation research, is an important skill of health planners. These techniques encourage use of all available information to understand and address a given health problem. They also promote careful and deliberate decision making. In addition to analytic skills, planning also requires specialized interactive skills in group process, community development, and leadership, essential tools for working with communities, forging partnerships, and maintaining critical relationships.

The knowledge and skills required to attack a specific health problem are usually obtained by assembling teams of carefully selected participants very early in the process. As needs for new information and points of view evolve, however, new members should be added to assure the best possible program for the problem at hand. Traditionally, official public health organizations at the federal, state, and local levels have carried out program planning. Health service organizations, such as acute care hospitals and long-term care facilities, have also engaged in program planning for specific population groups and health problems. In the 21st century, new players are joining this group of "traditional" public health planners. Recognizing that the determinants of health problems are much broader than biological and other individual factors and that interventions to address those problems must emerge from this broader universe, the IOM and others have identified a network of individuals and organizations that should be full partners in population health planning. These include academia, media, employers and business, and communities at all levels (Bruce & McKane, 2000; IOM, 2003; McKnight, 2000).

Program planning methods are often presented under different names in order to emphasize particular components or highlight significant advances in technology. Such well-known applications as Assessment Protocol for Excellence in Public Health (National Association of County Health Officials, 1991), Community Health Improvement Process (Durch, Bailey, & Stoto, 1997), Mobilizing for Action through Planning and Partnerships (National Association of County and City Health Officials, 2000), Perinatal Periods of Risk (2003), Preceed-Procede (Green & Kreuter, 1999), and Intervention Mapping (Bartholomew, Parcel, & Kok, 1998) are examples of such advances. The framework underlying each of them is the rational planning model described in this chapter. Mastery of the basic framework is the foundation necessary to tackle any new or existing program planning method with confidence. In this chapter, the first five steps of the program planning process are reviewed. The logic of each step and its relationships to other steps are explored, and some tools for conducting specific activities are presented. The sixth step, evaluation, is sufficiently broad to warrant more extensive coverage in Chapters 16 and 17.

# ASSESSMENT OF HEALTH PROBLEMS

Assessment of health problems is the foundation step for the entire planning process. This step involves recognition and analysis of health conditions that appear to have reached unacceptable levels. Assessing health problems draws extensively on basic public health concepts and methods, especially an ecological view of the determinants of health and epidemiologic methods. An ecological view promotes consideration of many types of determinants, including factors in biomedical, behavioral, social, economic, and physical environment domains (IOM, 2003). Two types of epidemiologic studies contribute to an understanding of health problems: analytic studies and descriptive studies (Friis & Sellers, 1999). Analytic or etiologic studies identify the determinants of disease in specific population groups. Reports of analytic studies found in the professional literature are used to formulate an understanding of a health problem for planning purposes. Descriptive studies are then conducted to characterize the amount and distribution of a health problem and its determinants in a population of concern. Assessment of health problems has four dimensions: perception, verification, prioritization, and analysis (Peoples-Sheps, Farel, & Rogers, 2001a).

## Problem Perception

The planning process begins when someone recognizes a health problem. A "problem" may be defined as an unacceptable gap between the real (what is) and the ideal (what should be). In the field of MCH, a health problem is identified when the actual level of health status of a population of mothers or children is different from the ideal level. What constitutes an ideal level varies according to who sets this standard and the methods that they employ.

Perception of a health problem usually occurs in one of the following ways:

- Routine surveillance of specific health indicators, often carried out to monitor progress on national or state level health objectives, indicates an adverse trend. An excellent example of this process is the tracking of childhood overweight rates during the 1990s, which led to recognition that they were increasing rapidly.
- A statewide or community assessment illuminates a problem. Health departments, community agencies, and advocacy groups carry out

these assessments frequently. State-level MCH programs conduct needs assessments at least every 5 years to comply with MCH Block Grant application requirements (Maternal and Child Health Bureau, 2003). A variety of health problems, risk factors, and services are examined for the purpose of identifying MCH problems. Routine surveillance of health indicators is one method used for these assessments. Focus groups and key informant interviews are also important contributors.

- An individual or a community develops an impression that there is too much of an adverse health condition (e.g., several cases of an unusual birth defect in a neighborhood). The actual level of the condition is compared with the standards of the perceiver, and an unacceptable gap between the real and the ideal is identified.
- Health services become inundated with requests for care. This might lead to the conclusion that more services are needed, but before that conclusion is reached, it is helpful to consider that a population-wide health problem may be emerging or increasing.

In general, it is important not to define a health service deficiency (e.g., lack of services for . . .) as a health problem. When a health service deficiency is identified as a problem, the only logical response is to provide the missing services, which may not be the most effective or appropriate way to improve health status. By focusing on health as the problem, opportunities to intervene in a variety of ways can be illuminated.

### Problem Verification

Before taking action on a perceived problem, it is important to verify that the original perception is correct. Several objective aspects of the problem are examined for the purpose of determining whether observed levels really constitute a departure from expected levels. You should address the following questions to verify that a perceived departure from expectations is really a health problem:

- Extent: What is the incidence or prevalence of the problem? How many people are affected?
- Variation: How does the problem vary across population groups (e.g., specific racial or age groups) and geographic areas? Does the problem affect some people more than others?

- Duration: How long has the problem been at the observed level? In what ways have the levels changed over time?
- Expected future course: What is likely to happen to the problem if no intervention takes place? How will sociodemographic changes in the community influence the problem over the next 5 or 10 years?

The existence of a health problem is supported if the incidence or prevalence of the condition is worse in the population of concern than it is in the general population or in another group serving as a standard for comparison (e.g., a subpopulation or a neighboring population group). Other evidence of a problem is found if the condition has worsened or has been at the same unacceptable level for some time and/or if it is likely to worsen in the future. Take, for example, the problem of overweight in children. In the National Health and Nutrition Examination Survey 1999–2000, 15% of children 6 to 11 years old and 12 to 19 years old were estimated to be overweight (Centers for Disease Control [CDC], 2003a; US Department of Health and Human Services [US DHHS], 2002). Fifteen percent of this population constitutes approximately 8.5 million children and adolescents, thus indicating that the *extent* of the problem is large. When one considers that the rate has been at this level for a short *duration* because it has been increasing steadily since 1963 to 1965, the *expected future course* of the problem assumes even greater concern. Finally, increasing rates over the past 4 decades have been observed for all race/gender combinations, but African American and Latino children showed troubling *variations* from the totals, with rates ranging from 17% to 28%. Thus, a review of extent, duration, expected course, and variations in rates of overweight suggest that the problem is real and that it harbors a distressing future if the trend is not reversed.

## Setting Priorities Among MCH Problems

Every local community, each state, and the nation usually have more MCH problems than they have human and/or financial resources to address them. This necessitates rank ordering of the problems in order to decide how to allocate resources. An agency or organization may set its own priorities, or they may be imposed by an outside body (e.g., funding agency, legislature, state health agency, managed-care organization). If an agency is setting its own priorities, it is most efficient for the process to occur before there has been too much of an investment in further analysis of the recognized problem.

In the process of setting priorities, it is important to include people who have an investment in the health problems. Representatives of state and local agencies, other public and private organizations, members of the MCH community, the media, relevant businesses, academia, and private citizens should be involved. When such groups convene, however, individuals with especially persuasive and/or persistent verbal skills may dominate. In such a milieu, important aspects of the problem may never emerge. To allow a variety of perspectives and criteria to be fully represented, a framework that encourages a balanced consideration of all of them is essential.

The development of a simple matrix can meet this need (Blum, 1974; McGinn, Maine, McCarthy, & Rosenfield, 1996; Spiegel & Hyman, 1991). Table 15–1 shows a matrix with several of the problems of contemporary concern to MCH programs in the left-most column. Heading the other columns are criteria that might be used to prioritize the problems. There is no ready-made set of criteria that will apply in all situations, and criteria will differ from place to place and over time, depending on the important issues of the day. Two perennially useful criteria are the seriousness of the consequences and the direction of trends (improving or worsening). Another important one is the extent of the problem (the proportion of people affected and/or at risk). Other criteria may be found in written and unwritten policies. For example, problems that have been identified in *Healthy People 2010* (US DHHS, 2000) are priorities for all federal agencies. The Maternal and Child Health Bureau develops a set of MCH priorities on an annual basis. Within state and local areas, sets of objectives or special reports may focus on certain problems, and these should be taken into account. The acceptability of addressing a problem may also be an appropriate criterion. For example, a controversial problem such as adolescent sexual behavior should be considered in light of the ability of the community to accept any interventions targeted to this problem.

As the ranking is carried out, variations on interpretation of criteria usually emerge. Most would agree, for example, that health problems with serious consequences are more important than those with less serious consequences, and problems that have been increasing in magnitude should have higher priority than those that are decreasing. However, each of these characteristics may not be so straightforward in practice. In the first case, the most serious problems may affect only a small proportion of the population. In the second situation, the rate of increase or decrease may modify

**Table 15–1  Priority Matrix of MCH Problems**

| Health Problem | Severe Consequences | Trends Increasing | Extent (High Incidence/ Prevalence) | Criteria In Healthy People 2010 | In State Priorities | Acceptability to Citizens | Total |
|---|---|---|---|---|---|---|---|
| Low birth weight | 1 | 1 | 1 | 1 | 1 | 1 | 6 |
| Infant mortality | 1 | 0 | 1 | 1 | 1 | 1 | 5 |
| Vision impairments | 0 | 0 | 0 | 0 | 0 | 1 | 1 |
| Hearing impairments | 0 | 0 | 1 | 1 | 0 | 1 | 3 |
| Overweight/obesity | 1 | 1 | 1 | 1 | 1 | 1 | 6 |
| Childhood communicable diseases | 1 | 1 | 0 | 1 | 1 | 1 | 5 |
| Adolescent pregnancy | 1 | 1 | 1 | 1 | 0 | 0 | 4 |
| Adolescent Smoking | 1 | 1 | 1 | 1 | 0 | 0 | 4 |

Scores: 0 = no/low, 1 = yes/high.
Source: Peoples-Sheps et al. (2001a).

conclusions about the trends. Discussion about how to incorporate these variations into the ranking process will enhance the results.

Using a matrix like Table 15–1, supplemented by discussion to guide the ranking of problems, places the decisions to be made within a broad framework that discourages a focus on irrelevant aspects of individual problems. A lively debate here may lead to new insights and much more informed decisions about which health problems to address. The matrix facilitates the discussion by providing for assignment of a yes/no or high/low score in each cell. The problems with the highest total scores are accorded highest priority according to the chosen criteria.

## Problem Analysis

Once the highest priority problems have been identified, each problem is analyzed to understand its precursors and consequences and the direction and strength of the relationships among them. This aspect of health problem assessment is crucial for linking the problems to appropriate interventions. If a problem is not well defined, it is not likely to be solved.

There are many ways to analyze public health problems, but they all share a special concern for the interconnections among biological, behavioral, social, and physical domains. The model in Figure 15–2 was adapted by the IOM Committee on Assuring the Health of the Public in the 21st Century (IOM, 2003) from a Swedish model (Dahlgren & Whitehead, 1991) to reflect the range of influences on health in the United States. It includes a wide array of domains that harbor determinants of health problems, emphasizing through dotted lines the extent of opportunities for interactions among them.

Figure 15–2 provides a broad framework that encourages a comprehensive problem analysis by guiding analysts to domains where determinants for specific problems may be found. For many public health problems, this search identifies scientifically tested causal relationships among the determinants and between determinants and the problem and suggests where well-respected theories of behavior might provide further illumination. A problem diagram, such as the one shown in Figure 15–3, is a useful tool that allows for consideration of all relevant domains in Figure 15–2 while also specifying the research- and theory-generated links necessary to understand a specific problem in depth.

Figure 15–3 is a diagram of selected precursors and consequences of childhood overweight. The diagram has four components: problem, precursors, consequences, and linkages (Blum, 1974) presented in a manner

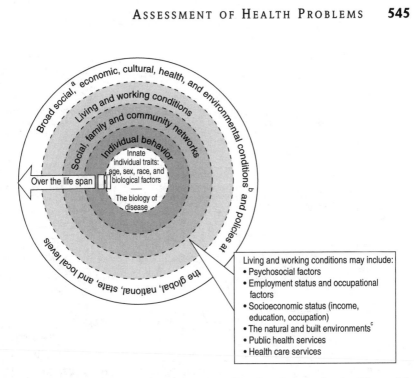

Adapted from Dahlgren and Whitehead (1991). The dotted lines between levels of the model denote interaction effects between and among the various levels of health determinants (Worthman, 1999).

[a]Social conditions include but are not limited to economic inequality, urbanization, mobility, cultural values, attitudes, and policies related to discrimination and intolerance on the basis of race, gender, and other differences.

[b]Other conditions at the national level might include major sociopolitical shifts, such as recession, war, and governmental collapse.

[c]The built environment includes transportation, water and sanitation, housing, and other dimensions of urban planning.

Reprinted with permission from the IOM (2003), by the National Academy of Sciences, courtesy of the National Academies Press, Washington, DC.

**FIGURE 15–2** A guide to thinking about the determinants of population health.

that reveals an image or map of the problem. The problem itself is placed in the middle, preceded by the precursors and followed by consequences. Arrows indicate linkages among these factors.

## Precursors

The precursors or determinants are factors that contribute to the problem. Some of them are directly related to the biological processes that lead to the problem. Others are not as directly linked; instead, they influence

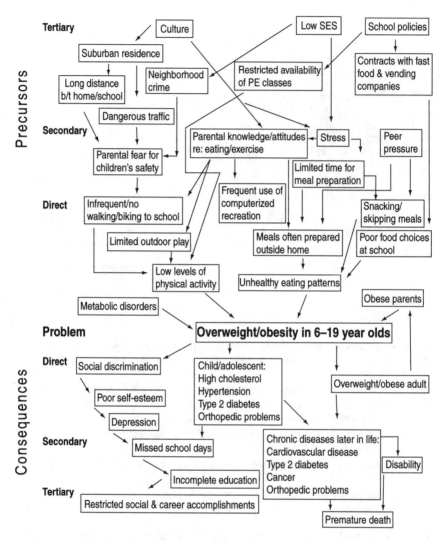

Sources: Centers for Disease Control and Prevention, 2003a; Dellinger & Staunton, 2002; Dietz, 1998; Goodman, Slap, & Huang, 2003; Haas, Lee, Kaplan, Sonneborn, Phillips, & Liang, 2003; Molloy, Kovach, Bors, Caldwell, Sommers, & Lebeuf, 2002; Ogden, Flegal, Carroll, & Johnson, 2002; Robinson, 1998; Troiano & Flegal, 1998; US DHHS, 2002.

**FIGURE 15–3** Diagram of selected precursors and consequences of overweight and obesity in children 6–19 years of age.[1]

---

[1]Innate characteristics that do not appear in this diagram include age (increasing), gender (female), and race/ethnicity (African-American/Hispanic).

the precursors that have a more direct effect. Still others are associated with the problem statistically, but they are considered markers for other unknown or unmeasured phenomena. When diagramming a health problem, it is helpful to consider precursors by proximity to the problem. These direct, secondary, and tertiary levels correspond with the circles in Figure 15–2.

At the direct level, the factors describe innate individual traits, such as biological and demographic characteristics, and individual behaviors. Although there may be two or more levels of these factors, they have the most immediate influence on the problem. In Figure 15–3, two of the major precursors of childhood overweight are behaviors: low levels of physical activity and unhealthy eating patterns. Each of these direct precursors has several behavioral precursors of its own, thus adding a few levels to the set of direct precursors.

Social, family, and community factors are often included at the secondary level. These secondary factors are usually precursors to the direct factors. In Figure 15–3, parental knowledge and attitudes, stress, and peer pressure are secondary precursors that affect those at the direct level. Innate characteristics, such as age, gender, and race/ethnicity, may also be included in the diagram at direct or secondary levels, as indicated in the footnote to Figure 15–3.

Tertiary factors usually include living and working conditions and the broader social and physical environment. Suburban location and school policies are tertiary precursors of overweight in children. Like direct factors, both the secondary and tertiary categories often have multiple levels.

Identifying the linkages among precursors and between the precursors and the problem requires familiarity with the analytic epidemiology literature and an understanding of the concept of relative risk. Relative risk, which is measured by an odds ratio, is an indicator of the strength of association between a risk factor and a health problem. It is the ratio of the incidence of the problem in the population of people with the risk factor to the incidence in the population without the risk factor (Friis & Sellers, 1999). Measures of relative risk can help in determining the potential impact of intervening at a specific precursor. For example, if overuse of video games and other sedentary recreation has a higher relative risk for overweight than eating meals outside of the home, an intervention intended to shift attention from video games to outside play would potentially have more of an impact on the problem than an intervention focused on eating at home.

To find evidence of linkages among factors, theories of human behavior can be very helpful. Many theories have been tested repeatedly, thus offering good evidence about determinants of certain behaviors and how these determinants relate to each other (Dignan & Carr, 1992; Glanz, Lewis, & Rimer, 1997). Theories used most frequently in MCH fall into one of the following categories (Peoples-Sheps, Foshee, & Bender, 2001c):

- Intrapersonal: theories that explain how beliefs, attitudes, perceptions, skills, attributions, and cognitions influence behavior and, ultimately, health.
- Interpersonal: theories that describe how interactions and dynamics with others influence health.
- Community organization: theories that describe processes of social change, steps in community development, and factors promoting community empowerment.
- Organizational change: theories that describe factors that influence organizational culture, climate, and communication between organizations.

### Consequences

Consequences are the effects of the problem on individuals, families, and society. They emphasize the significance of the problem. Figure 15–3, for example, demonstrates that being overweight or obese as a child can lead to serious chronic illness and premature death in adulthood. Like precursors, consequences can be categorized according to direct, secondary, and tertiary levels, each representing one or more domains that are increasingly removed from the problem. The consequences of one cycle of the problem may become precursors of the next, as indicated by the arrow connecting obese adults in the consequences to the obese parents in the precursors of Figure 15–3.

### Reality Checking

The diagram prepared so far may be derived from published literature. It is a solid beginning but not a finished product. A complete problem analysis is refined by discussions with people involved with the problem, by examination of extent, duration, and likely future course of the precursors and consequences, and through analysis of the precursors in that population. This refinement stage will allow identification of precursors and consequences that are especially prevalent in the population of concern as well as those that do not apply. For example, not walking or biking to school has been identified as a precursor of overweight. However, if most children in the population of concern do walk or bike to school, this precursor is not likely to contribute to this population's problem.

## Importance of Understanding Precursors and Consequences

Both precursors and consequences play critical roles in the rational planning process. Precursors

- Constitute a framework for identifying alternative interventions that either modify the risk factors or compensate for those that cannot be modified
- Identify the relationships from which a program hypothesis is developed
- Link the assessment phases of planning to program design and implementation

Moreover, by analyzing a broad range of precursors from different domains, programs with multiple interventions can be devised to attack several precursors simultaneously. These often harbor greater probabilities of success than single component interventions. They can assume even greater precision when directed towards target populations defined by innate precursors, such as age, race/ethnicity, and gender.

Precursors are the base from which program planning unfolds, whereas consequences serve a very different but equally important function. They encourage recognition of the problem, and if they are significant and/or extensive, they may form the rationale that convinces policy makers and funding agencies that the problem must be addressed.

## *Sources of Data for Assessing Health Problems*

Often the data required for assessment of health status problems are available from federal sources, such as those described in *From Data to Action: CDC's Public Health Surveillance for Women, Infants and Children* (Wilcox & Marks, 1995), the Agency for Healthcare Research and Quality *Child Health Toolbox* (2002), and the *HHS Directory of Health and Human Services Data Resources* (US DHHS, 2003). Data sources that are specific to states and local areas may be identified by state centers for health statistics. If data of acceptable quality are not available, collection of primary data should be considered. This is a decision that should be made carefully and in consultation with experts in qualitative and quantitative data collection, because collecting data is expensive and producing data of high quality depends on well-conceived and carefully executed methods.

# HEALTH SERVICES NEEDS ASSESSMENT

Recognizing a situation or condition as a "problem" implies that something should be done about it. The second step in the rational planning process begins to identify what to do. Health services needs assessment is a process for identifying needs for services that address specific precursors of a health problem. This assessment examines the adequacy of existing services to prevent the problem by attacking its precursors directly or compensating for their effects. If services that address the problem are available and used, needs for services are considered met. When services are unavailable or not used, unmet needs become apparent and interventions can then be developed to address them. Unfortunately, no single measure captures unmet need. Instead, needs are usually assessed from two or more of the following five perspectives (Peoples-Sheps, 2001a):

- Availability of recommended services
- Relative availability of services
- Demand for services
- Use of services by populations at risk
- Perceptions of service needs

## Availability of Recommended Services

The starting point for considering health service needs is an assessment of the extent to which appropriate services are available to prevent or ameliorate modifiable precursors of the health problem. Needs are met when recommended services are available and unmet when they are not. This assessment has three steps: (1) identifying effective interventions that could or should be available, (2) identifying services that are available, and (3) comparing the two lists to identify services that are not available. The last set represents unmet needs for services.

Because problem prevention must be directed toward the modifiable precursors of a problem, it is important to examine the problem diagram closely before attempting to locate appropriate interventions. For many MCH problems, recommendations for effective interventions have been developed. Public health and other professional organizations often promulgate these recommendations to foster adequacy and quality of care. Look to organizations such as the American College of Obstetricians and Gynecologists and the American Academy of Pediatrics for recommendations (sometimes called standards) for care of specific MCH medical problems. For broader programmatic interventions, the CDC and the Health Resources and Services Administration in the Department of Health and Human Services are excellent resources. These agencies develop interventions for emerging problems and sometimes offer funding to communities to implement them. Other recommendations are available from *The Guide to Community Preventive Services*, an Internet-based document developed by the independent Task Force on Community Preventive Services (2004). It summarizes current information about effectiveness and costs of a variety of population-based interventions. The goal of this process is to identify interventions that have either been shown to be effective through rigorous research methods or have been developed from well-accepted theories. Using resources such as those identified previously is a safe way of identifying such efforts. It is helpful to keep in mind, however, that intervention recommendations developed by specialized groups usually reflect the authors' points of view. Using a few different sources for recommendations tends to balance the perspectives represented.

Formal recommendations, such as those mentioned previously here, are often supplemented by recommendations developed by the local planning group, which should have a good sense of the community's culture and assets. By considering each precursor in light of local assets and issues, this group may identify (1) viable interventions that would not be appropriate in other areas or (2) important variations on the recommendations of professional groups. For example, one recommended approach to combating childhood overweight is for children to walk or bike to and from school (CDC, 2003b; MMWR, 2002; US DHHS, 2000). However, in a community where there are no crosswalks spanning major roads, walking or biking to school, even with adults, may not be prudent. In this case, the local planners may suggest building crosswalks or overpasses as a way of addressing this impediment in their community.

With a set of recommendations for interventions compiled, the next challenge is to inventory services that are actually available. Most communities have published inventories of community services. These guides are often general, however, and may not provide information of sufficient detail about interventions for specific health problems. As a result, some supplemental information may need to be collected through interviews with key informants, such as directors of relevant community agencies.

The final step in assessing availability of services involves comparing recommended with available interventions. The interventions that are recommended but not available to the population at risk, or are available only in part, represent unmet needs.

### Relative Availability of Services

Sometimes it is informative to assess service needs of the population of concern by comparing what is available to that group with the situation of another comparable population, such as people with similar risks in another area. The assumption underlying this approach is that the services available to the comparison population represent a desirable level. The emphasis is on equity so that unmet needs are defined as services that the comparison population has and the population of concern does not have. There are two ways to estimate relative need. The first is to compare a set of recommended interventions with the interventions available to the comparison group and with the population of concern. The recommended interventions available to the comparison group but not to the population of concern are considered unmet needs. The second approach is to use key informants in the comparison group to identify the services available for the problem and then determine whether they are also available to the population of concern. If not, these needs are unmet. The latter approach is sometimes easier than the former, but it is not recommended because of two important limitations. First, services in the comparison group, which constitute the standard, may not be theoretically derived or scientifically evaluated. Second, the services that establish the standard (i.e., the services in the comparison area) may not be the most appropriate ones to modify the extent of the problem. For example, in the comparison population, services for overweight or obese children may emphasize treatment once the problem exists rather than prevention of it in the first place. Using treatment services as the standard for comparison would bypass many preventive interventions and yield a biased estimate of needs.

### Demand for Services

The first two ways of assessing needs focus on availability of services. Whether available services are used is another question, addressed in part by an assessment of demand for services. With this measure, needs are reflected by the number of people who seek the recommended and available services. Those who receive the service are counted in use rates. The assumption underlying this perspective is that receipt of services signifies that needs are met. Those who do not receive the service presumably continue to have unmet needs. This approach has the appeal of producing an easy-to-understand proportion:

$$\frac{\text{Number of individuals not served}}{\text{Number of individuals who requested the service}}$$

Although measuring demand is attractive in its simplicity, it harbors some important limitations. First, those who do not seek services are omitted from this estimate. This group may not even know that appropriate interventions exist. In the case of overweight children, for example, parents may not seek help because they assume that being overweight is part of a stage their child is going through rather than a condition that puts him or her at risk for many subsequent health and social problems. Second, it is often difficult to access data on individuals not served because this type of "waiting list" information is not consistently retained by health care organizations.

Because of the second limitation, an alternative estimate of demand is in use. This involves comparing actual use of services to the maximum capacity of a service. If the service is consistently booked to capacity, it may be assumed that additional services would be used, if they were available. However, this conclusion should be tempered by recognition of the tendency of service utilization to expand to meet the level of available services.

## Use of Services by Populations at Risk

The fourth approach to measuring need is a variation on the demand measure. In this case, needs are considered met for the population at risk who receive a given intervention and unmet for those who do not. The population at risk is characterized by precursors in the problem diagram. Then the number of this group using (or not using) the service can be calculated as a proportion of the total number with a given risk factor. For example, if a school has developed a segment of the health curriculum that encourages children to be more active in their daily routines, proportions such as the following could measure the extent to which needs of the population at risk remain unmet:

$$\frac{\text{Number of children who ride in buses or cars to school}}{\text{but do not receive the curriculum}}$$
$$\text{Number of children who ride in buses or cars to school}$$

or

$$\frac{\text{Number of children who spend} >3 \text{ hours/day in sedentary activities}}{\text{but do not receive the curriculum}}$$
$$\text{Number of children who spend} >3 \text{ hours/day in sedentary activities}$$

Data on the use of each recommended intervention can be used to create informative measures, which, as a whole, yield a picture of needs for services of the population at risk. Needs are considered unmet when relatively large proportions of the population at risk are not receiving recommended and available services.

## Perceptions of Service Needs

Perceived needs are the services people say they need to prevent a health problem. Needs are unmet if the people are not receiving those services. Information about perceived need can be gathered through surveys, interviews and focus groups,[1] which can be designed to tap several important dimensions. People at risk, people with the problem, service providers, and community leaders may identify needed services that do not emerge through other means of assessing needs. They may also provide insight regarding the importance of some unmet needs in comparison to others and in identification of barriers to use of services. Barriers may be related to how the services are delivered or to cultural beliefs or expectations that inhibit use of services by the populations at risk. Equally important and often invaluable are informants' insights about community assets (e.g., infrastructure, organizations, associations, and individual talents) that can help meet perceived needs and serve as bases for launching interventions or as catalysts to make them successful (Kretzmann & McKnight, 1993; Tessaro, Eng, & Smith, 1994).

Information derived from perceptions of relevant informants personalizes health service assessments and makes the resulting information spe-

---

[1]Guidance on collecting and analyzing data for needs assessments can be found in Kettner et al. (1999) and Witkin and Altschuld (1995).

cific to the population and its community. Like the other perspectives of need, however, perceptions may harbor some limitations. The expectations of the individuals from whom perceptions are solicited can affect their responses. Needs may be underestimated if subjects are unaware of options that could be available to address the problem. They may be overestimated if the perceptions are based on unreasonable expectations.

## Assessing Other Characteristics of Services

Availability and use of services are the essential basic characteristics to examine in a needs assessment. Information about other qualities of services, however, can provide much deeper insight into service needs (Keppel & Freedman, 1995). Characteristics such as accessibility, acceptability, appropriateness, coordination, effectiveness, cost, and insurance coverage can be explored for further illumination of why certain deficiencies in availability and use exist.

## Summary of Unmet Needs

In the absence of a single measure of service need, planners must consider which of the alternative approaches to estimating need will generate the most useful information for their situations, with the fewest limitations. In general, it is rarely feasible to examine needs from all perspectives and rarely adequate to use only one. The wise approach is to use at least two perspectives, chosen carefully to generate the most useful information about the problem at hand.

Because the resulting set of unmet needs is generated from different perspectives/measures, some contradictory findings usually emerge. An assessment of recommended services, for example, may document numerous after school programs offering outdoor activities in the community, but the perceived needs assessment may indicate that most parents think there is an unmet need for such programs. Contradictions such as this provide an opportunity to explore the needs for service in greater depth. In this case, the true shortcomings may be in terms of knowledge about available programs, referrals to them, and/or financial coverage of those services.

## Setting Priorities Among Unmet Needs

If the list of unmet needs is long, it can be rendered more helpful to the planning process by setting priorities on the entries. This is a short process that involves considering the relative priority of each unmet need (or intervention) on the list, with highest priority given to interventions with (1) high prevalence of the precursor to which the service is addressed, (2) strong relationships between the precursor and the problem, and (3) relatively large extent of unmet need for the service. This prioritized list completes the health services needs assessment and serves as the starting point for the next step in the planning process.

### A Final Note on "Needs Assessment"

The two "assessment" steps—of health problems and of health services—are often grouped together under the rubric "needs assessment" (e.g., Petersen & Alexander, 2001). A distinction between these two steps is made here to explore the conceptual differences between them and the technical differences between their corresponding assessment methods. Both of these steps are essential components of the assessment required to understand the nature of the problem and to determine the extent to which existing services are addressing the problem. Where existing services fall short, unmet needs become apparent, and interventions can then be developed to meet these unmet needs.

## DEVELOPMENT AND SELECTION OF INTERVENTIONS

The third step in the planning process is development and selection of interventions. By this stage, the planning team has a good understanding of unmet needs for services to address the health problem. Services that are recommended but not available at all have been identified, as well as others that are in the community but not functioning well, or functioning well but covering only a portion of the people in need.

For many MCH problems, the set of unmet needs generated by a detailed needs assessment is a strong and adequate base from which to develop intervention options, as the set was derived from a large array of expert recommendations and the opinions of invested parties. However, a needs assessment does not always generate a complete list of alternative interventions. In some situations, interventions for key precursors may not be developed to the point of inclusion in professional recommendations or in the perceptions of involved individuals. For example, a traditional needs assessment of emerging diseases, such as severe acute respiratory syndrome (SARS) or long-standing problems that suddenly worsen, such as childhood overweight, may generate few or no ideas for promising interventions.

## Development of Interventions

Development of new interventions requires initiative and creativity on the part of the planners. It begins with a systematic review of each modifiable precursor, followed by brainstorming within the planning team for interventions that are likely to influence it. Table 15–2 shows how this process can produce multiple ideas for interventions for selected precursors of childhood overweight. Searching the literature for interventions that have been used to attack modifiable precursors in relationship to other health conditions can further refine this brainstormed list. A concurrent search for intervention theories that have been tested and found effective in modifying similar health problems and precursors may reveal additional alternatives. Over the past 2 decades, major advances in development of theories of human, organizational, and community behavior, and interventions to modify behavior, have been made (Glanz & Rimer, 1995). This work has been so productive

**Table 15–2** Relationship of Selected Precursors of Childhood Overweight to Potential Interventions

| Precursor | Potential Intervention |
|---|---|
| Restricted availability of physical education classes | In-service education for teachers/administrators about the importance of PE classes |
| | Add one to two PE class offerings per grade for each school |
| | Hire one additional PE teacher for each school |
| Parental limitations of knowledge and attitudes about eating and exercise | Educational intervention with parents using combinations of written materials, group meetings, postcard reminders, and rewards for participation |
| Parental fear for children's safety | Organized walking/biking groups with chaperones |
| | Identify and use "safe" routes between neighborhoods and schools |
| Infrequent/no walking or biking to school | Parental support and encouragement |
| | Rewards for walking or biking |
| Poor food choices at school | Modify cafeteria menus |
| | Modify vending machine contents |
| | Educational intervention using in-class student discussions and rewards for improved food choices |

that it is challenging for practitioners to keep track of the theories available to guide behavioral interventions. Intervention mapping (Bartholomew et al., 1998) provides a useful framework for linking precursors to appropriate intervention theories. Although interventions identified in this manner will not have been tested for effectiveness for the problem at hand, viable options can be evaluated in the future if they are chosen for implementation.

After completion of the needs assessment and a further identification of new intervention options, if warranted, planners should have a solid list of interventions that have been empirically tested and/or theoretically derived. If the list of options is relatively short, further development of each of them can begin at this point. However, if the list is fairly long, for example, more than five or six options, it is helpful to reduce the size of the pool. The basic idea here is to retain options that are the most likely to be selected for implementation. Depending on their specific situations, planners may consider retaining interventions that are

- Linked to precursors that are strongly associated with the problem
- Capable of serving the population most at risk
- Built on community strengths, interests, and priorities
- Considered essential in professional recommendations
- Consistent with mandates of agencies, organizations, and associations represented on the planning team
- Capable of showing effects sooner rather than later
- Likely to correspond with funding priorities

Although reducing the list of options is the goal, it is nevertheless wise to retain one or more interventions that address each level of the precursors (e.g., direct, secondary, tertiary, or behavioral, family network, social/physical environment). This permits a range of final options, as well as opportunity to combine options for multifaceted programs.

For the options retained, basic properties must be identified. Descriptions of interventions that have been tested in other settings can usually be obtained from their developers. For those under development by the planning team, this process is more complex. Discussion usually begins with the main activities of the program and then expands to administrative issues, as these two aspects of any intervention are basic and highly interdependent. For example, if changing meal options in schools is an intervention under consideration to prevent overweight in children, it could involve altering the menus prepared on site in school cafeterias or replacing the contents of vending machines with healthy products. Each of these interventions could require different administrative arrangements.

Once the basic features are decided, further discussion will help to flush them out. A brief (e.g., one-page) description of each program can capture these decisions. The description is actually a tool that informs the next several planning tasks. It should include major characteristics of the program (e.g., what the program will do, where activities will occur, who will be served), estimates of effectiveness in improving the health problem and in affecting other relevant outcomes, cost, administrative requirements, technical requirements, and any political controversies that may be anticipated.

### Criteria for Selection

The one-page descriptions characterize programs under consideration according to the major criteria to be used to select one program for implementation. The most frequently used criteria are effectiveness, cost, and feasibility (administrative, political, and technical).

The success of a public health program, of course, depends on its ability to ameliorate the health problem(s) of concern. The efficacy of the intervention is crucial. In addition to efficacy, this criterion should account for expected penetration of the target population, the time that might elapse before any effects are seen, and side effects. Ideally, effectiveness is estimated from evaluation studies of the effectiveness of this or a similar program on a similar population. If interventions were derived from professional recommendations, an estimate or direct evidence of effectiveness should be available from the same source. However, if the health problem is emerging and the intervention is a new recommendation or one developed by the planning group alone, evidence of effectiveness will not be available. In this case, estimates should be made, based on the known strength of the relationship between the targeted precursor and the health problem and of the estimated influence of the program on the precursor. If an intervention is based on one or more behavioral theories, research from applications to similar health problems may also inform estimates of effectiveness in this case.

Public health is moving more and more toward evidence-based interventions that have been shown to be effective for widespread application. New programs should be developed with sound theoretical underpinnings, implemented as small-scale demonstration projects and then evaluated with rigorous research methods before they are applied to large population groups. As a result, new programs serving small populations may not be able to produce competitive estimates of population effectiveness when compared with programs that can be dispersed to larger groups.

Effectiveness is a necessary criterion for selecting an intervention, but not a sufficient one. Even the most efficacious intervention cannot achieve its goals if staffing is inadequate, the clients and staff speak different languages, costs of services are beyond the means of intended recipients, or protesters ring the building in which the services are offered. All of these issues and many more must be considered. Even when an intervention with good marks in all of these areas is found, one must consider whether another option might be equally successful at a lower cost.

Cost is more easily measured than effectiveness, but some thought should be given to what costs are under consideration. Often in program planning, costs to the agency or organization (e.g., salaries, benefits, equipment, supplies, transportation, and communication) are the main considerations. However, instances exist in which costs to the client, family, or society are equally important. The degree to which costs are detailed at this point depends on the needs of the decision makers. Sometimes a ballpark figure that allows gross discrimination among alternative programs will suffice. Other times a detailed budget may be necessary to facilitate the decision.

Three feasibility criteria are frequently used to compare program options: administrative, political, and technical. Administrative feasibility refers to the extent to which a structure is in place to carry out such essential administrative tasks as organizing, monitoring, billing, personnel management, planning, and day-to-day oversight. If a structure is in place, can it absorb a new program? If there is no structure, is it feasible to develop one? Political feasibility, or the extent of support or opposition each program will encounter from various interests groups, authorities, and community members, is a critical factor for many MCH programs. Interventions that address adolescent sexual behavior, some family planning options, and ethical issues related to neonatal care and genetics are examples of ones that require careful consideration of political feasibility. Technical feasibility deals with the availability of human and technical resources required to carry out the program. Technical feasibility may be of consequence in rural areas of the United States and in developing countries where resources are very limited and technology may be difficult to obtain.

The five criteria described previously here are basic to most decisions. Another criterion of growing importance when addressing complex problems is the extent to which a program fosters organizational collaboration or partnerships among public agencies or between public and private organizations. MCH agencies and programs also place emphasis on the ability of the intervention to encourage development of systems of care, especially for children with special health care needs. If financial support from a third party is desirable, it is imperative to incorporate the funding agency's priorities into the criteria for selecting an intervention.

### Assessment of Program Alternatives According to the Criteria

Applying the criteria to program alternatives in order to select one for implementation is the third activity in this step of the planning process. There are many ways to do this, ranging from highly interactive discussions through highly quantitative analytic procedures. The most important ingredients for a sound decision are a systematic process and participation from many stake holders. The criteria-weighting method (Peoples-Sheps, 2001b; Spiegel & Hyman, 1991), described in part for prioritizing health problems, can be adapted for selecting interventions as well. This method promotes systematic consideration of each criterion, weighted according to its relative importance, and the process can be structured so that it encourages participation but allows verbal dominance to be controlled.

Table 15–3 is an example of criteria weighting. The criteria discussed previously here are listed in the left column of the matrix. Each criterion has been assigned a set of scores ranging from 1 (least consistent with the criterion) to 4 (most consistent). The next column indicates the weight assigned to each criterion. Weights are used when one or more criteria are considered more important than the others. In this case, the weights range from 1 (important) to 3 (most important). Technical feasibility is weighted 1, whereas both effectiveness and cost have been assigned weights of 3.

The next section of the matrix identifies three programs under consideration. Each program has two columns. The first includes a raw score on each criterion. A definition for each score, which can be modified according to the data available on each option, is given at the bottom of the table.

**Table 15–3** Criteria Weighting Method for Selecting a Program to Prevent Overweight in Children

| Criteria[1] | Weight[2] | Programs | | | | | |
| --- | --- | --- | --- | --- | --- | --- | --- |
| | | Physical Education Classes Three Times per Week | | Parent Education Classes | | Organized Walk to School Program | |
| | | Raw Score | Weighted Score | Raw Score | Weighted Score | Raw Score | Weighted Score |
| Effectiveness | 3 | 3 | 9 | 3 | 9 | 3 | 9 |
| Cost | 3 | 1 | 3 | 3 | 9 | 4 | 12 |
| Administrative feasibility | 2 | 4 | 8 | 4 | 8 | 4 | 8 |
| Political feasibility | 2 | 3 | 6 | 2 | 4 | 4 | 8 |
| Technical feasibility | 1 | 3 | 3 | 3 | 3 | 4 | 4 |
| Total | | 14 | 29 | 15 | 33 | 19 | 41 |

[1]**Criteria:**

Effectiveness:

4 = Highly effective, long-lasting
3 = Effective, duration of effects uncertain
2 = Good chance of improving the problem
1 = 50% chance of improving the problem

Cost:

4 = Very inexpensive
3 = Affordable
2 = Expensive
1 = Very expensive

Administrative feasibility:

4 = Fits easily in existing administrative unit
3 = Minor modifications in administrative unit required
2 = Difficult to administer
1 = Impossible to administer

Political feasibility:

4 = Acceptable to all constituents
3 = Acceptable to most constituents; little active opposition
2 = Acceptable to some constituents; little active opposition
1 = Unacceptable to most constituents

Technical feasibility:

4 = Technology and human resources readily available
3 = Technology available; human resources not available
2 = Technology not available; human resources available
1 = Technology and human resources not available

[2]**Weight:**

3 = Most important
2 = Very important
1 = Important

The second column under each program consists of weighted scores, that is, the product of the weight of each criterion and the corresponding raw score. The results of this analysis demonstrate the role that weights can play in the process. A one-point difference in the raw scores of the first two options becomes a four-point difference in weighted scores because parent education scored higher on the heavily weighted cost criterion.

The scores in Table 15–3 suggest that an organized walking to school program would be the best all-around choice. To increase the probability of success in improving a health problem, however, one might decide to combine interventions to address two or more precursors in a multifaceted program. This "ecological approach" (Gebbie, Rosenstock, & Hernandez, 2003) presents opportunities to affect several levels of precursors through a coordinated intervention strategy. With regard to childhood overweight, the planning team could decide to attack the problem on two or even three fronts by combining the interventions in Table 15–3 into one coordinated program.

Making a decision about which program to implement is one of the most important aspects of the planning process, on a par with defining the problem correctly in the first place. Regardless of whether a single intervention is selected or a few alternatives are ultimately combined into a broader spectrum initiative, the criteria-weighting method provides a useful framework for organizing the discussions that are essential to the ultimate decision.

## SETTING OBJECTIVES

In many ways, setting objectives is a process that starts when it is decided that a health problem should be addressed. Thus, either implicitly or explicitly, the main objective of the forthcoming program, *to improve the health problem*, is set very early in the process. Of course, other objectives, the ones that represent steps to be taken to ameliorate the problem, cannot be constructed until an intervention is selected. Also, in keeping with the iterative nature of the planning process, objectives continue to evolve as the program design and implementation plans are more fully developed.

Objectives are statements of purpose, which function primarily as a blueprint for the program (Peoples-Sheps, Byars, Rogers, Finerty, & Farel,

2001b). They communicate which problem is to be addressed, the activities that will be undertaken, precursors to be influenced by the program, the timeline for accomplishing specific activities, and the scope of the program and its intended effects. They are the first stop for anyone who wants to know what a proposal, plan, or program is all about. Objectives are also used as standards for comparison when assessing the program's progress. The resulting information can guide management decisions about program activities and resource allocation. If progress on one objective is poor, but other targets are met, resources may be diverted to improve performance on the lagging objective. If poor performance persists, either the activities or the targets may need to be modified. Thus, objectives are a framework around which the program is constructed and amended. There are two critical aspects to setting objectives: constructing a program hypothesis and developing the components of objectives.

### Program Hypothesis

A program hypothesis is the conceptual framework that links program activities to improvements in the health problem. The hypothesis is made up of a set of factors that includes one or more interventions and the expected modifications among the precursors that link the intervention to the health problem. Each of the factors in the hypothesis is the core content of one of the program's objectives. Program hypotheses are also known as logic models.

A framework for understanding the concepts behind a program hypothesis is in Figure 15–4. A program provides one or more activities or processes that are expected to produce results in the form of changes in specific risk characteristics of those who receive the intervention. Characteristics targeted for change by health programs might include knowledge, behavior, and biochemical measures. By altering these risk characteristics, it is expected that specific aspects of the health status of recipients, and subsequently, the larger community will improve, thus improving the general health status of the community. These higher levels of the hypothesis, representing improvements in the original health problem, are also called health outcomes. The population represented at each level may vary, but the principle that achievement of one level constitutes the means for achieving the next higher level is the core of a sound program hypothesis. A program hypothesis that corresponds to one chain of

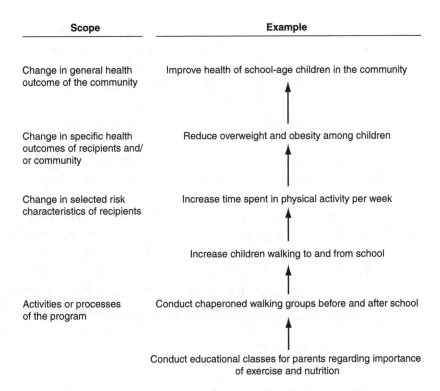

| Scope | Example |
|---|---|
| Change in general health outcome of the community | Improve health of school-age children in the community |
| Change in specific health outcomes of recipients and/ or community | Reduce overweight and obesity among children |
| Change in selected risk characteristics of recipients | Increase time spent in physical activity per week |
| | Increase children walking to and from school |
| Activities or processes of the program | Conduct chaperoned walking groups before and after school |
| | Conduct educational classes for parents regarding importance of exercise and nutrition |

**Figure 15–4** Program Hypothesis for a Childhood Overweight Prevention Program

precursors in the childhood overweight problem diagram in Figure 15–3 is shown in the example column of Figure 15–4. The program activities indicate that two interventions from Table 15–3 were combined into one program intended to attack precursors at two levels in the problem diagram: secondary, through parental knowledge and attitudes, and direct, through school transportation behavior.

## Components of Objectives

Each objective is composed of one measure of the performance of its underlying factor and one or more targets. A performance measure is "a specific quantitative representation (measure) of a capacity, process, or outcome deemed relevant to the assessment of program performance" (Perrin, Durch, & Skillman, 1999). Most programs create process (program activities) and outcome (risk characteristics and health status) measures for their objectives, consistent with the factors in the program hypothesis. You will often encounter more than one option for measuring a given factor. Issues related to selecting performance measures are discussed Chapter 16.

A decision about how performance will be measured must be made before the target of the objective can be set. A target is a numerical value that indicates the minimum desirable level of achievement for a particular activity or indicator. A target may have two parts: a quantity or amount (e.g., 20%) and a date of anticipated achievement (e.g., by the end of month 3). Usually outcome objectives are written for the life of the program, whereas the process objectives may have shorter, often 1-year, time frames. This is because program activities may change from year to year by design or because of developments encountered as the program is implemented. For example, a program may be designed so that recruitment of clients is a major activity in year 1, replaced in year 2 with service delivery activities. Alternatively, it may be found that by the end of year 1, recruitment has not been as productive as expected, and thus, different recruitment activities are added to the process objectives. In both cases, the process objectives would change from year 1 to year 2. Table 15–4 shows examples of how the objectives in Figure 15–4 can be structured with targets.

**Table 15–4** Selected Objectives of a Childhood Overweight Prevention Program, Year 1

| Performance Measure | Target |
| --- | --- |
| Percentage of children in Eastside School with gender- and age-specific BMI[1] within normal range | Seven-percent increase over baseline (estimated at 80%) |
| Percentage of children in the program with gender- and age-specific BMI[2] within normal range | Ten-percent increase over baseline (estimated at 80%) |
| Average amount of time spent in physical activity per week among children in the program | Four hours |
| Percentage of children in Eastside School who walk to and from school each day in chaperoned groups | Fifty percent of children in the school who walk in chaperoned groups 80% of the school days |
| Number of chaperoned walking groups of Eastside School students to and from school | Thirty neighborhood groups |
| Education classes for parents of Eastside School students: Number of classes | Four classes offered by October 1 |
| Percentage of parents attending at least one class | 70% |

[1]Body mass index: Body weight in kilograms divided by height in meters squared ($kg/m^2$).
[2]Children in the program: Eastside school students who walked to school in chaperoned groups 80% of school days.

Targets play a particularly important role in monitoring progress towards achievement of objectives. The most difficult aspect of setting targets is deciding on desirable levels of achievement. Help in this task can be found through a variety of sources. When targets are absolute numbers of program activities, such as the number of encounters with clients, individuals with experience delivering similar programs can provide useful insights. These sources may also be helpful when estimating the percentage of change for measures of outcome objectives. Relevant literature in the field, such as evaluations of similar programs, time studies and patient flow analyses, can also be helpful when these decisions are to be made. In addition, the targets in *Healthy People 2010* (US DHHS, 2000) and similar state and local objectives often correspond with outcome objectives for MCH programs. The targets proposed in these references are not universally transportable, but they provide benchmarks from which appropriate targets for a given program can be derived.

Availability of baseline data is another factor to consider when setting targets. Setting an absolute target, such as 87% for the measure "children at Eastside School with gender and age-specific body mass indices within normal range" does not indicate a starting point. The task is much larger if the current is 40% than if it is 80%. As the first objective in Table 15–4 shows, a more informative approach is to set the target as an amount of change from the baseline. Data for baseline comparisons should be available from the problem and needs assessments. If they are not available, baseline data can be collected before the program starts or early in its operational phase.

Other factors to consider in target-setting include the speed with which the program will become fully operational, whether some negative effects are expected before seeing positive ones (e.g., often programs that rely on reporting of cases see an increase in cases reported because the intervention is available before they see a decrease due to the intervention itself), and if there is a reason to set targets particularly high or low. In the end, the levels selected for targets are usually derived from a synthesis of the data and guidance available at the time. In the next round of planning, experience with the new program will inform these decisions.

# PROGRAMMING AND IMPLEMENTATION

Programming and implementation, the fifth step in the program planning process, starts with a set of objectives that form a blueprint for the program and a brief description of major characteristics developed to help decide which intervention to select. Through the processes of selecting interventions and setting objectives, ideas for program design are usually generated. Now the challenge is to harness those ideas into a logical design that will encourage achievement of the program's objectives. When the design of the program is fully developed, you can identify resources and action steps required to implement it successfully, and then construct a realistic budget.

## Program Design

Designing a program involves careful attention to four major design elements: program activities, client characteristics, organizational infrastructure, and human resources. A program's design should be developed by individuals with the knowledge and skills to incorporate relevant theories and practice standards appropriately. Often these individuals are members of the professions that will deliver the intervention. Hence, health educators may be best qualified to design behavior modification interventions because they are trained in this area; public health nurses are in a similar position with regard to infant health care interventions, and health administrators are likely to have greater expertise in efforts to modify organizational behavior. To change federal or state policies, laws, or regulations, experts in the specific change processes required should play major roles.

### Program Activities

Every detail of the program's operations should be considered at this point. If the intervention is to be offered in an agency setting, this would include space and scheduling issues. Interventions that are regulatory in nature, such as efforts to change laws or modify federal regulations governing activities that put children at risk of injury, would involve collaborating with key change agents, proposing the exact wording of the new regulation or law, and shepherding the proposal through appropriate channels. For a school-based program to encourage children to walk to school, size of the walking groups, timing and locations of rendezvous, and number of chaperones would be among the topics for discussion and decision.

Some MCH program activities are determined by theories underlying the selected intervention. As indicated previously, theories are used extensively throughout the planning process. For example, in the problem analysis stage, theories help to identify problem precursors and to specify links among them. In developing and selecting an intervention, some of the options may be theoretically derived, rather than interventions previously applied and evaluated for the problem at hand. Now, as the program is being fully designed, the theories underlying the intervention are operationalized.

The childhood overweight problem offers an example of how a theory could be applied to program design. To develop the content of the educational message the planners want to deliver to parents about walking or biking to school, they could use an intrapersonal theory, the Health Belief Model (Glanz & Rimer, 1995; Rosenstock, 1974). This theory describes the following six factors that influence a person's decision to take a preventive action:

- Perceived susceptibility: belief that they or their children are susceptible to getting a health problem (like overweight)
- Perceived severity: belief that the health condition and its sequelae are serious
- Perceived benefits: belief that the preventive action will reduce the risk and seriousness of the health problem
- Perceived barriers: perception of few tangible and psychological costs to taking the preventive action
- Cues to action: once motivated, cues to action may be needed to prompt the activity
- Self-efficacy: confidence in ability to take action

According to the Health Belief Model, the program's educational intervention with parents needs to address each of these factors in order to motivate parents to allow and encourage their children to walk or bike to school. Through written materials and discussions, perceived susceptibility could be addressed by describing the characteristics of children at risk: more than 3 hours/day playing video games and watching television, minimal outdoor exercise, and inadequate nutrition. Perceived severity could be addressed by describing the physical and emotional consequences of overweight on the child, as well as the long-term consequences as the child grows to adulthood. The materials could also point out the cyclical relationship between obese children, obese adults, and obese parents of the next generation of obese children. To address the benefits of walking or biking, the materials and classes can emphasize opportunities for children to get some physical activity, develop habits of taking some exercise each day, control weight, engage in social interaction with peers, and build healthy bones, muscles, and joints. Perceived barriers could be addressed by focusing on parents' biggest concern: safety. By designing the program so that children walk or bike along preselected safe routes in neighborhood groups with parental chaperones, the message to parents can emphasize that the children will be safe from dangerous traffic and neighborhood bullies. Parents who chaperone will have the same amount of control over their children's safety as those who drive their children to school and more control than those who send them on a school bus. Cues to action, such as reminders, thank you notes for chaperoning, or rewards and recognition for participation, can be developed to encourage and maintain involvement. Finally, self-efficacy can be addressed by coaching parents (1) in ways to overcome children's resistance to walking and (2) on managing disciplinary issues that may arise while chaperoning. Although each of these points may seem like common sense, the planners of this program may not have considered them specifically without the theory of the Health Belief Model to prompt their thinking.

This description involves both the contents, or methods, of the intervention (i.e., the messages to be delivered to parents) and the modes, or strategies, by which the methods will be delivered (i.e., classes and written materials). While designing a program, you should try out different combinations of methods and strategies until you find one that fits best with the target population and the parent organization's capabilities.

Descriptions of theories and applications relevant to different types of programs can be found in the literature (Glanz & Rimer, 1995; Glanz et al., 1997; Hochbaum, Sorenson, & Larig, 1992). If the chosen intervention is one that has been developed and recommended by a public health source, like CDC or Health Resources and Services Administration, its theoretical foundation should already be developed. Your role in this case may be limited to choosing activities that fit best with your populations' circumstances.

To specify details of program activities, it is helpful to consider when each activity will occur and where and how it will be done. Two tools that are helpful at this stage are written procedures and flow charts (Spiegel & Hyman, 1978, 1991). Written procedures are clear and concise statements about activities to be done, including exactly what tasks are involved, the sequence they should follow, and who is responsible for them. Flow charts offer another way of accomplishing the same result. These charts show the sequence of activities in diagrammatic form. They are especially useful when depicting several parallel sets of activities.

Another important aspect of program design is coordination of the program's activities. For a program to function smoothly, components must work together. For example, the personnel department and service delivery units or various service units, each providing a different type of service, must have specific mechanisms for assuring unimpeded interactions. These mechanisms should be detailed as procedures for routine coordination, like referral procedures from one clinic to another. In addition, there should be a procedure for handling the atypical problems that will arise.

## Client Characteristics

The program must fit with the characteristics of the clients in order for it to function well. If the first language of the target group is not English, then bilingual providers or interpreters should be hired. If the intervention is targeted to mothers of young children, provisions for child care should be taken into account. If the target group is school-age children, marketing materials should be designed to correspond with the interests and reading levels of that age group in its geocultural setting. Many of these characteristics were identified when the health problem was analyzed, but a more detailed understanding may require interviews or focus group discussions with members of the target population as the full program is designed.

## Organizational Infrastructure

When selecting an intervention, consideration was given to feasibility, both administrative and technical. The issue at that stage was the extent to which the administrative structure and technical capability to carry out the program existed or could be developed. Now these capabilities must be operationalized so that appropriate administrative support and control is available to assure that program objectives can be met. The organizational chart is the universal tool for depicting the structure of an organization and subunits within it (Breckon, 1997, Chapter 5). Most MCH programs are set up within existing agencies, where the location of a new program can facilitate or impede day-to-day operations. One possible location is within an existing organizational unit. There is often some economic advantage to this approach, but there is also a risk that the program will become indistinguishable from the other programs in the unit.

An alternative is to structure the program as a demonstration project by setting it up as an organizationally distinct, short-term initiative. One reason to take a demonstration project approach is to retain the totality of the intervention so that it can be rigorously evaluated. From an administrative perspective, demonstration projects often have high visibility, are not tied to the peculiarities of an ongoing bureaucracy, and are allowed considerable organizational autonomy. All of these characteristics tend to encourage creativity within the project. On the other hand, there are disadvantages of demonstration projects. Because they may require the same types of staff as ongoing units, functions may be duplicated and thus become wasteful and inefficient. High visibility may bring negative attention. Also, demonstration projects sometimes become elitist and entrenched in their own institutional culture, thereby losing the creativity and flexibility for which they are best known.

Traditionally, MCH programs have been offered in either the public or the private sector. As new types of health care organizations dominate the field and as public–private partnerships are encouraged from many sides, new challenges for organizational structure have emerged. In situations in which staff members are shared by partnering organizations, chains of authority and responsibility present emerging challenges.

## Human Resources

With the program's activities and organizational structure specified, the types and numbers of personnel can be determined. The planning team should discuss alternative types of providers so that the final selection represents the best fit of provider training and experience with the job to be done (Charns & Lockhart, 1997). The number of personnel required should be estimated by determining the proportion of total service each staff member can provide in light of the total amount that needs to be done. Supervisory responsibilities and time commitments are taken into account when estimating expected productivity of staff members. These estimates should be calculated as carefully as possible because underestimates could cause serious delays in achievement of process objectives. These delays, in turn, will have adverse effects on outcome objectives.

The universal tool for linking staff members to program activities and to organizational structure is the position description (Breckon, 1997)

(Chapter 8). Most organizations and agencies have standard formats for position descriptions, which include job title, minimum and desired qualifications, chain of command, and job functions and responsibilities. Because position descriptions reflect many decisions made in the process of program design, they are critical links in the planning process. They can also serve an important role for the individuals who fill the positions in that they link those individuals to the program's specific process objectives and, through them, to the overall program hypothesis.

Thoughtful attention to the program's activities, the target population, organizational structure, and program personnel will lead to a thorough explication of the program. Such extensive immersion in the complexities of the program often fosters emergence of new objectives, another manifestation of the iterative nature of the rational planning process.

## Implementation Planning

Implementation refers to a set of activities conducted in the time period between formal approval of the program and the program's actual start date. Implementation planning is the process of (1) identifying what needs to be done during that period of time and (2) scheduling those activities so that the program can be launched smoothly. The resources and activities required to implement a program are different from the design elements of an operating program (i.e., program activities, client characteristics, organizational infrastructure, and human resources). Implementation resources include equipment, personnel, arrangements, and other items required to begin program operations. Implementation activities are the tasks that must be done in order to have the resources available to start the program (Spiegel & Hyman, 1991). Once the program is fully designed, this is the logical next step. The distinction between ongoing activities of a program and the resources and implementation activities required to launch it is illustrated later here.

In a program in which children walk to school, ongoing program activities would include having chaperones meet the children at certain locations and times and then walk with small groups of them to school along certain routes. The resources needed to carry out these ongoing activities include chaperones, designated safe routes, and procedures covering rendezvous points, schedules, and numbers of children per group. Implementation activities are the tasks required to have these resources when and where they are needed. Parents must be contacted and their enthusiastic support obtained. Chaperones will have to be recruited and trained. Safe routes must be designated and schedules developed. Finally, preliminary tasks for each of these tasks may have to be identified.

Most implementation activities can be derived from the program's process objectives. Some key tasks, however, cut across the entire program:

- Obtaining administrative approvals to implement the program or some parts of it
- Identifying parties that can assist or hinder implementation and ways to communicate with them
- Anticipating side effects of the program and developing approaches to minimize resulting problems

In addition to these tasks, many unanticipated events between a program's approval date and actual start date can spawn more implementation activities. As a result, it is wise to allow for slack time during the implementation period.

Scheduling implementation activities to meet program start dates can be challenging. For each activity, the length of time required for completion and its sequence relative to the other activities must be determined. In addition, responsibilities for each activity should be assigned. If many people are working on implementation, several chains of activities can be carried out concurrently.

If the number of implementation activities is relatively small (approximately 20 to 40), they can be easily organized in a diagram that shows at a glance when each should start and be completed. Ordering the activities may be considerably more difficult when there are a great number, especially if many of them should be undertaken concurrently. In this case, a project management tool will facilitate the task. These tools are widely available in computer software. They are based on the Program Evaluation Review Technique (Frame, 1987; Spiegel & Hyman, 1991), which can also be accomplished by manual calculations. Whichever approach is used, the end result is a schedule that shows what needs to be done, when to start and stop, and who is responsible.

## Budgeting

The budget is one of the most essential components of the planning process. If the budget is omitted or poorly executed, all of the preceding work amounts to no more than wishful thinking. Like the objectives and program hypothesis, the budget provides a blueprint of the plan. It can also help to clarify roles and responsibilities and contribute to cost awareness among the participants in the process. Working through budget details may produce some fresh ideas or new perspectives on other parts of the plan, thus offering another opportunity for iteration.

Most organizations and funding sources have required formats for budgets. In general, the budget has two parts: personnel and nonpersonnel. The personnel section has entries for each type of personnel (by name if known), the number of each type, percentage of time devoted to the program, salary, and benefits. Nonpersonnel items include equipment, supplies, travel, communication, contractual arrangements, and other items specific to the program. A budget using these categories is called a line-item budget. It may be developed for the entire program or for each of the process objectives. When developed for each process objective, the cost of each program component is readily apparent, thus facilitating decisions about where to trim costs if it becomes necessary to do so.

Estimating the cost of each item is fairly straightforward. The key is to obtain costs from the correct source; for example, the personnel department of the organization is usually the best source for salaries and benefits, whereas distributors are more reliable sources for nonpersonnel items. Cost estimates for each item are then multiplied by the quantity required of that item. Changes in costs over the budget period, such as salary raises and airfare increases, must be built into the estimates. Some costs that may not be immediately obvious are (1) items that will be needed later in the budget period for phased-in services, (2) costs of evaluation, and (3) implementation expenses. All of these should be included in the budget.

In addition to cost estimates, it is sometimes necessary to distinguish between requested funds and donated funds. This distinction is used when a proposal for the program is being submitted to an outside funding source for consideration. Funding sources are often interested in the extent to which the applicant organization will support the program. The term "donated" refers to the applicant's contributions. "Requested" funds are those the applicant is requesting from an outside source.

The costs identified here are direct, that is, the costs expected to be incurred while implementing and conducting the program. However, the direct costs of a specific program or project may not represent all of its costs. For example, facilities, utilities, and equipment are often used by several programs and may not be included in the direct costs of any of them. Some funding agencies will pay a percentage of direct costs to compensate for the indirect costs incurred by the new program. Specifications for calculating indirect costs vary across agencies and should be obtained from them directly when needed (Frame, 1987; Kiritz, 1979).

## EVALUATION

The evaluation plan is the last step in the program planning process. Evaluation results inform the next round of planning, identify whether the program is going awry so that it can be corrected, and produce information useful for decision making by managers, policy makers, funding agencies, and the public. The evaluation plan should be an integral part of the program plan. If the planning process is conducted as described in this chapter, completing an evaluation plan is relatively straightforward because two of the key prerequisites for evaluation, a logical program hypothesis and measurable objectives, are already developed. The three major strategies for program evaluation—monitoring, performance appraisal, and evaluation research—are discussed in Chapters 16 and 17.

## CONCLUSION

For MCH professionals, the systematic steps of the program planning process sometimes seem to get lost amidst continually changing resources, legislative mandates, and administrative red tape. In the face of these realities of everyday life in busy agencies, however, mothers and children are encountering complex and multifaceted health problems. The challenge to MCH professionals is to develop and implement programs to prevent those problems. Program planning provides an ecological perspective and a problem-solving analytic framework for meeting this challenge. It promotes deliberate decision making and the development of creative and responsive programs of interventions, while operating comfortably in a social and political context. It uses many of the analytic, interactive, and managerial techniques available to the field of public health, thus serving as a bridge between research and practice. Program planning can be used at any jurisdictional level (e.g., local, state, and federal) and for any system of care (e.g., managed-care organizations and traditional public health systems). The process is dynamic, involving continuity and iteration, as well as the development of program plans that are intended to be changed. Over many years, MCH professionals have found that program planning skills are indispensable tools in their efforts to improve the health of mothers and children.

## *Acknowledgment*

Most of the content of this chapter is examined in more detail in a series of self-instructional manuals available for review or download at www.shepscenter.unc.edu/trainingMaterials.html. I am grateful to the co-authors of the manuals whose unique skills and perspectives have enriched my understanding of program planning in countless ways. I would like to extend special appreciation to Mary Rogers, DrPH, for helpful comments on the entire chapter and to Janice Dodds, PhD, RD, for guidance on the fine points of Figure 15–3.

# REFERENCES

Agency for Healthcare Research and Quality. (2002). *Child health toolbox: Measuring performance in child health programs.* Available March 14, 2004, from: http://www.ahrq.gov/chtoolbx

American Health Planning Association. (2005). Mission statement. Washington, DC. Last updated: 1/8/2005. Available February 9, 2005, from: http://www.ahpanet.org/Images/03%3DAHPAmission.pdf.

Bartholomew, L.K., Parcel, G.S., & Kok, G. (1998). Intervention mapping: A process for developing theory- and evidence-based health education programs. *Health Education and Behavior, 25,* 545–563.

Blum, H.L. (1974). *Planning for health: Development and application of social change theory.* New York: Human Sciences Press.

Breckon, D.J. (1997). *Managing health promotion programs: Leadership skills for the 21st century.* Gaithersburg, MD: Aspen Publishers.

Bruce, T.A., & McKane, S.U. (2000). *Community-based public health: A partnership model.* Washington, DC: American Public Health Association.

Centers for Disease Control and Prevention. National Center for Health Statistics. (2003a). *Prevalence of overweight among children and adolescents: United States 1999–2000.* Available February 10, 2004, from: http://www.cdc.gov/nchs/products/pubs/pubd/hestats/overwght99.htm

Centers for Disease Control and Prevention. (2003b). *Kids walk-to-school.* Available February 10, 2004, from: http://www.cdc.gov/nccdphp/dnpa/kidswalk/index.htm

Charns, M.P., & Lockhart, C.A. (1997). Work design. In S.M. Shortell & A.D. Kaluzny (Eds.), *Essentials of health care management*. New York: Delmar Publishers.

Dahlgren, G., & Whitehead, M. (1991). *Policies and strategies to promote social equity in health*. Stockholm: Institute for the Futures Studies.

Dellinger, A.M., & Staunton, C.E. (2002). Barriers to children walking and biking to school—United States, 1999. *Morbidity Mortality Weekly Report, 51*, 701–704.

Dietz, W.H. (1998). Childhood weight affects adult morbidity and mortality. *Journal of Nutrition, 128*, 411S–414S.

Dignan, M.B., & Carr, P.A. (1992). *Program planning for health education and health promotion* (2nd ed.). Philadelphia: Lea & Febiger.

Durch, J.S., Bailey, L.A., & Stoto, M.A. (Eds.). (1997). *Improving health in the community: A role for performance monitoring*. Washington, DC: National Academy Press.

Frame, J.D. (1987). *Managing projects in organizations: How to make the best use of time, techniques, and people*. San Francisco: Jossey-Bass Publishers.

Friis, R.H., & Sellers, T.A. (1999). *Epidemiology for public health practice* (2nd ed.). Gaithersburg, MD: Aspen Publishers.

Gebbie, K., Rosenstock, L., & Hernandez, L.M. (Eds.). (2003). *Who will keep the public healthy? Educating public health professionals for the 21st Century*. Washington, DC: National Academies Press.

Gilbert, N., & Specht, H. (1977). *Planning for social welfare*. Englewood Cliffs, NJ: Prentice-Hall.

Glanz, K., & Rimer, B. (1995). *Theory at a glance: A guide for health promotion practice*. Washington, DC: US Department of Health and Human Services. Public Health Service, National Institutes of Health, National Cancer Institute.

Glanz, K., Lewis, F.M., & Rimer, B.K. (Eds.). (1997). *Health behavior and health education: Theory, research and practice* (2nd ed.). San Francisco: Jossey-Bass Publishers.

Goodman, E., Slap, G.B., & Huang, B. (2003). The public health impact of socioeconomic status on adolescent depression and obesity. *American Journal of Public Health, 93*, 1844–1850.

Grason, H.A., & Guyer, B. (1995). *Public MCH functions framework: Essential public health services to promote maternal and child health in America*. Baltimore, MD: The Child and Adolescent Health Policy Center. The Johns Hopkins University.

Green, L.W., & Kreuter, M.W. (1999). *Health promotion planning: An educational and ecological approach* (3rd ed.). New York: McGraw Hill Higher Education.

Haas, J.S., Lee, L.B., Kaplan, C.P., Sonneborn, D., Phillips, K.A., & Liang, S-Y. (2003). The association of race, socioeconomic status, and health insurance status with the prevalence of overweight among children and adolescents. *American Journal of Public Health, 93*, 2105–2110.

Hochbaum, G.M., Sorenson, J.R., & Larig, K. (1992). Theory in health education practice. *Health Education Quarterly, 19*, 295–313.

Institute of Medicine. (1988). *The future of public health.* Washington, DC: National Academy Press.

Institute of Medicine. (2003). *The future of the public's health in the 21st century.* Washington, DC: National Academies Press.

Keppel, K.G., & Freedman, M.A. (1995). What is assessment? *Journal of Public Health Management and Practice, 1*, 1–7.

Kettner, P.M., Moroney, R.M., & Martin, L.L. (1999). *Designing and managing programs: An effectiveness-based approach* (2nd ed.). Thousand Oaks, CA: Sage Publications.

Kiritz, N.J. (1979). Program planning and proposal writing, *The Grantsmanship Center NEWS*: 71–79.

Kretzmann, J.P., & McKnight, J.L. (1993). *Building communities from the inside out: A path toward finding and mobilizing a community's assets.* Evanston, IL: Institute for Policy Research.

Maternal and Child Health Bureau. (2003). *Understanding Title V of the Social Security Act: A guide to the provisions of the federal Maternal and Child Health Block Grant.* Washington, DC: Maternal and Child Health Bureau, Health Resources and Services Administration, US Department of Health and Human Services.

McGinn, T., Maine, D., McCarthy, J., & Rosenfield, A. (1996). *Setting priorities in international reproductive health programs: A practical framework.* New York: Center for Population and Family Health.

McKnight, J.L. (2000). Rationale for a community approach to health improvement. In T.Q. Bruce & S.U. McKane (Eds.), *Community-based public health: A partnership model.* Washington, DC: American Public Health Association.

MMWR. (2002). Editorial note following barriers to children walking and biking to school: United States, 1999. *Morbidity Mortality Weekly Report, 51*, 701–704.

Molloy, M., Kovach, K., Bors, P., Caldwell, D., & Sommers Lebeuf, J. (2002). The epidemic of childhood overweight and obesity: Extent of the problem and prospects for change. *North Carolina Medical Journal, 63*, 291–299.

National Association of County and City Health Officials. (2000). *Mobilizing for action through planning and partnerships (MAPP).* Available January 24, 2004, from: http://www.naccho.org/tools.cfm

National Association of County Health Officials. (1991). *APEXPH: Assessment protocol for excellence in public health.* Washington, DC: National Association of County Health Officials.

Ogden, C.L., Flegal, K.M., Carroll, M.D., & Johnson, C.L. (2002). Prevalence and trends in overweight among US children and adolescents, 1999–2000. *Journal of the American Medical Association, 288*, 1728–32.

Peoples-Sheps, M.D. (2001a). *Health services needs assessment.* Washington, DC: Maternal and Child Health Bureau, Health Resources and Services Administration, US Department of Health and Human Services. Available

August 28, 2004 from: http://www.shepscenter.unc.edu/trainingMaterials. html.

Peoples-Sheps, M.D. (2001b). *Development and selection of interventions.* Chapel Hill: School of Public Health, University of North Carolina. Available August 28, 2004, from: http://www.shepscenter.unc.edu/trainingMaterials.html.

Peoples-Sheps, M.D., Farel, A., & Rogers, M.M. (2001a). *Assessment of health status problems.* Washington, DC: Maternal and Child Health Bureau, Health Resources and Services Administration, US Department of Health and Human Services. Available August 28, 2004, from: http://www. shepscenter.unc.edu/trainingMaterials.html.

Peoples-Sheps, M.D., Byars, E., Rogers, M., Finerty, E., & Farel, A. (2001b). *Setting objectives.* Chapel Hill: School of Public Health, University of North Carolina. Available August 28, 2004, from: http://www.shepscenter. unc.edu/trainingMaterials.html.

Peoples-Sheps, M.D., Foshee, V., & Bender, D. (2001c). *Programming and implementation.* Chapel Hill: School of Public Health, University of North Carolina-Chapel Hill. Available August 28, 2004, from: http://www. shepscenter.unc.edu/trainingMaterials.html.

*Perinatal periods of risk.* (2003). CityMatCH at the University of Nebraska Medical Center, Centers for Disease Control and Prevention, National March of Dimes Birth Defects Foundation, and Health Resources and Services Administration/Maternal and Child Health Bureau. Available February 10, 2004, from: http://www.citymatch.org.

Perrin, E.B., Durch, J.S., & Skillman, S.M. (Eds.). (1999). *Health performance measurement in the public sector: Principles and policies for implementing an information network.* Washington, DC: National Academy Press.

Petersen, D.J., & Alexander, G.R. (2001). *Needs assessment in public health: A practical guide for students and professionals.* New York: Kluwer Academic/ Plenum Publishers.

Robinson, T.N. (1998). Does television cause childhood obesity? *Journal of the American Medical Association, 279,* 959–60.

Rosenstock, I.M. (1974). The health belief model and preventive health behavior: *Health Education Monographs, 2,* 354–386.

Spiegel, A.D., & Hyman, H.H. (1978). *Basic health planning methods.* Germantown, MD: Aspen Systems.

Spiegel, A.D., & Hyman, H.H. (1991). *Strategic health planning: Methods and techniques applied to marketing and management.* Norwood, NJ: Ablex Publishing.

Task Force on Community Preventive Services. (2004). The guide to community preventive services. Available August 28, 2004, from: http://www. thecommunityguide.org.

Tessaro, I., Eng, E., & Smith, J. (1994). Breast cancer screening in older African-American women: Qualitative research findings. *American Journal of Public Health, 8,* 286–293.

Troiano, R., & Flegal, K.M. (1998). Overweight children and adolescents: Description, epidemiology, and demographics. *Pediatrics, 101,* 497–503.

Turnock, B.J. (1997). *Public health: What it is and how it works.* Gaithersburg, MD: Aspen Publications.

US Department of Health and Human Services. (2000). *Healthy people 2010* (conference edition, in two volumes). Washington, DC: US Department of Health and Human Services.

US Department of Health and Human Services. (2002). *Health, United States 2002.* Table 71: Overweight children and adolescents 6–19 years of age, according to sex, age, race, and Hispanic origin: United States, selected years 1963–65 through 1999–2000. Available January 18, 2005, from: http://www.cdc.gov/nchs/data/hus/hus02.pdf.

US Department of Health and Human Services. (2003). *HHS directory of health and human services data resources.* Available February 17, 2004, from: http://www.aspe.hhs.gov/datacncl/datadir/

Wilcox, L.S., & Marks, J.S. (1995). *From data to action: CDC's public health surveillance for women, infants and children.* Atlanta, GA: Centers for Disease Control and Prevention, US Department of Health and Human Services.

Witkin, B.R., & Altschuld, J.W. (1995). *Planning and conducting needs assessments.* Thousand Oaks, CA: Sage Publications.

Worthman, C.M. (1999). Epidemiology of human development. In C. Panter-Brick & C.M. Worthman (Eds.), *Hormones, health, and behavior: A socioecological and lifespan perspective.* Cambridge: Cambridge University Press.

# CHAPTER 16

# Maternal and Child Health Program Monitoring and Performance Appraisal

*Mary D. Peoples-Sheps and Joseph Telfair*

*Organizations that measure the results of their work—even if they do not link funding or rewards to those results—find that the information transforms them.* (Osborne & Gaebler, 1992, p. 146)

## INTRODUCTION

Program monitoring and performance appraisal are two of three types of program evaluation used in maternal and child health (MCH). Basically, evaluation involves a comparison of a program's processes and outcomes with selected standards in order to assess its accomplishments. In program monitoring, this is carried out by assessing the extent to which a program is implemented as designed. Monitoring is a relatively low-tech, inexpensive, administrative function that involves tracking progress toward achievement of a program's objectives. Performance appraisal, or performance measurement, is a process that has grown rapidly in the last decade to meet needs for accountability, especially on the part of government agencies. It involves tracking a selected set of indicators of program performance, with special emphasis on broad-based programs and community or higher levels of assessment that are not addressed by the other evaluation methods. Evaluation research involves the application of social science research methods to determine whether a program is the cause of observed results. It relies on both qualitative and quantitative research methods, and often a triangulation of the two, to produce informative results. Evaluation research is the strategy to use when the effectiveness of a new program or the relative usefulness of one program over another must be determined.

Evaluations are approached from two distinct professional traditions: planning and research. Professional planners take the first approach, and professional evaluators sometimes take the second. Although both groups ultimately use the same methods, the two see evaluation through different lenses. To a program planner, evaluation is the sixth step in the rational program planning process described in Chapter 15. This is a crucial step whose primary function is to produce information that feeds directly into the assessment of the health problem and service needs in the next round of the planning cycle. From the planner's perspective, program evaluation always involves monitoring. Whether performance appraisal is necessary depends on outside demands for information. Similarly, evaluation research is warranted when there is a specific rationale, such as when the effectiveness of an intervention has not been previously demonstrated. In this case, the evaluation research plan is developed with the program staff and a professional evaluator is expected to be involved from the beginning.

An evaluator often comes to the evaluation task, however, after the program has been developed, possibly after it is well underway. The evaluator's job is to use evaluation research methods to determine the impact of the overall program or to investigate specific aspects of it. Although the evaluator's major focus is evaluation research, monitoring and performance appraisals also fit into the evaluator's framework. They are used to explore the dimensions of a program in order to understand what it is and how well it was implemented. This information informs selection of research methods and measures and helps to explain the results of evaluation research. Because research is the primary focus for professional evaluators, monitoring and performance appraisal are considered preliminary steps, or pre-evaluation, from their perspective.

Program evaluation is an integral part of MCH practice. Whether you are reviewing literature, determining your program's impact, or planning an attack on an emerging health problem, program evaluation skills are invaluable. The field of evaluation has expanded greatly in recent decades, as new methods have been developed to serve a correspondingly broad array of purposes, from assessing whether a small service program is operating as it should to determining the effectiveness of a large multisite teen pregnancy prevention trial. Because evaluation is such a large and complex topic, it is covered in two chapters. Program monitoring and performance appraisal are examined in this chapter, and evaluation research is explored in Chapter 17.

At the heart of both program monitoring and performance appraisal is the measurement of performance of a program or intervention (Wholey, 1997). In this chapter, aspects of performance measurement that are common to both types of evaluation are examined first. This provides a foundation for exploring ways in which performance measures are analyzed, interpreted, and used in program monitoring and performance appraisal. Throughout the chapter, major distinctions between the two processes are highlighted.

# MEASURING PERFORMANCE

Both program monitoring and performance appraisal depend on strong, meaningful measures of program performance. A performance measure is "a specific, quantitative representation (measure) of a capacity, process, or outcome deemed relevant to the assessment of program performance" (Perrin, Durch, & Skillman, 1999, p. 19). *Relevance to program performance* is what distinguishes a performance measure from any other health indicator. For example, the measure, *percentage of adolescents who use illegal substances,* is an indicator of risk for a number of health problems, but it is only a performance measure when it is used to assess the performance of a relevant intervention. To construct performance measures, three tasks must be undertaken: identifying concepts to be measured, selecting or constructing measures, and locating or developing data sources.

## Identifying Performance Concepts

The aspects of a program that are measured attract attention and generate action (Hatry, 1999). Conversely, aspects that are not measured may go unnoticed until a crisis brings them to the surface. Even though it is tempting to go straight to available data sources to find performance measures, deciding what to measure is an essential first step—worthy of serious attention. If you take the time to think through what you need, you are much less likely to miss something important. To cover all of the bases, start with the program's hypothesis to identify the main program events and expected outcomes. A program hypothesis (Peoples-Sheps, Byars, Rogers, Finerty, & Farel, 2001),[1] also called a logic model or outcome sequence chart (Hatry, 1999), is a narrative or diagram that states the sequence of processes and outcomes that make up the theoretical foundation of a program. In a well-designed program, the relationships among processes and outcomes are supported by empirical evidence and/or accepted theory. Figure 16–1 is an example of one hypothesis for a program to prevent overweight in children derived from CDC recommendations for walking to school (CDC, 2004c). Most public health programs have multiple hypotheses underlying their activities and outcomes. A program hypothesis helps to identify three distinct categories of performance used in public health: capacity, process, and outcome (Perrin & Koshel, 1997). Capacity represents the ability to provide specific services. This includes both infrastructure and specific resources, such as size

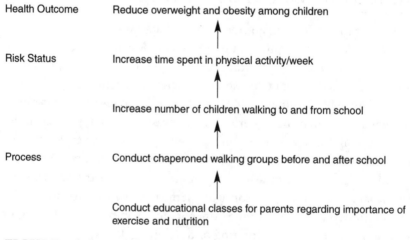

**FIGURE 16–1** A childhood overweight prevention program hypothesis.

---

[1]For a discussion of the derivation of a program hypothesis, see Chapter 15.

and qualifications of the workforce, information technology, quality of facilities and equipment, administrative capability, organizational relationships, financial capacity, and the clinical infrastructure necessary to carry out a given intervention, such as having relevant protocols in place. Capacity is not always explicit in a program hypothesis, but it can be deduced from a program's activities (Chen, 1990).

Process refers to "what is done to, for, with, or by defined individuals or groups as part of the delivery of services" (Perrin & Koshel, 1997, p. 3). Traditional examples of process are the activities of a program, such as providing well-child checkups or offering an educational service. In public health agencies and MCH programs, however, process also refers to essential MCH services, such as surveillance, investigation, and planning (Grason & Guyer, 1995; Handler, Issel, & Turnock, 2001).

Outcomes are divided into two groups: risk status and health outcomes. Risk status represents intermediate outcomes, the changes in risk levels that are expected from an intervention before any change in health status should occur. Risk status is very important because it represents the immediate results of a program. These are results over which a program has greater control than it has over health status. For example, if a program offers education to parents about using child restraints in automobiles correctly, the expectation is that appropriate use of restraints (an aspect of risk) will improve in the population that receives the service. The health outcome in this case would be motor vehicle crash occupant injuries for children, which can be affected by other factors such as social influences, roadway engineering, and driving skills, over which the program has no control. Risk status is also important because it serves as a link between program processes and outcomes. When measures can be developed in process, risk outcome, and health outcome categories, changes in risk status help to explain both positive and negative changes in health outcomes. Finally, because changes in risk status are expected to occur fairly soon after receipt of program processes, they can often be measured in the short timeframes of budget cycles and annual reports.

Health outcomes can be represented in three different ways: health status, social functioning, and consumer satisfaction (Perrin & Koshel, 1997). Positive states of physical and mental health, as well as diseases and deaths, are reflected in health status. In MCH, social functioning usually refers to the functional abilities of children with special health care needs, including their ability to perform activities of daily living.

Customer satisfaction, of course, is not exactly a health outcome, but it is an outcome of MCH interventions that is influenced by the services offered and received.

An example of performance measures in each of these categories for the part of the overweight reduction program in Figure 16–1 is shown in Table 16–1. As the table suggests, measuring performance of an intervention in each of the categories gives depth to the results and direction to further investigation.

Locating program hypotheses may be challenging. Sometimes they can be found in narrative or diagram form in program documents. When performance measures are developed in conjunction with development of a program (the recommended approach), the hypotheses are usually in the program's plan. However, when performance measures are developed after the program has been operating for a while, clear hypotheses may not be available. In these cases, they must be constructed. Even if a model of an operating program is available, it may not be a true reflection of the current program. Sometimes programs are not implemented as planned. In other cases, program processes and outcomes shift over time in response to changing circumstances. Both of these situations require modification to the original program hypothesis.

The information necessary to construct a hypothesis or model of an ongoing program can be acquired from key informants, such as high-level

**Table 16–1** Sample Performance Measures for a Childhood Overweight Prevention Program

| Type of Performance Measure | Example |
| --- | --- |
| Health status outcome | Percentage of children with a body mass index (BMI) within the normal range |
| Risk status outcome | Average time spent in a physical activity per week |
| | Percentage of children who walk to and from school each day |
| Process | Number of chaperoned walking groups before and after school |
| | Number of education classes for parents |
| | Percentage of parents who attend classes |
| Capacity | Percentage of schools with walk-to-school programs in place |
| | Number of walk-to-school coordinators hired |

administrators, providers, and others who might have had a hand in design of the program or in its current operations. Interviews, focus groups, and surveys of these individuals may be used to generate the information. If the program is supported or delivered by a consortium of partners, it is important to obtain their input as well. Useful information may also be obtained from enabling legislation, mission statements, budget documents, program descriptions, annual reports, and program evaluations.

The program hypotheses offer a solid foundation for identifying what to measure, but it is also wise to consider other events and factors that reflect program performance. Both positive and negative potential side effects should be anticipated in order to avoid unexpected crises, such as overburdening diagnostic and treatment services by implementing a new screening program. If left unchecked, this side effect could result in a lower standard of care for all clients. In addition to side effects, other aspects of a program that should be considered for measurement of performance are quality of care elements such as accessibility and acceptability, costs to consumers and the program, reimbursements, and equity in service delivery and outcomes.

## Selecting or Constructing Measures

Once you have decided what you would like to measure, decisions about which measures to use can be made. At the local level, measures of some program activities, such as the number of encounters between providers and patients, or capacity, such as the availability of physical facilities, can be constructed with minimal difficulty. However, for complex measures, such as asthma attacks among children in a statewide program, several steps are required and numerous choices must be considered. Regardless of the size or complexity of the program, the process begins by searching for measures that correspond to the capacity, processes, and outcomes in the program hypotheses.

Performance measures can be formulated in many different ways. They may be numbers (number of maternal deaths), rates (neonatal mortality rate), proportions or percentages (percentage of days missed at school among children with asthma), averages (average number of emergency department visits per child 1 to 4 years of age in a given year), or categories (meetings held, services available). Numbers, percentages, and rates are the most frequently used in public health. It is often helpful to include numbers along with rates and percentages so that the latter measures can be understood in the context of the size of the population from which they were derived.

Regardless of how it is formulated, a measure should have very precise wording, a specific timeframe, and a clearly defined population. The need for precision in wording often means that each measure taps only one aspect of a larger condition or event, possibly generating a need for additional measures to represent other relevant aspects.

To select or develop high-quality performance measures, candidate measures are generally assessed according to criteria that represent both scientific rigor and practical relevance. A performance measure should be meaningful, valid, reliable, responsive, and understandable and should allow for risk adjustments (Agency for Healthcare Research and Quality [AHRQ], 2002; Durch, Bailey, & Stoto, 1997; Hatry, 1999; McGlynn, 2003; Perrin et al., 1999; Wholey, 1997). To be meaningful, a measure should generate useful and important information about the program. If an indicator corresponds to one of the categories that we already reviewed (capacity, process, outcome), this criterion will be met at a minimal level. All aspects of a program, however, are not equally important. When measures are selected for performance appraisal, for example, the ones that produce information of particular relevance to consumers assume greater importance than others. The Performance Measurement Coordinating Council[2] has identified three categories of important measures: high priority for maximizing the health of persons or populations, financially important (high per person costs or affects a large number of people), or has demonstrated variation in care (across health systems, for example) and/or potential for improvement (Performance Measurement Coordinating Council, 1999). These recommendations fit well with performance measures at the national level. At a local or agency level, on the other hand, the most important indicators may be the ones that are capable of suggesting specific program modifications, such as key services or risk factors.

A valid measure is one that measures what it intends to measure. Validity, like all of the qualities in this list, is measured on a continuum, meaning that some measures have greater validity than others. For exam-

---

[2]The Performance Measurement Coordinating Council is a collaborative venture with the American Medical Association, the Joint Commission on the Accreditation of Healthcare Organizations, and the National Committee for Quality Assurance.

ple, a high validity measure of severe asthma in a population of children would be the incidence of severe asthma attacks in children 6 to 12 years of age in a given time period. This population-based measure, however, is difficult to obtain. An alternative is to measure the hospitalization rate for asthma among children in the same age group and within the same time-frame. This has lower validity because all severe asthma attacks are not treated in the hospital, but it may be the only feasible option because hospital data are more likely to be available than population-based data.[3]

Reliable performance measures can be reproduced regardless of who collects the data or when they are collected (assuming the true results have not changed). Like validity, reliability is viewed as a continuum. In general, the most reliable measures are made with instruments that have little susceptibility to human interference. Weights, for example, are considered highly reliable, whereas opinion surveys are lower on the reliability continuum.

Responsive measures are able to detect a change. This is a subtle point, as you would be unlikely to select a performance measure that you did not think was able to detect a change. The measure *infant mortality* offers an example of this point. The infant mortality rate is a good measure to track for changes in a state's infant death rate over time and across population groups. However, it is unlikely to be responsive (able to detect a change) when used to assess the effects of a prenatal counseling program serving a segment of a community that accounts for a small proportion of the community's infant deaths (Perrin et al., 1999).

Measures need to be understandable to the audience to whom they will be presented. Because the audiences for program monitoring are different from the audiences for performance appraisal, somewhat different measures may have to be selected for each purpose. This is further explored in subsequent sections of this chapter. Finally, some outcome measures should be amenable to stratification[4] or adjustment[5] by relevant risk factors (Performance Measurement Coordinating Council, 1999). Again,

---

[3]The role of data availability in the development of performance measures is discussed later in this chapter.

[4]Stratification involves analyzing performance measures within specific categories of risk factors (Dever, 1991, pp. 241–247).

[5]Adjustment is the process of calculating summary measures in which statistical procedures have been applied to remove the effect of differences in risk composition of the populations included in the measure (Friis & Sellers, 1999, p. 95).

the extent to which this is necessary depends on the use of the measure. If the measure is used primarily for program monitoring, risk adjustment or stratification may not be necessary. However, if the measure is to be used to compare across population groups or for accountability to an external stake holder, then adjusting for factors other than the program that are known to affect the measure is wise. Stratification may be even more informative in these cases because you can see exactly how the groups differ on the measure of interest.

Fortunately, several professional groups and health organizations have recognized the need for good quality performance measures with clear standard definitions that allow for comparisons. A selected group of measurement sets relevant to MCH is briefly described in Table 16–2. Other sources of measures of relevance to MCH, such as the AHRQ Quality Indicators, can be found at the AHRQ Child Health Toolbox website (2002) and the National Quality Measures Clearinghouse website (AHRQ, 2005). In most cases, measures in these sets are presented with detailed specifications that support applications to many programs and jurisdictional levels. However, using them is not always appropriate. Your program or health problem may not be addressed by the measures in a particular set. Alternatively, measures related to your program may be included; however, they may be worded to serve a purpose that deviates considerably from yours, or they may be appropriate for one level of measurement (e.g., national or community) but not for others. In addition, some of the measures, such as the AHRQ Quality Indicators and Consumer Assessment of Health Plans measures (AHRQ, 2002), were developed for specific data sources. If these sources are not available to you, constructing the measures may not be possible.

If you are unable to find the measures that you need in standard measurement sets, then you can either modify existing measures to meet your needs or create your own measures of important concepts. Two helpful resources for developing measures are AHRQ's *Child Health Toolbox* (AHRQ, 2002) and Monahan and Sykora's (1999) *Developing and Analyzing Performance Measures*. This step may be greatly facilitated if you also collaborate with experts in the field.

### Sources of Data

The selection of measures is closely tied to the data available to construct them. Data sources should be of high quality, with standardized definitions and data collection methods and acceptable levels of validity and

## Table 16-2 Selected Sources of Performance Measures for MCH Programs

| | |
|---|---|
| Maternal and Child Health Bureau Measures | The Maternal and Child Health Bureau has developed a set of national measures that includes 9 capacity, 18 process, and 6 outcome indicators. These measures are relevant to major Maternal and Child Health Bureau priorities, activities, programs, and funds (www.mchb.hrsa.gov). |
| *Healthy People 2010* | *Healthy People 2010* (US Department of Health and Human Services [US DHHS], 2000) includes 10 leading health indicators reflecting major public health concerns in the United States, all of which are related to MCH. It also has 467 objectives, which include measures for tracking progress. |
| The Health Plan Employer Data and Information Set | The Health Plan Employer Data and Information Set (HEDIS), developed by the National Committee for Quality Assurance, includes a set of standardized measures designed to ensure that the public has appropriate information to compare the performance of managed care plans. Almost 90% of all health plans measure their performance using the Health Plan Employer Data and Information Set (NCQA, n.d., www.ncqa.org/Programs/HEDIS). Many HEDIS measures relate to MCH problems and interventions. A national database of HEDIS measures for managed care organizations that enroll Medicaid beneficiaries has been also developed (www.cmwf.org/programs/quality/partridge_aphsa_hedis_1999.pdf). |
| The Consumer Assessment of Health Plans | The Consumer Assessment of Health Plans (CAHPS), a research tool of the AHRQ, has developed composite measures of health care access, use, and quality for Medicaid and commercial health plans. Data for the child health measures are obtained via survey of parents. The Consumer Assessment of Health Plans measures emphasize identification of children with chronic conditions and measures of their special health care needs. A database of multiple users is also available for benchmarking purposes (www.ahrq.org/chtoolbx/measure2). |
| Community Health Improvement Process | The Institute of Medicine Committee on Using Performance Monitoring to Improve Community Health (Durch et al., 1997) developed several prototype sets of performance indicators that emphasize accountability for participating agencies' contributions to performance. These prototypes include process and outcome measures for immunizations and infant health. |
| National Public Health Performance Standards Program | The National Public Health Performance Standards Program has developed tools for measuring performance of state and local public health systems. Measures that focus on capacity and process include optimal standards for performance associated with the 10 essential public health services (www.phppo.cdc.gov/nphpsp). |

Sources: United States Department of Health and Human Services (2000) and Durch et al. (1997).

reliability on the items of interest. In addition, they should be available within your timeframe, and the cost should conform to your budgetary constraints. In general, it is more efficient to construct measures from existing, or secondary, data sources, rather than to collect new, or primary, data specifically for a given set of performance measures.

Numerous secondary data sources are available. They fall into at least four broad categories (Monaghan & Sykora, 1999; Perrin et al., 1999; Stroup, Zack, & Wharton, 1994):

- Registries (e.g., vital statistics, birth defects, and communicable disease registries), which attempt to collect data on all events within their purview
- Surveys (e.g., National Health and Nutrition Examination Survey), which collect data from population samples
- Patient or client records, which include clinical information collected during the delivery of services
- Administrative data (e.g., insurance claims, characteristics of services and providers), which are collected routinely for administrative purposes

Large national databases with MCH-related data in them are collected and maintained by several national agencies, such as the Centers for Disease Control and Prevention, the AHRQ, the Food and Drug Administration, the Indian Health Service, and the National Highway Safety Administration (Agency for Health Care Policy and Research, 1997; AHRQ, 2002; Association of State and Territorial Health Officials, 2004; National Institute on Disability and Rehabilitation Research, n.d.; Perrin & Koshel, 1997; US DHHS, 2003; Wilcox & Marks, 1994[6]). In addition, most states maintain some registries, conduct surveys, and collect other types of MCH-related data that are available for performance measurement.

Finding the source that includes the precise data items required to construct a given measure for a specific population group is the challenge. For example, someone interested in pediatric asthma measures can find the items to create them in several sources, but the information in each database is slightly different. They could access hospital discharge data for dis-

---

[6]These references contain lists and descriptive information about many of the large databases available.

charges for asthma-related conditions, hospital admissions data for admissions and emergency department visits for asthma-related conditions, patient records for prescriptions written for appropriate medications for children with asthma (AHRQ, 2002), or clinic protocols to determine how pediatric asthma is expected to be managed in different settings.

In addition to locating data sources with the items required to construct specific measures, other characteristics of the data should be evaluated. Many data sets have been developed for specific populations, such as managed-care participants or Medicaid clients. It is important to ascertain that a data source includes and identifies the population you need. Another important aspect is whether the source allows comparisons across programs and population groups and whether it includes baseline data that can be tracked into the future.[7] User support is another consideration. Large databases harbor unique complexities that can befuddle even experienced data managers. The opportunity to consult with user support services about these issues as they arise is invaluable (AHRQ, 2002).

Two issues that are encountered frequently with large data sets are geographic availability and periodicity. Some of the large data sources are not uniformly available in every state. An example is the Pregnancy Risk Assessment Monitoring System (Centers for Disease Control, 2004b), which operates in 32 states. The number of participating states has grown over the years, but it still does not enjoy full coverage. Other data sources may be available within states, but they may not be accessible to the MCH professionals who need them (Maternal and Child Health Bureau, n.d.). Periodicity presents another hurdle. Outcome measures at the national and state levels are most likely to be available through surveys. However, surveys are usually conducted periodically, sometimes with several years elapsing between data collections. The periodicity of collection and dissemination of the data can have a major impact on whether a given source is appropriate for the measures you need.

The extent to which sources developed to generate data for measures at the national or state level apply to smaller jurisdictions depends on sample size and distribution. For example, data from the National Health and Nutrition Examination Survey (NHANES) can be used to follow trends in childhood and adolescent overweight at the national level (US DHHS,

---

[7]Telfair J. (2001). *8 Steps for project/program planning and monitoring/assessment leading to evaluation for state and community service agencies/programs*. Unpublished manual.

2002), but the sample is usually not large enough to support performance measurement for smaller geographic areas.

In seeking data sources for performance measures at the small program or community level, there are still other considerations. First, to construct performance measures for a specific local program, it must be possible to identify the population receiving the services of the program in the database. Most large national and state databases do not provide that level of detail, although it has become fairly common to link large population databases to program databases to achieve this goal. This can be done if there are unique identifiers (e.g., name, birth date) in each database. Second, as shown in the next section, program monitoring often requires a level of detail about the program that is not available in large databases. Third, managing large databases requires specific skills that may not be available within a specific program's human resource inventory.

Fortunately, for measures of program processes and outcomes within small geographic areas, local data sources are available or can be developed. Table 16–3 identifies six sources of data that are usually available within programs or can be collected from program participants, along with descriptive comments and examples.

Regardless of jurisdictional level, existing data can usually be obtained within shorter timeframes and at lower cost than primary data. Before deciding to use a secondary data source, however, consider carefully the completeness and accuracy of the data, the consistency of data collection across populations and geographic areas, and availability of the data. Attention should also be paid to the purpose for which the database was developed. Claims data, for example, are intended to monitor finances, not health care. Key aspects of care may be missing from claims databases (Grembowski, 2001).

If you are unable to find a suitable data source for the measures you need, three options are available:

- Consider adding the required data items to an existing data collection tool.
- Change the measure so that it conforms to existing data sources.
- Plan to develop a new data collection system.

The first option is the easiest, but it is only feasible if there is an existing data system on which to "piggy-back" and if appropriate permissions can be obtained. The second choice, changing the measure, is a compro-

**Table 16–3** Sources of Data for Performance Measures of Community Programs

| Potential Sources of Data | Remarks | Examples |
| --- | --- | --- |
| Client service or claims database | Usually used to track clients' use of services within a program. Recorded as the client uses the service. Usually aggregated daily. | Medical/clinical records<br><br>Use surveys |
| Client intake profile database | Excellent source of information on client descriptors (e.g., demographics). Recorded when client is first seen and periodically thereafter (usually annually) as long as client is in the program. | Claims applications<br><br>Direct observations |
| Interview documents or notes | Usually a structured interview containing both quantitative and qualitative data. Collected periodically for various purposes, such as gathering new information or confirming existing information on a client or as a supplement to the intake data form. | Satisfaction surveys<br><br>Stake holder surveys |
| Meeting documents or notes | A qualitative data source that is used primarily to document the program's day-to-day and overall decision-making activities. Recorded within a week of the meetings and summarized. May lack some specificity. | Minutes of relevant meetings |
| Pre, post, and follow-up tests | Usually structured measures of performance of individual clients. Used for assessment of knowledge or skill before, immediately after, and 3 to 6 months after a training or education session. | CME (Continuing Medical Education) training assessments<br><br>Follow-up knowledge retention or skills tests. |
| Program archives | Excellent source of information on service and program descriptors (e.g., personnel, audit results). Usually updated annually. | Log books<br><br>Access and use (service) records |

mise. It is a wise choice if starting a new data system is not possible. The third option is the most complex. Developing a new data collection system should be undertaken only after serious consideration of the other choices, if there are many measures that cannot be constructed from existing data, and if the time, funding, and expertise to carry out this task are available. Very specific methods are used to assure collection of high quality data. Discussion of these methods is beyond the scope of this chapter but is covered in Chapter 17 and in research and evaluation texts such as Miller's *Handbook of Research Design and Social Measurement* (Miller, 1991, pp. 115–230).

### Summary

Measuring performance is at the heart of both program monitoring and performance appraisal. Creating good quality measures begins with identifying the concepts to be measured in capacity, process, and outcome categories by examining a program's hypotheses. Once the concepts are identified, measures are found or developed to represent them. This involves careful consideration of scientific rigor, practical relevance, and availability of necessary data. Many existing data sources support performance measurement, but they do not meet all possible measurement requirements. In these cases, other alternatives, including selecting different measures and collecting new data, must be considered.

## PROGRAM MONITORING

Program monitoring is the process of assessing progress toward achievement of a program's objectives to determine whether the program was implemented as planned and whether expected changes occurred in health outcomes of the people served. It is a very traditional form of evaluation that is generally considered an administrative function and integral to the ongoing operations of every program (Kettner, Moroney, & Martin, 1999). Development of a monitoring system is an essential component of a program's plan. The information derived from program monitoring shows which objectives need more attention in the future and whether any of them require less intensive work. If the program has fallen short on some objectives, this information should trigger an in-depth search for the reasons the expected targets were not achieved. This search, in turn, is part of the health problem and service assessments in the next round of planning. The monitoring process described in this section identifies the program's objectives as the base from which formulas to measure progress are developed, relative weights are assigned as necessary, data collection plans are developed, and achievement scores are calculated at predetermined intervals.

## Start with the Program's Objectives

The objectives of a program, each of which consists of a performance measure and a target, serve as the foundation for program monitoring. A selected set of fully developed, measurable objectives that correspond with the hypothesis in Figure 16–1 and the performance measures in Table 16–1 is shown in Table 16–4. Objectives such as these are typically developed as a program is being planned.[8] Each of them should have an explicit date by which the target is to be achieved. In Table 16–4, the date by which the objectives should be achieved is one year from the start, as noted in the title of the table. With objectives clearly and precisely stated, the next challenge is to develop a system through which progress towards meeting the program's targets can be monitored.

**Table 16–4** Selected Objectives of a Childhood Overweight Prevention Program, Year 1

| Performance Measure | Target |
| --- | --- |
| Percentage of children in Eastside School with gender and age-specific BMI[1] within normal range | A 7% increase over baseline (estimated at 80%) |
| Percentage children in the program[2] with gender and age-specific BMI (body mass index) within normal range | A 10% increase over baseline (estimated at 80%) |
| Average amount of time spent in physical activity per week among children in the program | Four hours |
| Percentage of children in Eastside School who walk to and from school each day in chaperoned groups | Fifty percent of children in the school walk in chaperoned groups 80% of school days |
| Number of chaperoned walking groups of Eastside School students to and from school | Thirty neighborhood groups |
| Education classes for parents of Eastside School students: Number of classes | Four classes offered by October 1 |
| Percentage of parents attending at least one class | 70% |

[1]BMI: Body weight in kilograms divided by height in meters squared (kg/m$^2$).
[2]Children in the program: Eastside school students who walked to school in chaperoned groups 80% of school days.

[8]See Chapter 15 for information on developing objectives and setting targets.

## Developing a Monitoring System

Although monitoring can be done on a casual basis, a structured process with specific methods and timeframes for tracking progress is highly recommended. A structured process, like the one described later here, encourages regular monitoring, as well as consistency of measurement over time and across evaluators. Table 16–5 shows the components of a monitoring system. The first two columns are identical to those in Table 16–4, performance measures and targets. The remaining three columns represent the basic elements of a monitoring system, as it builds on the program's objectives.

### Formulas

The first step in developing a monitoring system is to construct formulas to reflect progress toward achievement of the objectives' targets. Three types of formulas can serve this purpose. Each one is based on the principle that a score of 1.00 is complete accomplishment (Guild, 1990). A score of 0.99 or lower signifies that the performance measure fell short of the target; a score that exceeds 1.00 indicates greater than expected achievement.

When the target is a percentage, proportion, or a simple count, the most informative and frequently used formula involves dividing the level of actual achievement at a specified time with the level given in the target.

$$\frac{\text{Actual value}}{\text{Targeted value}}$$

Several examples of this formula are shown in the third column of Table 16–5.

A second type of formula is used when the target is a date. A score of 1.00 is given if the activity is completed at the projected time. If the activity is completed ahead of schedule, 1.00 + the proportional equivalent of the number of months early is calculated. This involves multiplying the number of months early by 0.08, as 0.08 is the decimal equivalent of 1/12 of a year. If completion were late, 0.08 would be subtracted for each month. The same logic can be used for other time segments (e.g., weeks).

The third alternative can be used with any target, whether it is a percentage, proportion, number, or date. This is a simple process of scoring 1.00 if the target is reached and 0.00 if it is not reached. The simplicity of this method is compelling, and it can be very informative for tracking the occurrence of meetings or other events, as suggested by its use in

**Table 16–5  Year 1 Summary of Monitoring for Selected Objectives of a Childhood Overweight Prevention Program**

| Performance Measure | Target | Formula to Measure Progress | Results at End of Year 1 | Achievement Score |
|---|---|---|---|---|
| Percentage of children in Eastside School with gender and age-specific BMI[1] within normal range | A 7% increase over baseline (estimated at 80%) | Percentage over baseline with BMI within normal range / 7 | 1.75% | 0.25 |
| Percentage of children in the program[2] with gender and age-specific BMI within normal range | A 10% increase over baseline (estimated at 80%) | Percentage over baseline with BMI within normal range / 10 | 8% | 0.80 |
| Average amount of time spent in physical activity per week among children in the program | Four hours | Number of hours spent in physical activity / 4 | 3.2 hours | 0.80 |
| Percentage of children in Eastside School who walk to and from school each day in chaperoned groups | Fifty percent of children in the school who walk in chaperoned groups 80% of the school days | Percentage of children who walk 80% school days / 50 | 37% | 0.74 |
| Number of chaperoned walking groups of Eastside School students to and from school | Thirty neighborhood groups | Number of neighborhood groups / 30 | 21 | 0.70 |
| Education classes for parents of Eastside School students:    Number of classes | Four classes offered by October 1 | 1.00 or 0.00 | 1.00 | 1.00 |
| Percentage of parents attending at least one class | 70% | Percentage of parents attending one or more classes / 70 | 65.7% | 0.94 |

[1]BMI: Body weight in kilograms divided by height in meters squared ($kg/m^2$).
[2]Children in the program: Eastside school students who walked to school in chaperoned groups 80% of school days.

Table 16–5. However, it is not very informative when a percentage or a proportion is involved because it does not acknowledge partial progress toward achievement of the objective.

## Weights

When there are multiple objectives at each level of a program's hypotheses (e.g., process, risk status, health status), weights may be used to show that accomplishment of some objectives is relatively more important than accomplishment of others. The heavily weighted objectives usually address determinants that have stronger relationships to the health problem than others. Accomplishing them may be critical to improving the problem, and thus, they are assigned greater weight than others when assessing overall program accomplishments. Weights are assigned on a scale agreed on a priori by the planning group. Weights are not used in Table 16–5 because each of the objectives in this small set is considered essential—of equal weight—in achieving better BMIs for the students. However, most programs, including this one, have many other objectives. Consider how weights may be useful when monitoring a complete set of this program's objectives. An objective that does not appear in Table 16–5 is *increase the percentage of children who walk to and from school by themselves or with others, but not with the chaperone option offered by the program.* Walking, with or without chaperones, is the factor expected to contribute to more physical activity in general and, according to the program's hypothesis, to better BMIs among children in the school. However, the program developers may choose to assign greater weight to an objective addressing the chaperoned walking option because they expect that most parents will want their children to belong to these groups. They may reason that a change in walking behavior of a larger number (expected to be the chaperoned group) is likely to have a greater impact on the BMI objective for the entire school than an improvement in the smaller group of unchaperoned walkers.

## Data Collection Plan

The first three columns of Table 16–5 should be completed with the program's initial plan. To create a fully operational monitoring system, one more step is required: data items and sources necessary to construct performance measures should be identified. This step should not be missed even if some data sources seem obvious. It is far too common for otherwise careful planners and evaluators to discover that they had incorrectly assumed the necessary data would be available and accessible when they needed it.

To monitor the objectives in Table 16–5, systems must be in place to generate administrative data on parent meetings, chaperoned groups, and participating children. In addition, *the number of hours of physical activity/ week for children in the program* must be collected, as well as heights and weights (to construct BMIs) for all children in the school, or a representative sample of them. Because baseline BMI data have been collected in the past, it may not be too difficult to repeat the process.

## Monitoring Progress

Monitoring is usually done at frequent intervals so that any indicated program adjustments can be made, although results may be reported less frequently. Whatever the pace, when it comes time to consider what has occurred in the program, the formulas to measure progress are applied and achievement scores are calculated. Examples for the objectives of the childhood overweight prevention program are in the fourth and fifth columns in Table 16–5. The fourth column shows actual results at the end of the program's first year. The fifth column shows the score produced when the formula for the measure is applied. Looking at the first objective as an example, the target was 7% over the baseline value of 80%. During year 1, only a 1.75% improvement over baseline (i.e., 1.75/7) was documented. This indicates that the program fell far short of its target, with an achievement score of 0.25, although some progress was made.

In addition to calculating an achievement score for each objective, overall achievement scores can be calculated by summing the scores over all objectives and dividing by the number of objectives to obtain an average for the entire program. If the objectives are weighted, weights can be applied by multiplying the score for each objective by the weight before summing. To obtain a weighted average, the sum of all weighted scores is divided by the sum of the weights.

## Interpretation of Results

The information derived from monitoring shows which objectives need more attention in subsequent years and whether any of them require less intensive work. Adjustments in resource allocations can be based on the needs of specific objectives for more or less effort. Careful assessment of the reasons for shortfalls on objectives should be conducted before any reallocation decisions are made.

A review of end of year achievement scores in Table 16–5 provides helpful information for further investigation and subsequent program adjustments. As noted previously here, progress on the first objective was very limited; the achievement score was only 0.25. However, progress on the second objective, which is the same performance measure but specific to the group that received the intervention, was much more promising. It showed an 8% increase over baseline, yielding a score of 0.80. The expectation was that a substantial improvement in BMIs in the program group would contribute to a slightly more limited, but still substantial improvement, in the BMIs of the total population in Eastside School. This expectation was not met. Findings such as these invite further investigation. One possible explanation can be found deeper in the table. The number of chaperoned groups and the percentage of children in the school who walked 80% of the school days were considerably lower than targeted (achievement scores of 0.70 and 0.74, respectively). Therefore, whereas the children in the program did quite well in improving their BMIs, the program did not reach as many of them as anticipated. In other words, the program was not implemented as planned, and that may explain why the BMI objective for the entire school improved only a small amount. However, it is also possible that children who were more likely to engage in physical activity joined the walking groups, whereas those who prefer sedentary activities declined to participate. Thus, at least two plausible explanations exist for the findings that should be investigated further. Once a good understanding about the causes of the disappointing results for BMIs of all children is reached, appropriate programmatic adjustments should be made.

Programs may not reach their targets for a number of reasons. A primary reason is inadequate resources, which may take the form of insufficient funds across the board or misallocation of funds across objectives. It may be possible to detect misallocation if some targets are overachieved, whereas others fall short. Other commonly cited reasons why programs may fall short in achieving objectives include (1) a lack of adequate knowledge about feasible target levels, (2) external factors that make it difficult or impossible to reach the target (e.g., inability to find the required type of personnel), (3) inaccurate measurement of the objective, and (4) a conceptual error in the program hypothesis.

## *Advantages and Disadvantages of Monitoring*

Program monitoring is a valuable tool for planning and management decisions. The process is inexpensive and can be applied readily by anyone with entry-level training or experience. It includes a flexible set of methods that can be modified to accommodate the needs of each program. Monitoring requires program planners to develop objectives that serve as the basis of the process and then to plan for necessary data so that the capability for tracking progress is assured. Another important advantage is that it encourages the production of information for critical management decisions in both short- and long-term time frames and across all levels of program functioning. As a result, it is compatible with most governmental and private foundation proposal guidelines.

As an evaluation strategy, monitoring has three important shortcomings. First, it does not produce evidence of cause–effect relationships; only evaluation research can do that. Second, the results of monitoring are limited to a single program; they cannot be extrapolated from one program to another. Finally, there are no firm guidelines for interpretation of the scores. Although a score of 0.70 might be considered good and 0.90 might be superior, the most useful interpretations depend on the program's context (Peoples-Sheps, Rogers, & Finerty, 2002).

# PERFORMANCE APPRAISAL

Performance appraisal, which is also called performance measurement or performance monitoring, is the process of assessing accomplishments of very large programs, multiple related programs, and health care systems on a regular basis. It is an emerging form of evaluation that has gained considerable stature in the past several years. A major impetus was provided by the Government Performance and Results Act of 1993 (PL 103-62, 1993), which required the federal government to measure the performance of all federal programs. This was followed in 1995 by Federal Performance Partnership Grants (Perrin et al., 1999), which were intended to promote states' accountability for progress towards program goals in return for greater flexibility with regard to how the goals were met. These federal initiatives led to establishment of expert committees to examine issues related to development and collection of performance measures (Perrin & Koshel, 1997; Perrin et al., 1999) and to explore the role of performance appraisal as a means of promoting health at the community level (Durch et al., 1997). Concurrently, performance appraisal was growing in other fields, both governmental (Hatry, 1999; Morley, Bryant, & Hatry, 2001; Wholey & Hatry, 1992) and in the private sector, especially regarding the quality of care in managed care organizations (National Committee on Quality Assurance, n.d.).

Performance appraisal is based on the same principle as program monitoring, that is, using performance measures to track progress in relation to a defined standard. Until recently, the comparable data required to apply this principle to geographically dispersed, multicomponent programs were not available. Each program had its own information system, which made producing uniform, or common, measures extremely difficult. With widespread development and use of information technology, however, programs that span regions and agencies can construct an increasing number of uniform indicators.

## Distinctions Between Performance Appraisal and Program Monitoring

Performance appraisal and program monitoring share many characteristics, so much so that it is sometimes difficult to distinguish between them. Key similarities and differences between the two assessment methods are summarized in Table 16–6.

The scope of program monitoring is usually a single program, whereas the potential scope of performance appraisal is much broader, and its boundaries are still emerging. Performance appraisal, for example, is used to assess the broad-based, national programs of the Maternal and Child Health Bureau, whereas program monitoring is used within each constituent program as an administrative control mechanism to inform managers about the program's progress so that they can make adjustments to keep it on track. Performance appraisal, on the other hand, also may serve administrative control needs, but they are at a higher level (e.g., state MCH agency). More often, performance appraisal supports reporting to external stake holders on aspects of program performance, making comparisons among programs under a larger umbrella, triggering investigations of problem areas, and justifying requests for new funds to address a difficult problem.

Although both program monitoring and performance appraisal use measures of program capacity, process, and outcomes, monitoring tends to focus more heavily on processes, the factors that a specific program can

**Table 16–6** Distinguishing Characteristics of Program Monitoring and Performance Appraisal

| Characteristic | Program Monitoring | Performance Appraisal |
|---|---|---|
| Scope | Single program | Large sets of programs (e.g., MCHB) |
| | | Related programs (community or state level) |
| | | Health care systems |
| Purpose | Program management | External reporting for accountability and advocacy |
| | | Comparisons across programs |
| | | Identification of problem areas |
| | | Justification of new programs and budgets |
| | | Program management |
| Primary focus | Program processes | Outcomes, both risk status and health outcomes |
| Consumers | Administrators, providers | Government and private funders, elected officials, advocates, potential clients |
| Methods | Comparison between actual achievements and targets of objectives | Comparison with a variety of benchmarks: |
| | | Surveillance over time |
| | | Comparison with national and state health targets and/or means for the same measures |
| | | Comparison with other geographic areas, organizations, agencies, or programs |
| Usual sources of data | Program generated | Contributed by constituent programs |
| | | Large databases |
| Usual sources of performance measures | Program generated and standardized sets | Standardized sets |
| Number of performance measures | Depends on complexity of program | Relatively small number of key measures |
| | May be many detailed measures | |

modify on a daily basis. Performance appraisal tends to focus more on the outcomes of interest to its external stake holders, such as government and private funders, elected officials, advocates, and potential clients.

Program monitoring involves a comparison of a program's accomplishments with the targets in its objectives. The methods of performance appraisal also involve comparison with standards, including national and state health targets. However, comparisons over time, with national and state averages and among program locations, are also frequently conducted.

The data used in program monitoring are often generated by the program itself through its information system. However, programs may turn to other sources at the community, state, or national level to obtain data on outcomes, if those sources allow identification of the population served. The data used for performance appraisal tend to come from two sources. They may be contributed from a broad-based program's constituent programs, and/or they may be mined from any of several large national databases.

With regard to performance measures, individual programs are more likely to develop measures that meet their specific monitoring needs than to rely on the measurement sets that have been promulgated nationally, such as those described in Table 16–2, which offer a better fit for performance appraisal.

Finally, the number of measures used in program monitoring can be quite large and detailed to meet administrative control purposes. The number used in performance appraisal tends to be small, but the measures are selected very carefully in order to satisfy specific information needs of consumers.

### Selecting Performance Measures

As in program monitoring, the search for measures for performance appraisal begins with the program's hypotheses. In keeping with the wider scope of programs assessed with performance appraisal methods, however, additional investigation is usually needed to find all concepts that might be appropriate to measure. Searching for unintended effects and modifying the program's official hypotheses with input from partners, officials, and other involved parties can greatly expand the list of relevant concepts. This expanded set of concepts is then scrutinized to identify concepts that will carry the greatest meaning and importance with the external stake holders who comprise a major audience for performance appraisal.

An important consideration in selecting measures for performance appraisal is the extent to which they can be stratified by other relevant factors. Many public health problems, risk factors, and measures of program use vary across population groups. By examining data across groups, populations with different experiences in relationship to a particular performance measure can be identified. An analysis of stratified performance measures offers a deeper understanding of program performance, as well as direction for targeting subsequent modifications. Stratification factors may be innate characteristics (age, gender, and race/ethnicity), socioeconomic factors (income, family composition, language spoken in the home), geography (state, county, region), program characteristics (type, size, provider-mix), and risk factors in the population. Identifying which of these factors is most important for a given performance measure is a step that should be undertaken carefully. The decisions are based on research that identifies clear determinants of the concept in the performance measure as well as professional experience with the programs and populations of concern. A laundry list of stratification factors for each performance measure is unnecessary and inappropriate. Rather, the breakouts that are most likely to produce important information for the intended audience are key.

## Analyzing Measures for Performance Appraisal

The essence of performance appraisal is comparing actual results on performance measures with at least one benchmark. In the absence of comparisons, there is no way to know whether performance is good or bad. Thus, selecting benchmarks that will carry meaning and generate respect from the intended audience is imperative (Hatry, 1999; Morley et al., 2001). The benchmarks used most frequently in MCH are as follows:

- Previous time periods
- Other geographic areas
- Other organizations, agencies, or programs
- National or state means
- *Healthy People* targets (and similar objectives for each state)
- Targets set at the beginning of a performance period

Several examples of how benchmarks are used in analysis of performance measures are discussed later in this section.

Figure 16–2 is an example of a comparison with previous time periods and a *Healthy People 2010* objective[9] (US DHHS, 2000). This analysis shows that the percent of overweight children and adolescents (a health outcome measure) in the United States has increased steadily over the

---

[9] *Healthy People 2010* objective 19-3.

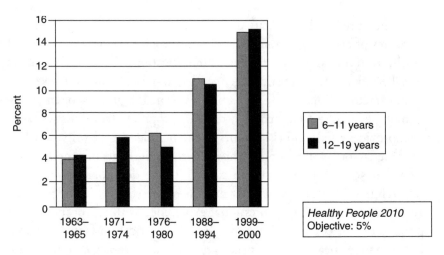

Source: US DHHS (2002).

**FIGURE 16–2** Overweight children and adolescents in the United States, selected time periods 1963–1965 through 1999–2000.

years, despite a nationwide effort to curb the trend since at least 1990[10] (US DHHS, 1990). The *Healthy People 2010* objective of 5% demonstrates how far the nation has to go to reach an acceptable level of this problem and that reaching it will be a challenge since it means reversing a 30-year trend.

An example of analysis across geographic areas is in Figure 16–3, which shows a comparison of folic acid awareness (a risk outcome measure) across selected states and over a 4-year timeframe. Awareness of the importance of folic acid supplements is a prerequisite for taking the supplements during the periconceptional period to prevent neural tube defects. During the period shown, numerous efforts, both nationwide and within individual states, were underway to promote awareness of folic acid (Ahluwalia & Daniel, 2001). This graph allows for two sets of comparisons that show differences across states and across time.

Tables 16–7 and 16–8 show how measures of immunization levels, which may be either process or risk measures, can be analyzed. Table 16–7 is taken from the Title V Information System (TVIS) of the Maternal and Child Health Bureau, US DHHS. It shows the performance measure, *percent of children 19–35 months who have received a full schedule of immu-*

---

[10]*Healthy People 2000* objective 2.3.

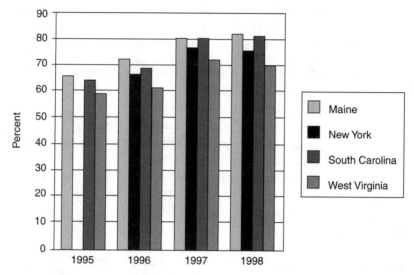

Source: Ahluwalia and Daniel (2001).

**FIGURE 16–3** Prevalence of folic acid awareness among Pregnancy Risk Assessment Monitoring System (PRAMS) participants, selected states 1995–1998.

*nizations* for the states in DHHS Region V. The TVIS offers three options for comparison: time periods, other states, and preset targets (called objectives in the TVIS). Table 16–8 is an example of using a stratification factor in analysis. In this case, a measure of immunizations from the Institute of Medicine Community Health Improvement Process prototype indicators (Durch et al., 1997) is stratified to allow comparison of immunization performance of two insurance options with the total population. This type of stratification works well at the community level.

A similar situation at the national level is shown in Table 16–9. In this table, four HEDIS (Health Plan Employer Data and Information Set) measures from the American Public Human Services Association Medicaid HEDIS Database Project are shown with national means calculated as benchmarks for Medicaid and commercial MCO patients (Partridge, 2001; Partridge & Szlyk, 2000). These benchmarks can be used by state Medicaid programs to assess their performance, as well as for the comparisons shown between the Medicaid and commercial MCO populations.

**Table 16–7** Percentage of 19 to 35 Month Olds Who Have Received Full Schedule of Age-Appropriate Immunizations

| State | Measure | 2000 | 2001 | 2002 | 2003 |
|---|---|---|---|---|---|
| Illinois | Indicator | 75.4 | 75.6 | 78.0 | |
| | Objective | 76.0 | 79.0 | 78.0 | 79.0 |
| Indiana | Indicator | 75.3 | 80.8 | 78.4 | |
| | Objective | 80.0 | 81.0 | 82.0 | 83.0 |
| Michigan | Indicator | 73.7 | 70.0 | | |
| | Objective | 90.0 | 90.0 | 92.0 | 85.0 |
| Minnesota | Indicator | 82.4 | 76.3 | | |
| | Objective | 90.0 | 90.0 | 90.0 | 90.0 |
| Ohio | Indicator | 71.8 | 71.7 | | |
| | Objective | 85.0 | 85.0 | 75.0 | 75.0 |
| Wisconsin | Indicator | 77.6 | 78.4 | 77.4 | |
| | Objective | 90.0 | 78.0 | 78.5 | 78.8 |

Source: Maternal and Child Health Bureau, (n.d.). *Title V Information System.*

Figure 16–4 is another example of using stratification factors, this time in combination with another relevant population and with a specified target for comparison. The figure shows up-to-date Pap tests (a process or risk measure) by race (a stratification factor) among women who use community health centers (CHCs) compared with the National Health Interview Survey population and a *Healthy People 2000* objective[11] (Figure 16–4).

**Table 16–8** Up-to-Date Immunization Rate for Children at 24 Months of Age

| Performance Measure | Percentage |
|---|---|
| Up-to-date immunization rate at 24 months of age for all children in the community | 65 |
| Up-to-date immunization rate at 24 months of age for children currently enrolled in MCOs | 75 |
| Up-to-date immunization rate at 24 months of age for children currently enrolled in Medicaid | 50 |

---

[11] *Healthy People 2000* objective 16.12.

**Table 16–9** Commercial and Medicaid MCO Means, HEDIS Benchmark Measures, 1999

| Measure | Description | Medicaid MCO Mean | Commercial MCO Mean |
|---|---|---|---|
| Childhood immunization | Percentage of children who reached the age of 2 years within the year who received 13 recommended immunizations | 52.2% | 62.8% |
| Adolescent well care visits | Percentage of members ages 12 through 21 years as of December 31 who had at least one comprehensive well-care visit | 29.3% | 28.9% |
| Prenatal care in the first trimester | Percentage of women ages 21 through 64 years who gave birth during the measurement year and who had a prenatal care visit in the first trimester | 59.2% | 84.5% |
| Check-ups after delivery | Percentage of women who had a postpartum visit 3 to 8 weeks after delivery | 47.9% | 72.3% |

Source: Partridge (2001), Table 2.

Finally, Table 16–10 demonstrates a comparison across substate regions and with targets set at the beginning of a time period. Similar to a program monitoring table, it shows a comparison of actual results for each region with preset targets for two measures of capacity to carry out prenatal screening for domestic violence.

These examples demonstrate not only how to analyze performance measures, but also the added information produced when multiple comparisons are made simultaneously. Even more information about the performance of a given program can be generated when a comprehensive view, with capacity, process, risk outcome, and health outcome measures for a program, is examined. Analysis may be further enhanced by selective use of statistical methods. Statistical procedures can be used to estimate the influence of stratification factors on performance measures, to adjust for the effects of those factors, and to estimate the probability that

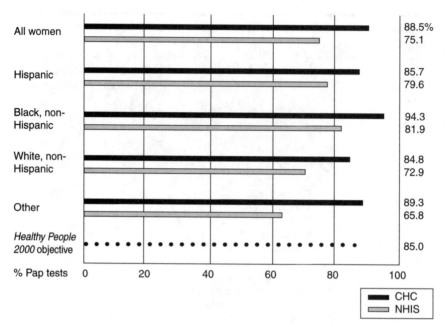

Source: Shekar (2003).

**FIGURE 16–4**  Up-to-date Pap tests by race: Women at community health centers (CHC), NHIS comparison group, and *Healthy People 2000* objective for up-to-date Pap tests.

differences in performance measures across stratified groups occurred by chance. Information about which procedures to use for each purpose can be found in methodological textbooks (e.g., Friis & Sellars, 1999). If you are unfamiliar with statistical procedures, it is wise to consult with a statistician in your health department or local university.

## Interpretation and Use

Analysis of performance measures produces a wealth of information that can be used in several ways. The most common uses are as follows:

- Informing stake holders of the program's progress
- Assessing program effectiveness
- Triggering investigations of problem areas
- Improving program performance
- Justifying budget requests (Hatry, 1999; Perrin et al., 1999)

**Table 16–10** Infrastructure for a Prenatal Domestic Violence Intervention by Region

| Performance Measure | Region | Target | Result |
|---|---|---|---|
| Percentage of prenatal clinics with | 1 | 80% | 35% |
| standardized protocols for screening | 2 | 80% | 84% |
| for domestic violence | 3 | 80% | 72% |
| | 4 | 80% | 50% |
| Percentage of prenatal clinics with | 1 | 75% | 27% |
| memoranda of understanding with | 2 | 75% | 78% |
| local agencies involved in prevention and | 3 | 75% | 64% |
| treatment of domestic violence | 4 | 75% | 56% |

The examples of different analysis strategies discussed previously also provide opportunities to explore options for interpretation and use.

### Informing Stake Holders of the Program's Progress

The CHC graph in Figure 16–4 makes a powerful statement, used by the Health Resources and Services Administration (Shekar, 2003), to call attention to the success of the CHC program model. The data show that women served by CHCs met or exceeded the *Healthy People 2000* objective for up-to-date Pap tests and also exceeded the general population in the National Health Interview Survey in each racial/ethnic group. Having *up-to-date Pap tests* is an important and meaningful measure for CHCs for three reasons:

1. If cervical cancer is caught early, it can be treated, but clients of CHCs who struggle under the effects of poverty usually do not seek health care until they feel sick. For cervical cancer to be controlled, this timeframe would be too late. CHCs have succeeded in overcoming a tendency to avoid preventive care in this population.
2. The primary audience for these data includes federal officials. The choice of two other federal undertakings, National Health Interview Survey and a *Healthy People 2000* objective, for comparison guarantees that the analysis will get the attention of the intended audience.
3. Results such as this provide very positive feedback to individual CHC staff at the local level, as well as demonstrating strong progress to stake holders. In addition, they suggest that the CHC model includes an example of "best practice" that might be exported to other programs.

### Assessing Program Effectiveness

Performance appraisal, like program monitoring, is not a research tool. Thus, it cannot generate evidence that a program caused a specific effect. However, it does offer information about what occurs within a program and progress on risk and health outcomes. The data on overweight children and adolescents shown in Figure 16–2 provide an assessment of the effectiveness of efforts in the 1990s to curb this problem. The 1988–1994 NHANES data were the only source available to assess performance near the end of the decade, and they were not encouraging. When the data for the 1999–2000 NHANES were released, it was clear that the initiatives of the 1990s were failing and that additional work needed to be done. Overweight and obesity subsequently became a high priority for public health agencies, leading to development and funding of a variety of interventions, such as the nutrition and physical activities programs of the Centers for Disease Control and Prevention.[12] As these new programs are implemented, a reversal of the trend in this performance measure will serve as the gold standard for effectiveness of the entire effort.

### Triggering Investigations of Problem Areas

Table 16–10 holds the type of information that should trigger an investigation of a problem. The table shows that Region 2 exceeded its targets for creating an infrastructure for domestic violence screening but that the other regions fell short, with Region 1 far below its goal. These findings raise questions about whether insufficient resources, staffing problems, issues outside the program (e.g., political turmoil locally), or other problems in prenatal service delivery might have contributed to the results. As these issues are investigated and conclusions are reached, modifications to the program should be made. Explanations for shortcomings like these and plans to correct them are part of the reporting package to external stake holders.

Table 16–9 also suggests further investigation. The national averages for three of the four HEDIS measures in the table are smaller for Medicaid than for commercial MCOs. This is not surprising as the demographics of the two groups are very different. However, the averages for adolescent well care visits are consistently low for both the Medicaid and

---

[12]Centers for Disease Control and Prevention. (2004c). *Nutrition and physical activity programs.* Available March 27, 2004, from: http://www.cdc.gov/nccdphp/dnpa

commercial groups, thus suggesting that access and/or use of preventive services for this age group are a problem (Partridge, 2001). This is a problem that invites further investigation.

## Improving Program Performance

Improving program performance usually occurs after further investigation of the causes of unexpected results in performance appraisal. Tables 16–7 and 16–8 provide examples of how this would occur. Both tables summarize immunization data. In Table 16–7, a reasonable expectation is that immunization rates would improve from year to year. This has not happened in some of the states, thus prompting them to reduce their targets. In addition, although some states were fairly close to their targets, Michigan, Minnesota, and Ohio were having difficulty meeting them in 2000 and 2001. These results indicate which states should work toward improving their values, but they do not provide any clues about what should be done. Each state involved has to examine immunization rates by relevant stratification factors, such as geographic area or population characteristics, to refine knowledge about the problem further. These results will lead to further questions until the reasons for the state-level shortcomings are understood. At that time, specific actions to improve performance in the future can be identified.

Table 16–8 presents a different scenario, but one that requires a similar approach. Here, the variation in rates suggests that children enrolled in Medicaid are not served as well as those in MCOs. With this information in hand, Medicaid officials and their partners who provide outreach to clients would first want to determine whether these results are due to a reporting problem, such as incomplete ascertainment or a miscalculation. If there is no reporting error, they would want to examine trends over time to see whether this represents a sudden change or is part of a steady decline. Surveys or focus groups with clients and providers may be launched to find explanations. Officials of the public health system may also talk with MCO managers about their techniques for assuring immunizations. The resulting information could contribute to modification of current practices.

## Justifying Budget Requests

Figure 16–3 offers an example of using performance appraisal results to justify budget requests. These Pregnancy Risk Assessment Monitoring

System data highlight differences across states but also show overall improvement in folic acid awareness until 1997, when a plateau, and even some reductions in awareness, occurred. At least two of the states, New York and West Virginia, used these data to show that higher levels of awareness could be reached in order to justify external funding to enhance their folic acid educational and outreach efforts (D'Angelo & Gilbert, 2002).

### Other Uses of Results of Performance Appraisal

The results of analysis of performance measures are often used to guide resource allocations. A frequently cited explanation for falling short on performance expectations is that inadequate resources were allocated in the first place. In these cases, reallocation of the budget can focus resources where they are needed most. A variation on this theme, performance-based budgeting, has emerged in recent years. In a performance-based budgeting system, programs that demonstrate strong performance are rewarded, whereas those with weaker performance can lose funding. Although it can be very effective to reward programs for doing well, there is an inherent danger in this approach. The weaker programs may not have the resources to improve. In such cases, removing funds can only make the problem worse. Providing technical assistance and other forms of instrumental support to weak programs has the potential to be more helpful in the long run to the populations affected.

## Strengths and Limitations of Performance Appraisal

Performance appraisal is an exciting and versatile evaluation tool that is changing standards of accountability for large, multicomponent MCH programs. However, that is only its first major contribution to the field. Because of its ability to support comparisons across programs, specific interventions, and insurance plans, it helps program managers understand the levels of results that are achievable and can also point to new ways of improving performance. Without external comparisons, this information is not available (Morley et al., 2001). The comparative capability of performance appraisal also allows for development of "report cards" and other educational tools that have transformed consumer education. In addition, performance appraisal offers insight into problem areas that are not responding to current interventions. This information, in turn, can lead to further investigation and evaluation research projects to unveil the reasons for poor performance and/or to development of new approaches to these difficult problems. Performance appraisal also provides the hard data to justify funding of the new efforts.

Like all good things, this compelling technique has limitations. The first major limitation is that it is not research and, therefore, cannot generate evidence that a program or intervention caused an outcome. This limitation cannot be overcome and is managed by using performance appraisal to answer appropriate questions, while deferring the cause and effect issues to evaluation research. The other major limitation is data related. Because performance appraisal is a data-driven activity that often requires large amounts of data collected across geographic and jurisdictional boundaries, it must continually accommodate to shortcomings in availability and comparability of data items and databases. Obtaining and managing large databases can be an expensive enterprise and one that requires a level of skill not yet uniformly available throughout the country. These problems can be overcome, and as they are mastered, performance appraisal is likely to emerge as an even more powerful evaluation tool.

## CONCLUSION

Program monitoring and performance appraisal play critical roles in the program planning and evaluation framework within which MCH programs flourish. Monitoring has been a linchpin of MCH program planning and management for many years. It is the essential evaluation component that must accompany any program plan, from a small inhouse proposal to an application for external funding of a statewide initiative, and it produces the information required to keep programs on track so they can reach the targets of their objectives.

Most MCH programs are also called on to contribute to performance appraisal in some way. They may be required to produce specific measures or to contribute raw data to a larger database from which measures are later constructed. The rapid development of performance appraisal in the past decade attests to the magnitude of need that went unmet in the past. This evaluation tool fills a void in assessment of large, multicomponent programs, whether they are geographically dispersed or community based. It produces a level of accountability for MCH program expenditures that has not previously been available on a widespread basis and holds tremendous potential for informed stewardship of MCH programs in the future.

# REFERENCES

Agency for Health Care Policy and Research. (1997). *A compendium of selected public health data sources.* Washington, DC: Author.

Agency for Healthcare Research and Quality. (2002). *Child health toolbox: Measuring performance in child health programs.* Available March 15, 2004, from: http://www.ahrq.gov/chtoolbx

Agency for Healthcare Research and Quality. (2005). *National quality measures clearinghouse.* Available January 17, 2005, from: http//www.qualitymeasures.ahrq.gov

Ahluwalia, I.B., & Daniel, K.L. (2001). Are women with recent live births aware of the benefits of folic acid? *MMWR, 50*(RR06), 3–14.

Association of State and Territorial Health Officials. (2004). *Public health data sources and assessment tools, Resources to measure access and health disparities, ASTHO resource compendium.* Available March 24, 2004, from: http://www.astho.org/templates/display_pub.php?pub_id=1093

Centers for Disease Control. (2004a). *National public health performance standards program.* Available February 23, 2004, from: http://www.phppo.cdc.gov/nphpsp.

Centers for Disease Control and Prevention. (2004b). *CDC's reproductive health information source, surveillance and research, Pregnancy Risk Assessment Monitoring System (PRAMS).* Available July 7, 2004, from: http://www.cdc.gov/reproductivehealth/srv_prams.htm.

Centers for Disease Control and Prevention. (2004c). *Nutrition and physical activity programs.* Available March 27, 2004, from: http://www.cdc.gov/nccdphp/dnpa.

Chen, H.T. (1990). *Theory-driven evaluation.* Newbury Park, CA: Sage Publications.

D'Angelo, D., & Gilbert, B.C. (Eds.). (2002). *From data to action: Using surveillance to promote public health: Examples from the Pregnancy Risk Assessment Monitoring System (PRAMS): Executive summary.* Atlanta, GA: Division of Reproductive Health, National Center for Chronic Disease Prevention and Health Promotion, Centers for Disease Control and Prevention.

Dever, G.E.A. (1991). *Community health analysis: Global awareness at the local level* (2nd ed.). Gaithersburg, MD: Aspen Publishers.

Durch, J.S., Bailey, L.A., & Stoto, M.A. (Eds.). (1997). *Improving health in the community: A role for performance monitoring.* Washington, DC: National Academy Press.

Friis, R.H., & Sellers, T.A. (1999). *Epidemiology for public health practice* (2nd ed.). Gaithersburg, MD: Aspen Publications.

Government Performance and Results Act of 1993. (1993). PL 103-62. Washington, DC: US Government Printing Office.

Grason, H.A., & Guyer, B. (1995). *Public MCH program functions framework: Essential public health services to promote maternal and child health in America.* Baltimore, MD: The Child and Adolescent Health Policy Center, The Johns Hopkins University.

Grembowski, D. (2001). *The practice of health program evaluation.* Thousand Oaks, CA: Sage Publications.

Guild, P.A. (1990). Goal-oriented evaluation as a program management tool. *American Journal of Health Promotion, 4,* 296–301.

Handler, A., Issel, M., & Turnock, B. (2001). A conceptual framework to measure performance of the public health system. *American Journal of Public Health, 91,* 1235–1239.

Hatry, H.P. (1999). *Performance measurement: Getting results.* Washington, DC: The Urban Institute Press.

Kettner, P.M., Moroney, R.M., & Martin, L.L. (1999). *Designing and managing programs: An effectiveness-based approach* (2nd ed.). Thousand Oaks, CA: Sage Publications.

Maternal and Child Health Bureau. (n.d.). *TVIS Home.* Available January 19, 2005, from: https://performance.hrsa.gov/mchb/mchreports/tvisreports.asp.

Maternal and Child Health Bureau. (n.d.). *Title V information system.* Available January 19, 2005, from: https://performance.hrsa.gov/mchb/mchreports/Search/search.asp.

McGlynn, E.A. (2003). Selecting common measures of quality and system performance. *Medical Care, 41*(Suppl.), I-39–I-47.

Miller, D.C. (1991). *Handbook of research design and social measurement* (5th ed.). Thousand Oaks, CA: Sage Publications.

Monahan, C.A., & Sykora, J. (1999). *Developing and analyzing performance measures: A guide for assessing quality of care for children with special health care needs.* Chicago: University of Illinois at Chicago, School of Public Health. Available March 3, 2004, from: http://www.uic.edu/sph/cade/qcmc/qcmc3/frontmatter.pdf.

Morley, E., Bryant, S.P., & Hatry, H.P. (2001). *Comparative performance measurement.* Washington, DC: The Urban Institute Press.

National Committee for Quality Assurance. (n.d.). *NCQA: Measuring the Quality of America's Healthcare.* Available January 19, 2005, from: http://www.ncqa.org.

National Committee for Quality Assurance. (n.d.). *HEDIS: Health plan employer data and information set.* Available March 9, 2004, from: http://www.ncqa.org/Programs/HEDIS/.

National Institute on Disability and Rehabilitation Research. (n.d.). *Research and statistics in NIDRR.* Available March 20, 2004, from: http://www.ed.gov/rschstat.

Osborne, D. & Gaebler, T. (1992). *Reinventing Government.* New York: Addison-Wesley.

Partridge L. (2001). *The APHSA Medicaid HEDIS database project: Report for the third year (data for 1999).* Available July 10, 2004, from: http://www.cmwf. org/programs/quality/partridge_aphsa_hedis_1999.pdf.

Partridge, L., & Szlyk, C.I. (2000). *National Medicaid HEDIS database/benchmark project: Pilot year experience and benchmark results.* Available July 10, 2004, from: http://www.cmwf.org/programs/quality/partridge_hedis_366.asp.

Peoples-Sheps, M.D., Byars, E., Rogers, M.M., Finerty, E.J., & Farel, A. (2001). *Setting objectives* (revised). Chapel Hill, NC: The University of North Carolina at Chapel Hill. Available July 10, 2004, from: http://www.shepscenter. unc.edu/trainingMaterials.html.

Peoples-Sheps, M.D., Rogers, M.M., & Finerty, E.J. (2002). *Evaluation: Monitoring progress towards achievement of objectives* (revised). Chapel Hill, NC: School of Public Health, The University of North Carolina at Chapel Hill. Available July 10, 2004, from: http://www.shepscenter.unc.edu/ trainingMaterials.html.

Performance Measurement Coordinating Council. (1999). *Desirable attributes of performance measures.* Available March 15, 2004, from: http://www.ahrq. gov/chtoolbx.

Perrin, E.B., & Koshel, J.J. (Eds.). (1997). *Assessment of performance measures for public health, substance abuse, and mental health.* Washington, DC: National Academy Press.

Perrin, E.B., Durch, J.S., & Skillman, S.M. (Eds.). (1999). *Health performance measurement in the public sector: Principles and policies for implementing an information network.* Washington, DC: National Academy Press.

Shekar, S. (2003). *Remarks to the National Association of Community Health Centers.* Washington, DC. Available February 8, 2004, from: http://newsroom. hrsa.gov/speeches/2003speeches/shekar-march2003.htm.

Stroup, N.E., Zack, M.M., & Wharton M. (1994). Sources of routinely collected data for surveillance. Chapter 3. In S.M. Teutsch & S.M. Churchill (Eds.), *Principles and Practice of Public Health Surveillance.* New York: Oxford University Press.

Telfair, J. (2001). *8 Steps for project/program planning and monitoring/assessment leading to evaluation for state and community service agencies/programs.* Unpublished manual.

US Department of Health and Human Services. (1990). *Healthy People 2000: National health promotion and disease prevention objectives* (full report with commentary). DHHS Publication No. (PHS) 91-50212. Washington, DC: US Government Printing Office.

US Department of Health and Human Services. (2000). *Healthy People 2010* (conference edition in two volumes). Washington, DC: January 2000.

US Department of Health and Human Services. (2002). *Health, United States 2002* (Table 71: Overweight children and adolescents 6–19 years of age, according to sex, age, race, and Hispanic origin: United States, selected years 1963–65 through 1999–2000). Available January 10, 2004, from: http://www.cdc.gov/nchs/data/hus/hus02pdf.

US Department of Health and Human Services. (2003). *HHS Directory of health and human services data resources.* Available March 17, 2004, from: http://www.aspe.hhs.gov/datacncl/datadir.

Wholey, J.S. (1997). Trends in performance measurement: Challenges for evaluators. In E. Chelimsky and W.R. Shadish (Eds.), *Evaluation for the 21st century: A handbook* (pp. 124–133). Thousand Oaks, CA: Sage Publications.

Wholey, J.S., & Hatry, H.P. (1992). The case for performance monitoring. *Public Administration Review, 52,* 604–610.

Wilcox, L.S. & Marks, J.S. (Eds.). (1994). *From data to action: Public health surveillance for women, infants and children.* Atlanta: US Department of Health and Human Services, Public Health Service, Centers for Disease Control and Prevention.

# 17

# The Practice of Evaluation Research in Maternal and Child Health

*Joseph Telfair*

> *Just because you can quantify something, doesn't mean you understand it.*
> (Aubel, 1993, p. 10)

## INTRODUCTION

Much of what drives the field of maternal and child health (MCH) are concerns about the effective delivery and assessment of services that are a part of programs for women, infants, children, adolescents, and families. Because of this service-based orientation, the process, utility, and implications of assessment become vital. In the field of MCH, evaluation plays a key role in determining the validity and reliability of programs and services. For the purpose of this chapter, evaluation research has a twofold definition: (1) the use of scientific methods and techniques for the purpose of marshaling and presenting objective evidence of the worth of a particular program or activity (Baker & Northman, 1981) and (2) the systematic application of this

**625**

$$Y_{\text{Evaluation Practice}} = \alpha + \beta_1 X1 \text{ social} + \beta_2 X2 \text{ political} + \beta_3 X3 \text{ technical} + e$$

**FIGURE 17-1** Regression equation of evaluation in practice.

evidence to inform the decision-making process of the development, implementation, or continuation of a program or service activity (Carter, 1994; Patton, 1997; Rossi, Lipsey, & Freeman, 2004; Wholey, 1994).

This definition implies that evaluation research, like other applied research, is primarily concerned with two substantive activities: (1) the assessment of the effectiveness of MCH program interventions and (2) the outcome data from these assessments and the use of these data to influence program and policy development and change. Rossi and Freeman (1993) suggested that in practice there should be a focus on "evaluation research as a robust area of activity devoted to collecting, analyzing, and interpreting information on the need for, implementation of, and effectiveness and efficiency of intervention efforts to better the lot of humankind" (p. 3). In MCH practice, the emphasis is on activities and approaches that will provide information needed to make judgments about a program. These determinations are not made without consideration of the social, political, and cultural contexts in which programs are developed and implemented, as well the nature and scope of collaborations with other agencies and programs and the level of participation of stake holders (Brunner & Guzman, 1989; Peoples-Sheps, 1997; Roberts & Evans, 1997; Rosin, Whitehead, Tuchman, Jesien, & Begun, 1993; Telfair & Mulvihill, 2000). As such, the practice of evaluation research in MCH is a product that is partly social, partly political, and *only* partly technical (Chelimsky, 1997; Herman, Morris, & Fitz-Gibbon, 1987) (Figure 17-1).

# CONTEXT FOR THE PRACTICE OF MCH EVALUATION RESEARCH

It is critical that evaluators recognize and act on the reality that many MCH programs engage in evaluation activities because they are asked to so by funders or other stake holders. For a number of reasons, program administrators often fulfill this request by engaging an outside "expert" or hiring a temporary staff person to design and implement these assessment activities, generally within a single year. Thus, evaluation-like service delivery is conceptualized as necessary to meet a need or address a problem and is completed when the need is met.

In addition, this reality has existed because of the funders' or stake holders' general expectations and/or satisfaction with the evaluation process and results (e.g., expecting reports of only process or indicator data and less often something more rigorous such as outcome assessments) and the temporary working relationship of staff with the "expert" or assessment staff member.

As a result, viewing evaluation as a part of the service delivery process, maintaining on staff a person or persons with at least elementary evaluation skills, focusing on the use of evaluation results beyond the funding period, and viewing evaluators as collaborators on the service delivery team are rare. Thus, for those engaged in setting policies and planning programs to be implemented at the community level and for program administrators being faced with new demands for more rigorous accountability (e.g., the United Way's focus on outcomes), this reality is very frustrating.

What is needed is to challenge the existing reality by engaging in evaluation at the program level that allows for the needs of all involved (clients, staff members, administrators, planners, and policy makers) to be met without feeling they are at risk of giving something up (e.g., staff members taking time away for providing services) or of losing something (e.g., planners not having the opportunity to get information that would help in long-term decision making).

Given the challenging contexts for evaluation, this chapter provides an overview of the practice and art of evaluation research as applied to the field of MCH and will cover three main areas: (1) content focus, purpose, types, and procedures; (2) establishment of parameters; and (3) key problems and issues. Special attention is paid to an applied as opposed to a theoretical or a "how to" approach to evaluation. Readers wishing to understand more about evaluation theory are referred to an excellent text by Shadish, Cook, and Leviton (1991). Those wishing more of the "how-to's" of evaluation are referred to two excellent texts by Fitz-Gibbon and Morris (1987) and Isaac and Michael (1997).

# CONTENT FOCUS, PURPOSE, TYPES, AND PROCEDURES

## Content Focus

From the outset, it is important to understand the fundamental difference between evaluation research (both terms will be used) and basic (social)

research. These differences are outlined in Table 17–1 developed by
Miller (1991). Table 17–1 illustrates that basic research, often defined as
*pure research*, is primarily concerned with seeking new knowledge and
explanation of observed phenomena, whereas interventions to address a

**Table 17–1**  Research Design Orientations

| Defining Characteristic | Basic (Pure)* | Applied (Policy–Action–Useful)† | Evaluation (Assessment–Appraisal)‡ |
|---|---|---|---|
| Nature of the problem | Basic scientific investigation seeks new knowledge about social phenomena, hoping to establish general principles with which to explain them. | Applied scientific investigation seeks to understand a demanding social problem and to provide policy makers well-grounded guides to remedial action. | Evaluative research seeks to assess outcomes of the treatment applied to a social problem or the outcome of prevailing practices. |
| Goal of the research | To produce new knowledge, including discovery of relationships and the capacity to predict outcomes under various conditions. | To secure the requisite knowledge that can be immediately useful to a policy maker who seeks to eliminate or alleviate a social problem. | To provide an accurate social accounting resulting from a treatment program applied to a social problem. |
| Guiding theory | Selection of theory to guide hypothesis testing and provide reinforcement for a theory under examination. | Selection of a theory, guidelines, or intuitive hunches to explore the dynamics of a social system. | Selection of a theory to fit the problem under assessment. Watch for ways to hook findings to a new theory or an established one. |
| Appropriate techniques | Theory formulation, hypothesis testing, sampling, data collection techniques (direct observation, interview, questionnaire, scale measurement), statistical treatment of data, validation, or rejection of hypotheses. | Seek access to individual actions and inquire what actors are feeling and thinking at the time. Elicit the attributions and evaluation made about self, other, or situational factors. Regard crucial explanations as hypotheses to be tested. | Use all conventional techniques appropriate to the problem. |

*Dubin (1969) and Kaplan (1964).
†Argyris, Putnam, and Smith (1985); Coleman (1972); Freeman, Dynes, Rossi, and Whyte (1983); and Lawler and Associates (1985).
‡Juster and Land (1982); Lauffer (1994); and Luck (1955).

problem and a focus on outcomes are not (necessarily) of interest (Barnard, 2000; Miller, 1991; Rossi & Freeman, 1993). Evaluation, as a form of applied research, is concerned with providing information that is both useful and that can be applied to social problems faced by and/or being addressed by MCH agencies and programs. It has as its primary interest the results of the rigorous and systematic assessment of a program or agency's service-based intervention ability to produce change for the persons receiving the intervention. Attention is on the "outcome(s)" of the intervention (Schalock, 2001). As such, the focus of evaluation practice is the systematic use of social research methods and program outcomes "to judge and to improve the planning, monitoring, effectiveness, and efficacy of health, education, welfare and other human service programs" (Rossi et al., 2004, p. 21).

## Purpose of Evaluation

One purpose of evaluation is to answer some very basic, but often difficult, questions about the services provided by the agency or program in addressing both a target problem and the potential for producing change. Some of the difficult questions that arise involve the kind of change desired, the means by which the change is to be brought about, operationalizing the definition of the desired change, identifying indicators appropriate for the identification and measurement of the change, and the feasibility of the service to produce the desired change (Fitz-Gibbon & Morris, 1987; Isaac & Michael, 1997; Telfair, 1999). Several basic questions to be addressed are as follows (Herman et al., 1987; Patton, 1997):

1. Should the program be continued or discontinued?
2. What needs to be done to improve the practices and procedures of a program, and how can it be done?
3. What specific programmatic strategies or techniques need to be added or dropped?
4. Can the program be replicated elsewhere?
5. Are program resources being allocated/used appropriately within the program (are resources adequate)?
6. What is the nature and scope of the problem requiring action?
7. What program activities or interventions may be undertaken to improve the problem significantly?

8. What is the appropriate target population for the program or intervention?
9. Is the program or intervention effective?
10. What are program or intervention costs relative to their effectiveness and benefits?

A second purpose of evaluation research for MCH is to address the social and political accountability issues inherent in applied work. Many programs are instituted with the hope that they will effectively ameliorate a specific problem (e.g., teenage pregnancy) or address a long-standing issue. Nonetheless, the basis for assessing the short- and long-term outcomes of these programs is not always clearly defined or agreed on by those involved, the stake holders. This dilemma requires that the evaluation endeavor be comprehensive and flexible enough to anticipate and address a number of key accountability issues that define MCH programs (Telfair & Mulvihill, 2000). These would include the following:

1. To assure that the service-based intervention is adequate for addressing the problem that it was designed to target
2. To ensure that target program, with its cluster of services, is achieving maximum effectiveness
3. To assure that the program's or agency's mechanism for accountability is functioning as it should (such as meeting the requirements of its funders)
4. To influence policy and other decision makers
5. To enhance the standing of the target agency/program
6. To provide evidence that allows for stake holders to understand and appreciate the extent and effectiveness of the services provided to clients

Evaluation research has a range of primary stake holders that are invested in the products of its endeavors and are integral to the successful use of these products (Patton, 1997). These primary stake holders and descriptions of each include the following (Brunner & Guzman, 1989; Rossi et al., 2004, pp. 48–49):

1. *Policy makers and decision makers:* persons responsible for deciding whether a programs is to be instituted, continued, discontinued, expanded, or curtailed
2. *Program sponsors:* organizations that initiate and fund the program to be evaluated

3. *Evaluation sponsors:* organizations that initiate and fund the evaluation (sometimes identical with the program sponsors)
4. *Target participants:* persons, households, or other units who participate in the program or receive the intervention services under evaluation
5. *Program management:* the group responsible for overseeing and coordinating the intervention program
6. *Program staff:* personnel responsible for actual delivery of the intervention (e.g., teachers)
7. *Evaluators:* group or individuals responsible for the design and/or conduct of the evaluation
8. *Program competitors:* organizations or groups that compete with the program for available resources
9. *Contextual stake holders:* organizations, groups, individuals, and other units in the immediate environment of a program with interests in what the program is doing or what happens to it (e.g., other agencies or programs, public officials or citizens' groups in the jurisdiction in which the program operates)
10. *Evaluation and research community:* evaluation professionals who read evaluations and pass judgment on their technical quality and credibility and researchers who work in areas related to a program

Depending on the demands and level of program involvement of the stake holders, the level of accountability may lead to a greater emphasis on the social and political elements of the evaluation process. Technical rigor remains a crucial part of the work of evaluators, particularly in determining and implementing the type of evaluation approach most suitable for addressing key program problems and issues. Therefore, it is crucial that the evaluator determine beforehand what are the minimal allowable methodologic or technical adjustments that can be made to accommodate the programmatic and stake holder demands. This minimum is dependent on the type of evaluation to be engaged in.

## Types and Procedures of Evaluation

Weiss (1991) stated, "Evaluations are used in many ways; one must do different things to facilitate different uses" (p. 179). To accommodate these "differences," evaluation designs often use a broad band of methodologic methods and procedures (the evaluator's "toolbox"), most notably triangulation method (integration of quantitative and qualitative methods) as discussed by Miller (1991), Morse (1991), Patton (1990), and Datta (1997). Determination of the type of evaluation approach to be used in the assessment of MCH agencies and programs must be based on a joint review and understanding of the goals and objectives of the program/ agencies by the participants, staff, administrators, and the evaluator. Once this understanding is achieved, one or a combination of the following types of evaluation designs can be used:

1. *Needs and assets assessment,* as part of the pre-evaluation assessment (Leviton, Collins, Laird, & Kratt, 1998; Wholey, 1987), involves the identification process of describing problems of a target population, the assessment of the importance and relevance of the problems, and the determination of the agency or program's capacity to engage, not to engage, or to delay engagement in the evaluation (Kretzman & McKnight, 1993). A needs and assets assessment answers these questions: What do we need to do? What do we need to obtain? What do we have in place?

2. *Monitoring* does not necessarily involve a formalized evaluation schedule or set of procedures but allows for the assessment of whether or not an intervention or program is operating in conformity to its design reaching its specified target population. Based on the results of the needs and assets assessment, monitoring may be the only type of assessment some agency or programs are able to engage in at the time when an evaluation is being considered. An advantage of monitoring is that it allows for the understanding of the gap between actual and expected levels of achievement and when corrective action (such as increased transportation support to assist women in getting to care or the early identification of depressive symptoms leading to appropriate treatment for the child) may be warranted (Peoples-Sheps, 1997; Wholey & Hatry, 1992; Wholey & Newcomer, 1997).[1]

3. *Formative evaluation* refers to evaluation activities related to the provision of information that allows program/intervention planners and implementers to make decisions regarding the improvement or refinement of a developing or ongoing program. This type of evaluation is ongoing and allows for the design and implementation of

---

[1]Monitoring is covered in greater detail in Chapter 16.

mechanisms to test for the maximum effectiveness of a program. A process evaluation answers this question: Which aspect or component of the service-based intervention works better?

4. *Process evaluation,* as a type of formative evaluation, refers to evaluation activities related to target identification and assessment of the appropriateness of services, programs, or interventions. Process evaluation allows for the verification of what program aspects are/were delivered to the target population and if in the intended dose. The advantage of this method for the agency or program is that it allows for an assessment of the variations in program delivery and provides information of what components contribute to the achieved short- and long-term outcome differences between recipients and nonrecipients. It is the latter focus on clearly identified short- and long-term outcomes based on key, targeted questions about recipients and nonrecipients that distinguish process evaluation from monitoring (Scheirer, 1994). Process evaluations answer these questions: What services are actually being delivered and to whom? Is there a discernible change in the clients participating in the program? Is this change as planned?

5. *Summative evaluation* refers to evaluation activities related to the provision of information that allows program/intervention planners and implementers to assess the overall quality and impact of a program for the purposes of accountability and policy. Summative evaluation answers these questions: Did the program make a difference? What immediate changes did clients experience?

6. *Outcome evaluation,* a form of summative evaluation, determines the current and desired person- and program-referenced outcomes and their uses, the extent to which a program met its intended goals and objectives, and whether a program made a difference compared with either no program or an alternative program (impact) (Schalock, 2001). Outcome evaluation also answers this question: Did the program make a difference? However, here the evaluator's interest is in the program's *ultimate* impact, that is what longer term changes occurred.

7. *Cost-effectiveness or cost benefit evaluation* compares the outcomes of decision options in terms of their monetary cost per unit of effectiveness. It is generally used to set priorities for the allocation of resources and to decide among one or more interventions. Cost

benefit/cost-effectiveness is most useful when it compares alternative interventions or approaches for the same type of program. Cost benefit/cost-effectiveness compares program costs with expected benefits or compares the cost differences of alternative programs or intervention strategies (Greenberg & Appenzeller, 1998; Petitti, 1994). Cost-effectiveness answers this simple question: At what price does program or intervention success or failure occur?

Besides obtaining clarity on the types of evaluation design needed to address MCH problems and issues, evaluators must have clarity in the basic terminology and definitions used in developing evaluation designs. Based on the program evaluation literature, the following are the basic definitions and terminology and examples of their application to MCH issues:

1. *Goal* is a broad statement of a desired health or social status outcome. The statement does not necessarily need to be in measurable terms. Goals are the ultimate purpose of the program. For example, "to reduce the teen pregnancy rate among adolescents (14–17 years old) in the North Charleston School District #4 through school and community prevention efforts" (Petitti, 1994) is a goal.

2. *Objectives* are mileposts that evaluators set out to pass on the way to achieving a goal. They must be written, clearly stated, measurable, unique to the program(s) or intervention(s) of focus, and specific to the time frame for their accomplishment. Objectives are of three primary types:
   - *Program level*: A specific, measurable statement of desired change in knowledge, behavior, biomedical measures, or other intermediate characteristics that are expected to occur because of the intervention. For example, "The proportion of unenrolled CSHCN in Roland County who are eligible for special insurance services will decrease by 10% by June 30, 1999."
   - *Process level*: A specific, measurable statement of activity (tasks) to be carried out by the program. For example, "50% of all CSHCN deemed eligible for special insurance services in Roland County will be enrolled in the regional center program."
   - *Outcome level*: A specific, measurable statement of desired change that is deemed the ultimate result or impact of the service or intervention. For example, "Eligible children in undeserved Roland County receiving special insurance services by 1999 will report 10% fewer problems in getting access to needed services."

3. *Intervention* is any planned effort designed to produce intended changes in a target population, for example, a school-based pregnancy prevention program.

4. *Tasks or program elements* are identifiable and discrete intervention activities carried out by designated program personnel (or others) for the purpose of achieving the program objective(s). Tasks or program elements are what the program will do to achieve the objective(s). It is important to remember that each task must be linked to a specific objective.

5. *Indicator* is a measure of the expected program outcome that corresponds to the cognitive, health, or social condition of the population targeted by the program for intervention. Indicators are what the evaluator is going to measure. An indicator is a measurement that reflects the status of a system and/or *something* that points to a problem or a condition. Indicators provide a means for talking about how current conditions do not match the desired state for any given system, context, or resource. For example, knowledge of HIV/AIDS, rates of violent behavior, and rates of unwanted/unintended pregnancies are indicators.

   The most important point about indicators is that they need to be as relevant as possible to the community they serve or to the program under observation, that they need to be used to spur constructive change, and that they are true measures of the condition or population. Characteristics of a good indicator (and the data they comprise) are

   - Relevant
   - Credible
   - Valid
   - Reliable over time
   - Comparable
   - Accessible and affordable
   - Understandable[2]

6. *Key indicator:* one of a number of primary indicators that when compiled gives an overall picture of the progress made toward achievement of the objective.

---

[2]In Chapter 16, performance measures of risk and health outcomes are noted as indicators as defined here.

7. *Supporting indicator:* a potentially more detailed or finely focused indicator, several of which may add up in a congregate fashion to support a key indicator.

8. *Index:* a collection or set of indicators that, when considered as a whole, provides an image of the overall health, well-being, and quality of life in the community. For example, an index of basic health services would include measures of the percentage of primary care providers for adolescents, the percentage of providers accepting Medicaid, the percentage of services for special needs populations, or the quality rating of local health services by consumers. *Categories* of indicators are a helpful ways to organize the index. One of the best examples of how to organize an index is from the Title V MCH Core Services (Direct Health Care Services indicators, Enabling Services indicators, Population-Based Services indicators, and Infrastructure Building Services indicators).

9. A *target* is a numerical *quantity* or amount (count) that indicates the minimum desirable level of achievement for a particular activity or indicator (outcome). A numeric target usually has two parts: (1) quantity or amount and (2) date of anticipated achievement. A target is also an agreed on (consensus) set of qualitative statements or observations that indicate the minimum desirable level of a particular activity or indicator to be reached. A *qualitative* target is usually part of mixed-method evaluation and has two parts: (1) an agreed on timeframe for the statements to be collected or observations to be made and (2) date of anticipated merging (mixing) with the numeric targets. As part of the operational level objective, a target is usually linked with a date of anticipated achievement, for example, a 10% increase in enrollment by the 12th month of the program's implementation.

10. *Target populations* are the persons, households, organizations, communities, or other units at which programs or interventions are directed. Evaluators must define target populations carefully. Target populations must be defined narrowly (if possible) and homogeneously. When considering the targets, the evaluator must ask this: Who is the program really designed to reach?

11. *Target problems* are conditions, deficiencies, or defects at which programs or interventions are designed or directed, for example,

"determining which children should be covered under an insurance program."

12. *A program impact model* is the formal statement about the expected relationships between a program or intervention and its designated goals and objectives. It is the strategy that outlines and operationalizes the process of evaluating the link between goals and objective set forth during the planning process and what is actually happening. Other terms for the Program Impact Model are the Logic Model and Program Hypothesis (Peoples-Sheps, Byars, Rogers, Finerty, & Farel, 2001; Perrin & Koshel, 1997).

13. *Measures* are tools and formulas for calculating the extent to which objectives are achieved. They are the means or "formula" to assess progress and outcomes. For qualitative objectives, for example, they are the extent to which consensus is reached on which components of the objective have been achieved.

14. *Qualitative measurement:* Expected changes are more often expressed in words rather than numbers. Qualitative data are usually collected by document review, observation, and interviews. However, qualitative data can also be expressed in numbers. For example, interview responses can be tallied to report the number of participants who respond in a particular way (i.e., consensus statements, observations) such as achieved composition of stake holder advisory groups, achieved agreement between groups or agencies on how to conduct project activities, achieved agreement on consistent participation of key players in focus or related decision-making groups.

15. *Quantitative measurement:* Information that is measured and expressed with numbers or percentages, as ranges or averages, and in tables and graphs. It can also be used to compare different groups or participants—girls and boys, clients from different socioeconomic or ethnic backgrounds, or clients in your program who are nonparticipants (counts, values, percentages, rates) according to such indicators as health status, health-related knowledge, skills, behavior, and satisfaction with care. For quantitative long-term monitoring or process evaluation, one might assess not only the number of people who participate but how their composition (age, race, or economic class) compares with the composition of a particular community.

16. *Outcome:* The result, effect, or impact (expected or unexpected, intended, or unintended) that can be reasonably attributed to the activities or actions of a program. This can be an intermittent (short-term/ongoing) or an ultimate (long-term or end-of-program) outcome. Of particular concern and interest to community and state-level programs are outcomes that follow directly from the initiation of program activities.

Once the participants, program staff, and evaluator have determined the type of evaluation to be used and have obtained a mutual understanding of the evaluation terminology and definitions, the last content and procedure issue to address is to decide what to actually measure and observe that will provide comprehensive data to catalogue the effectiveness of the program intervention. Herman et al. (1987) and Blalock (1990) noted five components of a program that could be assessed to provide broad-based data for evaluation. These program components are as follows:

1. *Context characteristics* require attention to the setting or context (framework) within which a program must operate. They include the complex network of sociopolitical factors that influence almost all programs (e.g., power, leadership, communication) as well as program specific factors, such as class size, time frame within which the program must operate, budget, and specific incentives. It is especially important to get accurate information about aspects of the context that you suspect might affect how a program operates and its success.

2. *Participant characteristics* require attention to such things as age, sex, socioeconomic status, language dominance, ability, attendance, attitudes, and background/experience. It is sometimes important if a program shows different effects with different groups of clients.

3. *Characteristics of program implementation* require attention to the program's principal activities, services, processes, materials, staffing, and administrative arrangements. In summative evaluations, these will usually be the processes and characteristics that distinguish the program from other similar ones. In formative evaluations, these will usually be those aspects of the program that are most problematic.

4. *Program outcomes:* In most evaluations, it is important to measure or observe the extent to which the program goals have been achieved.

This requires that the evaluator must be alert to unanticipated outcomes (*positive and negative*) and consider both long- and short-range outcomes that focus the evaluation on agreed upon goals and objectives.

5. *Program costs* address the question of what are the required resources and relative cost-effectiveness of competing alternatives. In considering program costs, Herman et al. (1987) stated that it is important to gather situation-specific data about obvious costs (staff time, materials, equipment, facilities) and indirect, opportunity, and other hidden costs.

## Establishing the Parameters of the Evaluation

Once the content focus, purpose, and types and procedures of an evaluation have been determined and agreed on, establishing the parameters (context and "boundaries") of the evaluation presents the next challenge (Herman et al., 1987; Isaac & Michael, 1997; Rossi & Freeman, 1993). Establishing parameters of the evaluation requires all involved in the evaluation process to outline the methodologic elements of the evaluation process and allows for all to have an agreed-on course of action that increases the probability of the success of the program/intervention and the usefulness of the outcome data. As such, the process of establishing the parameters includes establishing contextual and specification parameters (guidelines) as well as selecting of appropriate methods, design issues, and guidelines for data collecting and analysis.

### Establishing the Contextual Parameters

Constituting parameters for the evaluation of MCH programs or interventions involves (1) determining the program goals and objectives, (2) carefully defining the target population, (3) defining the program-specific tasks, that is, the principal activities or services to be provided to meet the objectives and the expected progress based on the implementation of these activities or services, (4) determining the resources available, including financial, personnel, agency, and other supports, as well as materials to be used, (5) determining the frequency and duration of the intervention to be provided, (6) determining the person(s) responsible for implementation of the overall program and/or specific intervention, and (7) developing the evaluation plan.

**Establishing Specifications**

In addition to setting up the context of the evaluation process, certain specifications must be adhered to in establishing the "boundaries" of the evaluation (Herman et al., 1987; Telfair & Mulvihill, 2000). These specifications are

1. The evaluation design should be reflective of a process that took into account both the need for enough rigor to demonstrate the effectiveness of the service or program and the unique requirements of the sociocultural context in which the service or program is to be implemented (e.g., which data questions to ask and of whom to ask them, training time for translators or indigenous persons to assist with the evaluation).
2. The evaluation should be tied to the overall goals of the program and specific interventions.
3. The evaluation should be broad based and take into consideration the range of desired outcomes, whether they are the stake holders' or the evaluator's or whether they are short or long term.
4. Goal attainment at all levels should be documented through the measurement of specific program and operational level objectives.
5. The evaluation should examine the process by which outcomes are achieved (particularly in relationship to the measurement of key indicators).
6. The data from the evaluation should be used in an ongoing fashion to improve services and programs. It is essential that the *data are understood and are useable.*
7. The data from the evaluation should be made available to stake holders and others in a manner that is simple and straightforward, such as charts, graphs, story boards, or simple tables.

As with the contextual parameters, these specifications will increase the probability that the social, political, and cultural components of the evaluation are addressed.

**Selecting the Appropriate Evaluation Methods**

Once the context and boundaries of the evaluation have been secured, the evaluator must determine the appropriate method and design (logistical) considerations that will guide the evaluation process. The primary method for these considerations include the following:

1. Tasks should be fleshed out into a clearly specified, program-sensitive set of data collection procedures and, where relevant, measurement instruments.
2. Attention must be paid to the specific aspects of program context, processes, and outcomes on which the assessment will focus.
3. Attention must be paid to the best feasible methods to measure or otherwise observe those program tasks (i.e., specific measurement instruments that you will purchase or develop and/or sources of information for other data collection methods).
4. Attention must be paid to the design and sampling plan for administering or enacting chosen assessment methods.
5. Attention must be paid to the logistical plan that will allow for the completion of evaluation tasks within a specified schedule.
6. Attention should be focused on collecting information of greatest interest and utility to primary users (targeted populations and stake holders) about the most significant aspects of the program or intervention and its outcomes in a way that ensures the quality, validity, and reliability of the information collected.

### Determining Design Issues

One of the methodological challenges in evaluation research is addressing the need for a control or comparison group. Having a control/comparison allows for some level of causality between the influencing and outcome variables to be determined (Rossi et al., 2004). However, often the context and circumstances in which evaluation takes place do not readily lend themselves to random selection, as would be required for true experimental designs and control groups. Despite its limitation, the use of quasi-experimental designs and comparison groups is more often the method of choice (Shadish et al., 1991).

In evaluation research, the use of a matched comparison group with at least three measurement points (e.g., before, after, and follow-up) is considered one of the strongest quasi-experimental deign models. By selecting and collecting the same information from a comparison sample that shares most of the characteristics of the persons or programs being evaluated allows for more control of threats to internal and external validity of the evaluation design. However, such a selection is not always such a straightforward process. Social and political factors are often at work in the delivery of MCH services. These factors influence decisions about who does and does not receive the program or its services, as well as what information can or cannot be collected and from whom. In such cases, evaluators are often challenged with the reality that program staff, often for very good reasons, are not comfortable with withholding services from one group for a period of time even if the reason for this withholding is critical to determining whether the services are as effective as they think.

The solution is to propose and negotiate alternative strategies that allow for comparison group selection and use as well as assurances that those in need of services will get them. One example of such a strategy is the delayed crossover design. This is a formative evaluation strategy that requires that those selected will be placed in either the group to initially receive the intervention or the group that will crossover and receive the intervention at a latter time after at least two periods of data collection (before and after) have passed. In this case, the early group will crossover and be followed to determine the long-term effect of the intervention, and after at least two data collection periods, the latter group will also be followed. The critical lesson here is that the evaluator in partnership with the program staff develop creative and scientifically sound strategies that allow for the attribution of program or service effectiveness.

Other less robust models are a part of the menu of choices for quasi-experimentation and address the issue of denial of service. Space does not allow for a full recitation here. The reader is referred to two volumes: the classic Cook and Campbell (1979) *Quasi-experimental Design and Analysis Issues for Field Settings,* and Miller (1991) Section B: Evaluation Research, in the *Handbook of Research Design and Social Measurement* (5th ed.).

Droitcour (1997), Cook (1991), Marcantonio and Cook (1994), and Rossi et al. (2004) advised that independent of the research design chosen by the evaluator (experimental or quasi-experimental) the validity and reliability of the design must be of primary concern. Concerns with insuring validity must address two questions:

1. To what extent is the program or intervention effects really due to the program or intervention rather than competing explanations (in basic research, this is an issue of causality)?
2. To what extent can results be generalized to other situations?

In addition, threats to the internal and external validity of the design must be addressed, particularly if a quasi-experimental design is chosen (Barnard, 2000; Miller, 1991). Concerns with insuring the reliability of the evaluation design must address this question: To what extent have the assessment of the measure(s) being used, the target of the intervention, costs, logistics, time, and previous appraisals of reliability been made? Further discussion of design reliability issues can be found in Chapter 14.

## Data Collecting and Analysis Parameters

Finally, given the applied nature of evaluation research and the emphasis on identifying and obtaining outcome data that are useful and relevant to stake holders connected to the program, delineating data collection and analysis guidelines is crucial. The following guidelines are suggested:

1. Focus data collection where it is most likely to uncover program effects (if any). Which objectives are most likely to show change?
2. Try to collect a variety of information, particularly if multiple methods are being used to achieve a similar objective (e.g., using both group and one-to-one counseling to increase the self-esteem of female teenagers).
3. Try to think of imaginative (and credible) ways to detect achievement of program objectives. What best illustrates the success of the innovative methods that we have developed to achieve our objectives?
4. Collect information to show that the program at least has done no harm to the target population.
5. Measure or observe what is essential, as well as what is thought to be in the interest of the sponsor and other stake holders.
6. Try to measure or observe things that will advance the development of target services or other outcomes linked to the target program(s).
7. Focus data collection where it is most likely to uncover program effects, if any.
8. Try to collect a variety of information (triangulation); that is, try to find useful qualitative (process) and quantitative (counts) information that is going to be collected anyway. This provides the advantage of presenting a thorough look at the program or intervention.
9. Try to be flexible by balancing the need for measures to be collected over time and adjustment with the natural changes in the program setting (understandably a difficult task) without hurting the integrity of the measure.

10. Try conducting data collection that is not susceptible to cultural differences, historical events, or other barriers that prevent accurate calculation of indicators or calibration of measures.

Involving the program staff and other relevant stake holders as collaborative partners in the process of implementing these guidelines will assist the evaluator in assuring their successful completion.

## Key Evaluation Problems and Issues

As discussed earlier in this chapter, evaluation research takes place in a dynamic social and political environment. As such, a myriad of logistical problems and issues must be recognized and addressed if the outcomes of the evaluation are to be useful, practical, and relevant. These problems and issues fall into two categories: (1) data and measurement specific and (2) program and stake holder specific problems and issues.

### Data and Measurement Specific Problems and Issues

Because evaluation often does not take place in a controlled environment, is very reliant on the participants and/or program staff for its implementation, and often uses more than one data collection method, ensuring scientific rigor becomes a real challenge. To ensure rigor, the evaluator must both anticipate and address (as part of the evaluation process) the following problems and issues: (1) establishing the parameters for a comparison group, (2) establishing a measurement design agreement between program staff and/or stake holders and evaluator, (3) establishing parameters of adequacy of program or intervention effects, (4) establishing accountability roles and tasks of persons involved in the data collection process, and (5) identifying data collection issues and strategies such as availability, use, and advantages/disadvantages of collected data (archival records, agency's administrative records, unobtrusive [qualitative] measures); original (routine, ongoing) data collection; use and advantages/disadvantages of interview questionnaires; use and advantages/disadvantages of self-administered questionnaires; use and advantages/disadvantages of telephone interviews; and establishing the parameters for data analysis and use.

### Program- and Stake Holder-specific Problems and Issues

Because of the emphasis on social and political accountability that surrounds the information produced by the evaluation endeavor, a number of logistical and reporting problems and issues arise. As Rossi and Freeman

(1993), Patton (1997), Bicknell and Telfair (1999), and Schalock (2001) pointed out, evaluators usually find themselves confronted with individuals, groups, and/or agencies that have competing views on the use and appropriateness of the evaluation process and its results. In order to conduct their work with a reasonable degree of rigor and effectiveness, evaluators must understand their relationship with stake holders and programs, as well as stake holder and program relationships with one another (Rossi & Freeman, 1993, p. 110). The following are stake holder- and program-specific problems and issues the evaluator must address at the outset (e.g., during the pre-evaluation phase) or as a part of the evaluation process:

1. Agreeing to a set of indicators that allows for the separation of program generalities from those describing program performance or effect
2. Agreeing to a set of specific outcomes that, if achieved, will allow for determining that programmatic objectives are being achieved
3. Agreeing to and delineating which important dimensions of program objectives need to be identified, including the following:
   - The nature or content of the objective (those areas the intervention is intended to change)
   - The level of specificity of the stated objectives
   - The number of objectives (most programs have more than one)
   - The expected short-term versus long-term effect(s)
   - The expected magnitude of an interventive effect(s) (how large an effect is expected?)
   - The stability of an interventive effect(s) (how long is/are the effect[s] intended to last?)
   - The level of interrelatedness of objectives (the objectives may be highly related and similar to each other or unrelated and dissimilar)
   - The hierarchy (importance) of each objective
   - The unexpected (unintended and unanticipated) consequences of the intervention

## CONCLUSION

The use of evaluation information is dependent on the social, cultural, and political contexts in which the endeavor takes place. As with all forms of applied research, evaluators must be vigilant in appraising the environment of those involved with the work (stake holders). Participation in the evaluation process by those being evaluated is a key tenet of MCH practice. Furthermore, the use of evaluation results for decision making and program development must be of primary concern if changes in these programs are to reflect the needs of its participants (e.g., women, children, youth, and families) and if the changes are to have the desired effect.

# REFERENCES

Argyris, C., Putnam, R., & Smith, D.M. (1985). *Action science.* San Francisco, CA: Jossey-Bass.

Aubel, J. (1993). *Participatory program evaluation: A manual for involving program stakeholders in the evaluation process.* The Gambia: Catholic Relief Services-USCC.

Baker, F., & Northman, J.E. (Eds.). (1981). *Helping: Human services for the '80s.* St. Louis: The C.V. Mosby Company.

Barnard, H.R. (2000). *Social research methods: Qualitative and quantitative approaches.* Thousand Oaks, CA: Sage Publications.

Bicknell, R.C., & Telfair, J. (1999). The process of selling a community evaluation to a community: The Cumberland County experience. *New Directions in Evaluation, 83,* 87–94.

Blalock, A.B. (1990). *Evaluating social programs at the state and local level.* Kalamazoo, MI: W.E. Upjohn Institute.

Brunner, I., & Guzman, A. (1989). Participatory evaluation: A tool to assess and empower people. In R.F. Connor & M.H. Hendricks (Eds.), *New directions for program evaluation: International innovations in evaluation methodology* (no. 42, pp. 9–17). San Francisco: Jossey-Bass Publishers.

Carter, R. (1994). Maximizing the use of evaluation results. In J.S. Wholey, H.P. Hatry, & K.E. Newcomer (Eds.), *Handbook of practical program evaluation* (pp. 576–589). San Francisco: Jossey-Bass Publishers.

Chelimsky, E. (1997). The political environment of evaluation and what it means for the development of the field. In E. Chelimsky & W.R. Shadish (Eds.), *Evaluation for the 21st Century* (pp. 53–68). Thousand Oaks, CA: Sage Publications.

Coleman, J.S. (1972). *Policy research in the social sciences.* Morristown, NJ: General Learning Press.

Cook, T.D., & Campbell, D.T. (1979). *Quasi-experimental design and analysis issues for field settings.* Skokie, IL: Rand McNally.

Cook, T.D. (1991). Clarifying the Warrant for Generalized Causal Inferences in Quasi-Experimentation. In M.W. McLaughlin & D. Phillips (Eds.), *Evaluation and Education: At Quarter Century,* 1991 Yearbook, National Society for the Study of Education. Chicago, IL: National Society for the Study of Education.

Datta, L. (1997). Multimethod evaluations: Using case studies together with other methods. In E. Chelimsky & W.R. Shadish (Eds.), *Evaluation for the 21st century* (pp. 344–359). Thousand Oaks, CA: Sage Publications.

Droitcour, J.A. (1997). Cross-Design Synthesis: Concept and Application. In E. Chelimsky & W.R. Shadish (Eds.), *Evaluation for the 21st Century* (pp. 360–372). Thousand Oaks, CA: Sage Publications.

Dubin, R. (1969). *Theory building.* New York: Free Press.

Fitz-Gibbon, C.T., & Morris, L.L. (1987). *How to design a program evaluation.* Newbury Park, CA: Sage Publications.

Freeman, H.E., Dynes, R.R., Rossi, P.H., & Whyte, W.F. (Eds.) (1983). *Applied sociology: Roles and activities of sociologists in diverse settings.* San Francisco: Jossey-Bass.

Greenberg, D.H., & Appenzeller, U. (1998). *Cost analysis step-by-step: A how-to-guide for planners of welfare-to-work and other employment and training programs.* San Francisco: MDRC.

Herman, J.L., Morris, L.L., & Fitz-Gibbon, C.T. (1987). *Evaluator's handbook.* Newbury Park, CA: Sage Publications.

Isaac, S., & Michael, W.B. (1997). *Handbook in research and evaluation* (3rd ed.). San Diego: EdITS.

Juster, F.T., & Land, K.C. (Eds.) (1982). *Social accounting systems: Essays on the state of the art.* New York: Academic Press.

Kaplan, A. (1964). *The conduct of inquiry.* San Francisco, CA: Chandler.

Kretzman, J.P., & McKnight, J.L. (1993). *Building communities from the inside out.* Chicago: ACTA Publications.

Lauffer, A. (1994). *Assessment tools* (Vol. 30). Beverly Hills, CA: Sage.

Lawler, E.E., III, & Associates (1985). *Doing research that is useful for theory and practice.* San Francisco, CA: Jossey-Bass.

Leviton, L.C., Collins, C.B., Laird, B.L., & Kratt, P.P. (1998). Teaching evaluation using evaluability assessment. *Evaluation, 4,* 389–409.

Luck, T.J. (1955). *Personnel audit and appraisal.* New York: McGraw-Hill.

Marcantonio, R.J., & Cook, T.D. (1994). Convincing quasi-experiments: The interrupted time series and regression-continuity designs. In J. Wholey, H. Hatry, & K. Newcomer (Eds.), *Handbook of Practical Program Evaluation.* (pp. 133–154). San Francisco, CA: Jossey-Bass Publishers.

Miller, D.C. (1991). *Handbook of research design and social measurement* (5th ed.). Newbury Park, CA: Sage Publications.

Morse, J.M. (1991). Approaches to qualitative-quantitative methodological triangulation. *Nursing Research, 40,* 120–122.

Patton, M.Q. (1990). *Qualitative evaluation and research methods* (2nd ed.). Newbury Park, CA: Sage Publications.

Patton, M.Q. (1997). *Utilization-focused evaluation* (3rd ed.). Thousand Oaks, CA: Sage Publications.

Peoples-Sheps, M.D. (1997). Planning and monitoring maternal and child health programs. In J.B. Kotch (Ed.), *Maternal and child health: Programs, problems and policy in public health* (pp. 423–460), Gaithersburg, MD: Aspen Publishers.

Peoples-Sheps, M.D., Byars, E., Rogers, M.M., Finerty, E.J., & Farel, A. (2001). *Setting objectives* (revised). Chapel Hill, NC: The University of North Carolina at Chapel Hill.

Perrin, E.B., & Koshel, J.J. (Eds.). (1997). *Assessment of performance measures for public health, substance abuse, and mental health*. Washington, DC: National Academy Press.

Petitti, D.B. (1994). *Meta-analysis, decision-analysis and cost-effectiveness analysis: Methods for quantitative synthesis in medicine*. New York: Oxford University Press.

Roberts, R.N., & Evans, J.E. (1997). Cultural competence. In H.M. Wallace, J.C. MacQueen, R.F. Biehl, & J.A. Blackman (Eds.), *Mosby's resource guide to children with disabilities and chronic illness: Cultural competency* (pp. 117–124). St. Louis: Mosby.

Rossi, P.H., & Freeman, H.E. (1993). *Evaluation: A systematic approach* (5th ed.). Newbury Park, CA: Sage Publications.

Rossi, P.H., Lipsey, M.W., & Freeman, H.E. (2004). *Evaluation: A systematic approach* (7th ed.). Thousand Oaks, CA: Sage Publications.

Rosin, P., Whitehead, A., Tuchman, L., Jesien, G., & Begun, A. (1993). Module I: Family centered care: Building partnerships between parents and service providers. In P. Rosin & L. Irwin (Eds.), *Partnerships in early intervention: A training guide on family centered care, team building, and service coordination*. Madison, WI: Wisconsin Family-Centered In-service Project of the Waisman Center Early Intervention Program.

Shadish, W.R., Cook, T.D, & Leviton, L.C. (1991). *Foundations of Program Evaluation: Theories of Practice*. Newbury Park, CA: Sage Publications.

Schalock, R.L. (2001). *Outcome-based evaluation* (2nd ed.). New York: Kluwer Academic/Plenum Publishers.

Scheirer, M. (1994). Designing and Using Process Evaluation. In J. Wholey, H. Hatry & K. Newcomer (Eds.), *Handbook of Practical Program Evaluation*. (pp. 40–68). San Francisco, CA: Jossey-Bass Publishers.

Telfair, J. (1999). Improving the prospects for a successful relationship between community and evaluator. *New Directions for Evaluation, 83,* 55–66.

Telfair, J., & Mulvihill, B.A. (2000). Bridging science and practice: The integrated model of community-based evaluation. *Journal of Community Practice, 7,* 37–65.

Weiss, C.H. (1991). Linking evaluation to policy research. In W. R. Shadish, T.D. Cook, & L.. Leviton (Eds.), *Foundations of program evaluation: Theories of practice* (pp. 179–224). Thousand Oaks, CA: Sage Publications.

Wholey, J.S. (1987). Evaluability assessment: Developing program theory. *New Directions for Program Evaluation, 33,* 77–92.

Wholey, J.S. (1994). Assessing the feasibility and likely usefulness of evaluation. In J.S. Wholey, H.P. Hatry, & K.E. Newcomer (Eds.), *Handbook of practical program evaluation* (pp. 15–39). San Francisco, CA: Jossey-Bass Publishers.

Wholey, J.S., & Hatry, H.P. (1992). The case for performance monitoring. *Public Administration Review, 5,* 604–610.

Wholey, J.S., & Newcomer, K.E. (1997). Clarifying goals and reporting results. *New Directions for Evaluation, 75,* 91–98.

# CHAPTER 18

# Advocacy and Policy Development in Maternal and Child Health

*Donna J. Petersen and Catherine A. Hess*

*Never doubt that a small group of thoughtful, committed citizens can change the world. Indeed it is the only thing that ever has.*
(Margaret Mead, 2005)[1]

## INTRODUCTION

In this chapter, we address an important skill area for maternal and child health (MCH) professionals, the skill of advocacy. Margolis, Cole, and Kotch (2005) in Chapter 1 provide an excellent framework for a discussion of advocacy, nesting it in the broader context of social justice and children's rights. Here we expand on this discussion by focusing on actions that can be taken as part of the policy development process for the purposes of promoting and protecting the health and well-being of children and families. Given the mission of Title V of the Social Security Act (US Congress, 1935), the legislative basis for MCH programs in the United States, to assure the health of all mothers and children, it is

---

[1]Courtesy of the Institute for Intercultural Studies, Inc., New York.

entirely appropriate that MCH professionals and constituents engage in advocacy. As a public health program, MCH engages in the core functions of public health—assessment, policy development, and assurance (Institute of Medicine, 1988). Advocacy draws on the scientific knowledge base generated through assessment activities to promote and influence policy development. Advocacy can also be a tool for assuring that policies are implemented effectively to achieve desired results. Advocacy is a fundamental element of nearly every essential public health service, including mobilizing partnerships to identify and solve MCH problems and providing leadership for priority setting, planning, and policy development (Grason & Guyer, 1999).

Although assessment and assurance functions are explicitly included within the statutory responsibility of Title V MCH programs (Health Resources and Services Administration, n.d.), this legislation is less direct in speaking to the policy development role. The legislation's emphases on assessing the need for and assuring access to care support contemporary priorities of key stake holders: federal and state legislators interested in accountability and constituents interested in social justice in the form of universal health insurance and equal access to quality health care. Still, the history of MCH in this country has its roots in active advocacy for program and policy development aimed at improving child health and welfare more broadly (Alexander et al., 2002; Hutchins, n.d.; Rosenbaum, 1983). Attention to advocacy and policy development remains important in current and future efforts to achieve the goals of MCH. In this chapter we define and discuss the nature of advocacy and policy development and why advocacy is an important MCH activity. We describe the nature of advocates and the various types of people and organizations that engage in advocacy. We then discuss the targets of advocacy efforts and how advocacy can be more successful while sharing some advocacy examples. Finally, we conclude with a brief overview of the policy development process and an encouraging word for those who might be willing to join with others in advocating for optimal MCH.

## WHAT IS ADVOCACY?

We define advocacy as urging action to effect change toward a desired end for a defined population. Advocacy in MCH is typically conducted in a policy development context and seeks to secure the authority, the resources, and the direction to support efforts on behalf of the health of the population of interest to MCH: women, children and youth (including those with special health care needs), and families. We advocate for the creation of new programs or policies that are needed for the benefit of the MCH population. We advocate for the elimination of policies and programs that are no longer needed or are potentially harmful, and we advocate for the amendment of existing policies and programs toward improving their reach, quality, or outcome. Assuming the necessary legislative, or policy, basis exists for our desired programs, we can advocate for effective implementation, for necessary resources, or for appropriate interpretation and enforcement. We can advocate for changes in program direction, for improved collaboration and cooperation, or to inform relevant audiences about important MCH issues and MCH work. Common synonyms for "advocate" (verb) include recommend, support, urge, lecture, or preach. For "advocate" (noun) we find such synonyms as counselor, proponent, or counselor-at-law. These words help us to understand the nature of advocacy and the role of advocates seeking change.

# WHY IS ADVOCACY IMPORTANT IN MCH?

The history of MCH is a chronicle of successful advocacy efforts on behalf of the nation's mothers and children. From the establishment of the early legislative basis for MCH (US Congress, 1912, 1935) to modern-day efforts to craft universal health insurance for children, MCH leaders have embraced advocacy as a fundamental responsibility and have viewed it as necessary to achieve MCH goals. Grace Abbott, Director of the Children's Bureau from 1921–1934, summed it beautifully in this quote, now familiar to most in the MCH professions:

> Sometimes when I get home at night in Washington, I feel as though I had been in a great traffic jam; the jam is moving toward the Hill where Congress sits in judgment on all the administrative agencies of the government. In that traffic jam there are all kinds of vehicles moving up toward the Capitol. . . . There are all the conveyances that the Army can put in the street. . . . There are the hayricks and the binders and the ploughs and all the other things the Department of Agriculture manages to put into the streets. . . . I stand on the sidewalk watching it become more and more congested and more difficult, and then, because the responsibility is mine and I must, I take a very firm hold on the handles of the baby carriage and I wheel it into the traffic. (Alexander et al., 2002, p. 1)

Because the MCH population is typically comprised of those who cannot speak for themselves, a voice is required, an advocate, someone speaking on behalf of children and their families to express their needs. Further justifications for advocacy in MCH include the vulnerability of the population, particularly during critical periods of growth and development, the dependence of children on families and institutions to assure their well-being, the disproportionate representation of the underserved, including minorities and the poor within the population of the nation's mothers and children, their persistent lack of representation in political arenas, and the known efficacy of preventive interventions directed at children in promoting healthy adulthood (Saunders, Hess, Nelson, & Petersen, 1995). In spite of these truths, or perhaps because of them, we now have in the United States myriad programs designed to address various aspects of child growth and development, pregnancy and childbearing, family stability, and community empowerment. The advocacy efforts that led to the establishment of a national public school system and what we know today as the MCH Services Block Grant, or the development of such programs as Aid to Families with Dependent Children (now Temporary Assistance for Needy Families), Head Start, Medicaid, and child protection programs all had their roots in society's desire to give every child and family an opportunity to achieve their greatest potential.

These are successes primarily of *legislative advocacy*, working through the legislative process to create the foundation, the authorization and the appropriation of funds for specific programs. Unfortunately, the resulting confusion over program eligibility, covered services, jurisdictional province, and fiscal responsibility has led to the development of a new kind of advocacy: *interagency or systems-level advocacy*. In this type of advocacy, MCH leaders work to forge partnerships across programs in order to lessen the administrative barriers so that resources and opportunities can be optimized. As an example of the distinction between the two, in the early 1990s in Minnesota, advocates were successful in securing legislative approval for the creation of a program within the state human services agency to provide mental health services to children. As the program was implemented, it quickly became apparent to advocates that unless the state departments of health and education contributed to the program by helping to identify, screen, and refer children, the program would never achieve its stated goal of improving child mental health status in the state. Having the program created in statute and funded with state appropriations is an example of legislative advocacy. Encouraging other state agencies to collaborate with the new program in order to promote its success is an example of systems-level or interagency advocacy.

The third type of advocacy in MCH is *judicial advocacy*, which is invoked when legislative and systems-level advocacy efforts are exhausted and the only remaining route of redress is through the courts. Judicial advocacy typically seeks to clarify the interpretation of a statute or a regulation, to force the implementation of a law, or to promote personal or group constitutional rights. This type of advocacy resulted, for example, in a 1998 Consent Decree for Medicaid-based Early Periodic Screening Diagnosis and Treatment Services on behalf of children in state custody who were being inadequately served in Tennessee.

We need also mention here that although we typically think of MCH advocacy as being directed *at* government policy makers and program directors, advocates for MCH can operate *from within* government MCH programs as well. As advocacy and policy development are part of the leadership functions of MCH professionals, it is not uncommon for government agency staff to advocate for MCH issues within their own agencies as well as with other public agencies whose work affects the health of MCH populations. Ideally, advocates outside public institutions work in concert with advocates inside these public agencies toward a collective agenda.

Advocacy is important in MCH because the policy development process is so complex, and policy makers must respond to competing and often conflicting demands. As stated in a public hearing on April 9, 2004, by Lee Hamilton, former Congressman from Indiana and Vice-Chair of the 9/11 Commission, "Policy makers face terrible dilemmas; information is incomplete, the in-box is huge, resources are limited, there are only so many hours in the day. The choices are tough, and none is tougher than deciding what is a priority and what is not." Advocates help to assure that the needs and desires of women, children, and families remain priority issues for policy makers.

## WHO ARE ADVOCATES?
## WHO CAN BE AN ADVOCATE?

Anyone can be an advocate, and everyone in the field of MCH should be an advocate. It is difficult, if not impossible, to achieve improvements in health without urging change in factors that affect health. Although the

Children Bureau's charge at the time of its establishment in 1912 was "to investigate and report on all matters pertaining to child life and welfare among all classes of people" (US Congress, 1912), it was the Bureau's activist interpretation of that charge that led to success in areas such as national birth registration, the national school lunch program, and child labor laws (Hutchins, n.d.; Rosenbaum, 1983). That interpretation, using data or evidence to stimulate action, has been a continuous thread woven through MCH success stories at local, state, and national levels over the past century.

Advocates come in all types, and organizations that engage in advocacy can take many forms. From the individual parent advocating in response to a personal tragedy (e.g., Megan's Law) and grass-roots coalitions assembled to address the needs of specific classes of individuals (e.g., children with special health care needs) to large, well-established national organizations with broad and varying agendas, such as the Children's Defense Fund, advocates share a desire to effect change. For some advocates, the role is a temporary one that can be abandoned once the pertinent situation is resolved. For others, such as the parent advocates who organize locally to maintain a focus on children with special health care needs and who collectively comprise the national organization Family Voices, the nature of the advocacy work usually results in a lifetime commitment. These types of advocates have a personal stake, a clear self-interest, in the results of their advocacy work, although clearly their successes result in benefits to large numbers of people.

Further along the advocacy continuum are the organizations that identify advocacy as an essential component of their mission. It is useful to consider the various types of organizations that typically advocate for MCH and to assess their relative strengths and weaknesses as advocates (Johnson, 1999). One type of organization that engages in advocacy is the trade association. These are membership organizations of individuals or agencies that are involved in the same line of work. Examples relevant to MCH are state and national associations of clinicians such as the American Academy of Pediatrics, the American College of Obstetricians and Gynecologists, the American Academy of Family Practitioners, or the American College of Nurse Midwives and associations of provider organizations such as the National Association of Children's Hospitals or state Primary Care Associations. Other key associations focus on public health broadly, including the American Public Health Association and related state associations; the Association of State and Territorial Health Officials; the National Association of County and City Health Officials; and the National Association of Local Boards of Health. Still others focus on MCH specifically, including CityMatCH, the Association of Teachers of Maternal and Child Health, and the Association of Maternal and Child Health Programs.

MCH professionals are eligible to join many of these trade associations and do so for purposes of professional development and affiliation or to benefit from opportunities to work with and learn from peers. All of these associations also play a key role in advocating for MCH directly and providing an important vehicle and support for individual advocacy. Most of these organizations provide fact sheets, policy news briefs and updates, and legislative contact information. They offer training and other tools for advocacy and organize opportunities for advocates to join others in collaborative efforts to influence state legislatures or Congress (see the references for a list of relevant websites).

These associations and others like them have played key and successful roles in advocacy at local, state, and national levels. Each brings with it the credibility of the expertise of its membership. These groups often serve as resources for policy makers seeking information and guidance on specific issues. On the other hand, these groups may be perceived as motivated by self-interest and therefore biased in the information they provide. We discuss ways to overcome these weaknesses in later sections of this chapter.

Another kind of organization that plays a key role in MCH advocacy is the voluntary organization. These organizations include groups such as The Arc and the March of Dimes. Strengths of these organizations are the extensive volunteer base that they enjoy and the passion that they bring to the issues that affect them directly. On the other hand, their focus within MCH tends to be narrowed to very specific issues. The National March of Dimes in 2004 is focused on preventing premature birth (www.modimes. org), whereas The Arc is urging support of the passage of a Lifespan Respite Care Act by the US Congress (http://thearc.org).

Some organizations are not membership/volunteer based but are established for the sole purpose of representing or speaking on behalf of certain groups or causes. The Children's Defense Fund at the national level is an example, and most states have child advocacy organizations represented nationally by Voices for America's Children. The strengths of these organizations include the depth of their knowledge about the subject matter of interest to them, their knowledge about the policy-making process, and their highly professional approach to their work. Like trade associations, however, these groups are believed to have strong political biases that may mute their overall effectiveness in the political arena.

Last, but not least, are public agencies. Although bound by official policies and procedures that often dictate who can advocate about what issues in public arenas, public agencies, their leaders, and staff carry an official mantle that carries its own weight in advocacy. For MCH professionals within public agencies, advocacy usually starts within with assembling the data, information, and arguments for the agency advancing certain policies and programs. When successful, such internal advocacy can result directly in new policies or programs, from those at the level of an administrative division to Gubernatorial or legislative initiatives. When agency resources or political constraints impede action to advance specific policies and programs, the information and arguments may be picked up by external partners who often have had a role in shaping them. For public agencies, having strong family and consumer involvement is essential not only for effective internal policy and program development but also for creating a knowledgeable constituency that will advocate for key programs and policy positions when needed.

The strategic question may not be who can be an advocate because anyone at any point in time can be an advocate whether operating alone, as part of a grass roots coalition, or as a member of a large organization. Rather, more important questions might be which type of advocate is more likely to be effective on a given issue with a particular target audience or what combination of advocates as private individuals, as official agency representatives, as members of associations, or as volunteers at local, state, and national levels are required to achieve advocacy success.

# WHERE ARE ADVOCACY EFFORTS DIRECTED?

As discussed earlier, MCH advocacy is aimed at achieving change to improve the health of women, children, and families. Where it is directed or targeted depends on who has the power to make the change or who can influence those with that power. Advocates for the prevention and reduc-

tion of tobacco use have succeeded in securing national legislation prohibiting tobacco advertising in broadcast media, restricting the sale of
tobacco products to underage youth, and requiring warning statements
on tobacco packaging and on print advertisements. Advocates were also
extremely important in the negotiations that led to the Master Settlement
Agreement of 1998. Still, these advocates know that it is unlikely that a
national prohibition on the sale or use of tobacco products will ever be
enacted by the US Congress, and as such, they have turned their attention
to the state level, where they have been effective in the establishment of
Clean Indoor Air Laws in most states, in the banning of vending
machines in others, and in the establishment of ever-increasing tobacco
taxes. In states where these efforts have been less successful, advocates
have turned their focus to the community level, recognizing the truth in
the old adage, "all politics is local." In Prattville, Alabama, the City
Council was persuaded to enact a local smoking ordinance based on the
work of a local youth group that conducted extensive public polling and
interviews with restaurant and bar owners in order to demonstrate strong
public sentiment for restrictions on smoking in public places. Spending
the time clarifying objectives, assessing the likelihood of success, and
securing the right blend of allies will determine the most appropriate target for advocacy work.

As another example, we can examine the persistent concern over uninsured children. According to our assessment of the problem, some of
these children are eligible for Medicaid but are not enrolled, some children are eligible for the State Children's Health Insurance Program
(SCHIP) but are not enrolled, and still others do not qualify for any federally funded program. This latter group includes certain immigrant children. If our advocacy goal is to increase the number of children with
insurance, should we advocate at the local level, the state level, or the federal level? Should we target our efforts at legislators, the courts, or the
agencies that operate at the systems level? Further analysis of the problem
and potential solutions should help to guide us, for in this instance and
many others, action may be appropriate and necessary at all levels in each
of these arenas. If our concern is primarily focused on immigrant children, our efforts are probably best directed at the federal level where the
prohibitions on their coverage originate. Although federal legislation sets
the parameters for these programs and provides the first dollars, states
must commit matching dollars in order to draw down federal funds and

make many of the decisions on eligibility, coverage, and enrollment systems. Advocating with state legislatures may be needed to assure that the state allocates the necessary resources and adopts state level legislation authorizing federal requirements or selected options. If children in our community or state are eligible for SCHIP or Medicaid but are not enrolled, our efforts may best be directed at the level at which enrollment and outreach for enrollment occur. Because states vary on their approach to matters such as these, determining what is needed and how to ask for it is part of the assessment and strategy development process that is critical to successful advocacy.

It is important to note that, regardless of the target of advocacy efforts, the involvement of professionals and constituents from the local level is critical to success at every level, be it local, state, or national. "Grass-roots support" may be an overused term, but the underlying meaning suggests strength in numbers and true constituent/public support for the advocacy agenda. Professional advocacy organizations and trade organizations have learned that the best way to get around the perceived bias that they bring to their advocacy is to involve a broad-based coalition specific to the issue being addressed. The power of the scientific and content expertise of the professionals within the organization, coupled with the power of local constituent support, is a potent force for change in advocacy efforts. Child safety experts in the State of Maryland were not successful in securing passage of a child safety seat law until they engaged the help and support of the obvious constituency group: parents of young children. Policy makers find it hard to ignore the demands of large blocks of voters who are passionate about an issue. Of course, this can work in the opposite direction as well. Despite the mounting scientific evidence in support of motorcycle helmet laws, until very recently, the Maryland legislature found more persuasive the message delivered every year by the hundreds of motorcycle enthusiasts who would circle the state capitol building and fill the hearing rooms than the testimony of the experts.

In terms of directing advocacy efforts in the early 21st century, targeting the state level will probably be most productive. A conservative political shift begun in the early 1980s and sustained for over 2 decades has brought with it an emphasis on devolution of responsibility from the federal level to the state level. Although advocates in the 1980s were quite successful directing their efforts at the US Congress to secure passage of successive pieces of federal legislation that have resulted in expanded

Medicaid eligibility and benefits for pregnant women and children that we still enjoy today, 1997 was the last year that any major legislation affecting Medicaid or creating other major coverage options was enacted at the federal level. Despite the history of legislative support for Medicaid expansions, Congress rejected expansion of the federal Medicaid program for children, instead creating the Children's Health Insurance Program. Within a limited amount of funding, this program gave considerable discretion to states. Congress later required that the word *state* be added to the program's name. The few major pieces of federal health legislation introduced subsequently to address MCH concerns failed to win enactment year after year. These included failed bills to allow children with special health care needs to "buy-in" to Medicaid and to entitle newly arriving legal immigrants to Medicaid coverage.

This conservative political shift has not only affected Congress but has resulted in stricter enforcement of rules governing "lobbying" on the part of governmental agencies or other organizations that receive government funds. The gagging or stifling of many professional associations coupled with a Congressional reticence to enact new or expanded legislation in the social welfare or health arenas has resulted in a shift of advocacy emphasis to the state level. This should not imply that national-level advocates have moved on to other activities. Just as local involvement is critical regardless of the level where advocacy is directed (local, state, or national), national-level advocates can be essential to success at the state or local level. In the early 1990s, MCH advocates toiling at the state level to assure that coverage and benefits provisions under various states' health reform laws would be adequate to meet the needs of MCH populations benefited enormously from the availability of national technical experts and from the expert policy briefs generated by national organizations. This critical "vertical dynamic," involving people working at local, state, and national levels, is important in advocacy efforts, wherever targeted.

# HOW IS ADVOCACY CONDUCTED? HOW CAN ADVOCACY BE MORE SUCCESSFUL?

Optimally, advocacy is an artful blend of education and action. Few problems in MCH have only one best solution. Information and education lay important groundwork for identifying policy options and advocacy strategies. There are often various ways to approach a particular problem, and given that public health interventions may involve infringements on liberty (e.g., seat belt laws and compulsory vaccinations) or challenge prevailing wisdom or tradition (e.g., dietary recommendations and methods of child discipline), information and education can be critical in garnering support for policies that will be effective. The odds of success of advocacy efforts can be enhanced by discussion with a broad constituency about the problem and about which approach is likely to work and be acceptable to the public and the elected or appointed officials who need to act. As such, the best advocacy is based on knowledge about a situation grounded in rigorous scientific data that leads to a shared understanding of the problem and an honest dialogue about the best approach for a particular community.

Common elements of successful advocacy include the following:

1. Sound assessment of the problem and possible solutions, sufficient to identify and justify the best clear alternative program or policy options that have strong odds of success in addressing the problem and improving outcomes.
2. The clear articulation of both the problem *and* the suggested program and policy strategies for resolving or addressing the problem.
3. The identification of key decision makers, those who can influence decision makers, other stake holders and constituents who have or should have interest in the problem, including both those who may agree and may disagree with the advocacy position.
4. The development of a strategy for achieving the goals of the advocacy efforts that may include the following:
   • Identifying an existing coalition or forming a new coalition to support the effort
   • Developing and executing a communication strategy to reach and educate key players in the desired action and to anticipate and address issues that may be raised in opposition; communication targets potentially include the decision makers, those who can influence them, other stake holders, the media, and the general public
   • Follow-up, follow-up and more follow-up including reminders, thank you notes, and communication about the results/successes of the advocacy effort

The intensity of any of these elements or whether they are included in an overall advocacy effort will depend on the nature of the advocacy (legislative, systems or judicial), the level at which it is being undertaken (federal, state, or local), and the scope of those involved in the advocacy (one individual, a few individuals, a small coalition, a large coalition). The extent to which each of these elements is used is also dependent on a realistic appraisal of the time frame and the political environment for action.

We have mentioned the term "coalition" several times in this chapter. It is true that no matter what your advocacy objective is, your chances of success will be enhanced if you partner with others. Forming coalitions, from informal alliances to formally organized groups, increases the odds for success in a number of ways. On a basic level, numbers matter. The more individuals and organizations that are working together to advocate, the more the effort may receive attention from certain target audiences, especially executive and legislative policy makers or the media that influence them. Partnering with others also increases the depth and breadth of expertise that is brought to bear on advocacy efforts. Furthermore, the inclusion of specific individuals or organizations can enhance the credibility of the effort. It can also have the opposite effect, depending on the issue and the target audience you are trying to reach. In one state, having the Catholic Archdiocese join in advocacy efforts to increase family planning funding paid big dividends. On the other hand, when the Ku Klux Klan offered their support for the males-only membership policy of the Augusta National Golf Club, the club's reception was less than enthusiastic. The larger and more diverse the coalition, the greater will be the effort necessary to organize the work, but the greater the ultimate success. Whether to form a coalition, who should be asked to join, and how it should operate are questions that should be considered in the context of the goal of the advocacy effort and a strategic analysis of the strengths, weaknesses, opportunities, and threats associated with this goal.

It may take decades to achieve some major policy changes, as it did with tobacco control efforts. Coalitions are important in sustaining energy and momentum in these instances. On the other hand, some policy actions can happen quickly, "in the dead of night" and with little public debate. The fact that policy change can happen quickly and without open discussion with stake holders argues for the importance of ongoing information sharing and education of key decision makers, stake holders, and constituents that they may be armed with solid information before action is required.

Standing coalitions and organizations with advocacy missions also need to be prepared to act quickly, proactively seizing opportunities and reactively addressing unanticipated counterproposals and actions.

In 1996, toward the end of the US Senate's consideration of legislation to overhaul the welfare system, some new language was added to the massive bill by one Senator. This provision, to authorize a new program within Title V of the Social Security Act of abstinence-only education for youth, was added without public hearing or debate. Although some advocates for more comprehensive approaches to sex education did discover that the provision had been added to the legislation, there was no time or opportunity to promote a full consideration of the merits of this relatively small provision within this major piece of legislation. Advocates succeeded only in changing the language to require new funding, rather than drawing funding away from core MCH programs, as was originally proposed.

An example of a successful, longer term effort at the national level was the advocacy that resulted in the 1997 enactment of the SCHIP. The foundation for the success of that advocacy can be traced back to the Maternal and Child Health Coalition formed in the 1980s to advocate for key programs providing health coverage and access, such as Title V, Medicaid, and Community Health Centers. Active leaders in this large coalition included the Children's Defense Fund, the March of Dimes, the Association of Maternal and Child Health Programs, the American Academy of Pediatrics, the National Association of Children's Hospitals, and the National Association of Community Health Centers. This coalition achieved advocacy successes in federal appropriations and in major legislative changes in Title V and Medicaid in the late 1980s.

When there seemed to be a real possibility of national health care reform in the early 1990s, the MCH Coalition and its members advocated for attention to the specific needs of children. Although the effort at national reform ultimately failed, these organizations and their state and local counterparts had done much of the work necessary to advocate for improved health care coverage for children and learned some valuable lessons for future advocacy on behalf of SCHIP.

After mourning the loss of the national health reform opportunity and licking their individual and collective wounds, these groups formed a new coalition in the mid 1990s to advocate specifically and more narrowly for federal legislation to expand health coverage for children. From the previous advocacy efforts, the information on the problems of uninsured children was available, clear, and compelling. The new Child Health Coalition also was clear about its objective to secure federal legislation to increase the numbers of children with health care coverage. Although many of the organizations individually had well-developed positions about such important issues as the vehicle for coverage (Medicaid or not), the benefits package, the providers, and other policy options, the coalition was united in agreeing that there were multiple ways to achieve improved coverage. The coalition made it clear that it would work with and support the efforts of those in Congress who shared the overall goal. The coalition developed materials, held briefings, and invited Congressional staffers from both branches and both parties to its meetings to inform and educate them about the problem of uninsured children and about important issues to consider in designing solutions. Although the 1997 legislation reflects the multiple compromises made to accommodate the various interests and political philosophies of those involved in its passage, today millions of children have benefited from SCHIP coverage. All of the components of advocacy outlined previously here came into play in this example, with coalition building, education, information sharing, and development and adjusting of strategy occurring over the course of a decade.

Lessons learned from this example are that successful advocacy often takes time and that what may appear to be an advocacy failure may in the long run be viewed as an important contributing step toward later success. Many major policy and systems changes have similar histories. At the very least, advocacy efforts communicate interest in an issue on the part of a group of concerned constituents, raise awareness of the level of interest in or concern for that issue, and encourage others to become involved. At their very best, such advocacy efforts enable policy and program creation or improvement toward the larger goals of promoting the health of women, children and youth, those with special health care needs, and their families. Advocacy is an essential element in successful policy development, implementation, and evaluation. As such, all MCH professionals must understand it.

## HOW DOES ADVOCACY RELATE TO THE POLICY DEVELOPMENT PROCESS?

Someone once said that laws were like sausages—no one should have to see how they are actually made. The truth is that the public policy process is indeed a messy one but one that we must be willing to engage in if we are to succeed in effecting change for MCH. Many good websites are available (www.house.gov) that describe the process of law making at the national and state levels, and it is important that one become familiar with how this process works at the level that advocacy efforts will be targeted in order that opportunities to influence the process not be missed. How bills are created and introduced, the various committees that hear certain types of bills, how floor votes are handled, how conference committees are formed, the role of the political parties in the process, and the role of the executive branch and the governor are all things one must understand. Beyond the mechanics of these processes, however, lie the nuances of the traditions and the culture within which they are executed. It is equally important that one understand these subtleties of the policy-making process in a given state to avoid undermining advocacy efforts inadvertently. Which hearings are open to public testimony? How can one sign up to testify? How long should someone be prepared to speak? What are the "rules" for addressing the members of the committee and for responding to questions? Should advocates testify alone or should whole groups attend hearings? Should handouts be distributed? Can written testimony be provided in addition to or in lieu of oral testimony? Do the committees have staff assigned? Do the individual members have staff assigned? Is it better to meet with the legislator or his or her staff member? Where do people park? All of these are important to successful advocacy efforts.

It is always a good idea to visit the state capitol and determine the lay of the land and how to get around before venturing there in a mad rush during the legislative session. It is essential that advocates learn the structure of the legislature; identify the committees that are likely going to be key to their efforts (usually a health or health and human services committee, the finance and appropriations committees, possibly the education committee, or maybe a special or select committee dedicated to issues relating to children and families); and learn the names, backgrounds, and political affiliations of key members of each chamber (the senate and the house), each committee of interest to the advocacy agenda, and any special legislative commission. It is important to determine the level of staff infrastructure that exists within the state and whether those staff are assigned to political parties, chambers, committees, committee chairs, or individual members. Some states have very well-developed staff structures in place, whereas in others, the legislators operate with little to no staff support. It is also important to learn the location of the local offices of key legislators outside of the capitol. It is often easier to reach them and to have more extensive conversations with them when the legislature is not in session.

It is also important to know the calendar for budget preparation and the process by which agencies develop their legislative agendas. Some states have biennial budgets, whereas others do budgets annually. Most legislatures meet in the winter and spring; agencies work on budgets and legislative agendas in the summer and fall. Clearly, advocacy is important year round.

## CONCLUSION

Although anyone and everyone can and should be an advocate, how one advocates and the strengths and weaknesses of one's advocacy vary by one's position, the type of advocacy, and its context. One can and should advocate as a private individual, separate from and regardless of any advocacy efforts that may be conducted in the context of one's work position. Advocating as an individual can be a way to build on or compensate for limitations on advocacy at work. Advocacy as an individual also can provide a vehicle for having an effect at a level different from that at which one generally works. For those MCH professionals working at the federal or national level, getting involved in advocacy at the local or state level can be a stimulating and rewarding effort, both for the individual and the issues on which he or she works. Similarly, for those working at a local or state level, national-level advocacy can be an invigorating and enlightening experience.

In any event, as an MCH professional engaging in advocacy, you should be prepared to follow a few simple rules to improve your chances of success while maintaining the integrity expected of your position.

1. Be prepared. Do your homework! It is your responsibility to bring the science base to advocacy efforts. Others will contribute plenty of politics, but as a professional, you must keep the advocacy responsible.
2. Never raise a problem without offering a solution, preferably a solution you believe will be effective, cost-efficient, and acceptable to the public.

3. Be inclusive. Numbers matter, and various points of view strengthen your position. It is better to identify your opposition early and to invite them to discuss issues with you directly rather than learn about them during a confrontation in front of the members of the legislature.

4. Be prepared for the long haul. Even at the state level, it can take years to affect policy change. Be willing to engage in critical self-assessment in order to determine possible areas of weakness and to modify your strategy accordingly.

5. Be consistent. If you have your facts lined up, your strategy prepared and your coalition assembled, it should be easy to stay on message and avoid confusion and contradiction. When you can, keep the message simple and direct.

6. Be respectful. Take the high road on the issues. Thank everyone who participates and contributes to your efforts. Respond to every enquiry. Follow-up with everyone who helps you, who requests information or who may need a reminder.

Our legacy is one of strong leadership, advocating for the structures, systems, and services that women, children, and their families need to achieve their optimal potential. Our future will be shaped by the advocacy efforts that we undertake today to continue to support an agenda that values women, children, and families and that promotes MCH. Best wishes!

# REFERENCES

Alexander, G.R., Chadwick, C., Petersen, D.J., Pass, M.A., Slay, M., & Shumpert, N. (2002). *Maternal and child health/public health milestones.* Birmingham, AL: The MCH Leadership Skills Training Institute, Department of Maternal and Child Health, University of Alabama at Birmingham.

Grason, H., & Guyer, B. (1999, December). *Public MCH program functions framework: Essential public health services to promote maternal and child health in America.* Baltimore, MD: The Johns Hopkins University, Child and Adolescent Health Policy.

Health Resources and Services Administration. (n.d.). *Understanding Title V of the Social Security Act.* Rockville, MD: US Public Health Service.

Hutchins, V.L. (n.d.). *Maternal and child health at the millennium.* Rockville, MD: Health Resources and Services Administration, Maternal and Child Health Bureau.

Institute of Medicine. (1988). *The future of public health*. Washington, DC: National Academy Press.

Johnson, K. (1999). Harnessing our energy: A counterpoint to "breaking away." *Maternal and Child Health Journal, 3,* 57–60.

Margolis, L., Cole G., & Kotch, J.B. (2005). Children's rights, social justice and advocacy in maternal and child health. In J. Kotch (Ed.), *Maternal and child health: Programs, problems and policy in public health* (2nd ed.). Gaithersburg, MD: Jones and Bartlett.

Mead, M. (2005, Jan. 6). The Institute for Intercultural Studies, Inc. Available Jan. 12, 2005, from: www.interculturalstudies.org.

Rosenbaum, S. (1983). The Maternal and Child Health Block Grant of 1981: Teaching an old program new tricks. *Clearinghouse Review, 17,* 400–414.

Saunders, S.E., Hess, C.A., Nelson, R., & Petersen, D.J. (1995). Health care reform and the MCH population. *Journal of Public Health Management and Practice, 1,* 78–85.

US Congress. (1912). *An act to establish in the Department of Commerce and Labor a bureau to be known as the Children's Bureau.* 37 US Statutes 79.

US Congress. (1935). Grants to states for maternal and child welfare. *Social Security Act.* 49 US Statutes 633, Title V.

# WEBSITES FOR FURTHER INFORMATION

www.modimes.org—National March of Dimes

www.amchp.org—Association of Maternal and Child Health Programs

www.aap.org—American Academy of Pediatrics

www.acog.org—American College of Obstetricians and Gynecologists

www.acnm.org—American College of Nurse Midwives

www.atmch.org—Association of Teachers of Maternal and Child Health

www.apha.org—American Public Health Association

www.astho.org—Association of State and Territorial Health Officials

www.naccho.org—National Association of City and County Health Officials

www.nalboh.org—National Association of Local Boards of Health

www.citymatch.org—CityMatCH

www.childrenshospitals.net—National Association of Children's Hospitals

www.nachc.com—National Association of Community Health Centers

http://thearc.org—The Arc

www.childrensdefense.org—Children's Defense Fund

www.cdfactioncouncil.org—Children's Defense Fund Action Council

www.childadvocacy.org—Voices for America's Children

www.familyvoices.org—Family Voices

www.familiesusa.org—Families USA

www.mchb.hrsa.gov—Maternal and Child Health Bureau, Health Resources and Services Administration, US Department of Health and Human Services

# INDEX

Page numbers in *italics* indicate figures and exhibits; those followed by t indicate tables

## A

Office of Child Health, 41
Office of Disability and Health, CDC, 369
Office of Economic Opportunity, 39
Office of Life Science, 424
Office of Management and Budget (OMB),
        Federal Statistical Policy Directive
        No. 15: "Race and Ethnic
        Standards for Federal Agencies
        and Administrative Reporting,"
        330
Office of Minority Health (OMH), 302,
        353, 498
Office of Research on Women's Health,
        NIH, 355
Office of Technology Assistance, US
        Congress, 266
Office on Child Abuse and Neglect, 223
Old Age Assistance, 77
Older women, 374–375
Olds, D.I., 185
Oleske, J.M., 226
Omnibus Budget Reconciliation Act
        (OBRA)
    1989, CSHCN programs and, 390–391
    MCH block grants and, 45–46
    Medicaid eligibility and, 44–45
Onanism, 100
Operational definitions, in research,
        502–503
Ordinal measures, 499
Organizational change theories, 548
Organizational infrastructure, program
        design and, 571–572
Organizations
    child advocacy, 11, 12–13
    MCH advocacy, 656–657
Osborne, N.G., 326, 327
Osteoporosis, 374
Osterholm, M.T., 226, 227
*Our Bodies, Ourselves* (Boston Women's
        Health Collective), 352
Outcome
    in evaluation research, 508, 509t, 633,
        638–639

as performance measure, 586, 587–588
Outcome level objectives, 634
Outcome sequence, performance measures
        and, 586
Out-of-range data, 518–519
Overpopulation, family planning and, 95,
        480
Overweight, 315, 426, 428

## P

Pacific Islanders, 304, 309, 310t, 328–329
Pan American Sanitary Bureau and code,
        464
Parent Survey of the National Household
        Education Surveys Program, 234
Parenting, of adolescents, 250–251
Parents
    adolescent, 283 (*See also* Pregnancy,
        adolescent)
    adolescent connectedness to, 265
    of adolescents, 247
    childhood obesity and, 430
    cohabiting, 61
    family resource programs' holistic view of,
        219
    rights of, 6, 12
    as (child) savers, 12
    working, 66–67
Participant characteristics, in evaluation
        research, 638
Partners in Program Planning in Adolescent
        Health, 273
Partnerships, 561. *See also* Coalitions
Pastore, A.L., 402
Patient records, performance measure data
        sources in, 594
Patton, M.Q., 632, 645
Pearl, M., 145
Peckham, C., 435
Pediatric Nutrition Surveillance System
        (PedNSS), 191
Pediatric Section of the Work Group on
        HIV/AIDS, 226